Carbon Quantum Dots from Natural Sources

Carbon quantum dots (CQDs) are a novel class of zero-dimensional carbon nanomaterials that are relatively nontoxic and cost-effective and offer desirable properties which make them excellent candidates for various applications. This book introduces the fundamentals of CQDs, natural sources, methods used for their synthesis, and characterization techniques. It addresses applications in biomedical, environmental, electrical, and other areas.

- Covers current research and future possibilities
- Details modern fabrication methods and their drawbacks
- Discusses applications in biomedical use, wastewater treatment, electrical and electronics, dye removal, 3D printing, and metal detection
- Provides insight into cytotoxicity and biocompatibility studies of these materials

The detailed insight into these nanomaterials in this book will benefit researchers, scientists, engineers, and advanced students in developing new methods and strategies in the advanced field of materials engineering.

Aswathy Jayakumar is a postdoctoral researcher at Kyung Hee University of Technology, Seoul, South Korea. She completed her Postdoctoral Fellowship at King Mongkut's University of Technology, Thailand. She received her Ph.D. in Biotechnology from School of Biosciences, Mahatma Gandhi University, Kottayam, India.

Sabarish Radoor received his Ph.D. (Chemistry) from National Institute of Technology, Calicut, India. He completed his Postdoctoral Research at King Mongkut's University of Technology, Thailand. He is a postdoctoral fellow at Department of Polymer Nano Science and Technology, Jeonbuk National University, Republic of Korea.

Jun Tae Kim is Associate Professor in the Department of Food and Nutrition, Kyung Hee University, Seoul, South Korea. He received his Ph.D. from Rutgers, The State University of New Jersey, USA, and worked as a Postdoctoral Research Associate at Cornell University.

Jyotishkumar Parameswaranpillai is Associate Professor at Alliance University, Bangalore, India. He received his Ph.D. in Chemistry (Polymer Science and Technology) from Mahatma Gandhi University, Kottayam, India.

Carbon Quantum Dots from Natural Sources

Properties, Development, and Emerging Applications

Edited by
Aswathy Jayakumar
Sabarish Radoor
Jun Tae Kim
Jyotishkumar Parameswaranpillai

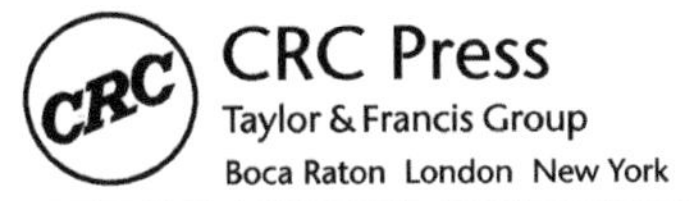

CRC Press
Taylor & Francis Group
Boca Raton London New York

CRC Press is an imprint of the
Taylor & Francis Group, an **informa** business

First edition published 2025
by CRC Press
2385 NW Executive Center Drive, Suite 320, Boca Raton FL 33431

and by CRC Press
4 Park Square, Milton Park, Abingdon, Oxon, OX14 4RN

CRC Press is an imprint of Taylor & Francis Group, LLC

Library of Congress Cataloging-in-Publication Data
Names: Jayakumar, Aswathy, editor.
Title: Carbon quantum dots from natural sources : properties, development, and emerging applications / edited by Aswathy Jayakumar, Sabarish Radoor, Jun Tae Kim, Jyotishkumar Parameswaranpillai.
Description: First edition. | Boca Raton : CRC Press, 2025. | Includes bibliographical references and index. |
Summary: "Carbon quantum dots (CQDs) are a novel class of zero-dimensional carbon nanomaterials that are relatively nontoxic and cost-effective and offer desirable properties that make them excellent candidates for various applications. This book introduces the fundamentals of CQDs, natural sources and methods used for their synthesis, and characterization techniques. It addresses applications in biomedical, environmental, electrical, and other areas. Covers current research and future possibilities. Details modern fabrication methods and drawbacks. Discusses applications in biomedical use, wastewater treatment, electrical and electronics, dye removal, 3D printing, and metal detection. Provides insight into cytotoxicity and biocompatibility studies on these materials. The detailed insight into these nanomaterials in this reference will benefit researchers, scientists, engineers, and advanced students in developing new methods and strategies in this advanced field of materials engineering" – Provided by publisher.
Identifiers: LCCN 2024032340 (print) | LCCN 2024032341 (ebook) | ISBN 9781032569581 (hbk) | ISBN 9781032569611 (pbk) | ISBN 9781003437857 (ebk)
Subjects: LCSH: Quantum dots. | Quantum dots–Industrial applications.
Classification: LCC TK7874.88 C37 2025 (print) | LCC TK7874.88 (ebook) |
DDC 621.3815/2–dc23/eng/20241115
LC record available at https://lccn.loc.gov/2024032340
LC ebook record available at https://lccn.loc.gov/2024032341

ISBN: 978-1-032-56958-1 (hbk)
ISBN: 978-1-032-56961-1 (pbk)
ISBN: 978-1-003-43785-7 (ebk)

DOI: 10.1201/9781003437857

Typeset in Times
by SPi Technologies India Pvt Ltd (Straive)

Contents

SECTION I   *Fundamentals*

M. Ramesh and R. Janani

Hao Xu, Long Chen, Zhengyu Jin and Ming Miao

*Subhanki Padhi, Ashutosh Singh, Valerie Orsat
and Winny Routray*

*Shristi Shefali Saraugi, Valerie Orsat, Ashutosh Singh
and Winny Routray*

Jeyakumar Saranya Packialakshmi and Jun Tae Kim

SECTION II   *Applications*

*Zohreh Riahi, Alireza Kaviani, Ajahar Khan,
Gholamreza Pircheraghi and Jun Tae Kim*

Preface

Nanotechnological innovations with environmentally friendly approaches have received great attention for various applications. Greener nanotechnology can offer superior-quality materials with high performance in every aspect of functionalities. Among the materials, carbon quantum dots (CQDs) are unique nanomaterials with a size range of <10 nm. These nanomaterials have high photoluminescence, large surface area, good solubility, and excellent biocompatibility along with antimicrobial features. This book gives a detailed insight into the introduction of CQDs, their properties, functions, and applications.

In this book, we have 17 chapters emphasizing the properties of CQDs and their applications. **Chapter 1** (Introduction to Carbon Quantum Dots) gives an overview of CQDs, their properties, and applications. **Chapter 2** (Natural Sources Used to Fabricate Carbon Quantum Dots) highlights the sources (plants and animals) utilized for the development of CQDs. Plant sources like grains, cereals, tubers, legumes, vegetables, and fruits, and animal sources like fish, shellfish, crustaceans, mammals, birds, and eggs are covered. **Chapter 3** (Methods Employed for the Development of Carbon Quantum Dots) gives an in-depth overview of the methods (top-down and bottom-up) used for the development of CQDs. **Chapter 4** (Characterization Techniques for Carbon Quantum Dots) discusses various characterization methods like UV-vis, FT-IR, XPS, Raman spectroscopy, SEM, TEM, AFM, DLS, XRD, PL spectroscopy, NMR, EDS, TGA, XPS, and zeta analyzer. **Chapter 5** (Antimicrobial Mechanisms Exhibited by Carbon Quantum Dots) discusses the antibacterial and antibiofilm activities of CQDs and their mode of action. **Chapter 6** (Antioxidant Properties and UV-blocking of Carbon Quantum Dots in Food Packaging Applications) highlights the antioxidant and UV blocking properties of CQDs. In addition, the mechanism behind the radical scavenging properties like adduct formation, hydrogen donation, and electron transfer is discussed in detail.

Chapter 7 (Anti-aging Properties and Utilization of Carbon Quantum Dots in Cosmetics) describes the application of CQDs in cosmetic products such as skin care, sunscreen, moisturizing lipstick, etc. Further, the major advantages and disadvantages associated with CQDs in cosmetics industries are elucidated. **Chapter 8** (Synergizing Carbon Quantum Dots for Biomedical Imaging, Targeted Drug Delivery, and Photodynamic Therapy) emphasizes the role of CQDs in biomedical imaging, their toxicity studies, pharmacokinetics, and biodistribution. Further the applications of CQDs in targeted drug delivery and photodynamic therapy and their role as photosensitizers for targeted cell death in cancer treatment are provided in detail. **Chapter 9** (Carbon Quantum Dots for Wound Healing and Wound Dressing) highlights the application of CQDs in the wound healing process and their application in wound dressings. The wound dressing materials like hydrogels, spray, sponges, and bandages are also reviewed in detail. **Chapter 10** (Carbon Quantum Dots for Treating Viral Infections) provides a detailed overview of CQDs in treating viral infections. The mechanisms behind the antiviral activity of CQDs are also emphasized in detail. **Chapter 11** (Carbon Quantum Dots and 3D Printing

Technology) highlights the diverse applications of CQDs in additive manufacturing technologies, especially in the field of sensing, imaging, and polymerization. In addition, the applications of CQDs as fluorescence/colorimetric sensors, optical imaging agents, and nano-photoinitiating catalysts to anti-counterfeiting are discussed in detail.

Chapter 12 (Carbon Quantum Dots for Bioimaging) provides an in-depth overview of CQDs in intracellular imaging of ions, organelles, and molecules and in imaging of various cells including cancer, stem cells, and neural cells. **Chapter 13** (Cytotoxicity and Biocompatibility Analysis of Carbon Quantum Dots) gives an overview of different cytotoxicity assessments and biocompatibility analysis of CQDs. In addition, the mechanism behind CQD-induced cell toxicity and the advancement in surface modification and functionalization strategies to enhance the biocompatibility of CQDs are given in detail. **Chapter 14** (Application of Carbon Quantum Dots in Dye Removal and Wastewater Treatment) highlights the use of CQDs in dye removal and treatment of wastewater. Removal of major dyes such as methylene blue, rhodamine B, crystal violet, and methyl orange is discussed in detail. Furthermore, this chapter covers the applications of CQDs in the detection of metal ions and organic matter in wastewater and adsorption of inorganic matter from wastewater, and the application of CQDs as disinfecting agents. **Chapter 15** (Application of Carbon Quantum Dots in Energy and Electronic Applications) systematically gives an in-depth overview of CQD-based composites and their application in energy and electronic applications. The major applications of CQD-based composites in supercapacitors, advanced batteries (as cathode and anode materials, separators), electrolytes, and advanced photovoltaics (dye and quantum dot-sensitized solar cells, solid-state nanostructured solar cells, etc.) are given in detail. **Chapter 16** (Carbon Quantum Dots for Metal Detection) gives an in-depth overview of CQDs in metal detection (mercury, copper, iron, lead, aluminum, arsenic, cadmium, cobalt, zinc, silver, and gold). Further, the major challenges, future perspectives, and the major strategies to enhance selectivity and sensitivity of metal ions are also discussed. **Chapter 17** (Environmental Issues Associated with Carbon Quantum Dots) emphasizes the major impact of CQDs on the environment and ecosystem, their hazards, and the major risk associated with them.

Dr. Aswathy Jayakumar, Republic of Korea
Dr. Sabarish Radoor, Republic of Korea
Dr. Jun Tae Kim Republic of Korea
Dr. Jyotishkumar Parameswaranpillai, India

Contributors

Shiji Mathew Abraham
Temple University
Philadelphia, Pennsylvania

Syed Ansar Ali
National Institute of Pharmaceutical
    Education and Research, Ahmedabad
Opp. Airforce Station
Gandhinagar, India

Srivalliputtur Sarath Babu
National Institute of Pharmaceutical
    Education and Research, Kolkata
Kolkata, India

M. K. Bera
Department of Physics
MM Engineering College
Maharishi Markandeshwar (Deemed to
    be University)
Haryana, India

Elyor Berdimurodov
Faculty of Chemistry
National University of Uzbekistan
Tashkent, Uzbekistan

Long Chen
School of Food Science and Technology
Jiangnan University
Wuxi, China

Karutha Pandian Divya
Bharathiar Cancer Theranostics
    Research Centre
Bharathiar University
India

Benny Harshitha
National Institute of Pharmaceutical
    Education and Research –
    Ahmedabad
Opp. Airforce station
Gandhinagar, Gujarat, INDIA

Bhawana Jain
Siddhachalam Laboratory
Raipur, India

R. Janani
Department of Physics
KIT-Kalaignarkarunanidhi Institute of
    Technology
Tamil Nadu, India

Zhengyu Jin
School of Food Science and
    Technology
Jiangnan University
Wuxi, China

Bony K. John
School of Chemical Sciences
Mahatma Gandhi University
Kerala, India

Govinda Kapusetti
National Institute of Pharmaceutical
    Education and Research –
    Kolkata
Kolkata, India

Chirantan Kar
Amity Institute of Applied sciences
Amity University Kolkata
Kolkata, India

Alireza Kaviani
Polymeric Materials Research Group
    (PMRG)
Department of Materials Science and
    Engineering
Sharif University of Technology
Tehran, Iran

Ajahar Khan
Department of Food and Nutrition
Kyung Hee University
Seoul, Republic of Korea

Jun Tae Kim
Department of Food and Nutrition
Kyung Hee University
Seoul, Republic of Korea

Muhammed Shukkoor Kondengaden
Escientificsolutions LLC
Atlanta, Georgia

Beena Mathew
School of Chemical Sciences
Mahatma Gandhi University
Kerala, India

Jincy Mathew
School of Chemical Sciences
Mahatma Gandhi University
Kerala, India

Ming Miao
School of Food Science and
    Technology
Jiangnan University
Wuxi, China

Reena Negi
Siddhachalam Laboratory
Raipur, India

Valerie Orsat
Department of Bioresource Engineering
Macdonald Campus
McGill University
Quebec, Canada

Jeyakumar Saranya Packialakshmi
Department of Food and Nutrition
Kyung Hee University
Seoul, Republic of Korea

Subhanki Padhi
Department of Food Process
    Engineering
National Institute of Technology
Rourkela, India

Ashutosh Pandey
Dr. C.V. Raman University
Bilaspur, India

Arpita Pandey-Tiwari
Department of Stem Cell and
    Regenerative Medicine and Medical
    Biotechnology
D. Y. Patil Education Society (Deemed
    to be University)
Maharashtra, India

Gholamreza Pircheraghi
Polymeric Materials Research Group
    (PMRG)
Department of Materials Science and
    Engineering
Sharif University of Technology
Tehran, Iran

Nagamony Ponpandian
Department of Nanoscience and
    Technology
Bharathiar University
India

Robert M. Pontrelli
Apex Development Foundation
New York, USA

M. Ramesh
Department of Mechanical
    Engineering
KIT-Kalaignarkarunanidhi Institute of
    Technology
Coimbatore, India

Zohreh Riahi
BioNanocomposite Research Center
Department of Food and Nutrition
Kyung Hee University
Seoul, Republic of Korea

Winny Routray
Department of Food Process
    Engineering
National Institute of Technology
Rourkela, India

S. Arun Sasi
Escientificsolutions LLC
Atlanta, Georgia, USA

Shristi Shefali Saraugi
Department of Food Process
 Engineering
National Institute of Technology
Rourkela, India

Tanvi Shingote
National Institute of Pharmaceutical
 Education and Research –
 Ahmedabad
Opp. Airforce station
Gandhinagar, Gujarat, INDIA

Ashutosh Singh
Food Engineering Research Lab
School of Engineering
University of Guelph
Ontario, Canada

Sanju Singh
Siddhachalam Laboratory
Raipur, India

Pradip Kumar Sukul
Amity Institute of Applied sciences
Amity University Kolkata
Kolkata, India

T. Saichand
National Institute of Pharmaceutical
 Education and Research – Kolkata
Kolkata, India

Vijay J. Upadhye
Department of Microbiology
Parul Institute of Applied Sciences (PIAS)
Parul University
Gujarat, India

Ravichandiran Velyutham
National Institute of Pharmaceutical
 Education and Research – Kolkata
Kolkata, INDIA

Anuja A Vibhute
Department of Stem Cell and Regenerative
 Medicine and Medical Biotechnology
D. Y. Patil Education Society (Deemed
 to be University)
Maharashtra, India

Hao Xu
School of Food Science and Technology
 Jiangnan Universityd
1800 Lihu Roa
Wuxi, 214122, China

Section I

Fundamentals

1 Introduction to Carbon Quantum Dots

M. Ramesh and R. Janani

1.1 INTRODUCTION

Quantum dots (QDs) are explored widely in various domains for their quantum confinement effect. Based on their size, semiconductor QDs will have tuneable optical properties including absorption and emission of different wavelengths. Nevertheless, their synthesis procedure involves usage of heavy metals like lead, mercury, cadmium, etc. which increase the toxicity even at low concentrations (Rasal et al. 2021). The accidental discovery of CQDs by Xu et al. (2004) gave solution to the toxicity dispute and substituted the usage of semiconductor QDs. Carbon-based nanoparticles with size less than 10 nm exhibiting strong fluorescence are generally known as CQDs. They are considered as a part of graphene-family having zero-dimension encompassing few layers of graphene oxide (GO) sheets. CQDs are superior to GO in terms of electronic and optical features as they possess edge effects and quantum confinement (Zhang et al. 2017). They are characterized with distinguished features like biocompatibility, low toxicity, high water solubility, enhanced surface functionalization, and superior specific surface area (El-Shabasy et al. 2021). These excellent physicochemical properties and ease of availability enable them to have great potential in many technical applications. The chapter is organized into three sections to provide an overall understanding about the carbon dots to the reader. Firstly, this chapter will explore the fundamental characteristics of carbon quantum dots. Followed by the exploration on diverse methodologies involving multiple techniques used for their production. Successively, a concise investigation on their vast range of applications including energy harvesting applications such as Li ion batteries, supercapacitors, photocatalysis, electrocatalysis, and biomedical applications such as bio-imaging and biosensing are presented.

1.2 PROPERTIES OF CQDs

CQDs are designated with a carbon core surrounded by organic functional groups which help in easy solubility compared to other carbon-based structures. CQDs hold several distinct properties such as extraordinary absorbance, tunable luminescence, infrared reception, excellent charge transportation, etc. They are recognized predominantly for their up-converted photoluminescence (UCPL) where fluorescence emission wavelength is shorter than the excitation wavelength (Wang et al. 2017). Bearing

DOI: 10.1201/9781003437857-2

in mind the astonishing properties of CQDs, it is no wonder to realize the progress of CQDs in the research and development for vast technical applications.

1.2.1 OPTICAL ABSORBANCE

CQDs exhibit absorption in the UV region between 230 nm and 320 nm and an extension to the visible region attributed to the π conjugated electrons. They show two different π transitions in their structure, namely π–π* transition of sp^2-conjugated carbon and n-π* transition of hybridized atoms, respectively. The absorption wavelength of CQDs could be tuned by surface passivation (Mitra et al. 2013; Wang et al. 2019). As an example, the absorption of CQDs has been narrowed down 46 nm to the visible region by acid treatment approach producing nitrogen-doped CQDs emitting multiple wavelengths (Oh et al. 2022). Shekarbeygi et al. (2020) reported a novel method of tuning the optical properties of CQDs by varying the method of extraction of carbon source from rose pigments. The alcoholic method of extraction resulted in highly stable quantum dots with high efficiency and good sensitivity for diazinon.

1.2.2 FLUORESCENCE

Carbon dots are emerging materials amidst several quantum dots attracting significant research interest with tunable fluorescence properties. The fluorescence behavior of CQDs is generated in either of the following two ways (Yuan et al. 2019):

1. Band to band transition between the conjugated π-domains
2. Surface defect-mediated emission.

The fluorescent nature and biocompatibility of the carbon dots have high potential in biomedical applications such as bio-imaging of damaged cells, drug delivery, biosensing, etc. There have been many efforts to improve the fluorescent intensity of the CQDs to enhance their performance in high-end applications. For instance, Ahmed et al. investigated the effect of duration of dialysis on the fluorescent intensity of the carbon dots. The CQDs synthesized with 3 h of hydrothermal treatment and dialysis showed 20 times enhanced fluorescence. Hence the carbon dots with superior fluorescence were explored as an excellent fluorescent marker for detection of metal ions and used as antimicrobial reagent (Ahmed et al. 2020). Jiang et al. (2020) proposed a novel technique of enhancing the fluorescence of CQDs through photoactivation method. The F- and N-doped CQDs showed elevated fluorescent intensity with ultraviolet irradiation for 30 minutes. The photoenhancement of carbon dots also enabled reduced photobleaching properties during probing.

1.2.3 PHOSPHORESCENCE

CQDs are being considered as next-generation nanomaterials for light-emitting diode (LED) displays because of their phosphorescence or delayed fluorescent properties. Nevertheless, the confinements of the triplet state transition in CQDs hinder the enhancement in the external quantum efficiency (EQE) of phosphorescence beyond a theoretical value of 5% (Shi et al. 2021). There are several attempts made to leap forward beyond the theoretical limitations. Shi et al. (2021) developed carbon dot organic frame works (CDOF) having monochromatic red emission with a quantum yield of 42.3%. The LEDs fabricated with CDOF had an EQE of 5.6% (Shi et al. 2021). On the other hand, Guo et al. (2019) proposed a novel approach of developing a solid film of CQDs that could overcome the aggregation-induced quenching of luminescence. This approach significantly promoted high photoluminescence simultaneously enabling the applicability in solid-state optoelectronic devices.

1.2.4 CHEMILUMINESCENCE

Chemical luminescence (CL) is generally defined as the emission of optical energy with the absorbed chemical energy. This type of luminescence is popular in optoelectronic applications because of their low background signal. With their efficient luminescence ability, CQDs can be considered for chemiluminescent applications also. Several efforts on exploring the chemiluminescent property of CQDs enabled their application in phototherapy, biosensing, and bioimaging (Jiang et al. 2022). A novel approach for generating CL in CQDs was developed by Yahyai et al. (2021). In their work, the sulfur and nitrogen-doped CQDs are oxidized by $KMnO_4$, resulting in enhanced emission at 510 nm. A similar approach of oxidizing the P- and Cl-doped CQDs with $KMnO_4$ exhibited linear quenching for logarithmic concentration of iodine ions (Figure 1.1). Hence, these heteroatom-doped CQDs are categorized as a novel class of materials for iodine detection (Jiang et al. 2022).

1.2.5 ANTIMICROBIAL PROPERTIES

All CQDs do not inherit antimicrobial properties in them. They are either functionalized by irradiation or through their compositional characteristics (Chatzimitakos and Stalikas 2020). They contain simpler carbon and oxygen groups in their structure depending on the precursor used for their synthesis and the heteroatoms that are doped with it. Moradlou et al. (2019) explored the antibacterial property of CQD-incorporated hematite's under both dark and light conditions. The antibacterial activity was observed for Gram-positive bacteria, while the Gram-negative showed

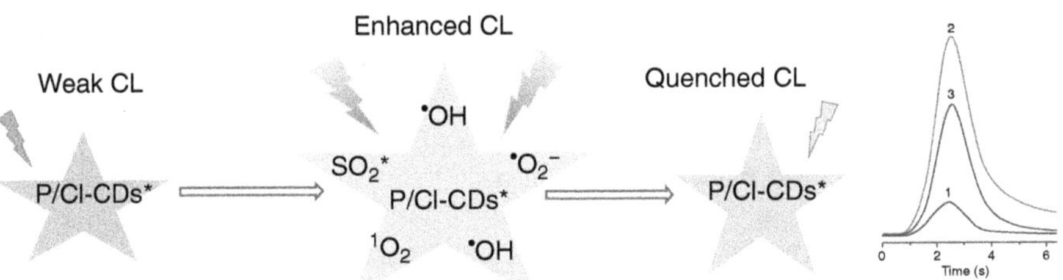

FIGURE 1.1 Chemical luminescence quenching in P/Cl-doped CQDS on I⁻ detection (Jiang et al. 2022).

resistance with its extra outer layer in its structure. The bactericidal study concluded that the observed method of disinfection was through the CQD-assisted quick mobility of iron cations inside the bacterial cell membrane which generated reactive oxygen species (ROS) required for the bacterial disinfection (Moradlou et al. 2019). Similarly, Pandiyan et al. (2020) investigated the antibacterial activity of CQDs synthesized from sugarcane bagasse pulp. The antimicrobial activity was examined with *Staphylococcus aureus*, *Bacillus cereus*, *Escherichia coli*, *Vibrio cholera*, and *Pseudomonas aeruginosa*. CQDs were found to attach with the bacterial cell wall through electron transfer. The functional groups present in the CQDs were found to generate ROS based on electrostatic interactions leading to the death of bacteria.

1.2.6 Antioxidant Properties

The presence of ROS plays a vital role in cell damage and formation of toxic elements in food products. Thus, the presence of antioxidants is essential for removing ROS in the products to preserve them for longer duration. Industries focus on synthesizing antioxidant agents from biodegradable sources for various applications related to food wrapping, packaging, beauty products, etc. (Sharma et al. 2020). The antioxidative properties of carbon dots can be attributed to their electron-accepting properties. CQDs synthesized from banana peel wastes exhibited extraordinary scavenging properties against superoxide anions, hydroxyl radicals, and hydrogen peroxide radicals (Rajamanikandan et al. 2021). Similarly, biocompatible CQDs synthesized from coconut husk exhibited antioxidative properties against DPPH (2, 2-diphenyl-1-picrylhydrazyl) assay (Chunduri et al. 2016).

1.2.7 UV-blocking Properties

Prolonged exposure to ultraviolet (UV) radiation is known to cause serious health-related effects in human body. On the other hand, the excessive exposure can also alter the properties of polymers. Hence, the necessity of developing a UV-resistant material coating is much needed for food packaging industries (Dong et al. 2019). CQDs possess high UV absorbing ability that can be useful in designing UV protective films. Ezati et al. (2022) combined CQDs as a filler in chitosan/gelatin-based films. The integration of CQDs enhanced the UV blocking property of the material without affecting its mechanical strength and water permeability. The CQD-incorporated film successfully inhibited the growth of fungus mold and increased the shelf life of avocado fruit more than 14 days. In their other work, Ezati et al. (2022) synthesized CQDs from glucose and used them to shield L929 fat cells from UV radiation. CQD-coated pectin film used in their study converted the incoming UV radiation into blue light which enhanced the UV blocking properties of the film. This enables the usage of the CQD/pectin film for protecting high fatty foods from radiation.

1.2.8 Biocompatibility

The biocompatibility is a critical property in utilization of a material in biological systems. CQDs synthesized from natural and bioorganic sources are often reported to be biocompatible and hence utilized for in vitro studies. Atchudan et al. (2021) synthesized CQDs from banana peel waste. The high fluorescent behavior and biocompatibility of the CQDs were beneficial in utilizing them for bioimaging of nematodes. Chandra et al. (2020) prepared nitrogen/sulfur-codoped carbon dots which possessed biocompatibility for HeLa cancer cells. Hence, it was used for picric acid detection in pathological environment. Similarly, CQDs synthesized from date palm fruit possessed high compatibility to zebra fish embryos and find application in drug delivery (Tungare et al. 2020).

1.2.9 CYTOTOXICITY

CQDs are considered as a potential candidate in the field of targeted diagnostic research, biomedicine, and biotechnology because of their unique properties such as fluorescence, low cytotoxicity, and biocompatibility. Song et al. studied the cytotoxicity of CQDs formed during the roasting process of Atlantic salmons. The CQDs generated at different roasting temperatures were taken for in vitro examination in rat kidney cell lines. The results suggested that the increase in the concentration of CQDs leads to change in metabolism from aerobic to glycotic (Song et al. 2019). Similarly, the cytotoxicity of CQDs synthesized from carbonization of citric acid was evaluated to be very low and hence utilized for targeted drug delivery to breast cancer cells (Mahani et al. 2021).

1.3 SYNTHESIS METHODS

CQDs are majorly synthesized by top-down or bottom-up approach. In the first method, CQDs are fabricated by physical or chemical methods involving destruction of macromolecules into smaller size, while in the second method, smaller organic molecules are used to produce CQDs through condensation or polymerization. It is observed that bottom-up technique is preferential as it is highly economical and time-saving and provides mild fabrication conditions. Carbon dots were fortuitously discovered during the purification process of single-walled carbon nanotubes (SWCNTs) by Xu et al. (2004). Since then, there have been so many methodologies explored for CQD synthesis in terms of cost-effectiveness, large-scale synthesis, simplicity, and sustainability. The synthesis methodologies adapted for preparation of CQDs could be briefly classified into two categories such as top-down method and bottom-up method. The top-down methodology encompasses the use of macro-level carbon sources such as graphite and charcoal and break the larger particles to nanoscale. Common top-down methods of preparing carbon dots are laser ablation (Hussein et al. 2019), arc-discharge (Shankar et al. 2020), ultrasonication (Das et al. 2021), chemical oxidation (Li et al. 2019), and plasma reactor method (Pho et al. 2023). Whilst the bottom-up strategy involves the carbonization of small organic molecules in the precursor to form carbon dots. Some of the bottom-up strategies include hydrothermal synthesis (Guo et al. 2020), microwave synthesis (Ganesan et al. 2022), thermal pyrolysis (Nallayagiri et al. 2021), waste-derived synthesis (Hanon et al. 2019), etc. CQDs have been considered as a very promising material in terms of non-toxicity especially when the synthesis procedure involves the usage of natural extracts as the precursor.

1.3.1 Top-Down Synthesis Routes

1.3.1.1 Laser Ablation

Recently, there have been a lot of investigations on the synthesis of CQDs using laser ablation technique. This facile and quick method facilitates easy control of morphology and hence is beneficial in preparation of nanomaterials. Cui et al. (2020) fabricated homogenous carbon dots by ablation of carbon cloth. In this work, with the assistance of a beam splitter, single beam of laser was split into two to cut down the ablation time. The CQDs thus prepared had good antijamming properties and hence utilized for bioimaging applications. Laser ablation technique was adapted to synthesize ligand-free highly fluorescent CQDs from carbon nanoparticles dispersed in colloidal solution. The bulk target immersed in the colloid was irradiated with a high-power laser beam which resulted in highly pure CQDs with meager byproducts (Donate-Buendia et al. 2020). This ligand-free highly pure CQDs are of greater demand in the field of nanomedicines. Sadrolhosseini et al. (2020) found that the interaction of gold nanoparticles with CQDs during laser ablation enhanced the photoluminescence properties of CQDs. Moreover, the presence of gold nanoparticles enriched the pyrene–CQD interaction in the system.

1.3.1.2 Arc Discharge

In arc discharge method, CQDs are synthesized from crude carbon nanotube sediments. Generally, carbon dots synthesized from this method are hydrophilic; however, during the process, many large-sized carbon molecules are also formed, which reduces the distribution of CQDs, leading to decreased specific surface area (Wang et al. 2019). Chao-Mujica et al. (2021) reported the synthesis of CQDs through submerged arc discharge method. Here pure graphite rods of different diameters are used as electrodes. The electrical arc discharge is carried out until the complete burning of the anode and the sediment is collected carefully for characterization. The obtained carbon dots were in the size between 1 and 5 nm with fluorescence band around 320–340 nm and 400–410 nm. The highly fluorescent dots possessed a fluorescent quantum yield of ~16% and were employed as fluorescent markers for in vitro studies.

1.3.1.3 Ultrasonic Synthesis

The pressure variation created in the liquid medium with ultrasonic waves produces vacuum bubbles through a process called cavitation. These vacuum bubbles with strong shearing forces could produce high-speed liquid jets that can cut macro-sized carbon molecules into smaller sizes. Huang et al. (2018) followed a one-pot strategy to synthesize highly functionalized carbon dots from cigarette ashes using ultrasonic waves (Figure 1.2).

These dots exhibited bright green fluorescence, biocompatibility, and excellent water dispersibility befitting biomedical applications (Huang et al. 2018). On similar grounds, the ultrasonic treatment of dopamine in dimethylformamide resulted in nitrogen-doped carbon quantum dots. Their stable temperature-dependent fluorescence, hydrophilicity, and cytotoxicity promoted their usage as nanothermometers to assess the temperature of cell walls (Lu and Zhou 2019).

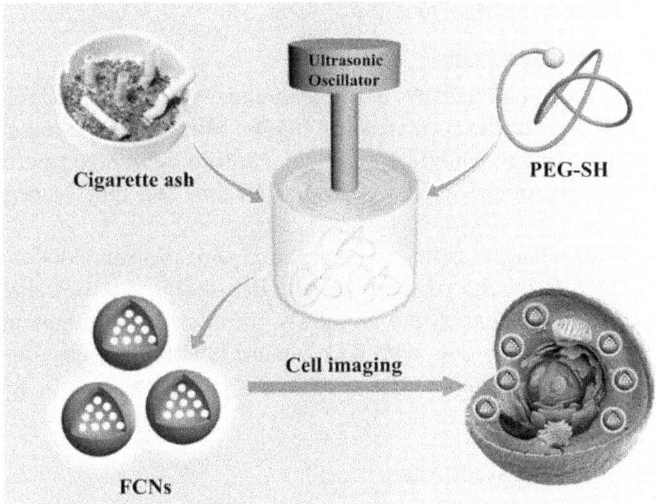

FIGURE 1.2 Ultrasonic synthesis of CQDs from cigarette ashes (Huang et al. 2018).

1.3.1.4 Chemical Oxidation

In chemical oxidation technique, carbon dots are prepared by fragmentation of carbon precursors such as graphite and graphene oxide, and reduction of graphene oxide by electrochemical oxidation process (Rasal et al. 2021). Blue luminescent nitrogen-doped carbon dots were prepared by exfoliation of graphite electrodes in inorganic nitrite-based salt solution by Tian et al. The synthesized carbon dots were of uniform dimension and morphology with an average diameter of around 3 nm. Besides, it is also proved that varying the electrolyte solution during the exfoliation process impacts the properties of the quantum dots (Tian et al. 2020). Similarly, a novel approach of exfoliation of g-C_3N_4 (GCN) with simultaneous formation of CQDs through hydrothermal treatment was reported by Wong et al. Herein, the effects of parameters of hydrothermal treatment played an essential role in the properties of GCN sheets and the carbon dots which were investigated through photocatalytic degradation of rhodamine B dye (Wong et al. 2019).

1.3.1.5 Plasma Reactor

This method is a simple, fast, and effective one-step technique that yields large-scale production of high-quality carbon dots. Weerasinghe et al. (2021) effectively synthesized dual emissive carbon dots using atmospheric air plasmas. They have also shown that the dual emissive nature of the quantum dots can be widely applied in many biomedical applications such as detection of Cu^{2+} ions. Gao et al. (2022) studied the influence of the flow rate of Ar gas during plasma-mediated synthesis of carbon dots. This study opens up a new way in understanding the formation of carbon dots using gas-liquid plasma reactors.

1.3.2 BOTTOM-UP SYNTHESIS ROUTES

1.3.2.1 Microwave Synthesis

In this technique, organic precursors are treated under microwave to breakdown the chemical bonds, allowing the formation of CQDs. Microwave-treated synthesis of CQDs from carbon linter exhibited excellent multifluorescent properties (Figure 1.3). The average size of the dots was around 10 nm, and they were utilized for cancer cell imaging.

The results reveal that the cells were able to absorb the nanodots within 2 h of exposure, and the cytotoxicity of the dots inhibited the growth of cells depending upon the dosage (Eskalen et al. 2020). Similarly, the microwave treatment of roasted chickpeas resulted in carbon dots with high intense blue fluorescence and excellent hydrophilicity. The synthesized CQDs exhibited selective sensitivity for Fe^{3+} ions (Basoglu et al. 2020).

1.3.2.2 Hydrothermal Synthesis

This is an easy and low-cost process where the CQDs are synthesized by carbonization of aqueous organic precursors confined in an enclosure called autoclave at high temperatures up to 200 °C (Xie et al. 2019). The hydrothermal treatment of glucose and m-phenylenediamine resulted in highly fluorescent nitrogen-doped carbon dots emitting strong blue luminescence. The carbon dots have graphene crystallization in their structure with a quantum yield of 17.5%. These dots emitted a strong fluorescent probe for sensing CrO_4^{2-} and Fe^{3+} ions (Shen et al. 2021). In the same way, nitrogen and sulfur co-doped carbon dots were synthesized by hydrothermal process

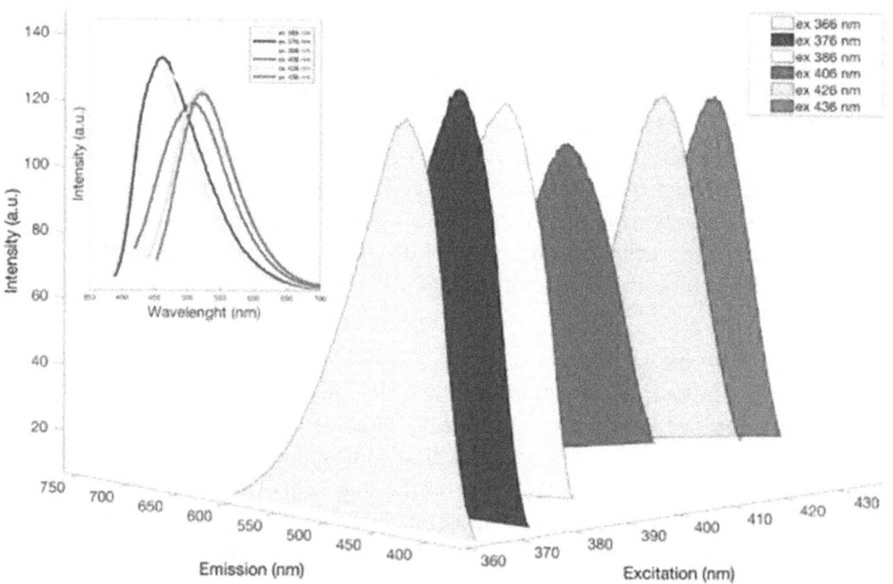

FIGURE 1.3 Photoluminescence spectra of microwave-synthesized CQDs (Eskalen et al. 2020).

of L-Lysine and thiourea. The synthesized carbon dots exhibited a high quantum efficiency of 53% and were able to detect picric acid in tap water with high selectivity (Khan et al. 2020).

1.3.2.3 Thermal Pyrolysis

This method allows one-step large-scale production of CQDs in a very short time. In this method, one or more salts are taken as precursors and heated at elevated temperatures. The precursor salts heated at higher temperatures undergo carbonization to generate CQDs. Jian et al. reported on the synthesis of CQDs through thermal pyrolysis of polyamine and dopamine at 270 °C. The generated carbon dots were combined with spermine to increase antibacterial properties and quick adhesion to surfaces like glass and contact lens material. The antibacterial coating made on the surface of contact lens and other biomedical instruments with spermine-treated CQDs could protect the material surface from contamination (Jian et al. 2020). Similarly, carbonization of citric acid and urea generated CQDs with controlled fluorescence through infrared pyrolysis. The produced dots had a uniform size distribution of 5–10 nm with a quantum yield of 22%. Here the crystallinity, surface functionalization and fluorescence properties were controlled by précising the weight ratios of the precursors (Gu et al. 2020).

1.3.2.4 Synthesis from Waste

Recently, the researchers have been fascinated about the readily available carbon sources from nature. In this method of synthesis, biomass wastes including fruit peels, leaves, bark of the trees, etc., are used as carbon sources for synthesizing CQDs. The main advantage of this technique is that the source of carbon used is eco-friendly and economical. Hence, biomass waste has been widely used as a carbon source for CQD synthesis. For example, Wang et al. used orange peel, leaves of ginkgo biloba, leaves of paulownia tree, and magnolia flower as a carbon source to synthesize CQDs. The obtained highly fluorescent CQDs exhibited sensitivity to Fe^{3+} ions in water resources (Wang et al. 2020). Similarly, Kasinathan et al. (2022) synthesized multifluorescent CQDs using sugarcane waste as the carbon source. The quantum dots obtained were having uniform spherical shape with size ranging from 2 to 8 nm. These multifluorescent dots were utilized for several applications including Hg^{2+} detection in water and live cancer cell imaging.

1.4 APPLICATIONS OF CQDs

1.4.1 SUPERCAPACITORS

Supercapacitors are energy storage devices which have received a lot of recognition with high power output, compatibility, and durability. Supercapacitors are chiefly known for their faster performance in energy storage, for which the materials chosen for their electrodes should possess quick charging capacity, wide surface area, and high energy densities as well as being highly economical and eco-friendly (Rasal et al. 2021). CQDs have been explored widely for energy storage applications recently. Naushad et al. (2021) developed a facile hydrothermal route to synthesize nitrogen-doped carbon dots coupled with cobalt oxide as an electrode material for supercapacitors. The nanocomposite developed exhibited an astounding specific capacitance value of 1867 Fg^{-1} at 1 Ag^{-1} current density. Similarly, a composite of nickel sulfide with carbon dots were reported for electrochemical energy storage application. The nanocomposite displayed tremendous stability up to 2000 charge–discharge cycle with a specific capacitance of 880 Fg^{-1} at 1 Ag^{-1} current density (Sahoo et al. 2018).

1.4.2 PHOTOVOLTAICS

Photovoltaic technologies are a greater boon to the rising energy demand globally. Sunlight is considered as the dynamic source among all forms of renewable energy. To achieve more sustainability, widespread research on efficient energy harvesting materials is much needed. Ali et al. (2021) have designed an efficient electrocatalyst integrating multiwalled carbon nanotubes (MWCNTs) with nitrogen-doped CQDs for energy storage applications. The high surface area of the carbon dots enhanced the dispersion of MWCNTs in the electrolyte. Moreover, the high charge carrier transportation of the carbon dots shows 50% enhancement in the photovoltaic performance when compared to pristine MWCNTs. In the same way, the introduction of N-doped carbon dots in the photoanode of CdS quantum dot-sensitized solar cell magnified the photovoltaic performance up to 40.9%. The efficiency improvement is attributed to the broad absorption, recombination resistance, and suitable band alignment provided by CQDs (Huang et al. 2020).

1.4.3 LI-ION BATTERIES

Li-ion batteries (LIBs) are of high commercial demand due to their advantages such as high energy density and high durability. Though they have gained a lot of commercial attention, several LIB electrodes suffer from fast discharge due to self-aggregation and increased charge carrier recombination. CQDs with excellent conductivity are being researched to address the challenges of LIB electrodes. To improve the conductivity of Bi_2O_3, CQDs were introduced into the oxide matrix through facile hydrothermal technique. The existence of the conducting carbon network in the Bi_2O_3-CQDs nanocomposite facilitated good reversibility and a high specific capacitance of 343 Cg^{-1} at 0.5 Ag^{-1} (Prasath et al. 2019).

1.4.4 BIOIMAGING

The attractive properties of CQDs including cytotoxicity, photostability, and good optical absorption have several advantages over other semiconductor quantum dots for in-vitro and in vivo visualization of biological structures (Lim et al. 2015). CQDs synthesized from banana peel waste without any chemical agent showcased excellent fluorescent stability. The lower toxicity and biocompatibility of the CQDs were employed to stain the whole body of nematodes (Figure 1.4) at an elevated concentration of 200 $\mu g \ mL^{-1}$ (Atchudan et al. 2021). Heteroatoms such as chlorine and fluorine were added to the surface of CQDs through the one-step hydrothermal process

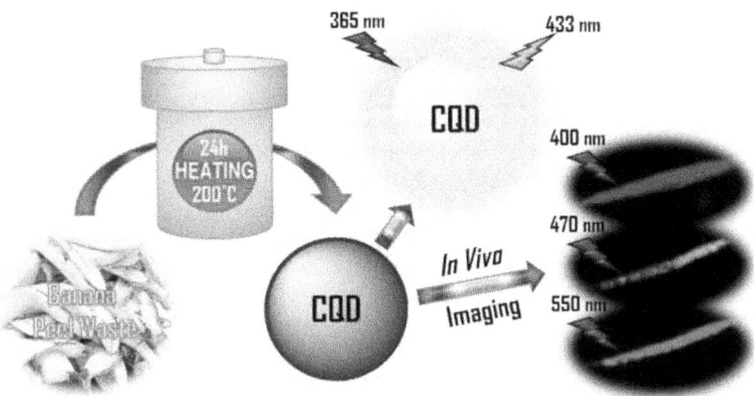

FIGURE 1.4 Bio-imaging of nematodes with CQDs derived from banana peel waste (Atchudan et al. 2021).

to enhance the optical properties of CQDs. The functionalized CQDs produced blue fluorescence with extraordinary antioxidant properties and used as fluorescent probes for cell imaging (Markovic et al. 2020).

1.4.5 BIOSENSING

The need of less-toxic high-fluorescent nanomaterial replacing conventional organic dyes as a tool for biodetection is posing a great challenge for the scientists. The tunable optical properties and biocompatibility of CQDs make them a potential candidate for biosensing. Carbon nanodots with tunable fluorescence were synthesized from biomass waste with a quantum yield up to 14 %. These CQDs were able to surpass cell membranes and emit fluorescence up to cytoplasm (Janus et al. 2020). According to Chellasamy et al. (2022), CQDs prepared from natural sources show higher biocompatibility compared to the ones synthesized with chemical agents. The attempt to synthesize CQDs from maple tree leaves through hydrothermal synthesis resulted in blue-emitting carbon nanodots with a size range of 1–10 nm. The as-synthesized quantum dots possessed stable fluorescence for nearly 100 days when used for cesium detection.

1.4.6 PHOTOCATALYSIS

The realization of solar energy as a boundless source of renewable energy that could meet the global demands has motivated the development of several photocatalytic materials to harvest solar energy efficiently. Many oxides and sulfide-based photocatalysts suffer from poor charge separation ability. CQDs with their excellent charge transportation capacity are widely incorporated as cocatalysts to enhance the photocatalytic behavior of the photocatalysts. On similar grounds, CQDs were used to improve the photoresponse of ZnO hollow spheres in degrading methylene blue dye (Figure 1.5).

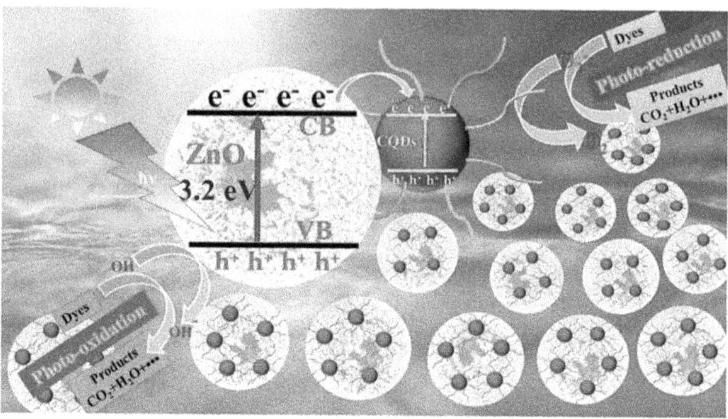

FIGURE 1.5 CQD-supported ZnO hollow spheres for dye degradation (Velumani et al. 2020).

The as-synthesized nanocomposites exhibited 96% efficiency in degradation of methylene blue dye (Velumani et al. 2020). Likewise, the photocatalytic activity of $K_2Ti_6O_{13}$ was enhanced by introducing CQDs into the lattice. The efficiency of the nanocomposite was evaluated by degrading amoxicillin under visible light irradiation. It was observed that the introduction of CQDs in the lattice of $K_2Ti_6O_{13}$ enhanced the electron-hole separation time and improved the degradation efficiency several times than pristine $K_2Ti_6O_{13}$ (Chen et al. 2019).

1.4.7 ELECTROCATALYSIS

Electrocatalysts play a major role in clear energy production through well-known hydrogen evolution reaction (HER) and oxygen evolution reaction (OER). The exceptional conductivity of carbon dots could be effectively used to fabricate electrodes for HER/OER systems. Moreover, CQDs could be a replacement for conventional noble metal-based electrodes such as 'Pt' and 'Rh' in terms of affordability (Peng et al. 2019). Heteroatom-doped carbon dots synthesized from vinegar residues were integrated with vertically aligned graphene sheets (VG) and used as electrocatalysts for HER. The developed catalyst showed excellent potential in HER activity when compared to bare VG electrodes (Jiang et al. 2023). A novel heterojunction of graphene and CQDs was built to serve as an electrode for electrocatalytic HER. The synergetic effect between defect-rich surface of CQDs and the graphene flakes exhibited superior activity in HER (Zhao et al. 2019).

1.5 CONCLUSION

To summarize, fluorescent carbon dots are new upcoming materials with fascinating properties that could be beneficial for next-generation applications. Despite numerous benefits and exceptional properties of CQDs, some drawbacks and limitations remain unaddressed yet. The origin of the fluorescence of CQDs still remains surreptitious, and research is much needed in terms of improving the quantum yield efficiency. There is a growing concern among the scientific researchers on utilizing green conversion technologies. It is observed that among various synthesis methodologies utilized for CQDs, there has been a wider exploration for synthesis of CQDs from natural sources such as fruits, leaves, barks of the tree as they are eco-friendly and economical. Next to them, hydrothermal techniques and chemical oxidation take upper hand, as in these techniques, it is feasible to control the composition and size of the dots. CQDs being a revolutionary material have taken a leap in biomedical applications. The intense fluorescence property and cytotoxicity of CQDs enable their usage as fluorescent probes and biosensors. The unique charge transportation property of CQDs efficiently fits for enhanced energy storage and environmental applications. Hence with the overview of the advancements in synthesis of CQDs and their applicability in various streams of engineering and technology, it is clear that CQDs remain a promising material for the future.

REFERENCES

Ahmed, H.B. et al. "Environmentally exploitable biocide/fluorescent metal marker carbon quantum dots", *RSC Adv.*, 2020, 10, 42916–42929, https://doi.org/10.1039/D0RA06383E

Ali, M. et al. "Microwave-assisted ultrafast in-situ growth of N-doped carbon quantum dots on multiwalled carbon nanotubes as an efficient electrocatalyst for photovoltaics", *J. Colloid Interface Sci.* 2021, 586, 349–361, https://doi.org/10.1016/j.jcis.2020.10.098

Atchudan, R. et al. "Sustainable synthesis of carbon quantum dots from banana peel waste using hydrothermal process for in vivo bioimaging", *Phys. E: Low-Dimens. Syst.*, 2021, 126, 114417. https://doi.org/10.1016/j.physe.2020.114417

Basoglu, A. et al. "Synthesis of microwave-assisted fluorescence carbon quantum dots using roasted–chickpeas and its applications for sensitive and selective detection of Fe^{3+} ions", *J. Lumin.*, 2020, 30, 515–526. https://doi.org/10.1007/s10895-019-02428-7

Chandra, S. et al. "Nitrogen/sulfur-co-doped carbon quantum dots: A biocompatible material for the selective detection of picric acid in aqueous solution and living cells", *Anal. Bioanal. Chem.*, 2020, 412, 3753–3763. https://doi.org/10.1007/s00216-020-02629-1

Chao-Mujica et al. "Carbon quantum dots by submerged arc discharge in water: Synthesis, characterization, and mechanism of formation", *J. Appl. Phys.*, 2021, 129, 163301. https://doi.org/10.1063/5.0040322

Chatzimitakos, T. and Stalikas, C., 2020. "Antimicrobial properties of carbon quantum dots", in *Nanotoxicity* (pp. 301–315). Elsevier. https://doi.org/10.1016/B978-0-12-819943-5.00014-2

Chellasamy, G. et al. "Green synthesized carbon quantum dots from maple tree leaves for biosensing of Cesium and electrocatalytic oxidation of glycerol", *Chemosphere*, 2022, 287(1), 131915, https://doi.org/10.1016/j.chemosphere.2021.131915

Chen, Q. et al. "Photocatalytic degradation of amoxicillin by carbon quantum dots modified $K_2Ti_6O_{13}$ nanotubes: Effect of light wavelength", *Chin. Chem. Lett.*, 2019, 30(6), 1214–1218. https://doi.org/10.1016/j.cclet.2019.03.002

Chunduri, L.A.A. et al., "Carbon quantum dots from coconut husk: Evaluation for antioxidant and cytotoxic activity", *Mater. Focus*, 2016, 5(1), 55–61. https://doi.org/10.1166/mat.2016.1289

Cui, L. et al. "Synthesis of homogeneous carbon quantum dots by ultrafast dual-beam pulsed laser ablation for bioimaging", *Mater. Today Nano.*, 2020, 12, 100091. https://doi.org/10.1016/j.mtnano.2020.100091

Das, P. et al. "Acoustic cavitation assisted synthesis and characterization of photoluminescent carbon quantum dots for biological applications and their future prospective", *Nano-Struct. Nano-Objects.*, 2021, 25, 100641. https://doi.org/10.1016/j.nanoso.2020.100641

Donate-Buendia, C. et al. "Pulsed laser ablation in liquids for the production of gold nanoparticles and carbon quantum dots: From plasmonic to fluorescence and cell labelling", *J. Phys.: Conf. Ser.*, 2020, 1537 012013. https://doi.org/10.1088/1742-6596/1537/1/012013

Dong, L. et al. "Synthesis of carbon quantum dots to fabricate ultraviolet-shielding poly(vinylidene fluoride) films", *J. Appl. Polym. Sci.*, 2019, 2019, 47555 (1–6). https://doi.org/10.1002/APP.47555

El-Shabasy, R.M. et al. "Recent developments in carbon quantum dots: Properties, fabrication techniques, and bio-applications", *Processes*, 2021, 9, 388. https://doi.org/10.3390/pr9020388

Eskalen, H. et al. "Microwave-assisted ultra-fast synthesis of carbon quantum dots from linter: Fluorescence cancer imaging and human cell growth inhibition properties", *Ind. Crops Prod.*, 2020, 147, 112209. https://doi.org/10.1016/j.indcrop.2020.112209

Ezati, P. and Rhim, J.W. "Pectin/carbon quantum dots fluorescent film with ultraviolet blocking property through light conversion", *Colloids. Surf. B Biointerfaces*, 2022, 219, 112804 https://doi.org/10.1016/j.colsurfb.2022.112804

Ezati, P. et al. "Carbon quantum dots-based antifungal coating film for active packaging application of avocado", *Food Packag. Shelf Life*, 2022, 33, 100878. https://doi.org/10.1016/j.fpsl.2022.100878

Ganesan, S. et al. "Microwave-assisted green synthesis of multi-functional carbon quantum dots as efficient fluorescence sensor for ultra-trace level monitoring of ammonia in environmental water", *Environ. Res.*, 2022, 206, 112589. https://doi.org/10.1016/j.envres.2021.112589

Gao, J. et al. "Synthesis of carbon quantum dots by gas-liquid plasma using ethanol as precursor", *IEEE 5th International Electrical and Energy Conference (CIEEC)*, 2022, 3385–3389. https://doi.org/10.1109/CIEEC54735.2022.9846313

Gu, S. et al. "Fluorescence of functionalized graphene quantum dots prepared from infrared-assisted pyrolysis of citric acid and urea", *J. Lumin.*, 2020, 217, 116774. https://doi.org/10.1016/j.jlumin.2019.116774

Guo, Y. et al. "Aggregation-induced emission enhancement of carbon quantum dots and applications in light emitting devices", *J. Mater. Chem. C*, 2019, 7, 5148–5154. https://doi.org/10.1039/C9TC01138B

Guo, Y. et al. "Hydrothermal synthesis of highly fluorescent nitrogen-doped carbon quantum dots with good biocompatibility and the application for sensing ellagic acid", *Spectrochim. Acta A Mol.*, 2020, 240, 118580. https://doi.org/10.1016/j.saa.2020.118580

Hanon et al. "Green synthesis of highly luminescent carbon quantum dots from lemon juice", *J. Nanomater.*, 2019, 2852816. https://doi.org/10.1155/2019/2852816

Huang, H. et al. "A one-step ultrasonic irradiation assisted strategy for the preparation of polymer-functionalized carbon quantum dots and their biological imaging", *J. Colloid Interface Sci.*, 2018, 532, 767–773. https://doi.org/10.1016/j.jcis.2018.07.099

Huang, P. et al., "Carbon quantum dots improving photovoltaic performance of CdS quantum dot-sensitized solar cells", *Opt. Mater.*, 2020, 110, 110535. https://doi.org/10.1016/j.optmat.2020.110535

Hussein, N.L. et al. "Simulation of optical energy gap for synthesis carbon quantum dot by laser ablation", *Iraqi J. Sci.*, 2019, 60, 52–56 https://doi.org/10.24996/ijs.2019.60.S.I.9

Janus, L. et al. "Facile synthesis of surface-modified carbon quantum dots (CQDs) for biosensing and bioimaging", *Materials*, 2020, 13(15), 3313. https://doi.org/10.3390/ma13153313

Jian, H.J. et al. "Highly adhesive carbon quantum dots from biogenic amines for prevention of biofilm formation", *Chem. Eng. J.*, 2020, 386, 123913. https://doi.org/10.1016/j.cej.2019.123913

Jiang, B. et al. "Electrocatalytic activity analysis of vinegar residue-based heteroatom-doped carbon quantum dots integrated on vertically aligned graphene arrays for hydrogen evolution reaction", *Int. J. Hyd. Energy*, 2023. https://doi.org/10.1016/j.ijhydene.2023.06.092

Jiang, L. et al. "Photoactivated fluorescence enhancement in F,N-doped carbon dots with piezochromic behavior", *Angew. Chem. Int. Ed.*, 2020, 59, 9986. https://doi.org/10.1002/anie.201913800

Jiang, Y. et al. "A novel carbon quantum dots-enhanced chemiluminescence method for the sensitive determination of iodide ion", *Dyes Pigm.*, 2022, 203, 110318. https://doi.org/10.1016/j.dyepig.2022.110318

Kasinathan, K. et al. "Green synthesis of multicolour fluorescence carbon quantum dots from sugarcane waste: Investigation of mercury (II) ion sensing, and bio-imaging applications", *Appl. Surf. Sci.*, 2022, 601, 154266. https://doi.org/10.1016/j.apsusc.2022.154266

Khan, Z.M.S.H. et al. "A facile one step hydrothermal synthesis of carbon quantum dots for label -free fluorescence sensing approach to detect picric acid in aqueous solution", *J. Photochem. Photobiol. A*, 2020, 388, 112201. https://doi.org/10.1016/j.jphotochem.2019.112201

Li, J. et al. "Three-dimensional nitrogen and phosphorus co-doped carbon quantum dots/reduced graphene oxide composite aerogels with a hierarchical porous structure as superior electrode materials for supercapacitors", *J. Mater. Chem. A*, 2019, 7, 26311–26325. https://doi.org/10.1039/C9TA08151H

Lu, M. and Zhou, Li "One-step sonochemical synthesis of versatile nitrogen-doped carbon quantum dots for sensitive detection of Fe^{2+} ions and temperature in vitro", *Mater. Sci. Eng. C*, 2019, 101, 352–359. https://doi.org/10.1016/j.msec.2019.03.109

Mahani, M. et al., "Doxorubicin delivery to breast cancer cells with transferrin-targeted carbon quantum dots: An in vitro and in silico study", *J. Drug Deliv. Sci. Technol.*, 2021, 62, 102342. https://doi.org/10.1016/j.jddst.2021.102342

Markovic, Z.M. et al. "Highly efficient antioxidant F- and Cl-doped carbon quantum dots for bioimaging", *ACS Sustainable Chem. Eng.*, 2020, 8(43), 16327–16338. https://doi.org/10.1021/acssuschemeng.0c06260

Mitra, S. et al., "Room temperature and solvothermal green synthesis of self passivated carbon quantum dots", *RSC Adv.*, 2013, 3, 3189–3193. https://doi.org/10.1039/C2RA23085B

Moradlou, O. et al., "Antibacterial effects of carbon quantum dots@hematite nanostructures deposited on titanium against Gram-positive and Gram-negative bacteria", *J. Photochem. Photobiol. A Chem.*, 379, 2019, 144–149 https://doi.org/10.1016/j.jphotochem.2019.04.047

Nallayagiri, A.R. et al. "Tuneable properties of carbon quantum dots by different synthetic methods", *J. Nanostructure Chem.*, 12, 2021, 565–580. https://doi.org/10.1007/s40097-021-00431-8

Naushad, M. et al., "Nitrogen-doped carbon quantum dots (N-CQDs)/Co_3O_4 nanocomposite for high performance supercapacitor", *J. King Saud Univ. Sci.*, 2021, 33, 101252. https://doi.org/10.1016/j.jksus.2020.101252.

Oh, G.H. et al., "Acid treatment to tune the optical properties of carbon quantum dots", *Appl. Surf. Sci.*, 2022, 605, 154690. https://doi.org/10.1016/j.apsusc.2022.154690.

Pandiyan, S. et al., "Biocompatible carbon quantum dots derived from sugarcane industrial wastes for effective nonlinear optical behavior and antimicrobial activity applications", *ACS Omega*, 2020, 5, 30363–30372. https://doi.org/10.1021/acsomega.0c03290

Peng, Z. et al. "Hollow carbon shells enhanced by confined ruthenium as cost-efficient and superior catalysts for the alkaline hydrogen evolution reaction", *Mater. Chem. A*, 2019, 7, 6676–6685. https://doi.org/10.1039/C8TA09136F

Pho, Q.H. et al. "Process intensification for gram-scale synthesis of N-doped carbon quantum dots immersing a microplasma jet in a gas-liquid reactor", *Chem. Eng. J.* 2023, 452(1), 139164. https://doi.org/10.1016/j.cej.2022.139164

Prasath, A. et al., "Carbon quantum dot-anchored bismuth oxide composites as potential electrode for lithium-ion battery and supercapacitor applications", *ACS Omega* 2019, 4, 3, 4943–4954. https://doi.org/10.1021/acsomega.8b03490

Rajamanikandan, S. et al., "Blue emissive carbon quantum dots (CQDs) from bio-waste peels and its antioxidant activity", *J. Clust. Sci.*, 2021, 33, 1045–1053. https://doi.org/10.1007/s10876-021-02029-0

Rasal, A.S. et al., "Carbon quantum dots for energy applications: A review", *ACS Appl. Nano Mater.* 2021, 4, 6515–6541. https://doi.org/10.1021/acsanm.1c01372

Sadrolhosseini, A.R. et al., "Enhancement of the fluorescence property of carbon quantum dots based on laser ablated gold nanoparticles to evaluate pyrene", *Opt. Mater. Express*, 2020, 10(9), 2227–2241. https://doi.org/10.1364/OME.396914

Sahoo et al., "Incorporation of carbon quantum dots for improvement of supercapacitor performance of nickel sulfide", *ACS Omega*, 2018, 3, 17936–17946. http://doi.org/10.1021/acsomega.8b01238

Shankar, S.S. et al. "Carbon quantum dots: A potential candidate for diagnostic and therapeutic application", *Nanobiomater. Eng.* 2020. https://doi.org/10.1007/978-981-32-9840-8_3

Sharma, N., et al., "Green synthesis of multipurpose carbon quantum dots from red cabbage and estimation of their antioxidant potential and bio-labeling activity", *Appl. Microbiol. Biotechnol.*, 2020, 104, 7187–7200. https://doi.org/10.1007/s00253-020-10726-5.

Shekarbeygi, Z. et al. "The effects of rose pigments extracted by different methods on the optical properties of carbon quantum dots and its efficacy in the determination of Diazinon", *Microchem. J.*, 2020, 158, 105232. https://doi.org/10.1016/j.microc.2020.105232

Shen, T.Y. et al. "Hydrothermal synthesis of N-doped carbon quantum dots and their application in ion-detection and cell-imaging", *Spectrochim. Acta A.*, 2021, 248, 119282. https://doi.org/10.1016/j.saa.2020.119282

Shi, Y. et al. "Red phosphorescent carbon quantum dot organic framework-based electroluminescent light-emitting diodes exceeding 5% external quantum efficiency", *J. Am. Chem. Soc.*, 2021, 143(45), 18941–18951. https://doi.org/10.1021/jacs.1c07054

Song, Y. et al., "Carbon quantum dots from roasted Atlantic salmon (Salmo salar L.): Formation, biodistribution and cytotoxicity", *Food Chem.*, 2019, 293, 387–395. https://doi.org/10.1016/j.foodchem.2019.05.017

Tian, L. et al., "The influence of inorganic electrolyte on the properties of carbon quantum dots in electrochemical exfoliation", *J. Electroanal. Chem.*, 2020, 878, 114673. https://doi.org/10.1016/j.jelechem.2020.114673

Tungare, K. et al., "Synthesis, characterization and biocompatibility studies of carbon quantum dots from Phoenix dactylifera", *Biotech*, 2020, 10, 540. https://doi.org/10.1007/s13205-020-02518-5

Velumani, A. et al., "Carbon quantum dots supported ZnO sphere based photocatalyst for dye degradation application", *Curr. Appl. Phys.*, 2020, 20(10), 1176–1184. https://doi.org/10.1016/j.cap.2020.07.016

Wang, C. et al. "Facile synthesis of novel carbon quantum dots from biomass waste for highly sensitive detection of iron ions", *Mater. Res. Bull.* 2020, 124, 110730. https://doi.org/10.1016/j.materresbull.2019.110730

Wang, R. et al., "Recent progress in carbon quantum dots: Synthesis, properties and applications in photocatalysis", *J. Mater. Chem. A*, 2017, 5, 3717. https://doi.org/10.1039/c6ta08660h

Wang, X. et al., "A mini review on carbon quantum dots: Preparation, properties, and electrocatalytic application", *Front. Chem.* 2019, 7, 671. https://doi.org/10.3389/fchem.2019.00671

Weerasinghe, J. et al. "Monochromatic blue and switchable blue-green carbon quantum dots by room-temperature air plasma processing", *Adv. Mater. Technol.* 2021, 7, 2100586. https://doi.org/10.1002/admt.202100586

Wong, K.T. et al., "Critical insight on the hydrothermal effects toward exfoliation of g-C$_3$N$_4$ and simultaneous in-situ deposition of carbon quantum dots", *Appl. Surf. Sci.*, 2019, 471, 703–713. https://doi.org/10.1016/j.apsusc.2018.12.064

Xie, F. et al., "Unveiling the role of hydrothermal carbon dots as anodes in sodiumion batteries with ultrahigh initial coulombic efficiency", *J. Mater. Chem. A* 2019, 7(48), 27567–27575. https://doi.org/10.1039/C9TA11369J

Xu, X. et al., "Electrophoretic analysis and purification of fluorescent single-walled carbon nanotube fragments", *J. Am. Chem. Soc.*, 2004, 126(40), 12736–12737. https://doi.org/10.1021/ja040082h

Yahyai, I.A. et al., "A paper-based chemiluminescence detection device based on S, N-doped carbon quantum dots for the selective and highly sensitive recognition of bendiocarb", *Anal. Methods*, 2021, 13, 3461–3470. https://doi.org/10.1039/D1AY00728A

Zhang, Y. et al. "Graphene oxide membranes for nanofiltration", *Curr. Opin. Chem. Eng.*, 2017, 16, 9–15. https://doi.org/10.1016/j.coche.2017.03.002

Zhao, M. et al., "Facile in situ synthesis of a carbon quantum dot/graphene heterostructure as an efficient metal free electrocatalyst for overall water splitting", *Chem. Commun.*, 2019. https://doi.org/10.1039/c8cc09368g

2 Natural Sources Used to Fabricate Carbon Quantum Dots

Hao Xu, Long Chen, Zhengyu Jin and Ming Miao

2.1 AN OVERVIEW OF NATURAL SOURCE CARBON QUANTUM DOTS

Carbon quantum dots (CQDs) are novel carbon materials with diameters less than 10 nm and they exhibit excellent fluorescence properties. They were first reported as an impurity during the preparing process of single-walled carbon nanotubes and could be separated and purified by preparative electrophoresis (X. Xu et al., 2004). Sun et al. (2006) prepared luminescent CDs by using laser ablation and surface passivation techniques. After that, a dramatically increased amount of research focused on exploring the practical properties of CDs.

Compared to traditional semiconductor quantum dots, organic dyes, and upconverting nanoparticles, CDs exhibit unique superiorities on high photostability, aqueous dispersity, excellent chemical inertness, and ability of modification. In addition, CDs display low toxicity and good biocompatibility, enabling their application in bioimaging, biosensing, and drug-delivery systems (H. Xu et al., 2022a). Moreover, CDs show outstanding electronic properties that make them as available electron donors and acceptors which are applied in catalysis and optronics (Xiang & Tan, 2022).

Based on the different carbon sources used for CD fabrication, CDs are classified as man-made and natural CDs (Humaera, Fahri, Armynah, & Tahir, 2021; X. Zhang et al., 2018b). Common man-made carbon sources include graphite, candle soot, fullerene C60, ammonium glucose, citrate, ammonium hydroxide, ethylenediamine, etc. While natural carbon sources for CDs contains a much wider variety of materials, in which biopolymers were the most popularly researched materials because of their advantages of abundance and low-cost. The environmentally effective natural materials show superiority on synthesizing natural-product-derived CDs (Y. Wang, Li, & Feng, 2020). Currently, the most frequently researched natural carbon sources for CDs were obtained from plants and animals. The processing of natural-product-derived CDs could contribute to high-value utilization of those biomaterials. Additionally, heteroatoms (N, S) that existed in natural biomaterials show advantages in the preparation of heteroatom-doped CDs, which avoided additional use of other ingredients containing N/S elements (Koshy et al., 2021).

DOI: 10.1201/9781003437857-3

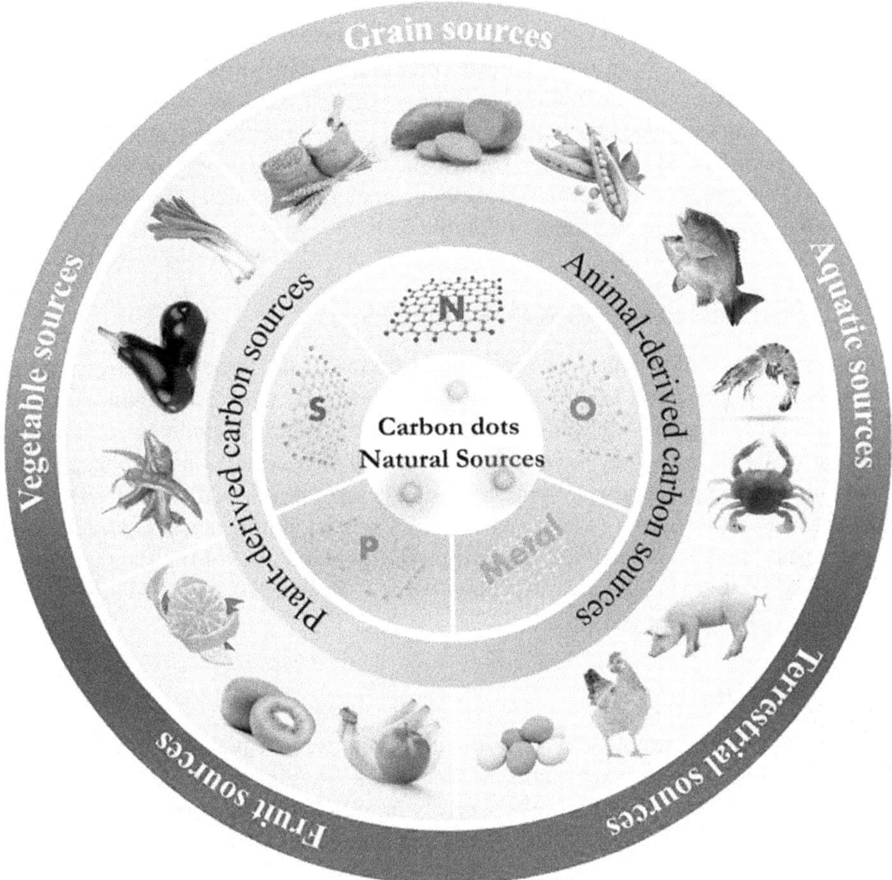

FIGURE 2.1 The natural sources and elemental composition of carbon dots.

With the increasing attention by researchers on natural-product-derived CDs, novel approaches were gradually developed for the preparation of CDs, which varied from those adopted for preparing CDs from man-made carbon sources. Since few publications provide a comprehensive analysis on the up-to-date preparation methods of natural-product-derived CDs, it is necessary to give an overview of the recent developments in CDs specifically from the perspective of raw material types, thereby promoting the development of CDs in industries (Figure 2.1).

2.2 PLANT-DERIVED CARBON SOURCES

Plants consist of up to 40–50% of carbon and are abundant in nature, which makes them superior natural sources for the preparation of CDs. Various types of plants have been researched as excellent raw materials for CD preparation, such as rose, lentil, leaf, and ginger, etc. (Amjadi, Hallaj, & Mayan, 2016). Quantum yield (QY) is an essential character for the preparation of CDs. Though CDs prepared using the aforementioned plant carbon sources exhibited uniformly distributed sizes of 2–10 nm, the QY of the prepared CDs was less than 15% because of high carbon content of the precursors. It has been reported that components consisting of heteroatoms that exist in the precursors are beneficial to improve the QY, such as vitamins and minerals. When using sweet pepper, ginkgo leaves, or cabbage as the raw material, the QY of the as-prepared CDs showed a significant improvement from 16.5% to 21.7%. While a QY of 18.98% was achieved by Wang et al. (2012) when using papaya as the carbon source of water- and ethanol-soluble CDs.

2.3 GRAIN BASED CARBON SOURCES

Grains cover a wide range and are usually divided into three categories, including Cereals, Tubers, and Legumes. Cereals include rice, wheat, sorghum, corn, etc. Legumes include peas, soybeans, broad beans, etc. Tubers include sweet potatoes, cassava, potatoes, etc. They have the advantages of easy collection and cheap as raw materials for CD preparation. Some researchers have developed several CDs using grains as a carbon source, such as rice, wheat, corn, sorghum, cassava, potato, sweet potato, peas, etc. (Jorn-am et al., 2021; Haochi Liu et al., 2019; Min, Ezati, & Rhim, 2022; Qiu, Li, Li, Ma, & Li, 2021; Sangubotla & Kim, 2019; Shi et al., 2022; Jing Wang, Ng, Lim, & Ho, 2014).

2.3.1 CEREALS

Cereals, as people's staple food, are mainly composed of high levels of carbohydrates and contain other rich nutrients, including protein, unsaturated fatty acids, B vitamins, and some inorganic salts. Cereals-based-CDs can be prepared by one-pot hydrothermal method (Figure 2.2a). Sabet and Salmeh (2020) dispersed milled rice powder in 100 ml distilled water, followed by high-pressure treatment at 180°C for 4.5 h to prepare rice CDs. The structure of this carbon material has dual characteristics of CDs and graphene oxide nanostructures, which has an emission wavelength of around 510 nm. The band gap of 2.41eV also indicates its photocatalytic activity. In addition, rice husks were also effective carbon sources for CDs. Wongso et al. (2021) cleaned the rice husks and carbonized them at a high temperature of 700°C for 2 h to produce rice husk ash. Then, combined with hydrothermal reactions, silicon containing rice husk-based CDs were prepared. With increasing hydrothermal temperature, CDs with smaller size were obtained, and its QY reaches a maximum of 19.11% (Wongso, Sambudi, Sufian, & Isnaeni, 2021). Hui et al. (2021) prepared CDs from rice husk and modified by using nitrogen and bismuth. The sizes of nitrogen- and bismuth-modified CDs were around 8 nm and 5 nm, respectively.

Similarly, bran, straw, and other parts of wheat have been used to fabricate CDs. John et al. (2020) collected the wheat bran and treated under hydrothermal conditions (180°C, 3 h); CDs with an average diameter of 4.9 nm were obtained. The CDs exhibit blue-green fluorescence and the excitation-dependent emission, and the QY was about 7.5%. Additionally, wheat straw was also utilized as the starting material of CDs. Under a hydrothermal reaction at 180°C for 12 h, wheat straw was degraded to form blue fluorescent CDs, whose emission also have excitation-dependent effect,

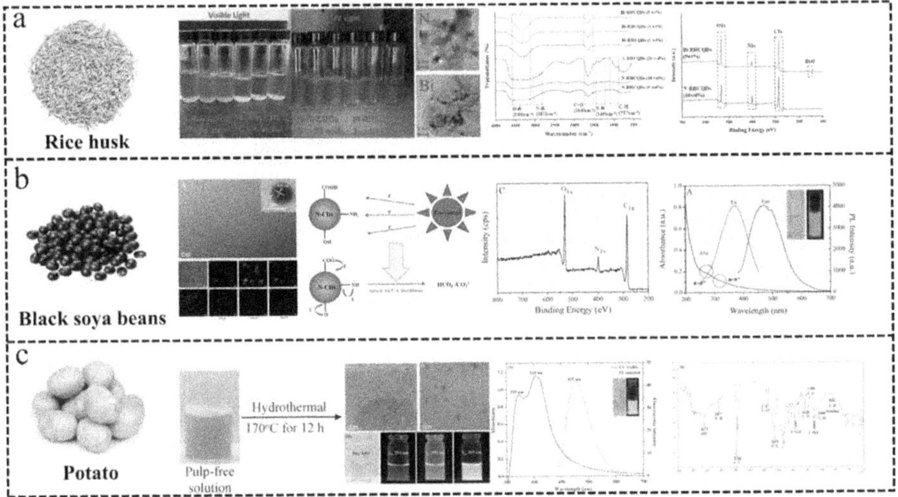

FIGURE 2.2 Carbon dots and their structural composition from grain sources. (a) Rice husk-derived carbon dots (Chung Hui, Lun Ang, & Soraya Sambudi, 2021). (b) Black soya beans-derived carbon dots (Jia et al., 2019). (c) Potato-derived carbon dots (Mehta, Jha, Singhal, & Kailasa, 2014).

and the size was about 5.7 nm (S. Liu et al., 2021b). When the hydrothermal temperature increases to 250°C for 10 h, the wheat straw formed smaller blue fluorescent CDs (1.7 nm) with a QY of around 9.2%, which can be applied in labeling, imaging, and sensing materials (M. Yuan et al., 2015).

Corn is also a promising carbon source in cereal plants for the preparation of CDs. Rajendran et al. (2019) prepared a corn-based carbon dot (CD) with blue-green fluorescence using sweet corn kernels as the carbon source. The prepared CDs had a small size of <2.4 nm, exhibiting excellent fluorescence stability and selective identification of sulfur ions. Corn straw was also used to hydrothermally develop CDs as a carbon source. These CDs have a diameter of 5 nm, a QY of 4.6%, and used in the detection of Cu^{2+} (Yang, Guo, & Yue, 2021). Zheng et al. (2023) used corn cob as the carbon source of CDs, with a QY of 1.9%. After modification by ionic liquid, the QY of CDs was increased to 15.15%, and the size was around 1.5 nm.

2.3.2 Tubers

Tubers are a general term for rhizome crops, including potatoes, sweet potatoes, taro, yams, etc., which also can be applied as carbon sources for CDs. Mehta et al. (2014) developed high fluorescence CDs with a size of 0.2–2.2 nm using potatoes by one-step hydrothermal method at 170°C for 12 h (Figure 2.2c). These CDs exhibit blue fluorescence at 365nm. Sinha et al. (2019) also choose the potato as a carbon source to fabricate CDs with a size of around 5.79 nm and a QY of 6.08%, which exhibited sensitivity to Cr^{6+} and Fe^{3+}. Similarly, sweet potato is one of the main agricultural crops distributed around the world, which means it can provide rich carbon source to develop CDs. Sweet potatoes are first crushed into a mixed juice and then subjected to hydrothermal reaction at 180°C for 18 h to prepare a blue fluorescent carbon dots (Shen, Shang, Chen, Wang, & Cai, 2017b). The as-prepared CDs have a diameter of about 3.4 nm, and a QY of 8.64%. Some researchers use sweet potato peel to prepare functional CDs using the hydrothermal approach. Liu et al. (2018) fabricated CDs with a size of about 2 nm using sweet potato peel and further modified it to obtain a carbon dot fluorescence probe capable of detecting oxytetracycline. Using such carbon source with the benefit of being abundant in nature greatly reduces the cost of safety monitoring probes. Interestingly, some researchers directly isolated CDs from the carbon residue of baked sweet potato; the isolated CDs exhibited superior aqueous solubility and they were able to prepare carbon dot probes that can detect Fe^{3+} successfully (Abdella & El-Malla, 2023). The CDs with an average diameter of 3.5 nm show a QY of 54%. In addition, cassava was also researched for its possibility as a carbon source for CDs. Jorn-am et al. (2022) mixed nitric acid and cassava peel and the mixture was subjected to a hydrothermal reaction at 200°C for 5 h to prepare CDs with a size of about 9 nm and with a negative surface charge. Other researchers choose cassava stems to fabricate lignocellulosic biomass–CDs. By modifying with nitric acid, the QY and fluorescence efficiency of lignocellulosic biomass–CDs were increased by 36% and 80%, respectively (Qiu et al., 2023).

2.3.3 LEGUMES

There are a wide variety of legumes with rich nutrients and a wide distribution area, including faba beans, peas, soybeans, black beans, red beans, etc. Many researchers also choose beans to prepare CDs. Fallah et al. (2023) developed CDs with strong blue fluorescence using faba beans by hydrothermal methods at 160°C for 24 h. These CDs have a size of 0.85nm, a QY of 5.94%, and exhibited sensitivity to Hg^+. Pea was as carbon source used to fabricate blue-emission CDs that contain three elements (C, N, and O) and have an average size of 1.91nm and a QY of 18.6%. A fluorescence detection method for Cu^{2+} and EDTA analysis has been established based on the performance of this carbon dot (W. Xu, Hao, Li, Dai, & Fang, 2021). N-doped CDs were developed by a pyrolysis method using black soya beans as carbon sources at 200°C for 4 h; their size was about 5.2 nm, and they exhibited strong photoluminescence properties with a QY of 38.7% (Jia et al., 2019). These CDs were Fe^{3+} sensitive, showing great potential in cellular imaging. Zhang et al (2019) developed CDs from black soybeans with treatment under hydrothermal conditions at 180°C for 18 h. These CDs showed a size of 10 nm and a QY of 5.6%. Compared with the black bean CDs mentioned above, different preparation methods can contribute to various performance of CDs from the same carbon source. Zulfajri et al. (2019) developed blue fluorescent CDs from cranberry beans source; these CDs were about 3.96 nm in size, showed a QY of 10.86%, and exhibited sensitivity to Fe^{3+}. Additionally, soya bean grounds were also reported as carbon sources to prepare CDs. A blue fluorescent carbon dot with a diameter of 3 nm was prepared using the hydrothermal approach from soya bean grounds, with a QY at around 13% (W. Li, Yue, Wang, Zhang, & Liu, 2013).

2.4 VEGETABLE CARBON SOURCES

Vegetables are one of the indispensable food types for human beings, with a wide variety and cultivation range. Vegetables contain a large amount of nutrients, including extremely high levels of vitamin C, vitamin A, and a large amount of plant-active ingredients. Many vegetables and their waste are used to prepare CDs, such as garlic, carrot, ginger, Momordica charantia, spinach, cabbage, etc. (Y. Chen, Wu, Weng, Wang, & Li, 2016; Dong, Zhang, Zhi, Yang, & Yao, 2021; R. Lin, Cheng, & Tan, 2022; Z. Liu et al., 2021a; Long et al., 2020; Jing Wang et al., 2014).

2.4.1 LEAFY VEGETABLES

Leafy vegetables contain a large amount of natural substances such as chlorophyll and vitamins, which can be naturally doped with other elements or are sensitive to certain elements, such as iron, during the preparation of CDs. Kaur et al. (2023) used spinach juice and different grades of Soxhlet extracts to prepare CDs. However, under the same hydrothermal reaction conditions (200°C for 6h), only spinach juice formed CDs with blue fluorescence, while Soxhlet extract only formed carbon nanoparticles. CDs prepared from spinach are almost noncytotoxic, have high fluorescence QY, and show superior aqueous solubility (Ren, Tang, Chai, & Wu, 2018). Usually, the fluorescence emission range of CDs synthesized by vegetables is limited from blue to green. Some researchers synthesized fluorescent CDs emitting red light when spinach was utilized. Xu et al. (2020) extracted chlorophyll from spinach leaves as a carbon source and prepared red-emissive CDs; these CDs had a size of 3 nm, and they were prepared through hydrothermal reactions at 140°C for 4 h.

Since scallions contain abundant C, N, O, and S elements, CDs doped with N and S atoms can be prepared using scallions as precursors. Gu et al. (2018) chopped scallions and heated them under 800W microwave for 4 min, and obtained blue fluorescent CDs successfully, with a fluorescence QY of 18.6% and a size of 3.23nm (Figure 2.3a). Some researchers synthesized N-doped CDs using cabbage as the precursor (Maruthapandi, Saravanan, Luong, & Gedanken, 2021; Sharma, Das, & Yun, 2020). Alam et al. (2015) crushed cabbage and then treated it in water at 140°C for 5 h to prepare blue light CDs with a QY of 7% and a size range of of 2–6 nm. Leek and celery are also used as precursors for carbon dot synthesis (Hu, Li, & Li, 2019; Qu, Yu, Zhu, Chai, & Su, 2020; Z. Shen et al., 2017a). Wu et al. (2020) synthesized dual and single emission fluorescent CDs using leek as precursors, with the average sizes of the two CDs of about 5.6 nm and 7.7 nm, respectively, and the QYs of 1.7% and 1.14%, respectively. Shasha et al. (2019) developed N-doped CDs that were sensitive to copper ions using celery stems as carbon sources.

2.4.2 RHIZOMES

In daily food, rhizomes are also a major category of vegetables, such as garlic, carrots, ginger, radishes, onions, etc. Many researchers choose rhizomes vegetable to prepare CDs. Zhao et al. (2015) prepared blue fluorescent CDs with a diameter of

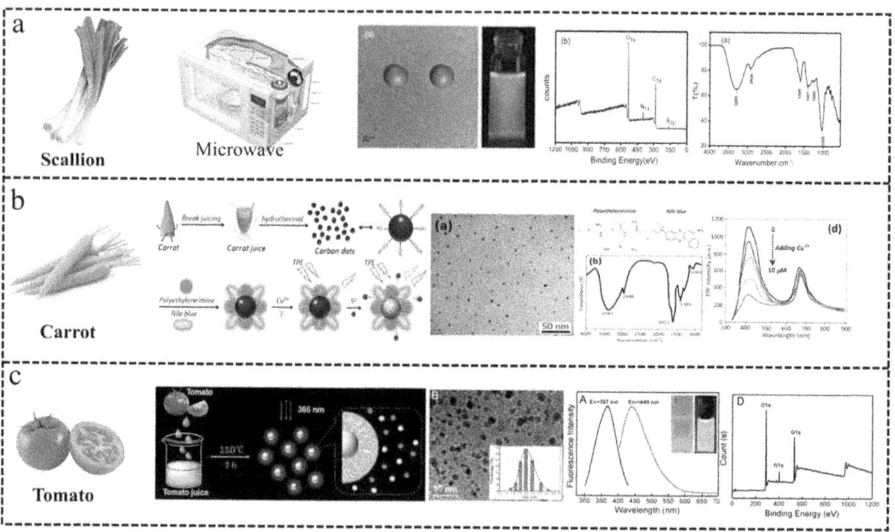

FIGURE 2.3 Carbon dots and their structural composition from vegetables. (a) Scallion-derived carbon dots (Gu, Hong, Zhang, Liu, & Shang, 2018). (b) Carrot-derived carbon dots (Jin, Gui, Wang, & Sun, 2017). (c) Tomato-derived carbon dots (Miao, Wang, Zhuo, Zhou, & Yang, 2016).

11 nm and a QY of 17.5%; garlic was used as the carbon source and after a 200°C hydrothermal processing for 5 h, the CDS were prepared. The obtained CDs contain four elements: C, N, O, and S. Carrots were used as precursors to prepare CDs upon treatment at 180°C under hydrothermal conditions for 5 h, and the prepared CDs showed a size of 4.8 nm (Figure 2.3b) (Jin, Gui, Wang, & Sun, 2017). Similarly, upon treatment with 800W microwave for 6 min, lotus roots can be processed into CDs with a QY of 19% and a diameter of 9.41 nm, which can be used for Hg^{2+} detection (Gu, Shang, Yu, & Shen, 2016). Interestingly, *Asparagus racemosus* root was also chosen to prepare CDs. Blue fluorescent CDs of size 4.6 nm with a QY of 2.46% were prepared by hydrothermal reaction at 160°C for 8 h in a high-pressure reactor (Naik et al., 2022). Li et al. (2023) CDs with a strong blue fluorescence using ginger aqueous solution, the average size of the CDs was 2.3 nm, and the CDs had been proven to show anti-inflammatory activity and wound healing property. Wang et al. (2018) prepared a 4–8 nm carbon quantum dot using beetroot powder without adding other reagents. It has been demonstrated that functional groups such as carboxyl groups existed on the surface of the CDs enable it to generate strong fluorescence. The red beet pigment can also be used to prepare CDs. Cao et al. (2022) used a one-step hydrothermal approach to prepare CDs from betaine. The obtained CDs showed an average diameter of 4.66 nm, and were rich in amino, carboxyl, and hydroxyl groups, which enable them to be used to detect tetracycline residues in food. Additionally, onions can also be used as precursors for carbon dot synthesis. SalimiShahraki et al. (2023) fabricated CDs with a QY of 12% by mixing onion peel extract with EDA and hydrothermal reaction at 120°C for 2.5 h. The material can be used to remove Congo red and methyl orange pigments.

2.4.3 SOLANACEAE AND FRUIT VEGETABLE

There are over 3000 species and approximately 90 genera in the Solanaceae family. The fruits of Solanaceae plants are an indispensable part of human vegetables. The well-known Solanaceae and fruit vegetables include tomatoes, eggplants, chili peppers, bitter gourds, and luffa (X. Song et al., 2024). Hoang et al. (2019) prepared blue fluorescent CDs with a diameter of 2–5 nm using eggplant as the carbon source by hydrothermal reaction at 220°C for 8 h. These carbon dots have potential application value in the preparation of three-dimensional porous materials for energy storage. Tomato was also used as the carbon source by some researchers. Rodríguez-Varillas et al. (2022) obtained CDs from tomato juice by the hydrothermal method. These CDs showed a size of 9 nm with a QY of 1%–1.2%. Owing to the surface functional groups and structure of the CDs, they have an antioxidant activity of up to 63% against DPPH. Other researchers have prepared blue fluorescent CDs with a QY of 13.9% and a size of 3 nm using tomato juice by hydrothermal processing (150°C, 2 h) (Figure 2.3c) (Miao, Wang, Zhuo, Zhou, & Yang, 2016). Using the same method, researchers prepared a carbon dot of size 2.6 nm with a QY of 53% at 200°C for 6 h (Haijian Liu et al., 2022). *Momordica charantia L.* can also be made into CDs after removing the seeds followed by processing at 180°C under hydrothermal conditions for 5 h, and the obtained CDs can be used to detect p-aminoazobenzene (Y. Liu et al., 2021c). *Luffa acutangula* was reported to be a carbon source to synthesize CDs (Chandrasekaran et al., 2022). The CDs were obtained upon reaction at 180°C for 12 h, which show a size of 4.4 nm and a QY of 14%.

2.5 FRUIT

Fruits, as a more widely distributed and diverse type of food, such as apple, orange, lemon, pear, grapefruit, cherry tomatoes, etc., are widely applied as carbon sources by many researchers for the fabrication of multifunctional CDs due to their easy availability and rich element content (Borna, Sabzi, & Pirsa, 2021; Dias et al., 2019; He et al., 2018; Huo et al., 2020; Sahu, Behera, Maiti, & Mohapatra, 2012; P. Wang et al., 2016b). Most organ parts of fruits can also serve as carbon dot precursors, including peel, seeds, pulp, etc. (Kang et al., 2023).

2.5.1 ORANGE FRUITS

Citrus fruits, including lemons (Figure 2.4a), pomelos, and oranges, are also commonly used as carbon sources. Aslan and Eskalen (2021) squeezed oranges into juice and subjected the juice under hydrothermal conditions at 170°C for 12 h to obtain CDs, and the resulting CDs were around 1.9 nm in size with a QY of 3.1%. Tangerine peel was also able to be used as carbon sources for CDs after being dried and ground into powder. A hydrothermal reaction at 140°C for 6 h enabled tangerine peel powder forming yellow fluorescent CDs with an average diameter of 3 nm (Ezati, Khan, Rhim, Kim, & Molaei, 2023). After 12 h of hydrothermal treatment at 240°C, lemon juice could be processed into green fluorescent CDs, which has photostability and dielectric properties and can be used for V5+detection in serum (Hoan et al., 2019).

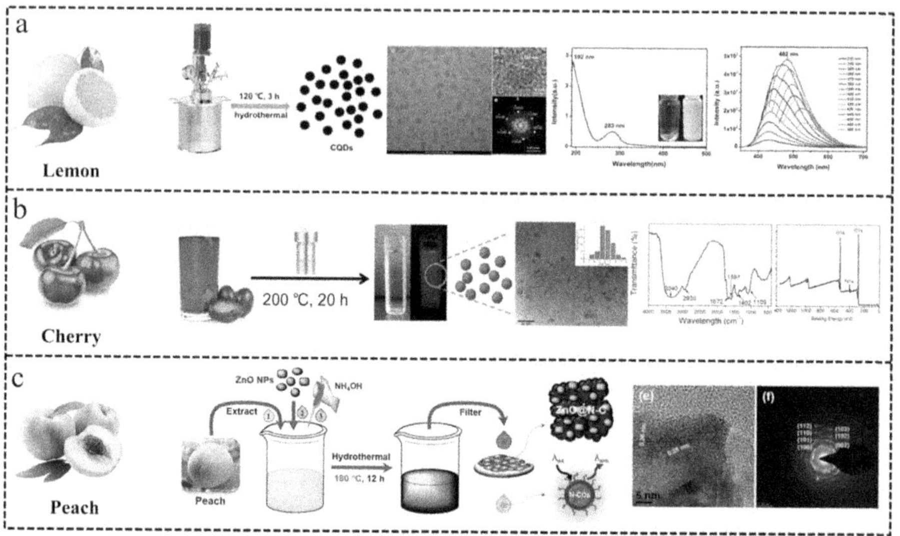

FIGURE 2.4 Carbon dots and their structural composition from fruit sources. (a) Lemon-derived carbon dots (He et al., 2018). (b) Cherry-derived carbon dots (Ma et al., 2019). (c) Peach-derived carbon dots (Atchudan et al., 2018).

Xiao et al. (2018) converted grapefruit peel extracts to green fluorescent CDs of size around 4.2 nm, and achieved sustainable and high value utilization of such fruit waste. Grapefruit juice has also been chosen as a carbon dot precursor. A blue light carbon dot containing N and S elements with a size of about 3.8nm and a QY of up to 84.9% can be prepared by mixing grapefruit juice with urea and undergoing a 180-degree hydrothermal reaction for 6 h (S. Wang et al., 2022a).

2.5.2 BERRIES FRUITS

Berry fruits are chosen as precursors of CDs due to their rich pigment substances. Yang et al. (2017) dried strawberries and prepared them into powder upon hydrothermal reaction at 170°C to prepare carbon dot materials. The size of the CDs was in the range of 1.5–2.5 nm, and the CDs were used in the development of photovoltaic devices. Salimi et al. (2020) prepared CDs using white mulberry upon treatment at 160°C under hydrothermal conditions for 6 h. The prepared CDs had a size of around 4.9 nm, and exhibited UV shielding and antibacterial properties. Aslandas et al. (2015) prepared a blueberry carbon dot using liquid nitrogen assisted centrifugation, which can be used for detecting Fe^{3+}. As is well known, kiwifruit is rich in amino acids, vitamin C, and many mineral elements including K, Se, Zn, etc. Xu et al. (2022) developed three types of CDs with different sizes using ultrasound combined with additives of EA, EDA, and acta. These three CDs exhibited green, yellow green, and pink fluorescence, respectively, and have the potential to be applied in anti-counterfeiting technology. Interestingly, grape seeds can also be collected to prepare CDs. Grape seeds can form green fluorescent CDs with a size of 4 nm after being baked at 300°C for 1 h (Parvathy & Praseetha, 2022). In addition, mulberry juice and grape skins were also processed into CDs with fluorescent property which were available for biological imaging applications (Salih Ajaj, Sadiq, & Schneider, 2023; Tang et al., 2022).

2.5.3 POME FRUITS

Liu et al. (2018) reported CDs with a size of 10 nm prepared from pear juice after undergoing hydrothermal processing at 150°C for 2 h. Upon 360 nm ultraviolet excitation, the CDs could emit blue fluorescence at a wavelength of 455 nm and have sensitivity for Cu^{2+}. Similarly, Mondal and Srivastava (2018) also prepared a carbon dot with blue fluorescence using pear juice by the same approach at 165°C for 3 h. This carbon dot has a similar emission wavelength (453 nm) to the aforementioned pear juice CDs upon 360 nm ultraviolet excitation, but its average size is only 1.1 nm. Apples, as a very common fruit, are also used as carbon dot precursors. After cutting the apple into pieces and directly reacting with hydrothermal solution at 200°C for 1 day, blue fluorescent CDs with an average size of 5 nm can be obtained, which can be used to detect efavirenz (Mohammadi, Haghnazari, & Karami, 2023). Some researchers separate fruit peels and juice to prepare apple-based CDs and obtain CDs with different functional properties. For example, Aggarwal et al. (2020) carbonized discarded apple peels at high temperatures into ash and isolated a carbon dot that can degrade pigments. Other researchers used apple juice hydrothermal synthesis to prepare a blue fluorescent carbon dot that can be used for microbial cell imaging (Mehta, Jha, Basu, Singhal, & Kailasa, 2015). Wang et al. (2022) attempted to prepare CDs from loquat through the hydrothermal method, and spherical blue fluorescent CDs of 4.46 nm were obtained with a QY of 10.36%. Some other pome fruits can also serve as carbon dot precursors, such as plums, mangosteens, peaches (Figure 2.4c), prickly pears, etc. (Atchudan, Edison, & Lee, 2016; Bhatt, Vyas, & Paul, 2022; R. Yang et al., 2017a; Zhu, Chu, Shen, Wang, & Wei, 2021).

2.6 ANIMAL-DERIVED CARBON SOURCE

Animals are another natural precursor material required for carbon dot preparation, covering a wide range of marine and terrestrial organisms, including fish, shellfish, crustaceans, mammals, birds, and eggs (Xiang & Tan, 2022). Animal-derived precursor substances mostly come from waste generated after slaughter or food processing. The reuse of these waste materials can be done to produce functional CDs for application in biological imaging, as fluorescent probes, in intelligent detection, as antioxidants, catalysts, etc. This is of great significance for environmental protection and economic value enhancement.

2.6.1 AQUATIC ANIMAL

2.6.1.1 Fish

Fish scales are composed of proteins, chitin, mineral elements, as well as lipids and pigments (Figure 2.5a). Therefore, by using them to prepare CDs, it is beneficial to obtain element-doped CDs without adding other elements. Campalani et al. (2021) prepared biomass CDs using scale waste generated from fish processing as a carbon

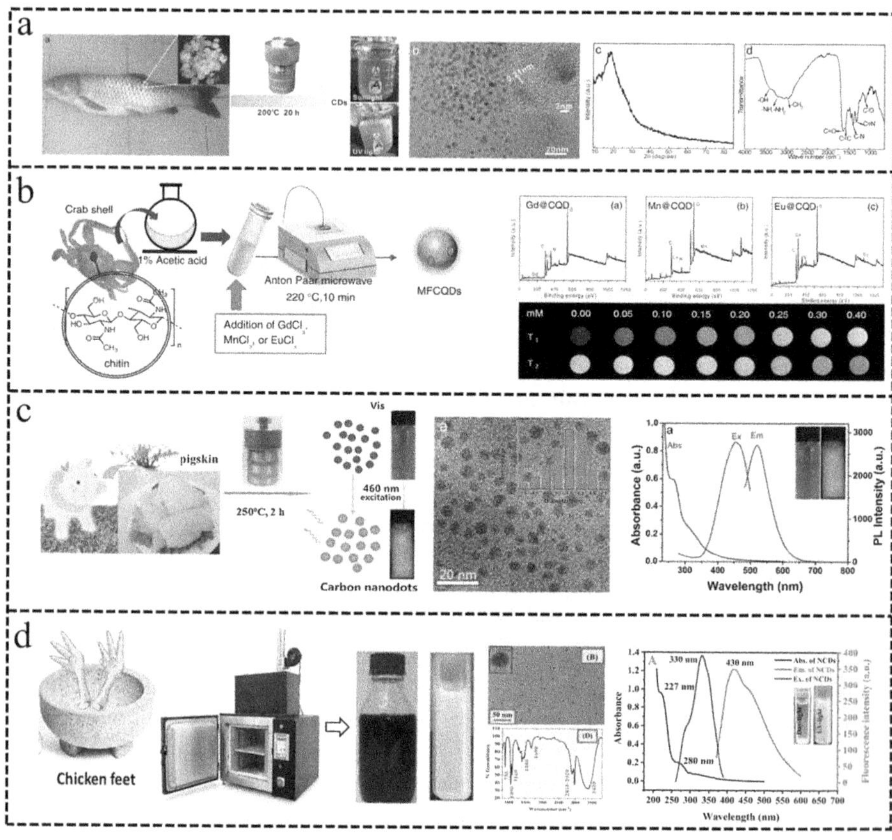

FIGURE 2.5 Carbon dots and their structural composition from animal sources. (a) Fish scales-derived carbon dots (Y. Zhang et al., 2018a). (b) Crab-shell-derived carbon dots (Yao et al., 2017). (c) Pigskin-derived carbon dots (Wen et al., 2016). (d) Chicken feet-derived carbon dots (Alkahtani, Mahmoud, Alqahtani, Ali, & El-Wekil, 2023).

source, the prepared CDs have a N content of 9%, an average size of 13 nm, and a QY of 6%. Some researchers used fish skin to prepare blue fluorescent CDs with a diameter of 6–8 nm upon hydrothermal reaction at 180°C for 7 h (Gopika, Ashraf, & Binsi, 2023). This carbon dot has been proven to have multiple fluorescent groups and can be used as an anti-corrosion material. Interestingly, other researchers have found that foodborne CDs are generated during food heat treatment, particularly in heat-treated foods such as barbecue. Cui et al. (2022) isolated foodborne CDs from grilled fish and studied their toxic effects on cells. They investigated the potential influence of foodborne CDs on human health and found that these CDs have certain effects on six metabolic pathways in mouse kidney cells.

2.6.1.2 Crustaceans

Crustaceans are famous for their hard shells scattered throughout their bodies. Most crustaceans are rich in nutrients and have a delicious taste, making them an important source of food for humans, such as shrimp and crabs. Crustaceans contain abundant natural substances such as chitin and astaxanthin, and using them to prepare CDs has inherent advantages in element doping. For example, crab shell waste is an excellent carbon source for the fabrication of CDs due to its rich content of chitin. Yao et al. (2017) dried and ground the shell of the blood red swimming crab (*Portunus sanguinolentus*) into powder as a carbon source material (Figure 2.5b). By doping metal ions, a blue fluorescent carbon dot was prepared in a microwave reactor. Various varieties of crabs have been reported to prepare CDs. Pourmahdi et al. (2019) used blue crab shell as a carbon source, heated it in a 210°C oven for 20 minutes, and extracted a spherical carbon quantum dot with a QY of 14.5% and the size range of 6-9 nm. Other researchers processed crab shells into green fluorescent CDs of size 10 nm upon treatment at 180°C for 12 h using a one-step hydrothermal method (Elango, Saranya Packialakshmi, Manikandan, & Jayanthi, 2022). Interestingly, this carbon dot has antibacterial properties and can detect Cd^{2+}. This antibacterial performance may mainly come from the action of reactive oxygen species at the photocatalytic sites on the surface of CDs. Some researchers used shrimp to prepare various CDs. Tai et al. (2019) obtained shrimp shells for preparing CDs from local agricultural markets, subjected them to a dry heat reaction at 230°C for 2 h, and then separated yellow fluorescent CDs with the size range of 3–5 nm. Shrimp eggs were also used as carbon source raw materials for developing carbon dot materials. Blue fluorescent CDs with a QY of 18.5% and a size of 3.25 nm were extracted upon heat treatment of shrimp eggs in a 180°C oven for 25 minutes and cold water extraction (P. Y. Lin et al., 2014). Other researchers have used shrimp waste to prepare a N containing carbon dot with photocatalytic performance under hydrothermal reaction without adding a N source, which can be used for catalytic hydrogen production (Wei, Wang, Zhang, & Li, 2015).

2.6.2 Terrestrial Animal

There are various types of terrestrial animals, including well-known livestock, poultry, etc., the vast majority of which are the main food sources for humans. Some researchers have explored their potential to fabricate CDs and developed various carbon dot materials with different properties to demonstrate their feasibility.

2.6.2.1 Livestock

Researchers have prepared blue fluorescent CDs from pork by treating at 180°C for 10 h using a hydrothermal method, and the QY of CDs was of 17.3%. The fluorescent carbon dots have an amino group and can undergo fluorescence quenching when uric acid existed (C. Zhao, Jiao, Hu, & Yang, 2018). Green fluorescent CDs could be prepared when using pig skin as the carbon source alone, and in this case, the QY reached 24.1% (Figure 2.5c). This fluorescent carbon dot can undergo fluorescence quenching in the presence of Co^{2+}, and thus, it can be applied for Co^{2+} detection in cells (Wen et al., 2016). Chen et al. (2021) innovatively fabricated blue fluorescent CDs with a fluorescence QY of 11.74% using pig liver as the carbon source, and the resulting CDs can be used for 6-thioguanine detection. Some researchers have explored the CDs and their properties present in grilled meat. Tan and his team isolated spherical CDs from roasted lamb, with a QY of 10% and a diameter of 2 nm, which can be used to quantify the glucose content in beverages (H. Wang et al., 2017). The antioxidant activity of CDs in baked lamb was further studied, and it was found that the baking temperature was closely related to the fluorescence QY and antioxidant activity of the CDs (H. Wang et al., 2019). Tan's team also studied the possible interaction between CDs isolated from roasted beef and human serum albumin (K. Liu, Song, & Tan, 2020). The carbon dot size of the roasted beef is between 1 and 5 nm and has a N content of 10.6%. Research has shown that the carbon dot can spontaneously form a protein crown between it and human serum albumin. Interestingly, some researchers have prepared blue fluorescent CDs with a QY of 16.3% using wool as a carbon source and by microwave pyrolysis method. The CDs were sensitive to glyphosate, with a detection limit as low as 12 ng/mL (L. Wang et al., 2016a). Song et al. (2022) reported CDs with the diameter range of 2–6 nm prepared from wool keratin. Unlike wool CDs, these CDs contain not only C and O elements, but also N and S doping elements, which allows the CDs to detect Cr^{6+} and Fe^{3+} contamination.

2.6.2.2 Poultry

Poultry is also a great carbon source for CDs. Some researchers make full use of postmortem chicken and their various parts to prepare CDs. Chicken leg meat can be treated by hydrothermal method at 180°C for 5 h to obtain blue fluorescent CDs with a QY of up to 32.86%. The CDs were able to detect ceftriaxone, with a detection limit of 0.44 nM (Narimani & Samadi, 2021). Some researchers use discarded chicken bones as carbon dot precursors. CDs with different fluorescence properties were prepared by different pyrolysis methods. Ye et al. (2022) synthesized blue fluorescent CDs with an excitation wavelength of 380 nm and an emission wavelength of 465 nm. Dwandaru, & Sari (2020) developed fluorescent CDs with dual fluorescent groups, emitting green fluorescence at 499.57 nm and red fluorescence at 673.52 nm, respectively. Other researchers have screened chicken cartilage as the carbon source to prepare CDs through hydrothermal method, resulting in blue fluorescent CDs with a size of 7.6 nm and an absolute QY of 10.3% (Lei Wu, Pan, Ye, Liang, & Zhao, 2022). Yuan et al., (2020) prepared CDs from chicken blood through hydrothermal method, and prepared blue fluorescent CDs. This carbon dot has been used for sensitive detection of thiol groups, and has been successfully utilized for CySH detection in human serum. Other researchers used chicken feet waste to develop CDs through microwave pyrolysis, and obtained blue fluorescent CDs with a fluorescence QY of up to 42.9% (Figure 2.5d) (Alkahtani, Mahmoud, Alqahtani, Ali, & El-Wekil, 2023). The prepared CDs were further used to detect the content of rutin with a detection limit of 5.3 nmol/L. Interestingly, Dhandapani et al. (2023) selected chicken feathers as carbon dot precursors and prepared a green fluorescent carbon dot with a size of 5 nm and a QY of up to 77.2% after a hydrothermal reaction at 180°C for 1 day. Goose feather was also reported for CDs preparation by microwave hydrothermal method, and blue fluorescent CDs with a size of 21.5 nm and a QY of 17.1% were synthesized (R. Liu et al., 2015). The CDs are rich in O, S, and N elements and exhibit high sensitivity to Fe^{3+} ions.

2.6.2.3 Eggs

The various parts of the egg have been used by some researchers as precursors for CD preparation. Wang et al. (2012) used egg liquid as a carbon source to obtain fluorescent CDs with a QY of 5.96% through plasma induction. Other researchers directly processed egg white into blue fluorescent CDs with a QY of up to 43% and a size of 3.3 nm using a one-step pyrolysis approach at 200°C (Baig & Chen, 2017). Because eggshell membrane is rich in protein, it becomes an ideal precursor for preparing CDs. Some researchers developed blue fluorescent CDs with a QY of 19.5% by microwave-assisted pyrolysis of eggshell membranes, which are highly sensitive to Hg^{2+} (H. Zhang, Wu, Xing, & Wang, 2021). Ke et al. (2014) directly synthesized N doped CDs with a N content of 4% and a size of 2.6 nm using discarded eggshells as carbon sources in one step.

2.7 OUTLOOK AND CHALLENGES

Nature is a treasure trove of raw materials required for material synthesis, especially abundant natural raw materials with renewable non-toxic, and environmentally friendly properties. These raw materials collected from nature can be used to prepare carbon dot materials with controllable optical properties, good biocompatibility, and multielement doping. Moreover, compared to other artificially synthesized carbon dot precursors, CDs synthesized using natural materials as carbon sources have significant advantages such as low cost.

This chapter provides a detailed summary of various natural source carbon dot precursors that have been studied in recent years. These carbon sources cover the entire biosphere, with plant carbon sources including various grains, vegetables, and fruits, and animal carbon sources including various marine and terrestrial organisms.

Although CDs from natural sources have many advantages, there are still many urgent problems to be resolved for the preparation of CDs using natural raw materials. These issues seriously limit their widespread application and efficient production. (1) Raw materials: Most carbon dot precursors from natural sources have complex components, complex elemental compositions, and different structural characteristics. During the preparation process, these complex factors lead to unstable properties and significant performance differences of the synthesized CDs, such as varying quantum yields. (2) Preparation methods: Due to the different properties of raw materials, the preparation methods and control strategies of CDs are not unified. In particular, the pretreatment methods of solid and liquid are different, such as the pretreatment methods of bone and animal blood. Moreover, the complexity of natural carbon sources makes it difficult to analyze the synthesis mechanism of CDs, so it is very difficult to formulate an appropriate preparation strategy of CDs. (3) Security risks: Some researchers have found that some CDs not only have good fluorescence properties, but also can produce ROS and have catalytic properties. However, ROS production has a certain negative impact on cell safety. Some researchers also found that CDs can pass through the gastrointestinal mucosa, thus further affecting cell metabolism. These factors make CDs have potential safety risks. Exploring the formation mechanisms of CDs from different sources and gaining a deeper understanding of their structure-activity relationships is the primary prerequisite for specifying precise regulation of carbon dot performance and formulating suitable synthetic strategy. Preventing CDs from being ingested by the human body through appropriate encapsulation and embedding techniques, and studying appropriate biodegradable or excretory strategies, are potential methods to address their safety issues.

REFERENCES

Abdella, A. A., & El-Malla, S. F. (2023). Environmentally benign sensing platform for label free detection of Fe^{3+} and tobramycin using highly fluorescent carbon dots valorized from sweet potato roasting residues. *Microchemical Journal*, 191.

Aggarwal, R., Saini, D., Singh, B., Kaushik, J., Garg, A. K., & Sonkar, S. K. (2020). Bitter apple peel derived photoactive carbon dots for the sunlight induced photocatalytic degradation of crystal violet dye. *Solar Energy*, 197, 326–331.

Alam, A.-M., Park, B.-Y., Ghouri, Z. K., Park, M., & Kim, H.-Y. (2015). Synthesis of carbon quantum dots from cabbage with down- and up-conversion photoluminescence properties: Excellent imaging agent for biomedical applications. *Green Chemistry*, 17(7), 3791–3797.

Alkahtani, S. A., Mahmoud, A. M., Alqahtani, Y. S., Ali, A. B. H., & El-Wekil, M. M. (2023). Selective detection of rutin at novel pyridinic-nitrogen-rich carbon dots derived from chicken feet biowaste: The role of bovine serum albumin during the assay. *Spectrochimica Acta Part A: Molecular and Biomolecular Spectroscopy*, 303, 123252.

Amjadi, M., Hallaj, T., & Mayan, M. A. (2016). Green synthesis of nitrogen-doped carbon dots from lentil and its application for colorimetric determination of thioridazine hydrochloride. *RSC Advances*, 6(106), 104467–104473.

Aslan, M., & Eskalen, H. (2021). A study of carbon nanodots (carbon quantum dots) synthesized from tangerine juice using one-step hydrothermal method. *Fullerenes, Nanotubes and Carbon Nanostructures*, 29(12), 1026–1033.

Aslandaş, A. M., Balcı, N., Arık, M., Şakiroğlu, H., Onganer, Y., & Meral, K. (2015). Liquid nitrogen-assisted synthesis of fluorescent carbon dots from Blueberry and their performance in Fe^{3+} detection. *Applied Surface Science*, 356, 747–752.

Atchudan, R., Edison, T. N. J. I., & Lee, Y. R. (2016). Nitrogen-doped carbon dots originating from unripe peach for fluorescent bioimaging and electrocatalytic oxygen reduction reaction. *Journal of Colloid and Interface Science*, 482, 8–18.

Atchudan, R., Edison, T. N. J. I., Perumal, S., Karthik, N., Karthikeyan, D., Shanmugam, M., & Lee, Y. R. (2018). Concurrent synthesis of nitrogen-doped carbon dots for cell imaging and ZnO@nitrogen-doped carbon sheets for photocatalytic degradation of methylene blue. *Journal of Photochemistry and Photobiology A: Chemistry*, 350, 75–85.

Baig, M. M. F., & Chen, Y. C. (2017). Bright carbon dots as fluorescence sensing agents for bacteria and curcumin. *Journal of Colloid and Interface Science*, 501, 341–349.

Bhatt, S., Vyas, G., & Paul, P. (2022). Microwave-assisted synthesis of nitrogen-doped carbon dots using prickly pear as the carbon source and its application as a highly selective sensor for Cr(vi) and as a patterning agent. *Analytical Methods*, 14(3), 269–277.

Borna, S., Sabzi, R. E., & Pirsa, S. (2021). Synthesis of carbon quantum dots from apple juice and graphite: Investigation of fluorescence and structural properties and use as an electrochemical sensor for measuring Letrozole. *Journal of Materials Science: Materials in Electronics*, 32(8), 10866–10879.

Campalani, C., Cattaruzza, E., Zorzi, S., Vomiero, A., You, S., Matthews, L., …Perosa, A. (2021). Biobased carbon dots: From fish scales to photocatalysis. *Nanomaterials*, 11(2).

Cao, Y., Wang, X., Bai, H., Jia, P., Zhao, Y., Liu, Y., …Yue, T. (2022). Fluorescent detection of tetracycline in foods based on carbon dots derived from natural red beet pigment. *LWT*, 157.

Chandrasekaran, P., Sivaraman, G., Rasala, S., Sethuraman, M. G., Kotla, N. G., & Rochev, Y. (2022). Quercetin conjugated fluorescent nitrogen-doped carbon dots for targeted cancer therapy application. *Soft Matter*, 18(30), 5645–5653.

Chen, W., Fan, J., Wu, X., Hu, D., Wu, Y., Feng, Z., ...Xie, J. (2021). Facile synthesis of nitrogen-doped carbon dots from pork liver and its sensing of 6-thioguanine based on the inner filter effect. *New Journal of Chemistry*, 45(11), 5114–5120.

Chen, Y., Wu, Y., Weng, B., Wang, B., & Li, C. (2016). Facile synthesis of nitrogen and sulfur co-doped carbon dots and application for Fe(III) ions detection and cell imaging. *Sensors and Actuators B: Chemical*, 223, 689–696.

Chung Hui, K., Lun Ang, W., & Soraya Sambudi, N. (2021). Nitrogen and bismuth-doped rice husk-derived carbon quantum dots for dye degradation and heavy metal removal. *Journal of Photochemistry and Photobiology A: Chemistry*, 418.

Cui, G., Zhang, L., Zaky, A. A., Liu, R., Wang, H., Abd El-Aty, A. M., & Tan, M. (2022). Protein coronas formed by three blood proteins and food-borne carbon dots from roast mackerel: Effects on cytotoxicity and cellular metabolites. *International Journal of Biological Macromolecules*, 216, 799–809.

Dhandapani, E., Maadeswaran, P., Mohan Raj, R., Raj, V., Kandiah, K., & Duraisamy, N. (2023). A potential forecast of carbon quantum dots (CQDs) as an ultrasensitive and selective fluorescence probe for Hg (II) ions sensing. *Materials Science and Engineering: B*, 287.

Dias, C., Vasimalai, N., Sárria, M. P., Pinheiro, I., Vilas-Boas, V., Peixoto, J., & Espiña, B. (2019). Biocompatibility and bioimaging potential of fruit-based carbon dots. *Nanomaterials*, 9(2).

Dong, Y., Zhang, Y., Zhi, S., Yang, X., & Yao, C. (2021). Green synthesized fluorescent carbon dots from momordica charantia for selective and sensitive detection of Pd^{2+} and Fe^{3+}. *ChemistrySelect*, 6(1), 123–130.

Dwandaru, W. S. B., & Sari, E. K. (2020). Chicken bone wastes as precursor for C-dots in olive oil. *Journal of Physical Science*, 31(2), 113–131.

Elango, D., Saranya Packialakshmi, J., Manikandan, V., & Jayanthi, P. (2022). Synthesis of crab-shell derived CQDs for Cd^{2+} detection and antibacterial applications. *Materials Letters*, 313.

Ezati, P., Khan, A., Rhim, J.-W., Kim, J. T., & Molaei, R. (2023). pH-Responsive strips integrated with resazurin and carbon dots for monitoring shrimp freshness. *Colloids and Surfaces B: Biointerfaces*, 221.

Fallah, S., Baharfar, R., & Samadi-Maybodi, A. (2023). Simple and green approach for photoluminescent carbon dots prepared from faba bean seeds as a luminescent probe for determination of Hg^+ ions and cell imaging. *Luminescence*, 38(11), 1929–1937.

Gopika, R., Ashraf, P. M., & Binsi, P. K. (2023). Epoxy polymers reinforced with phosphorus-doped carbon dots for enhanced corrosion protection of carbon steel in marine environments. *Materials and Corrosion*.

Gu, D., Hong, L., Zhang, L., Liu, H., & Shang, S. (2018). Nitrogen and sulfur co-doped highly luminescent carbon dots for sensitive detection of Cd (II) ions and living cell imaging applications. *Journal of Photochemistry and Photobiology B: Biology*, 186, 144–151.

Gu, D., Shang, S., Yu, Q., & Shen, J. (2016). Green synthesis of nitrogen-doped carbon dots from lotus root for Hg(II) ions detection and cell imaging. *Applied Surface Science*, 390, 38–42.

He, M., Zhang, J., Wang, H., Kong, Y., Xiao, Y., & Xu, W. (2018). Material and optical properties of fluorescent carbon quantum dots fabricated from lemon juice via hydrothermal reaction. *Nanoscale Research Letters*, 13(1).

Hoan, B. T., Thanh, T. T., Tam, P. D., Trung, N. N., Cho, S., & Pham, V.-H. (2019). A green luminescence of lemon derived carbon quantum dots and their applications for sensing of V5+ ions. *Materials Science and Engineering: B*, 251.

Hoang, V. C., Dinh, K. N., & Gomes, V. G. (2019). Iodine doped composite with biomass carbon dots and reduced graphene oxide: a versatile bifunctional electrode for energy storage and oxygen reduction reaction. *Journal of Materials Chemistry A*, 7(39), 22650–22662.

Hu, Y., Li, J., & Li, X. (2019). Leek-derived codoped carbon dots as efficient fluorescent probes for dichlorvos sensitive detection and cell multicolor imaging. *Analytical and Bioanalytical Chemistry*, 411(29), 7879–7887.

Humaera, N. A., Fahri, A. N., Armynah, B., & Tahir, D. (2021). Natural source of carbon dots from part of a plant and its applications: A review. *Luminescence*, 36(6), 1354–1364.

Huo, X., He, Y., Ma, S., Jia, Y., Yu, J., Li, Y., & Cheng, Q. (2020). Green synthesis of carbon dots from grapefruit and its fluorescence enhancement. *Journal of Nanomaterials*, 2020, 1–7.

Jia, J., Lin, B., Gao, Y., Jiao, Y., Li, L., Dong, C., & Shuang, S. (2019). Highly luminescent N-doped carbon dots from black soya beans for free radical scavenging, Fe^{3+} sensing and cellular imaging. *Spectrochimica Acta Part A: Molecular and Biomolecular Spectroscopy*, 211, 363–372.

Jin, H., Gui, R., Wang, Y., & Sun, J. (2017). Carrot-derived carbon dots modified with polyethyleneimine and nile blue for ratiometric two-photon fluorescence turn-on sensing of sulfide anion in biological fluids. *Talanta*, 169, 141–148.

John, T. S., Yadav, P. K., Kumar, D., Singh, S. K., & Hasan, S. H. (2020). Highly fluorescent carbon dots from wheat bran as a novel drug delivery system for bacterial inhibition. *Luminescence*, 35(6), 913–923.

Jorn-am, T., Praneerad, J., Attajak, R., Sirisit, N., Manyam, J., & Paoprasert, P. (2021). Quasi-solid, bio-renewable supercapacitor with high specific capacitance and energy density based on rice electrolytes and rice straw-derived carbon dots as novel electrolyte additives. *Colloids and Surfaces A: Physicochemical and Engineering Aspects*, 628.

Jorn-am, T., Supchocksoonthorn, P., Pholauyphon, W., Manyam, J., Chanthad, C., & Paoprasert, P. (2022). Quasi-Solid, bio-renewable supercapacitors based on cassava peel and cassava starch and the use of carbon dots as performance enhancers. *Energy & Fuels*, 36(14), 7865–7877.

Kang, K., Liu, B., Yue, G., Ren, H., Zheng, K., Wang, L., & Wang, Z. (2023). Preparation of carbon quantum dots from ionic liquid modified biomass for the detection of Fe^{3+} and Pd^{2+} in environmental water. *Ecotoxicology and Environmental Safety*, 255.

Kaur, H., Sareen, S., Mutreja, V., & Verma, M. (2023). Spinach-derived carbon dots for the turn-on detection of chromium ions (Cr^{3+}). *Journal of Inorganic and Organometallic Polymers and Materials*.

Ke, Y., Garg, B., & Ling, Y.-C. (2014). Waste chicken eggshell as low-cost precursor for efficient synthesis of nitrogen-doped fluorescent carbon nanodots and their multi-functional applications. *RSC Advances*, 4(102), 58329–58336.

Koshy, R. R., Koshy, J. T., Mary, S. K., Sadanandan, S., Jisha, S., & Pothan, L. A. (2021). Preparation of pH sensitive film based on starch/carbon nano dots incorporating anthocyanin for monitoring spoilage of pork. *Food Control*, 126, 108039.

Li, J., Fu, W., Zhang, X., Zhang, Q., Ma, D., Wang, Y., …Zhu, D. (2023). Green preparation of ginger-derived carbon dots accelerates wound healing. *Carbon*, 208, 208–215.

Li, W., Yue, Z., Wang, C., Zhang, W., & Liu, G. (2013). An absolutely green approach to fabricate carbon nanodots from soya bean grounds. *RSC Advances*, 3(43).

Lin, P. Y., Hsieh, C. W., Kung, M. L., Chu, L. Y., Huang, H. J., Chen, H. T., …Hsieh, S. (2014). Eco-friendly synthesis of shrimp egg-derived carbon dots for fluorescent bioimaging. *Journal of Biotechnology*, 189, 114–119.

Lin, R., Cheng, S., & Tan, M. (2022). Green synthesis of fluorescent carbon dots with antibacterial activity and their application in Atlantic mackerel (Scomber scombrus) storage. *Food & Function*, 13(4), 2098–2108.

Liu, H., Ding, L., Chen, L., Chen, Y., Zhou, T., Li, H., …Huang, N. (2019). A facile, green synthesis of biomass carbon dots coupled with molecularly imprinted polymers for highly selective detection of oxytetracycline. *Journal of Industrial and Engineering Chemistry*, 69, 455–463.

Liu, H., Li, Z., Zhang, W., Liu, Y., Pan, R., & Huang, G. (2022). Facile synthesis of tomato-based carbon nanodots and its utilization in sensitive detection of tartrazine. *Journal of the Indian Chemical Society*, 99(12).

Liu, K., Song, Y., & Tan, M. (2020). Toxicity alleviation of carbon dots from roast beef after the formation of protein coronas with human serum albumin. *Journal of Agricultural and Food Chemistry*, 68(36), 9789–9795.

Liu, L., Gong, H., Li, D., & Zhao, L. (2018). Synthesis of carbon dots from pear juice for fluorescence detection of Cu^{2+} Ion in water. *Journal of Nanoscience and Nanotechnology*, 18(8), 5327–5332.

Liu, R., Zhang, J., Gao, M., Li, Z., Chen, J., Wu, D., & Liu, P. (2015). A facile microwave-hydrothermal approach towards highly photoluminescent carbon dots from goose feathers. *RSC Advances*, 5(6), 4428–4433.

Liu, S., Liu, Z., Li, Q., Xia, H., Yang, W., Wang, R., …Tian, B. (2021b). Facile synthesis of carbon dots from wheat straw for colorimetric and fluorescent detection of fluoride and cellular imaging. *Spectrochimica Acta Part A: Molecular and Biomolecular Spectroscopy*, 246.

Liu, Y., Su, X., Chen, L., Liu, H., Zhang, C., Liu, J., …Zhu, G. (2021c). Green preparation of carbon dots from Momordica charantia L. for rapid and effective sensing of p-aminoazobenzene in environmental samples. *Environmental Research*, 198.

Liu, Z., Li, B., Shi, X., Li, L., Feng, Y., Jia, D., & Zhou, Y. (2021a). Target-oriented synthesis of high synthetic yield carbon dots with tailored surface functional groups for bioimaging of zebrafish, flocculation of heavy metal ions and ethanol detection. *Applied Surface Science*, 538.

Long, R., Tang, C., Li, T., Tong, X., Tong, C., Guo, Y., …Shi, S. (2020). Dual-emissive carbon dots for dual-channel ratiometric fluorometric determination of pH and mercury ion and intracellular imaging. *Microchimica Acta*, 187(5).

Ma, H., Sun, C., Xue, G., Wu, G., Zhang, X., Han, X., …Zhang, J. (2019). Facile synthesis of fluorescent carbon dots from Prunus cerasifera fruits for fluorescent ink, Fe^{3+} ion detection and cell imaging. *Spectrochimica Acta Part A: Molecular and Biomolecular Spectroscopy*, 213, 281–287.

Maruthapandi, M., Saravanan, A., Luong, J. H. T., & Gedanken, A. (2021). Polydopamine decorated carbon dots nanocomposite as an effective adsorbent for phenolic compounds. *Journal of Applied Polymer Science*, 139(10).

Mehta, V. N., Jha, S., Basu, H., Singhal, R. K., & Kailasa, S. K. (2015). One-step hydrothermal approach to fabricate carbon dots from apple juice for imaging of mycobacterium and fungal cells. *Sensors and Actuators B: Chemical*, 213, 434–443.

Mehta, V. N., Jha, S., Singhal, R. K., & Kailasa, S. K. (2014). Preparation of multicolor emitting carbon dots for HeLa cell imaging. *New Journal of Chemistry*, 38(12), 6152–6160.

Miao, H., Wang, L., Zhuo, Y., Zhou, Z., & Yang, X. (2016). Label-free fluorimetric detection of CEA using carbon dots derived from tomato juice. *Biosensors and Bioelectronics*, 86, 83–89.

Min, S., Ezati, P., & Rhim, J.-W. (2022). Gelatin-based packaging material incorporated with potato skins carbon dots as functional filler. *Industrial Crops and Products*, 181.

Mohammadi, A., Haghnazari, N., & Karami, C. (2023). Green synthesized fluorescent carbon dots from oak apple for detection of efavirenz. *Journal of Materials Science: Materials in Electronics*, 34(6).

Mondal, J., & Srivastava, S. K. (2018). Green synthesis of carbon dot weak gel from pear juice: Optical properties and sensing application. *ChemistrySelect*, 3(29), 8444–8457.

Naik, G. G., Minocha, T., Verma, A., Yadav, S. K., Saha, S., Agrawal, A. K., …Sahu, A. N. (2022). Asparagus racemosus root-derived carbon nanodots as a nano-probe for biomedical applications. *Journal of Materials Science*, 57(43), 20380–20401.

Narimani, S., & Samadi, N. (2021). Rapid trace analysis of ceftriaxone using new fluorescent carbon dots as a highly sensitive turn-off nanoprobe. *Microchemical Journal*, 168.

Parvathy, C. R., & Praseetha, P. K. (2022). Carbon quantum dot induced hemolysis and anti-angiogenesis in proliferating cancers with Vitis vinifera as the source material. *Vegetos*, 36(3), 890–898.

Pourmahdi, N., Sarrafi, A. H. M., & Larki, A. (2019). Carbon dots green synthesis for ultra-trace determination of ceftriaxone using response surface methodology. *Journal of Fluorescence*, 29(4), 887–897.

Qiu, Y., Li, D., Li, Y., Ma, X., & Li, J. (2021). Green carbon quantum dots from sustainable lignocellulosic biomass and its application in the detection of Fe^{3+}. *Cellulose*, 29(1), 367–378.

Qiu, Y., Wang, F., Ma, X., Yin, F., Li, D., & Li, J. (2023). Carbon quantum dots derived from cassava stems via acid/alkali-assisted hydrothermal carbonization: Formation, mechanism and application in drug release. *Industrial Crops and Products*, 204.

Qu, Y., Yu, L., Zhu, B., Chai, F., & Su, Z. (2020). Green synthesis of carbon dots by celery leaves for use as fluorescent paper sensors for the detection of nitrophenols. *New Journal of Chemistry*, 44(4), 1500–1507.

Rajendran, K., Rajendran, G., Kasthuri, J., Kathiravan, K., & Rajendiran, N. (2019). Sweet Corn (Zea mays L. var. rugosa) derived fluorescent carbon quantum dots for selective detection of hydrogen sulfide and bioimaging applications. *ChemistrySelect*, 4(46), 13668–13676.

Ren, G., Tang, M., Chai, F., & Wu, H. (2018). One-Pot synthesis of highly fluorescent carbon dots from spinach and multipurpose applications. *European Journal of Inorganic Chemistry*, 2018(2), 153–158.

Rodríguez-Varillas, S., Fontanil, T., Obaya, Á. J., Fernández-González, A., Murru, C., & Badía-Laíño, R. (2022). Biocompatibility and antioxidant capabilities of carbon dots obtained from tomato (Solanum lycopersicum). *Applied Sciences*, 12(2).

Sun, Y.-P., Zhou, B., Lin, Y., Wang, W., Fernando, K. S., Pathak, P. M., Meziani, J., Harruff, B. A., Wang, X., Wang, H. (2006). Quantum-Sized carbon dots for bright and colorful photoluminescence. *Jouranl of the American Chemical Society*, 128, 7756–7757.

Sabet, M., & Salmeh, F. (2020). Green synthesis of highly fluorescent graphene oxide/carbon quantum dot colloid from rice. *Journal of Electronic Materials*, 49(6), 3947–3955.

Sahu, S., Behera, B., Maiti, T. K., & Mohapatra, S. (2012). Simple one-step synthesis of highly luminescent carbon dots from orange juice: Application as excellent bio-imaging agents. *Chemical Communications*, 48(70).

Salih Ajaj, C., Sadiq, D., & Schneider, R. (2023). Mulberry juice-derived carbon quantum dots as a Cu^{2+} ion sensor: Investigating the influence of fruit ripeness on the optical properties. *Nanomaterials and Nanotechnology*, 2023, 1–11.

Salimi, F., Moradi, M., Tajik, H., & Molaei, R. (2020). Optimization and characterization of eco-friendly antimicrobial nanocellulose sheet prepared using carbon dots of white mulberry (Morus alba L.). *Journal of the Science of Food and Agriculture*, 101(8), 3439–3447.

Salimi Shahraki, H., Qurtulen, & Ahmad, A. (2023). Synthesis, characterization of carbon dots from onion peel and their application as absorbent and anticancer activity. *Inorganic Chemistry Communications*, 150.

Sangubotla, R., & Kim, J. (2019). A facile enzymatic approach for selective detection of γ-aminobutyric acid using corn-derived fluorescent carbon dots. *Applied Surface Science*, 490, 61–69.

Sharma, N., Das, G. S., & Yun, K. (2020). Green synthesis of multipurpose carbon quantum dots from red cabbage and estimation of their antioxidant potential and bio-labeling activity. *Applied Microbiology and Biotechnology*, 104(16), 7187–7200.

Shasha, P., Kim, J. H., & Park, S. J. (2019). Celery stalk-derived carbon dots for detection of copper ions. *Journal of Nanoscience and Nanotechnology*, 19(10), 6077–6082.

Shen, J., Shang, S., Chen, X., Wang, D., & Cai, Y. (2017b). Facile synthesis of fluorescence carbon dots from sweet potato for Fe^{3+} sensing and cell imaging. *Materials Science and Engineering: C*, 76, 856–864.

Shen, Z., Guo, X., Liu, L., Sunarso, J., Wang, G., Wang, S., & Liu, S. (2017a). Carbon-dot/natural-dye sensitizer for TiO2 solar cells prepared by a one-step treatment of celery leaf extract. *ChemPhotoChem*, 1(10), 470–478.

Shi, J., Zhou, Y., Ning, J., Hu, G., Zhang, Q., Hou, Y., & Zhou, Y. (2022). Prepared carbon dots from wheat straw for detection of Cu^{2+} in cells and zebrafish and room temperature phosphorescent anti-counterfeiting. *Spectrochimica Acta Part A: Molecular and Biomolecular Spectroscopy*, 281.

Sinha, R., Bidkar, A. P., Rajasekhar, R., Ghosh, S. S., & Mandal, T. K. (2019). A facile synthesis of nontoxic luminescent carbon dots for detection of chromium and iron in real water sample and bio-imaging. *The Canadian Journal of Chemical Engineering*, 98(1), 194–204.

Song, X., Zhang, Y., Li, C., Li, N., Shen, S., Yu, T., …Guo, D. (2024). Two major duplication events shaped the transcription factor repertoires in Solanaceae species. *Scientia Horticulturae*, 323.

Song, Y., Qi, N., Li, K., Cheng, D., Wang, D., & Li, Y. (2022). Green fluorescent nanomaterials for rapid detection of chromium and iron ions: Wool keratin-based carbon quantum dots. *RSC Advances*, 12(13), 8108–8118.

Tai, D., Liu, C., & Liu, J. (2019). Facile synthesis of fluorescent carbon dots from shrimp shells and using the carbon dots to detect chromium(VI). *Spectroscopy Letters*, 52(3–4), 194–199.

Tang, X., Wang, H., Yu, H., Bui, B., Zhang, W., Wang, S., …Chen, W. (2022). Exploration of nitrogen-doped grape peels carbon dots for baicalin detection. *Materials Today Physics*, 22.

Wang, H., Xie, Y., Liu, S., Cong, S., Song, Y., Xu, X., & Tan, M. (2017). Presence of fluorescent carbon nanoparticles in baked lamb: Their properties and potential application for sensors. *Journal of Agricultural and Food Chemistry*, 65(34), 7553–7559.

Wang, H., Xie, Y., Na, X., Bi, J., Liu, S., Zhang, L., & Tan, M. (2019). Fluorescent carbon dots in baked lamb: Formation, cytotoxicity and scavenging capability to free radicals. *Food Chemistry*, 286, 405–412.

Wang, J., Ng, Y. H., Lim, Y.-F., & Ho, G. W. (2014). Vegetable-extracted carbon dots and their nanocomposites for enhanced photocatalytic H2production. *RSC Advances*, 4(83), 44117–44123.

Wang, J., Wang, C. F., & Chen, S. (2012). Amphiphilic egg-derived carbon dots: rapid plasma fabrication, pyrolysis process, and multicolor printing patterns. *Angewandte Chemie International Edition in English*, 51(37), 9297–9301.

Wang, K., Ji, Q., Xu, J., Li, H., Zhang, D., Liu, X., …Fan, H. (2018). Highly sensitive and selective detection of amoxicillin using carbon quantum dots derived from beet. *Journal of Fluorescence*, 28(3), 759–765.

Wang, L., Bi, Y., Hou, J., Li, H., Xu, Y., Wang, B., …Ding, L. (2016a). Facile, green and clean one-step synthesis of carbon dots from wool: Application as a sensor for glyphosate detection based on the inner filter effect. *Talanta*, 160, 268–275.

Wang, P., Zhong, R.-B., Yuan, M., Gong, P., Zhao, X.-M., & Zhang, F. (2016b). Mercury (II) detection by water-soluble photoluminescent ultra-small carbon dots synthesized from cherry tomatoes. *Nuclear Science and Techniques*, 27(2).

Wang, P. P., Wang, J. X., Liu, T. T., Sun, Z. P., Gao, M., Huang, K., & Wang, X. D. (2022b). Loquat fruit-based carbon quantum dots as an "ON-OFF" probe for fluorescent assay of MnO_4^- in waters based on the joint action of inner filter effect and static quenching. *Microchemical Journal*, 178.

Wang, S., Huo, X., Zhao, H., Dong, Y., Cheng, Q., & Li, Y. (2022a). One-pot green synthesis of N,S co-doped biomass carbon dots from natural grapefruit juice for selective sensing of Cr(VI). *Chemical Physics Impact*, 5.

Wang, Y., Li, Y., & Feng, L. (2020). Exploring solvent-related reactions and corresponding band gap tuning strategies for carbon nanodots based on solvothermal synthesis. *The Journal of Physical Chemistry Letters*, 11(24), 10439–10445.

Wei, J., Wang, H., Zhang, Q., & Li, Y. (2015). One-pot hydrothermal synthesis of N-Doped carbon quantum dots using the waste of shrimp for hydrogen evolution from formic acid. *Chemistry Letters*, 44(3), 241–243.

Wen, X., Shi, L., Wen, G., Li, Y., Dong, C., Yang, J., & Shuang, S. (2016). Green and facile synthesis of nitrogen-doped carbon nanodots for multicolor cellular imaging and Co^{2+} sensing in living cells. *Sensors and Actuators B: Chemical*, 235, 179–187.

Wongso, V., Sambudi, N. S., Sufian, S., & Isnaeni. (2021). The effect of hydrothermal conditions on photoluminescence properties of rice husk-derived silica-carbon quantum dots for methylene blue degradation. *Biomass Conversion and Biorefinery*, 11(6), 2641–2654.

Wu, L., Long, R., Li, T., Tang, C., Tong, X., Guo, Y., …Tong, C. (2020). One-pot fabrication of dual-emission and single-emission biomass carbon dots for Cu^{2+} and tetracycline sensing and multicolor cellular imaging. *Analytical and Bioanalytical Chemistry*, 412(27), 7481–7489.

Wu, L., Pan, W., Ye, H., Liang, N., & Zhao, L. (2022). Sensitive fluorescence detection for hydrogen peroxide and glucose using biomass carbon dots: Dual-quenching mechanism insight. *Colloids and Surfaces A: Physicochemical and Engineering Aspects*, 638.

Xiang, S., & Tan, M. (2022). Carbon dots derived from natural sources and their biological and environmental impacts. *Environmental Science: Nano*, 9(9), 3206–3225.

Xiao, P., Ke, Y., Lu, J., Huang, Z., Zhu, X., Wei, B., & Huang, L. (2018). Photoluminescence immunoassay based on grapefruit peel-extracted carbon quantum dots encapsulated into silica nanospheres for p53 protein. *Biochemical Engineering Journal*, 139, 109–116.

Xu, H., Cheng, H., McClements, D. J., Chen, L., Long, J., & Jin, Z. (2022a). Enhancing the physicochemical properties and functional performance of starch-based films using inorganic carbon materials: A review. *Carbohydrate Polymers*.

Xu, J., Cui, K., Gong, T., Zhang, J., Zhai, Z., Hou, L., … Yuan, C. (2022b). Ultrasonic-Assisted synthesis of N-Doped, multicolor carbon dots toward fluorescent inks, fluorescence sensors, and logic gate operations. *Nanomaterials*, 12(3).

Xu, W., Hao, X., Li, T., Dai, S., & Fang, Z. (2021). Dual-mode fluorescence and visual fluorescent test paper detection of copper ions and EDTA. *ACS Omega*, 6(43), 29157–29165.

Xu, X., Cai, L., Hu, G., Mo, L., Zheng, Y., Hu, C., … Zhuang, J. (2020). Red-emissive carbon dots from spinach: Characterization and application in visual detection of time. *Journal of Luminescence*, 227.

Xu, X., Ray, R., Gu, Y., Ploehn, H. J., Gearheart, L., Raker, K., & Scrivens, W. A. (2004). Electrophoretic analysis and purification of fluorescent single-walled carbon nanotube fragments. *Journal of the American Chemical Society*, 126(40), 12736–12737.

Yang, J., Guo, Z., & Yue, X. (2021). Preparation of carbon quantum dots from corn straw and their application in Cu^{2+} detection. *BioResources*, 17(1), 604–615.

Yang, J., Tang, Q., Meng, Q., Zhang, Z., Li, J., He, B., & Yang, P. (2017b). Photoelectric conversion beyond sunny days: All-weather carbon quantum dot solar cells. *Journal of Materials Chemistry A*, 5(5), 2143–2150.

Yang, R., Guo, X., Jia, L., Zhang, Y., Zhao, Z., & Lonshakov, F. (2017a). Green preparation of carbon dots with mangosteen pulp for the selective detection of Fe^{3+} ions and cell imaging. *Applied Surface Science*, 423, 426–432.

Yao, Y.-Y., Gedda, G., Girma, W. M., Yen, C.-L., Ling, Y.-C., & Chang, J.-Y. (2017). Magnetofluorescent carbon dots derived from crab shell for targeted dual-modality bioimaging and drug delivery. *ACS Applied Materials & Interfaces*, 9(16), 13887–13899.

Ye, H., Liu, B., Wang, J., Zhou, C., Xiong, Z., & Zhao, L. (2022). A hydrothermal method to generate carbon quantum dots from waste bones and their detection of laundry powder. *Molecules*, 27(19).

Yuan, C., Qin, X., Xu, Y., Li, X., Chen, Y., Shi, R., & Wang, Y. (2020). Carbon quantum dots originated from chicken blood as peroxidase mimics for colorimetric detection of bio-thiols. *Journal of Photochemistry and Photobiology A: Chemistry*, 396.

Yuan, M., Zhong, R., Gao, H., Li, W., Yun, X., Liu, J., ... Zhang, F. (2015). One-step, green, and economic synthesis of water-soluble photoluminescent carbon dots by hydrothermal treatment of wheat straw, and their bio-applications in labeling, imaging, and sensing. *Applied Surface Science*, 355, 1136–1144.

Zhang, H., Wu, S., Xing, Z., & Wang, H. B. (2021). Turning waste into treasure: chicken eggshell membrane derived fluorescent carbon nanodots for the rapid and sensitive detection of Hg(2+) and glutathione. *Analyst*, 146(23), 7250–7256.

Zhang, X., Jiang, M., Niu, N., Chen, Z., Li, S., Liu, S., & Li, J. (2018b). Natural-Product-Derived carbon dots: From natural products to functional materials. *ChemSusChem*, 11(1), 11–24.

Zhang, Y., Gao, Z., Zhang, W., Wang, W., Chang, J., & Kai, J. (2018a). Fluorescent carbon dots as nanoprobe for determination of lidocaine hydrochloride. *Sensors and Actuators B: Chemical*, 262, 928–937.

Zhang, Y., Wang, J., Wu, W., Li, C., & Ma, H. (2020). A green, economic "Switch-On" sensor for cefixime analysis based on black soya bean carbon quantum dots. *Journal of AOAC International*, 103(5), 1230–1236.

Zhao, C., Jiao, Y., Hu, F., & Yang, Y. (2018). Green synthesis of carbon dots from pork and application as nanosensors for uric acid detection. *Spectrochim Acta A Mol Biomol Spectrosc*, 190, 360–367.

Zhao, S., Lan, M., Zhu, X., Xue, H., Ng, T.-W., Meng, X., ... Zhang, W. (2015). Green synthesis of bifunctional fluorescent carbon dots from garlic for cellular imaging and free radical scavenging. *ACS Applied Materials & Interfaces*, 7(31), 17054–17060.

Zheng, Y., Hao, J., Arkin, K., Bei, Y., Ma, X., Shang, Q., & Che, W. (2023). H_2O_2-assisted detection of melamine using fluorescent probe based on corn cob carbon dots-Ionic Liquid-Silver nanoparticles. *Food Chemistry*, 403.

Zhu, J., Chu, H., Shen, J., Wang, C., & Wei, Y. (2021). Green preparation of carbon dots from plum as a ratiometric fluorescent probe for detection of doxorubicin. *Optical Materials*, 114.

Zulfajri, M., Gedda, G., Chang, C.-J., Chang, Y.-P., & Huang, G. G. (2019). Cranberry beans derived carbon dots as a potential fluorescence sensor for selective detection of Fe^{3+} Ions in aqueous solution. *ACS Omega*, 4(13), 15382–15392.

3 Methods Employed for the Development of Carbon Quantum Dots

Subhanki Padhi, Ashutosh Singh, Valerie Orsat and Winny Routray

3.1 INTRODUCTION

Carbon is commonly acknowledged as a substance with dark appearance, and until recent years, there was reluctance to acknowledge its potential solubility in water and its ability to demonstrate significant fluorescence. Nanoscience has the potential to generate remarkable prospects for scientific and technological progress. For instance, the production of nanosized carbon structures results in materials with entirely distinct properties compared to macroscopic materials. Carbon quantum dots (CQDs) are nanosized carbon materials that were first time synthesized in 2004 from single-walled carbon nanotubes (Xu et al., 2004). The CQDs were named in 2006 as "carbon dots" for the first time by Sun et al. (2006) only two years after their first synthesis. The CQDs are well-known to have dimensions in the range of 1–10 nm and exhibit extraordinary fluorescence characteristics (Shen et al., 2012). In the recent decade, the CQDs have gained momentum in the field of research owing to their properties like optical stability, fluorescence emissions, lower toxicity, biocompatibility, and small nanosized particles. These characteristics of CQDs have enabled them to expand their applicability in optronics, biomedicines, bioimaging, drug delivery, and metal detection (Yang et al., 2022).

CQDs can be synthesized from various sources of carbon. Basically, synthesis techniques are broadly divided into two categories: top-down approach and bottom-up approach methods (Lim et al., 2015). Top-down methods refer to the breakdown of carbon bulk materials into smaller particles, whereas bottom-up method includes the development of nanosized CQDs from smaller carbon precursors (El-Shabasy et al., 2021). Figure 3.1 shows an overall process of synthesis of CQDs by bottom-up and top-down approaches. After synthesis, the properties of the obtained CQDs are enhanced by the addition of functional groups onto the surface of CQDs or by developing doped-CQDs (Tejwan et al., 2020). In this chapter, we have focussed only on various synthesis techniques.

The synthesis of CQDs using simpler, cost-effective and eco-friendly methods is the need of the hour. This chapter deals with the top-down and bottom-up approaches for the production of CQDs from different carbon sources. Further, various top-down

DOI: 10.1201/9781003437857-4

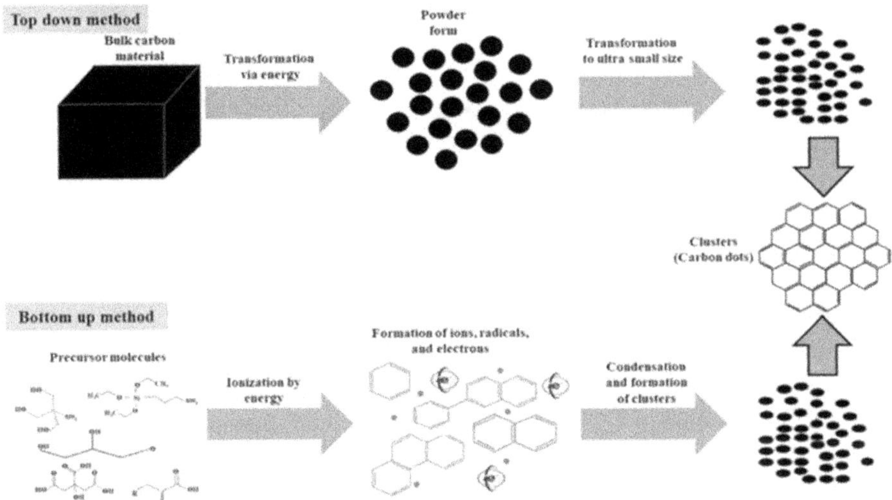

FIGURE 3.1   Schematic presentation of the top-down and bottom-up approaches for the synthesis of CQDs.

Used with permission from the Royal Society of Chemistry, from Desmond et al. (2021); permission conveyed through Copyright Clearance Center, Inc.

approaches such as arc discharge, laser ablation, and oxidation techniques and bottom-up approaches such as microwave, thermal routes, template method, and hydrothermal treatment have been discussed in detail. The main focus of this chapter is to list the various techniques that are in-trend for the production of CQDs and to briefly discuss on their efficiency in rendering the CQDs with desirable size and fluorescence properties to scale up their application in various fields. Also, the advantages and disadvantages of each method have been briefly discussed.

3.2   SYNTHESIS OF CARBON QUANTUM DOTS

In the past decades, a lot of techniques have been applied for the synthesis of CQDs from various raw materials. Broadly, the synthesis techniques can be classified into two types: top-down approach and bottom-up approach (Yang et al., 2022). CQDs having outstanding photoluminescence properties with better stability can be produced with either of these synthesis approaches. The type of synthesis used for producing CQDs depends upon the raw material used. Figure 3.2 shows different synthesis techniques of CQDs. Therefore, detailed techniques for synthesis of CQDs from various sources are further discussed below.

3.2.1   TOP-DOWN APPROACH METHODS

In the top-down approach method, the carbon materials are broken down to smaller particles i.e., carbon nanoparticles with the help of different chemical and physical

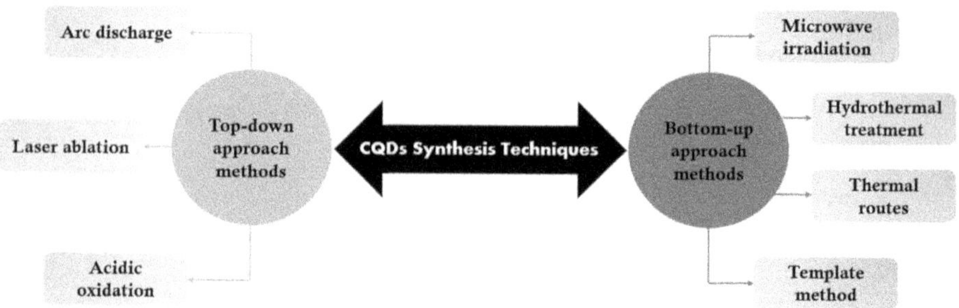

FIGURE 3.2 Different synthesis techniques of CQDs.

routes. The formation of CQDs in the top-down method depends upon the chemical bonds present between the carbon atoms (Lim et al., 2015). Some of the commonly used top-down methods are arc discharge, laser ablation, and oxidation methods. Top-down methods use strong oxidants like sulphuric acid, nitric acid, or a mixture of both to produce CQDs from activated carbon, graphite rods, carbon fibres, and nanotubes.

3.2.1.1 Laser Ablation

Laser ablation is an eco-friendly, hassle-free, and effective technique for the synthesis of CQDs from various carbon sources. The principle of this technique is based on the high-energy laser irradiation of the carbon target surface. The laser pulse irradiates the target surface to generate high pressure and temperature which leads to rapid heating of the surface and evaporation to a plasma state. The vapour formed gets crystallized to develop nanoparticles. Li et al. (2011) synthesized CQDs from carbon sources by laser ablation method using ordinary solvents like water, ethanol, and acetone. The developed CQDs had visible and tunable photoluminescence properties. Figure 3.3 shows the experimental setup used by Li et al. (2011) for their laser ablation process. Further, the properties of obtained CQDs can be improved by the use of effective solvents during the laser ablation process. Gonçalves et al. (2010) synthesized CQDs using UV pulsed laser irradiation technique from carbon targets. The obtained CQDs were functionalized using nitric acid, polyethylene glycol (PEG), and N-acetyl-L-cysteine (NAC). The functionalized CQDs exhibited better florescence properties and could be used for detection of Hg(II) and Cu(II) ions. Also, these CQDs could be used for applications in *in vivo* fluorescence sensing. Cui et al. (2020) synthesized homogeneous CQDs from low-cost carbon cloth by using dual-beam pulsed laser ablation technique (schematic representation of the setup is given in Figure 3.4). The yield of CQDs was reported to be 35.4% having better stability and photoluminescence effect that would be helpful for bioimaging. The use of double beam helped in reducing the time of laser ablation and thus increased the yield. Although the synthesis of CQDs using laser ablation technique is an effortless procedure, the requirement of a huge quantity of carbonaceous matter initially to develop the carbon target surface is a limitation.

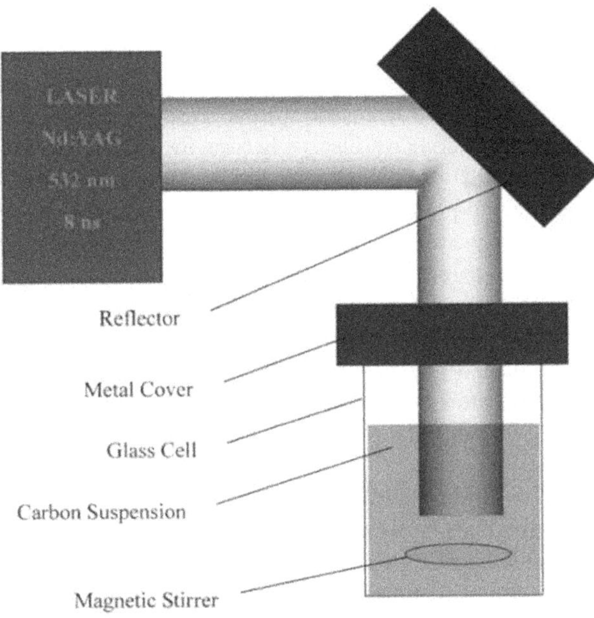

FIGURE 3.3 A schematic representation of the setup used for laser ablation by Li et al. (2011).

Used with permission from Royal Society of Chemistry; permission conveyed through Copyright Clearance Center, Inc.

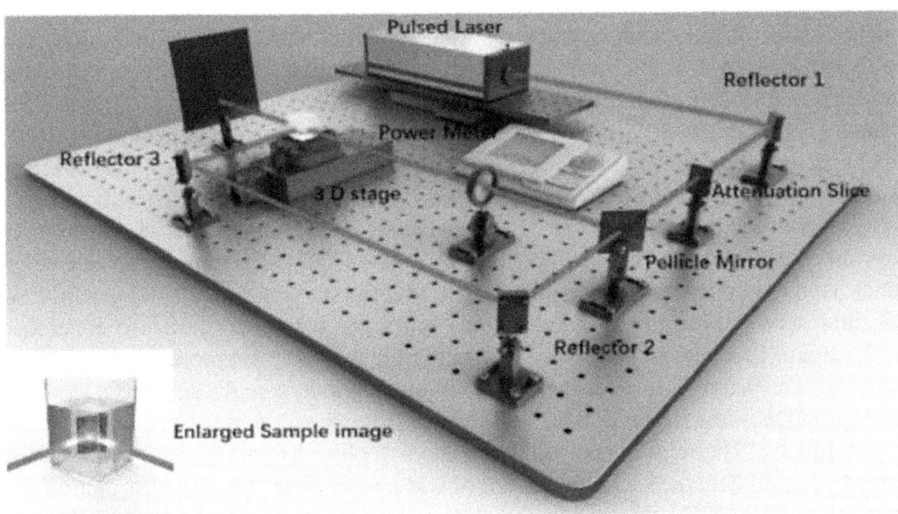

FIGURE 3.4 Schematic presentation of the dual-beam pulsed laser ablation technique for synthesis of CQDs.

Reprinted from Cui et al. (2020) with permission from Elsevier.

3.2.1.2   Arc Discharge

In the arc discharge method, the carbon atoms that get deposited in the anionic electrode are rearranged due to the generation of plasma gas within the reactor. This high-energy plasma gas is generated when the reactor temperature is higher i.e., 4000 K. The carbon vapours in the cathode collectively form the CQDs. The method of formation of CQDs by arc discharge was first reported by Xu et al. (2004). While using arc discharge synthesis technique for developing carbon nanotubes having single wall, Xu et al. (2004) found that carbon nanoparticles have fluorescence characteristics and varying relative molecular mass. They reported that at a wavelength of 365 nm, the obtained carbon nanoparticles (referred as CQDs) were observed to exhibit fluorescence of orange, yellow, and blue-green colour. Further experimentation showed the presence of hydrophilic carboxyl groups on the surface of CQDs. Although the CQDs were found to exhibit better water solubility, the size distribution range was large enough, which could further reduce the surface area of the obtained CQDs.

3.2.1.3   Acidic Oxidation Technique

Acidic oxidation method has been broadly utilized for exfoliation and decomposition of carbon precursors into carbon nanoparticles. This technique also includes the attachment of hydrophilic groups like carboxyl or hydroxyl groups onto the surface of the carbon nanoparticles, and thus, they are considered as CQDs (Shen & Xia, 2014). These developed CQDs have better fluorescence properties and water solubility. Q. Zhang et al. (2017) discovered the capacity of fullerene carbon shoots as a carbon precursor for obtaining CQDs while synthesizing fullerene. They concluded that a higher fluorescence quantum yield of CQDs i.e., around 3%–5% was obtained from fullerene carbon shoots by using a mixture of two concentrated acids like sulphuric acid and nitric acid. Additionally, they also found that the CQDs exhibited emission in the yellow range of the visible spectra, had photostability across a broad pH range, and were resistant towards long-term exposure to UV radiation and ionic strength. Another research team, Yang et al. (2014), developed a technique for producing CQDs that are heavily doped and have good photoluminescence characteristics. The synthesis method includes oxidation and simultaneous cutting of the carbon nanoparticles obtained from Chinese ink to get oxidized CQDs. Subsequently, the doped heteroatom (with Nitrogen (N), Sulphur (S), or Selenium (Se)) CQDs were acquired through hydrothermal reduction and *in situ* doping process. These heavily doped CQDs have dimensions of 1–6 nm and exhibited enhanced photoluminescence at different wavelengths, longer lifetime of fluorescence, better photostability and higher yield. Further, they also concluded that sulphur and nitrogen-doped CQDs were able to detect the presence of Hg^{2+} and Cu^{2+} ions, respectively. Despite being a common method for synthesis of CQDs, acidic oxidation has some disadvantages that restrict its application as a large-scale synthesis technique. The requirement of strong acids for the oxidation process is a major drawback as it generates a huge amount of waste acid water. The size distribution and structure of the CQDs obtained by this technique is also not uniform throughout.

3.2.2   Bottom-up Approach Methods

Bottom-up methods involve methods in which the smaller organic molecules are subjected to carbonization or pyrolysis in organic solvents or water to transform them into nanoparticles (Das et al., 2018). The various methods included in bottom-up synthesis are hydrothermal, microwave pyrolysis, thermal and combustion routes, and template methods. As the bottom-up methods do not use much of strong oxidizing agents, this method is considered as a green synthesis technology for CQDs. The bottom-up approach methods provide an enhanced ability to monitor the surface chemistry, characteristic properties, and dimensions of the synthesized CQDs. Therefore, the obtained CQDs through these methods have a wide range of applications in the fields of biotechnology and nanotechnology.

3.2.2.1 Microwave Irradiation

Microwaves encompass electromagnetic waves that have a wavelength span of 1 mm–1 m. Usually, materials containing carbohydrate and water can easily absorb microwave and dissipate the microwave energy as heat. Thus, this technique is preferred as a green synthesis technique for obtaining CQDs by heating the organic molecules with microwave energy that leads to carbonization (Vinoth Kumar et al., 2021). The CQDs synthesized by microwave irradiation exhibit a higher quantum yield and photoluminescence. Carbonaceous materials have the capacity to effectively interact with electromagnetic waves in a substantial manner. This particular characteristic has greatly improved the efficacy and precision of the heating process, thereby leading to enhanced carbonization procedures and simplified generation of distinctive morphologies in nanostructures (Tejwan et al., 2020). Numerous scientific investigations have been conducted to explore the environmentally friendly synthesis of quantum dots using this advanced technique. Wang et al. (2012) synthesized CQDs using microwave irradiation from eggshell membrane ash. The obtained CQDs had a 14% fluorescence quantum yield and exhibited emission peak of fluorescence at 450 nm. They also developed a fluorescent probe for the purpose of sensitive turn-on sensing of glutathione. This probe demonstrated a linear range that was deemed favourable and selectivity that was considered satisfactory. The fluorescence assay, which is based on CQDs, holds considerable potential in the fields of biotechnology and bioassay applications. Fluorescent CQDs doped with nitrogen (5.23%) were synthesized from lotus roots using microwave irradiation technique by Gu et al. (2016). The obtained CQDs had 19% quantum yield with 9.41 nm average diameter. These CQDs doped with nitrogen had the ability to detect Hg^{2+} ions and can also be used for cell imaging. Bajpai et al. (2019) utilized milk protein i.e., casein as a natural source of nitrogen and carbon for synthesizing nitrogen-doped CQDs using microwave irradiation. The synthesized CQDs had a quantum yield of 18.7% and emitted a blue spectrum of fluorescence under ultraviolet radiations. The various combinations of microwave power, heating time, and solvents used for microwave-assisted synthesis of CQDs from various carbon sources are summarized in Table 3.1.

3.2.2.2 Hydrothermal Technique

Hydrothermal processing is one of the bottom-up method for synthesizing CQDs exhibiting good fluorescent properties from carbon precursors. Mostly, organic compounds such as glucose, citric acid, or biobased materials containing carbon atoms are used as carbon sources for hydrothermal treatment to obtain CQDs (X. Zhang et al., 2017). Hydrothermal treatment is carried out in a closed aqueous medium under high temperature and pressure (Shen, 2020). Carbonization followed by fragmentation

TABLE 3.1

Synthesis of CQDs using Microwave Irradiation Technique from Various Carbon Sources

Sl. No.	Carbon Source	Microwave Power	Time	Solvent Used	Quantum Yield	References
1	*Calotropis gigantea* (crown flower) leaves	900 W	–	Water	4.24%	Sharma et al. (2022)
2	Chickpeas	350 W	2 min	Water	1.8%	Başoğlu et al. (2020)
3	Citric acid and thiourea	550 W	5 min	Water	26%	Pajewska-Szmyt et al. (2020)
4	Citric acid and urea	700 W	0–300 s	Water	–	Kumar et al. (2020)
5	Jackfruit seed	600 W	1 min 30 s	Phosphoric acid	17.91%	Raji et al. (2019)
6	L-arginine	750 W	3 min	Phosphoric acid and water	12–32%	Omer et al. (2019)
7	Gelatin	600 W	10 min	Water and polyethylene glycol	34%	Arsalani et al. (2019)
8	m-phenylenediamine and glucose	240 W	5 min	Ethylene glycol solution	11.2%	Guo et al. (2018)
9	Albumin (egg white)	700 W	5 min	Water	6.6 ± 0.1%	Hu et al. (2016)
10	Raw cashew gum	800 W	30–40 min	Water	8.7 ± 2%	Pires et al. (2015)

of the raw materials due to the application of high pressure and temperature leads to the synthesis of CQDs with nanometre dimension. The pressure, time, and temperature during the hydrothermal process can be controlled to obtain the CQDs with desired size and properties (Hu et al., 2010). The obtained CQDs using hydrothermal technique have higher fluorescence quantum yields, better photoluminescence, and distinct crystalline structure. Thus, all these properties make them an excellent material for various applications. The low cost, simple experimental setup, and easy maintenance are some of the advantages that make hydrothermal synthesis a widely used technique for obtaining CQDs (Titirici & Antonietti, 2010). Many researchers have used the hydrothermal approach to synthesize CQDs from various carbonaceous materials. Some of these works are reported in the following paragraphs.

Yang et al. (2012) synthesized fluorescent CQDs from chitosan using a hydrothermal carbonization technique. Chitosan was mixed with acetic acid and was subjected to hydrothermal carbonization for 12 h at 180°C, and the fluorescence quantum yield was 7.8%. Bioimaging using the synthesized CQDs exhibited good biocompatibility with human lung cells. Another study demonstrated the use of hydrothermal treatment for synthesis of CQDs from orange peel waste. An aqueous solution of oxidized orange peel waste was subjected to 180°C for 12 h in an autoclave (Prasannan & Imae, 2013). The yield was 12.3%, and the hydrothermal treatment enhanced the luminescence characteristics, which enables its application as catalysts and fluorescent markers in various biological fields. Misra et al. (2019) synthesized CQDs from groundnut by hydrothermal treatment for 6 h at 250°C in an autoclave. The CQDs had 7.8% quantum yield with high water solubility and 2.5 nm as their average size. Hydrothermal carbonization technique for 5 h at 180°C was applied for obtaining CQDs from *Boswellia ovalifoliolata* bark (Venkatesan et al., 2019). The CQDs synthesized in this study had a quantum yield of 10.2% and exhibited greater stability in aqueous medium. The CQDs had an average size of 4.16 ± 0.22 nm with green fluorescence emission. The CQDs synthesized from the bark can be utilized for Fe^{3+} detection because of their selectiveness and sensitivity towards metal ion sensing. Li et al. (2021) synthesized CQDs from corn stalk shell by hydrothermal treatment employed for 10 min at 270°C temperature and 5 MPa pressure. In this case, the stability, fluorescence ability, and biocompatibility of the synthesized CQDs using hydrothermal process were reported to be excellent, enabling their potential application in bioimaging and as sensors. The quantum yield was 16% with the emission of the blue fluorescence spectrum and the average size range was between 1.2 and 3.2 nm. Another interesting work by Alamdari et al. (2023) investigated the applicability of hydrothermal treatment for the synthesis of CQDs from agro-based wastes such as sugar beet vinasse and date seeds. The treatment was applied for 12 h at a temperature of 160°C. Both the obtained CQDs exhibited green fluorescence spectra with quantum yields of 20.64% and 5.16% from vinasse and date seeds, respectively. The CQDs synthesized from vinasse and date seeds had an average size of 6.82 and 2.37 nm, respectively. Another recent study showed the application of hydrothermal technique for the synthesis of CQDs from *Curcuma zedoaria* (Zhang et al., 2023). The hydrothermal treatment was conducted at 220°C for 12 h in aqueous medium. The CQDs exhibited blue fluorescence and had a diameter of 4.8 nm. It helped in detecting the presence of Fe^{3+} ions and also exhibited a radical scavenging activity.

Additional examples of the synthesis of CQDs using hydrothermal method from different carbon precursors are given in Table 3.2.

Thus, it can be concluded that the hydrothermal method of synthesizing CQDs can be considered as a green technique that develops CQDs with superior water solubility, stability, biocompatibility, and excellent fluorescence properties. The simple operating procedure, low-cost, and less time requirement for synthesizing CQDs are an additional benefit offered by this synthesis approach.

3.2.2.3 Thermal/Combustion Method

The carbon precursors undergo carbonization or pyrolysis at a high temperature to synthesize CQDs by thermal method. The process of pyrolysis/carbonization usually occurs at a temperature range of 200–1000°C in a controlled environment, i.e., without oxygen. The carbon source for thermal decomposition could be any organic compound containing carbon. These carbon sources are forced to rapid heating under a controlled environment for synthesizing CQDs. Due to greater temperatures during the reaction process, the chemical bonds within the source material break down to form smaller clusters of carbon particles which further nucleate and grow to develop into CQDs having sizes within nanometre dimension and good photoluminescence properties. The various advantages of this thermal method of CQD synthesis are its low cost, ease and simplicity of operation, which enables its applicability on a larger scale. Also, by controlling the concentration of raw materials, the reaction atmosphere, temperature, and time, CQDs with desired structure, dimension, and optical properties can be synthesized. The CQDs doped with nitrogen, phosphorus, or sulphur can also be developed through this thermal method. They help in improving the characteristic properties of the CQDs. The thermal or combustion technique also provides a scope for further modifications on the surface of CQDs, which can enhance their stability, biocompatibility, and solubility for various applications in the fields of biomedical sciences and technology.

Finger millet ragi (*Eleusine coracana*) was used as a carbon precursor for the formation of CQDs by the pyrolysis route and its sensitivity towards the detection of Cu^{2+} ions was evaluated (Murugan et al., 2019). The finger millet powder was subjected to heating at 300°C temperature for 3 h in a tubular furnace. This resulted in the development of CQDs with an average size of 3–8 nm that exhibited a blue fluorescence spectrum under UV light. Another researcher synthesized CQDs from fennel seeds using pyrolysis technique (Dager et al., 2019). Pyrolysis was conducted at a temperature of 500°C for 3 h, and the obtained CQDs were stable at different pHs and exhibited good fluorescence properties. Peanut shells were used as carbon precursors to synthesize CQDs at high temperatures of 340–420°C by thermal method (or pyrolysis) (Ma et al., 2017). The CQDs exhibited a blue fluorescence spectrum under UV-light exposure and had a quantum yield of 10.58% of. Xue et al. (2015) studied the synthesis of CQDs from lychee seeds by thermal decomposition technique at 300°C for 2 h. The obtained CQDs exhibited blue fluorescence with a quantum yield and an average particle size of 10.6% and 1.12 nm, respectively. The CQDs possess good solubility with less cytotoxicity and higher biocompatibility for application in living cell imaging.

TABLE 3.2

CQD Synthesis using Hydrothermal Method from Different Carbon Precursors

Sl. No.	Carbon Source	Temperature (°C)	Time (h)	Fluorescence Emission	Quantum Yield (%)	Average Size/ Diameter (nm)	References
1	Elm seeds	200	20	Blue	6.15	3.83 ± 1.03	Zhang et al. (2022)
2	Ascorbic acid	180–190	1–8	Blue	6.3	5.9	Shabbir et al. (2021)
3	Tangerine juice	170	12	–	3.1	1.1–2.6	Aslan and Eskalen (2021)
4	Dwarf banana peel	200	24	Blue	23	2.5–5.5	Atchudan et al. (2020)
5	Fish scale	180	24	Green	–	6 ± 1	Dhandapani et al. (2020)
6	Lemon juice	120–280	12	Green	14.86–24.89	3–5	Hoan et al. (2019)
7	*Phyllanthus acidus*	180	8	Blue	14	4.5	Atchudan et al. (2018)
8	Garlic	200	3	Blue	17.5	11	Zhao et al. (2015)
9	Apple juice	150	12	Blue	4.27	4.5 ± 1.0	Mehta et al. (2015)
10	*Saccharum officinarum* juice	120	3	Blue	5.67	2.71	Mehta et al. (2014)
11	Ginger juice	300	2	Blue	13.4	8.2 ± 0.6	Li et al. (2014)
12	Orange juice	120	2.5	Green	26	16	Sahu et al. (2012)

Overall, the thermal/combustion/pyrolysis technique is considered as a good sturdy method for synthesizing CQDs from different carbon precursors owing to its simple operating steps, affordability, and applicability on a large scale. Despite these advantages, there are a few limitations that challenge the process. These include explicit control over processing parameters such as high temperature that can lead to the synthesis of CQDs with the desired characteristics. Therefore, further research is required to confirm the consistent and reproducible results of thermal synthesis method for application on a larger scale.

3.2.2.4 Template Technique

One of the novel and flexible methods of synthesizing CQDs is the template approach. With the help of scaffolds/templates, this method synthesizes CQDs having sizes in nanorange and exceptional optical surface characteristics, making them potential materials for application in biobased imaging and as sensors (Perumal et al., 2021). Different organic and inorganic materials such as silica nanoparticles, zeolites, and polymers are used as templates for CQD synthesis. The main principle behind this synthesis method is that the carbon precursors get impregnated to the template surface and the template controls the size of the obtained CQDs. After impregnation, pyrolysis is carried out that leads to the formation of CQDs with morphology similar to that of the template material, wherein the template material is separated from the obtained CQDs. Since the CQDs are formed in a controlled environment provided by the template, they have a uniform size distribution and good optical properties for suitable/specific application purposes. Zhang et al. (2015) utilized the template method for obtaining CQDs. Acrylic acid and N-acryloyl were used to develop copolymers that further assembled to form a micellar template. The micellar template is then subjected to carbonization at 170°C to develop CQDs. The average size of the CQDs formed by this method was 2–5 nm, and the quantum yield was 22%. Another study reported on the use of mesoporous silica spheres as nanoreactors for synthesizing CQDs through the template method (Zong et al., 2011). The developed CQDs had a quantum yield and an average size of 23% and 1.5–2.5 nm, respectively. The obtained CQDs possessed good photostability and emitted blue colour fluorescence under UV light. Although the template method helped in developing monodisperse CQDs with well-defined sizes, the process is quite costly and requires more time. Another limitation is the separation of the template from the CQDs after the pyrolysis process that is carried out at a very high temperature. These limitations restrict its applicability on a larger production scale.

3.3 LIMITATIONS OF DIFFERENT SYNTHESIS TECHNIQUES

In this chapter, two major synthesis techniques of CQDs from different carbon precursors have been discussed in detail, namely the top-down and bottom-up approach techniques. Both techniques have some major advantages as well as some limitations that restrict their application on a larger production scale. Some pros and cons of different top-down and bottom-up approach methods are summarized in Table 3.3.

The top-down method synthesizes CQDs by breaking larger molecules into nanosized particles. One of the major challenges in this method is the uniform size

TABLE 3.3

Advantages and Disadvantages of Different Top-down and Bottom-up Approach Methods

	Method	Advantages	Disadvantages
Top-down approach	Laser ablation	Photoluminescence and size of the CQDs can be controlled easily by altering the processing parameters like time of irradiation.	Low quantum yield, poor control over size of CQDs, and it is not a green synthesis method.
	Arc discharge	Produces multi-walled carbon nanotubes that can be further broken down to generate CQDs.	The nanotube shoots have a large number of impurities. The oxidative stability of the graphitic sheets in the shoot is higher as compared to the nanotubes. It has low quantum yield and the method is composite.
	Acidic oxidation	The obtained CQDs exhibit tuneable photoluminescence characteristics, high quantum yield, and longer fluorescence lifetime.	The heavily doped heteroatoms can affect the PL properties due to the electronegativity of N, S, and Se.
Bottom-up approach	Microwave irradiation	A rapid and green synthesis technique, can be easily commercialized, has a simple operation method, and is environment friendly.	Poor control over size.
	Hydrothermal treatment	Facile green synthesis technique, has good quantum yield, and is non-toxic and cost-effective.	Poor control over size of CQDs, losses can occur via the reactor walls.
	Thermal treatment	Easy approach technique, can be scalable for larger productions, uniform particle size distribution.	Smaller polycyclic aromatic hydrocarbons (PAHs) are generated in soot formation; can cause environmental hazards.
	Template method	Produces monodisperse CQDs that possesses higher colloidal stability and biocompatibility.	Expensive technique, time-consuming, and lower quantum yield.

distribution of the obtained CQDs. This method does not allow the attachment of a wide range of functional groups onto the surface of the CQDs, which can further restrict their application in various fields of biosensors and cell imaging (Wang & Hu, 2014). Top-down approach method such as acidic oxidation uses several strong acids for the reaction process, which have a negative impact on the environment. The fluorescence quantum yield of the top-down approach methods is lower, which directly affects its optical properties and its applications in bioimaging and as sensors for detecting metal ions.

The bottom-up approach method works on the principle of developing nanosized CQDs from small carbon precursors. The major limitation of this technique is the complexity on the synthesis process. The bottom-up techniques require different steps for synthesizing CQDs, which consume more time and as it involves multiple steps, it becomes difficult to control the processing parameters to obtain CQDs with desirable properties (Wang et al., 2019).

3.4 CONCLUSION

The synthesis of CQDs has been a widely discussed topic owing to their excellent and precise applications in various fields. These CQDs have a size distribution in the range of nanosize i.e., 1–10 nm. They possess outstanding photoluminescence properties and biocompatibility, which enhances their potential application in bioimaging, and as sensors for detecting metal ions and for drug delivery. The various top-down and bottom-up methods of obtaining CQDs that have been discussed in this chapter have their own advantages and disadvantages. The method used for synthesizing CQDs from various carbon precursors majorly depends upon the required characteristic properties of the CQDs. Thermal/pyrolysis technique provides the development of CQDs in a controlled environment, which helps to obtain CQDs with desirable target characteristics. The template method helps in producing monodisperse CQDs having a uniform size distribution. On the other hand, hydrothermal method is a large-scale production technique because of its simplicity in operation and well-defined properties of obtained CQDs for various applications. Microwave irradiation is a simple, hassle free, and green synthesis technique that requires less time. Although several synthesis techniques have been in use, a particular method that can have a control over size as well as possess excellent optical properties is yet to be explored.

Different on-going research studies on this trending area of CQD have led researchers to develop precise techniques for synthesizing CQDs. Although many synthesis techniques have been developed by many researchers, the process of CQD synthesis is costly, requires a lot of time, and is not eco-friendly. Further research in this area will help in eliminating the limitations and developing green synthesis techniques that will not only take less time for production but will also be environment friendly, of low cost, and easily scalable for different applications. For industrial applications of CQDs in different imaging sensors and detection of metal ions, the production process of CQDs should consume less time and be cost-effective so that it can contribute towards economic development. Therefore, there should be more progress in research towards developing effective, efficient green synthesis techniques for obtaining CQDs from various precursor materials with desirable properties for vast applications in the fields of nanoscience and biotechnology.

REFERENCES

Alamdari, N. G., Almasi, H., Moradi, M., & Akhgari, M. (2023). Characterization of carbon quantum dots synthesized from vinasse and date seeds as agro-industrial wastes. *Waste and Biomass Valorization*, *14*(11), 3689–3703. https://doi.org/10.1007/s12649-023-02087-7

Arsalani, N., Nezhad-Mokhtari, P., & Jabbari, E. (2019). Microwave-assisted and one-step synthesis of PEG passivated fluorescent carbon dots from gelatin as an efficient nano-carrier for methotrexate delivery. *Artificial Cells, Nanomedicine, and Biotechnology*, 47(1), 540–547. https://doi.org/10.1080/21691401.2018.1562460

Aslan, M., & Eskalen, H. (2021). A study of carbon nanodots (carbon quantum dots) synthesized from tangerine juice using one-step hydrothermal method. *Fullerenes, Nanotubes and Carbon Nanostructures*, 29(12), 1026–1033. https://doi.org/10.1080/1536383x.2021.1926452

Atchudan, R., Edison, T. N. J. I., Aseer, K. R., Perumal, S., Karthik, N., & Lee, Y. R. (2018). Highly fluorescent nitrogen-doped carbon dots derived from *Phyllanthus acidus* utilized as a fluorescent probe for label-free selective detection of Fe^{3+} ions, live cell imaging and fluorescent ink. *Biosensors and Bioelectronics*, 99, 303–311. https://doi.org/10.1016/j.bios.2017.07.076

Atchudan, R., Edison, T. N. J. I., Perumal, S., Muthuchamy, N., & Lee, Y. R. (2020). Hydrophilic nitrogen-doped carbon dots from biowaste using dwarf banana peel for environmental and biological applications. *Fuel*, 275, 117821. https://doi.org/10.1016/j.fuel.2020.117821

Bajpai, S. K., D'Souza, A., & Suhail, B. (2019). Blue light-emitting carbon dots (CDs) from a milk protein and their interaction with *Spinacia oleracea* leaf cells. *International Nano Letters*, 9(3), 203–212. https://doi.org/10.1007/s40089-019-0271-9

Başoğlu, A., Ocak, Ü., & Gümrükçüoğlu, A. (2020). Synthesis of microwave-assisted fluorescence carbon quantum dots using roasted–Chickpeas and its applications for sensitive and selective detection of Fe^{3+} Ions. *Journal of Fluorescence*, 30(3), 515–526. https://doi.org/10.1007/s10895-019-02428-7

Cui, L., Ren, X., Wang, J., & Sun, M. (2020). Synthesis of homogeneous carbon quantum dots by ultrafast dual-beam pulsed laser ablation for bioimaging. *Materials Today Nano*, 12, 100091. https://doi.org/10.1016/j.mtnano.2020.100091

Dager, A., Uchida, T., Maekawa, T., & Tachibana, M. (2019). Synthesis and characterization of Mono-disperse Carbon Quantum Dots from Fennel Seeds: Photoluminescence analysis using Machine Learning. *Scientific Reports*, 9(1). https://doi.org/10.1038/s41598-019-50397-5

Das, R., Bandyopadhyay, R., & Pramanik, P. (2018). Carbon quantum dots from natural resource: A review. *Materials Today Chemistry*, 8, 96–109. https://doi.org/10.1016/j.mtchem.2018.03.003

Desmond, L. J., Phan, A. N., & Gentile, P. (2021). Critical overview on the green synthesis of carbon quantum dots and their application for cancer therapy. *Environmental Science: Nano*, 8(4), 848–862. https://doi.org/10.1039/d1en00017a

Dhandapani, E., Duraisamy, N., & Periasamy, P. (2020). Highly green fluorescent carbon quantum dots synthesis via hydrothermal method from fish scale. *Materials Today: Proceedings*, 26, A1–A5. https://doi.org/10.1016/j.matpr.2021.04.396

El-Shabasy, R. M., Farouk Elsadek, M., Mohamed Ahmed, B., Fawzy Farahat, M., Mosleh, K. N., & Taher, M. M. (2021). Recent developments in carbon quantum dots: Properties, fabrication techniques, and bio-applications. *Processes*, 9(2), 388. https://doi.org/10.3390/pr9020388

Gonçalves, H., Jorge, P. A. S., Fernandes, J. R. A., & Esteves da Silva, J. C. G. (2010). Hg(II) sensing based on functionalized carbon dots obtained by direct laser ablation. *Sensors and Actuators B: Chemical*, 145(2), 702–707. https://doi.org/10.1016/j.snb.2010.01.031

Gu, D., Shang, S., Yu, Q., & Shen, J. (2016). Green synthesis of nitrogen-doped carbon dots from lotus root for Hg(II) ions detection and cell imaging. *Applied Surface Science*, 390, 38–42. https://doi.org/10.1016/j.apsusc.2016.08.012

Guo, L., Li, L., Liu, M., Wan, Q., Tian, J., Huang, Q., Wen, Y., Liang, S., Zhang, X., & Wei, Y. (2018). Bottom-up preparation of nitrogen doped carbon quantum dots with green emission under microwave-assisted hydrothermal treatment and their biological imaging. *Materials Science and Engineering: C*, 84, 60–66. https://doi.org/10.1016/j.msec.2017.11.034

Hoan, B. T., Tam, P. D., & Pham, V.-H. (2019). Green synthesis of highly luminescent carbon quantum dots from lemon juice. *Journal of Nanotechnology, 2019*, 1–9. https://doi.org/10.1155/2019/2852816

Hu, B., Wang, K., Wu, L., Yu, S. H., Antonietti, M., & Titirici, M. M. (2010). Engineering carbon materials from the hydrothermal carbonization process of biomass. *Advanced Materials, 22*(7), 813–828. https://doi.org/10.1002/adma.200902812

Hu, X., An, X., & Li, L. (2016). Easy synthesis of highly fluorescent carbon dots from albumin and their photoluminescent mechanism and biological imaging applications. *Materials Science and Engineering: C, 58*, 730–736. https://doi.org/10.1016/j.msec.2015.09.066

Kumar, P., Bhatt, G., Kaur, R., Dua, S., & Kapoor, A. (2020). Synthesis and modulation of the optical properties of carbon quantum dots using microwave radiation. *Fullerenes, Nanotubes and Carbon Nanostructures, 28*(9), 724–731. https://doi.org/10.1080/1536383x.2020.1752679

Li, C.-L., Ou, C.-M., Huang, C.-C., Wu, W.-C., Chen, Y.-P., Lin, T.-E., Ho, L.-C., Wang, C.-W., Shih, C.-C., Zhou, H.-C., Lee, Y.-C., Tzeng, W.-F., Chiou, T.-J., Chu, S.-T., Cang, J., & Chang, H.-T. (2014). Carbon dots prepared from ginger exhibiting efficient inhibition of human hepatocellular carcinoma cells. *Journal of Materials Chemistry B, 2*(28), 4564. https://doi.org/10.1039/c4tb00216d

Li, X., Wang, H., Shimizu, Y., Pyatenko, A., Kawaguchi, K., & Koshizaki, N. (2011). Preparation of carbon quantum dots with tunable photoluminescence by rapid laser passivation in ordinary organic solvents. *Chem. Commun., 47*(3), 932–934. https://doi.org/10.1039/c0cc03552a

Li, Z., Wang, Q., Zhou, Z., Zhao, S., Zhong, S., Xu, L., Gao, Y., & Cui, X. (2021). Green synthesis of carbon quantum dots from corn stalk shell by hydrothermal approach in near-critical water and applications in detecting and bioimaging. *Microchemical Journal, 166*, 106250. https://doi.org/10.1016/j.microc.2021.106250

Lim, S. Y., Shen, W., & Gao, Z. (2015). Carbon quantum dots and their applications. *Chemical Society Reviews, 44*(1), 362–381. https://doi.org/10.1039/c4cs00269e

Ma, X., Dong, Y., Sun, H., & Chen, N. (2017). Highly fluorescent carbon dots from peanut shells as potential probes for copper ion: The optimization and analysis of the synthetic process. *Materials Today Chemistry, 5*, 1–10. https://doi.org/10.1016/j.mtchem.2017.04.004

Mehta, V. N., Jha, S., Basu, H., Singhal, R. K., & Kailasa, S. K. (2015). One-step hydrothermal approach to fabricate carbon dots from apple juice for imaging of mycobacterium and fungal cells. *Sensors and Actuators B: Chemical, 213*, 434–443. https://doi.org/10.1016/j.snb.2015.02.104

Mehta, V. N., Jha, S., & Kailasa, S. K. (2014). One-pot green synthesis of carbon dots by using Saccharum officinarum juice for fluorescent imaging of bacteria (Escherichia coli) and yeast (Saccharomyces cerevisiae) cells. *Materials Science and Engineering: C, 38*, 20–27. https://doi.org/10.1016/j.msec.2014.01.038

Murugan, N., Prakash, M., Jayakumar, M., Sundaramurthy, A., & Sundramoorthy, A. K. (2019). Green synthesis of fluorescent carbon quantum dots from Eleusine coracana and their application as a fluorescence 'turn-off' sensor probe for selective detection of Cu^{2+}. *Applied Surface Science, 476*, 468–480. https://doi.org/10.1016/j.apsusc.2019.01.090

Omer, K. M., Hama Aziz, K. H., Salih, Y. M., Tofiq, D. I., & Hassan, A. Q. (2019). Photoluminescence enhancement via microwave irradiation of carbon quantum dots derived from solvothermal synthesis of l-arginine. *New Journal of Chemistry, 43*(2), 689–695. https://doi.org/10.1039/c8nj04788j

Pajewska-Szmyt, M., Buszewski, B., & Gadzała-Kopciuch, R. (2020). Sulphur and nitrogen doped carbon dots synthesis by microwave assisted method as quantitative analytical nano-tool for mercury ion sensing. *Materials Chemistry and Physics, 242*, 122484. https://doi.org/10.1016/j.matchemphys.2019.122484

Perumal, S., Atchudan, R., Edison, T. N. J. I., & Lee, Y. R. (2021). Sustainable synthesis of multifunctional carbon dots using biomass and their applications: A mini-review. *Journal of Environmental Chemical Engineering, 9*(4), 105802. https://doi.org/10.1016/j.jece.2021.105802

Pires, N. R., Santos, C. M. W., Sousa, R. R., Paula, R. C. M. D., Cunha, P. L. R., & Feitosa, J. P. A. (2015). Novel and fast microwave-assisted synthesis of carbon quantum dots from raw cashew gum. *Journal of the Brazilian Chemical Society.* https://doi.org/10.5935/0103-5053.20150094

Prasannan, A., & Imae, T. (2013). One-Pot synthesis of fluorescent carbon dots from orange waste peels. *Industrial & Engineering Chemistry Research, 52*(44), 15673–15678. https://doi.org/10.1021/ie402421s

Raji, K., Ramanan, V., & Ramamurthy, P. (2019). Facile and green synthesis of highly fluorescent nitrogen-doped carbon dots from jackfruit seeds and its applications towards the fluorimetric detection of Au^{3+} ions in aqueous medium and in in vitro multicolor cell imaging. *New Journal of Chemistry, 43*(29), 11710–11719. https://doi.org/10.1039/c9nj02590a

Sahu, S., Behera, B., Maiti, T. K., & Mohapatra, S. (2012). Simple one-step synthesis of highly luminescent carbon dots from orange juice: Application as excellent bio-imaging agents. *Chemical Communications, 48*(70), 8835. https://doi.org/10.1039/c2cc33796g

Shabbir, H., Tokarski, T., Ungor, D., & Wojnicki, M. (2021). Eco friendly synthesis of carbon dot by hydrothermal method for metal ions salt identification. *Materials, 14*(24), 7604. https://doi.org/10.3390/ma14247604

Sharma, N., Sharma, I., & Bera, M. K. (2022). Microwave-assisted green synthesis of carbon quantum dots derived from calotropis gigantea as a fluorescent probe for bioimaging. *Journal of Fluorescence, 32*(3), 1039–1049. https://doi.org/10.1007/s10895-022-02923-4

Shen, J., Zhu, Y., Yang, X., & Li, C. (2012). Graphene quantum dots: Emergent nanolights for bioimaging, sensors, catalysis and photovoltaic devices. *Chemical Communications, 48*(31), 3686. https://doi.org/10.1039/c2cc00110a

Shen, P., & Xia, Y. (2014). Synthesis-modification integration: One-step fabrication of boronic acid functionalized carbon dots for fluorescent blood sugar sensing. *Analytical Chemistry, 86*(11), 5323–5329. https://doi.org/10.1021/ac5001338

Shen, Y. (2020). A review on hydrothermal carbonization of biomass and plastic wastes to energy products. *Biomass and Bioenergy, 134*, 105479. https://doi.org/10.1016/j.biombioe.2020.105479

Sun, Y.-P., Zhou, B., Lin, Y., Wang, W., Fernando, K. A. S., Pathak, P., Meziani, M. J., Harruff, B. A., Wang, X., Wang, H., Luo, P. G., Yang, H., Kose, M. E., Chen, B., Veca, L. M., & Xie, S.-Y. (2006). Quantum-sized carbon dots for bright and colorful photoluminescence. *Journal of the American Chemical Society, 128*(24), 7756–7757. https://doi.org/10.1021/ja062677d

Tejwan, N., Saha, S. K., & Das, J. (2020). Multifaceted applications of green carbon dots synthesized from renewable sources. *Advances in Colloid and Interface Science, 275*, 102046. https://doi.org/10.1016/j.cis.2019.102046

Titirici, M.-M., & Antonietti, M. (2010). Chemistry and materials options of sustainable carbon materials made by hydrothermal carbonization. *Chem. Soc. Rev., 39*(1), 103–116. https://doi.org/10.1039/b819318p

Roshni, V., Misra, S., Santra, M. K., & Ottoor, D. (2019). One pot green synthesis of C-dots from groundnuts and its application as Cr(VI) sensor and in vitro bioimaging agent. *Journal of Photochemistry and Photobiology A: Chemistry, 373*, 28–36. https://doi.org/10.1016/j.jphotochem.2018.12.028

Venkatesan, G., Rajagopalan, V., & Chakravarthula, S. N. (2019). *Boswellia ovalifoliolata* bark extract derived carbon dots for selective fluorescent sensing of Fe^{3+}. *Journal of Environmental Chemical Engineering, 7*(2), 103013. https://doi.org/10.1016/j.jece.2019.103013

Vinoth Kumar, J., Kavitha, G., Arulmozhi, R., Arul, V., Singaravadivel, S., & Abirami, N. (2021). Green sources derived carbon dots for multifaceted applications. *Journal of Fluorescence*, *31*(4), 915–932. https://doi.org/10.1007/s10895-021-02721-4

Wang, Q., Liu, X., Zhang, L., & Lv, Y. (2012). Microwave-assisted synthesis of carbon nanodots through an eggshell membrane and their fluorescent application. *The Analyst*, *137*(22), 5392. https://doi.org/10.1039/c2an36059d

Wang, X., Feng, Y., Dong, P., & Huang, J. (2019). A mini review on carbon quantum dots: preparation, properties, and electrocatalytic application. *Frontiers in Chemistry*, *7*. https://doi.org/10.3389/fchem.2019.00671

Wang, Y., & Hu, A. (2014). Carbon quantum dots: Synthesis, properties and applications. *Journal of Materials Chemistry C*, *2*(34), 6921. https://doi.org/10.1039/c4tc00988f

Xu, X., Ray, R., Gu, Y., Ploehn, H. J., Gearheart, L., Raker, K., & Scrivens, W. A. (2004). Electrophoretic analysis and purification of fluorescent single-walled carbon nanotube fragments. *Journal of the American Chemical Society*, *126*(40), 12736–12737. https://doi.org/10.1021/ja040082h

Xue, M., Zou, M., Zhao, J., Zhan, Z., & Zhao, S. (2015). Green preparation of fluorescent carbon dots from lychee seeds and their application for the selective detection of methylene blue and imaging in living cells. *Journal of Materials Chemistry B*, *3*(33), 6783–6789. https://doi.org/10.1039/c5tb01073j

Yang, S., Sun, J., Li, X., Zhou, W., Wang, Z., He, P., Ding, G., Xie, X., Kang, Z., & Jiang, M. (2014). Large-scale fabrication of heavy doped carbon quantum dots with tunable-photoluminescence and sensitive fluorescence detection. *Journal of Materials Chemistry A*, *2*(23), 8660. https://doi.org/10.1039/c4ta00860j

Yang, W., Li, X., Fei, L., Liu, W., Liu, X., Xu, H., & Liu, Y. (2022). A review on sustainable synthetic approaches toward photoluminescent quantum dots. *Green Chemistry*, *24*(2), 675–700. https://doi.org/10.1039/d1gc02964a

Yang, Y., Cui, J., Zheng, M., Hu, C., Tan, S., Xiao, Y., Yang, Q., & Liu, Y. (2012). One-step synthesis of amino-functionalized fluorescent carbon nanoparticles by hydrothermal carbonization of chitosan. *Chem. Commun.*, *48*(3), 380–382. https://doi.org/10.1039/c1cc15678k

Zhang, J., Abbasi, F., & Claverie, J. (2015). An efficient templating approach for the synthesis of redispersible size-controllable carbon quantum dots from graphitic polymeric micelles. *Chemistry: A European Journal*, *21*(43), 15142–15147. https://doi.org/10.1002/chem.201502158

Zhang, J., Zheng, G., Tian, Y., Zhang, C., Wang, Y., Liu, M., Ren, D., Sun, H., & Yu, W. (2022). Green synthesis of carbon dots from elm seeds via hydrothermal method for Fe^{3+} detection and cell imaging. *Inorganic Chemistry Communications*, *144*, 109837. https://doi.org/10.1016/j.inoche.2022.109837

Zhang, Q., Sun, X., Ruan, H., Yin, K., & Li, H. (2017b). Production of yellow-emitting carbon quantum dots from fullerene carbon soot. *Science China Materials*, *60*(2), 141–150. https://doi.org/10.1007/s40843-016-5160-9

Zhang, X., Jiang, M., Niu, N., Chen, Z., Li, S., Liu, S., & Li, J. (2017a). Natural-product-derived carbon dots: From natural products to functional materials. *ChemSusChem*, *11*(1), 11–24. https://doi.org/10.1002/cssc.201701847

Zhang, Y., Li, P., Yan, H., Guo, Q., Xu, Q., & Su, W. (2023). Green synthesis and multifunctional applications of nitrogen-doped carbon quantum dots via one-step hydrothermal carbonization of *Curcuma zedoaria*. *Analytical and Bioanalytical Chemistry*, *415*(10), 1917–1931. https://doi.org/10.1007/s00216-023-04603-z

Zhao, S., Lan, M., Zhu, X., Xue, H., Ng, T.-W., Meng, X., Lee, C.-S., Wang, P., & Zhang, W. (2015). Green synthesis of bifunctional fluorescent carbon dots from garlic for cellular imaging and free radical scavenging. *ACS Applied Materials & Interfaces*, *7*(31), 17054–17060. https://doi.org/10.1021/acsami.5b03228

Zong, J., Zhu, Y., Yang, X., Shen, J., & Li, C. (2011). Synthesis of photoluminescent carbogenic dots using mesoporous silica spheres as nanoreactors. *Chem. Commun.*, *47*(2), 764–766. https://doi.org/10.1039/c0cc03092a

4 Characterization Techniques for Carbon Quantum Dots

Shristi Shefali Saraugi, Valerie Orsat,
Ashutosh Singh and Winny Routray

4.1 INTRODUCTION

Carbon quantum dots (CQDs) are the nanomaterials category observed as zero-dimensional carbon-based nanoparticles. CQDs exhibit good chemical stability, fluorescence, and water solubility. Characterization of CQDs plays a vital role in scientific research and technological applications and advances, which encompasses their size, structure, composition, luminescence mechanism, surface chemistry, among other characteristics. Characterization of CQDs empowers researchers for a comprehensive study of their properties, facilitating improved synthesis methods and diversification of the applications in several fields, viz., bioimaging, environmental sensing, optoelectronics, 3-D printing technology, biomedical, metal detection, electronics, wastewater treatment, etc.

4.2 CHARACTERIZATION OF CARBON QUANTUM DOTS (CQDs)

Various techniques can be utilized for the structural and physical characterization of carbon dots, including transmission electron microscopy (TEM), atomic force microscopy (ATM), scanning electron microscopy (SEM), dynamic light scattering (DLS), X-ray diffraction (XRD), UV spectroscopy, Fourier transform infrared spectroscopy (FTIR), X-ray photoelectron spectroscopy (XPS), Raman spectroscopy, photoluminescence spectroscopy, nuclear magnetic resonance (NMR), energy dispersive spectroscopy (EDS), thermogravimetric analysis (TGA), zeta potential analysis, thin layer chromatography (TLC), quantum yield analyses, and cytotoxicity. These characterization techniques are summarized in Table 4.1, along with the parameters on which they are based (Dager et al., 2019).

4.2.1 MICROSCOPIC ANALYSIS-BASED TECHNIQUES

Microscopic analysis is generally practiced in assessing the morphology, structure, and particle aggregation. The dimensional, structural, morphological, and chemical constituents are the elemental aspects of the distinctive characterization of CQDs.

DOI: 10.1201/9781003437857-5

TABLE 4.1

Characterization Techniques for Carbon Quantum Dots (CQDs)

Sl. No.	Analysis Parameter	Characterization Parameters	Analytical Instruments
1.	Microscopic	Morphology (size, shape, and dispersion) and ultrastructure	TEM
		Surface topography, size, height, and particle structure	AMF
		Surface morphology (shape, texture, and distribution) and surface elemental composition	SEM
		Size distribution profile and hydrodynamic average diameter	DLS
2.	Diffraction	Crystallinity state, crystal structure, and crystallinity phase	XRD
3.	Spectroscopy and optical	Absorption peak, optical properties, bandgap energy	UV-vis absorbance spectroscopy
		Optical and electronic properties, fluorescence imaging, emission wavelength (λ_{em}), and excitation wavelength (λ_{ex})	Photoluminescence spectroscopy
4.	Spectroscopy	Chemical/functional group	FTIR spectroscopy
		Chemical state, elemental composition, functional moieties	XPS spectroscopy
		State of carbon	Raman spectroscopy
		Elements (C, N, and P), structural parameters, impurities	NMR spectroscopy
		Elemental composition	EDS
5.	Thermal	Thermal stability, phase transition, thermal decomposition	TGA
6.	Electrical charge	Surface charge and size distribution	Zeta-sizer
7.	Chromatography	Purity	Thin layer chromatography
8.	Quantum yield	Photophysical character	Quantum efficiency measurement system

Microscopic examination can be performed through transmission electron microscopy (TEM), atomic force microscopy (AFM), and other microscopic analysis methods.

4.2.1.1 Transmission Electron Microscopy (TEM)

TEM technique is utilized to examine the morphology (size, shape, and dispersion) and ultrastructure of the CQDs. TEM imaging is executed on samples when a higher-resolution image is the requisite (0.1 to 0.2 nm). A high-resolution TEM technique is used to evaluate the fine structure of carbon dots. The photon and electron signals are released when the incident electron beam strikes the surface of the CQDs. The emitted X-ray and auger electrons correspond to a surface-sensitive phenomenon and are used to retrieve the compositional information. Secondary electrons and the primary backscattered electrons assist in determining the topographic characteristics of CQDs. By extrapolating to the length scale, it is possible to estimate the average diameter and particle size of CQDs when using TEM imaging, which involves passing a beam of high-energy electrons via a specimen of carbon dots. TEM analysis is highly demanded in material sciences, pharmaceuticals, and various research and development sectors (Li et al., 2018). The crystalline form of carbon dots can be categorized based on the lattice fringes: (a) interlayer spacing −0.34 nm and (b) in-plane lattice spacing of 0.24 nm (Zuo et al., 2016).

Murru et al. (2020) investigated the morphological characteristics of CQDs obtained from organic sources. In Figure 4.1(a), it can be observed that carbon dots from glutathione/citric acid were mainly monodispersed and possessed an average diameter of 6 ± 0.8 nm. From Figure 4.1(b), it can be deduced that tea-based CQDs have an average diameter of 3.5 ± 0.6 nm, indicating the availability of crystalline graphite and amorphous phases. In grape pomace-based carbon dots of Figure 4.1(c), particles are monodispersed in nature with particle size diameters between 3 and 5 nm.

A research study was done by Sabet and Mahdavi (2019) on synthesizing nitrogen-doped CQDs from grass, and the corresponding TEM image is shown in Figure 4.2. From the TEM image, it can be noted that the produced CQDs are composed of very tiny particles. Various studies have been done to analyze the morphological characteristics of the CQDs synthesized from natural sources, some of these are mentioned in Table 4.2.

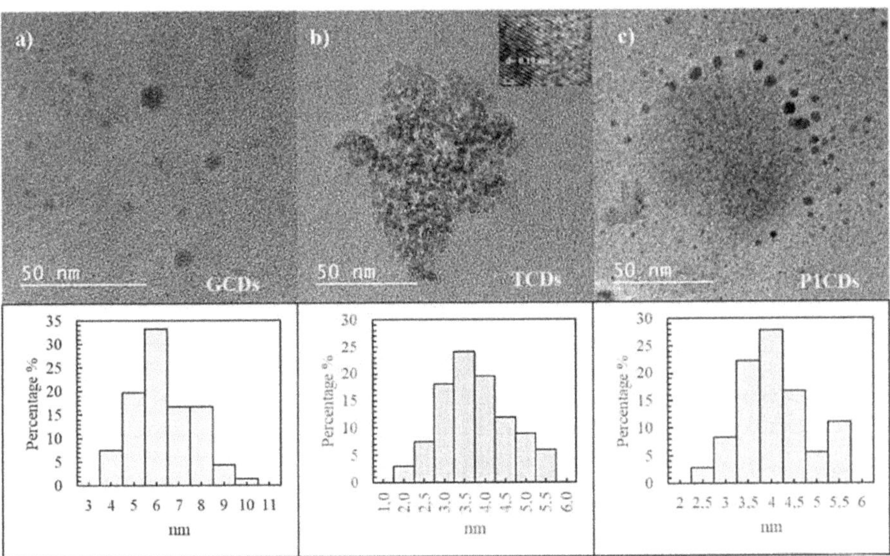

FIGURE 4.1 High-resolution TEM images of (a) carbon dots from glutathione/citric acid (GCQDs), (b) tea-based carbon dots (TCQDs), (c) grape pomace-based carbon dots (P1CQDs) and their corresponding size distribution histograms; n = 118 TCQDs, n = 106 GCQDs, and n = 144 P1CQDs (Murru et al., 2020).

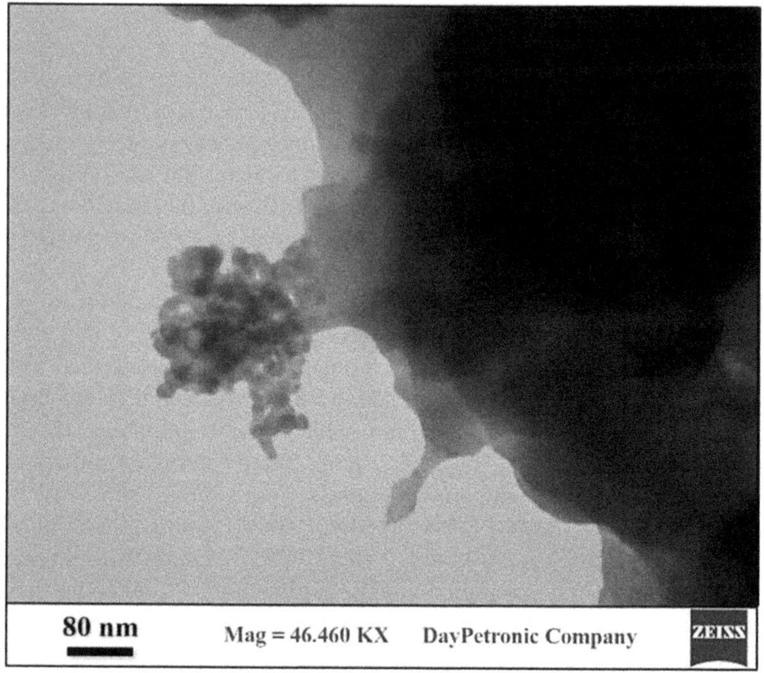

FIGURE 4.2 TEM image of nitrogen-doped CQDs from grass (Sabet & Mahdavi, 2019).

TABLE 4.2
Size Distribution/Average Size from TEM Images of Various CQDs

Source of Carbon	Size Distribution/Average Diameter (nm)	References
Garlic	10.7	Zhao et al. (2015)
Gram shell	3–5	Das et al. (2017)
Fennel seeds	3.9	Dager et al. (2019)
Sugarcane bagasse pulp	4.1±0.17	Thamiraj et al. (2016)
Flour	5–8	Zhang et al. (2015)
Lotus roots	9.41	Gu et al. (2016)
Tamarindus indica leaves	3–3.5	Bano et al. (2018)

4.2.1.2 Atomic Force Microscopy (AFM)

Atomic force microscopy is a powerful technique involving an imaging system utilized to analyze CQDs at the nanoscale. It is mainly used to investigate surface topography, quantitative measurement of size and height, and particle structure of CQDs. The principle of AFM is based on measuring the force between a sharp tip (detection of magnetic and electric properties of the sample) and the sample's surface. This sharp tip is utilized to image a sample through raster scanning across the surface line by line (Zainal et al., 2021).

Thambiraj et al. (2016) reported on the study of AFM of CQDs synthesized from sugarcane bagasse pulp, which was observed to be spherical and very small in size, as shown in Figure 4.3. The average diameter was between 3 and 5 nm, and the surface roughness was below 5 nm. The histogram obtained for the particles was studied in a ten-counting scale and an average roughness equivalent to 4.2 nm was observed.In a study, Sabet and Mahdavi (2019) investigated surface topography and roughness through AFM, as illustrated in Figure 4.4. It can be noticed that the particles of the CQDs are aggregated uniformly, and the surfaces of the CQDs are uniform in nature.

The CQDs were produced under a silicon substrate from the gram shell by Das et al. (2017), and the corresponding AFM is illustrated in Figure 4.5. From the two- (height profiles) and three-dimensional AFM images, it can be observed that the synthesized CQDs were well-dispersed and quasi-spherical in shape. Hence, depending on the source material and doping type, the CQDs' structure correspondingly affects different functional properties.

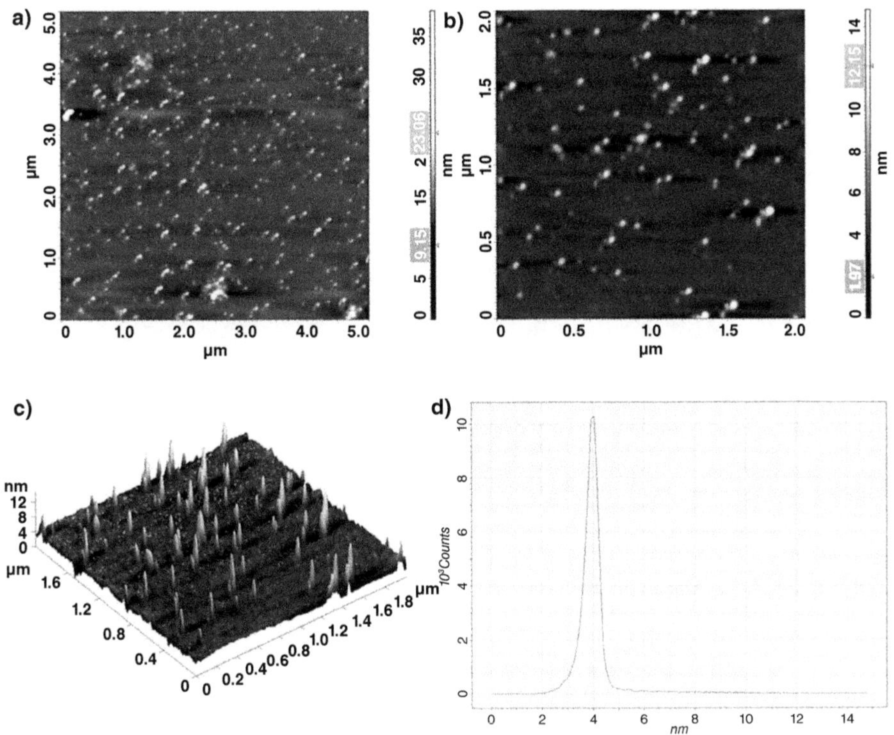

FIGURE 4.3 AFM image of CQDs synthesized from sugarcane bagasse pulp, (a) low magnification image (5 μm) of CQDs, (b) high magnification (2 μm) of CQDs, (c) three-dimensional images of CQDs correlated to image (b), (d) histogram image of the obtained CQDs with an average particle size of ~5 nm (Thambiraj, 2016).

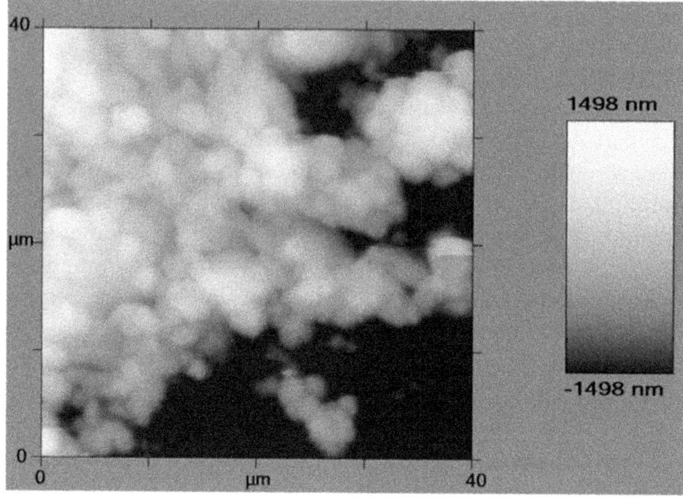

FIGURE 4.4 AFM image of the nitrogen-doped CQDs synthesized from grass (Sabet & Mahdavi, 2019).

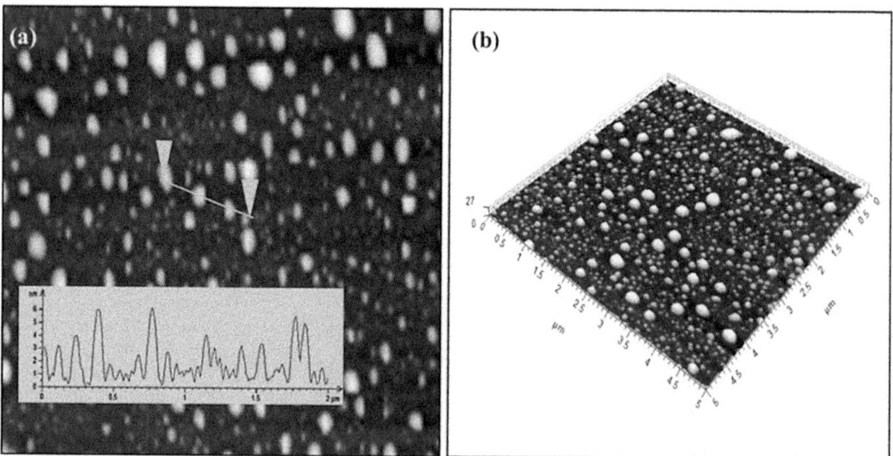

FIGURE 4.5 (a) Two-dimensional AFM of the gram CQDs and (b) three-dimensional AFM of the gram CQDs (Das et al. 2017).

4.2.1.3 Scanning Electron Microscopy (SEM)

Scanning electron microscopy (SEM) is an analytical imaging technique to inquisite surface morphology (shape, texture, and distribution), surface elemental composition, and contamination detection. The principle behind the SEM technique is that it develops largely magnified images through electrons instead of light to form an image; thus, it allows the generation of a high-resolution image of CQDs (Karatutlu et al., 2018).

During the study conducted by Sabet and Mahdavi (2019) on the SEM analysis of nitrogen-doped CQDs from grass, very small-sized carbon particles were identified, which carried high surface energy that could cause the aggregation of CQDs (Figure 4.6). To evaluate the size of the particles, the SEM images were assessed using Image J software. From Figure 4.6(b), it can be noticed that the synthesized CQDs are smaller than 10 nm. Moreover, the histogram curve in Figure 4.6(c) exhibits that the maximum particles were less than 10 nm in diameter.

Another study by Khalid et al. (2022) on the CQDs from grass for a fluorescent platform revealed the SEM analysis, characterizing the surface morphology and particle size of the produced CQDs as shown in Figure 4.7. The SEM micrograph shows that the produced CQDs were near-uniform and dot-shaped particles, confirming the

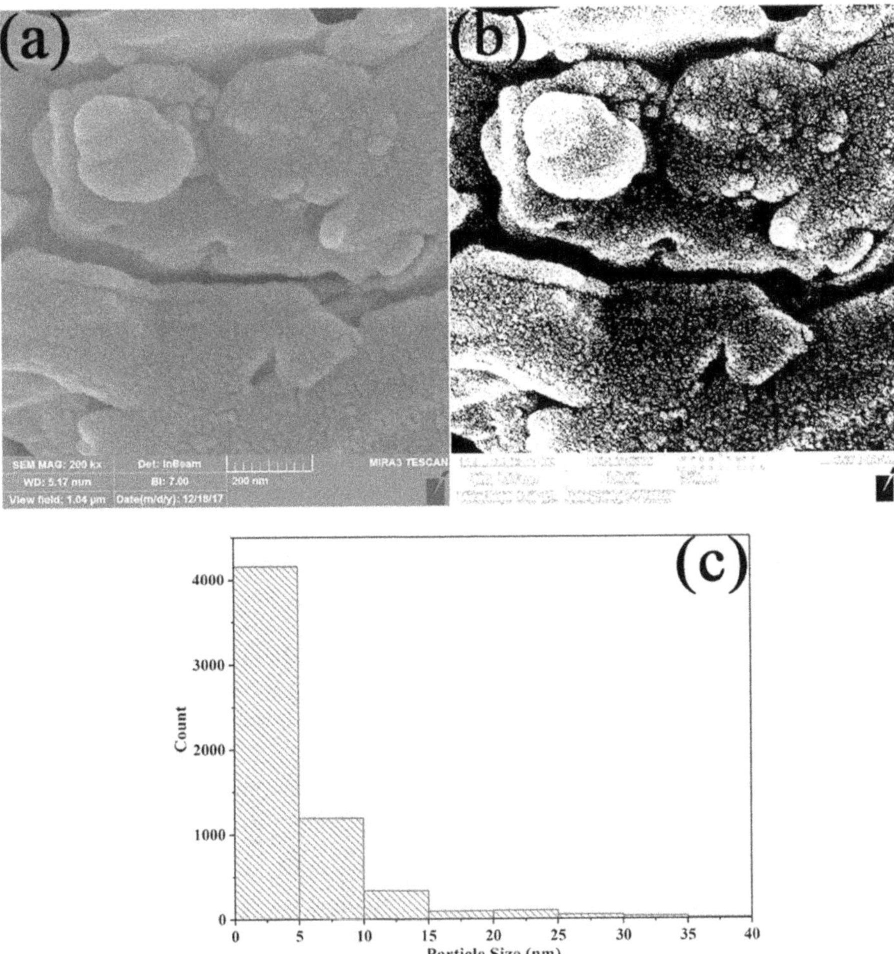

FIGURE 4.6 (a) SEM image of nitrogen-doped CQDs from grass, (b) SEM image employed under Image J software, (c) particle size histogram of the obtained CQDs by Sabet & Mahdavi. (2019).

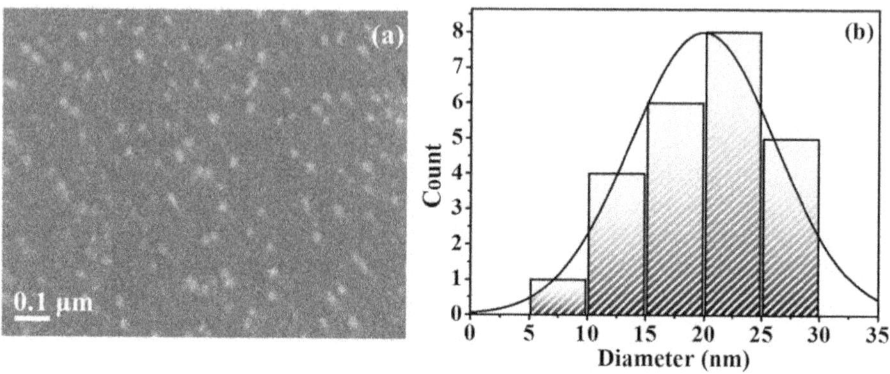

FIGURE 4.7 (a) SEM micrograph image and (b) particle size distribution graph of the produced CQDs (Khalid et al., 2022).

appropriate formation of the CQDs. It can also be observed that the size distribution ranged between 15 and 25 nm, and the average particle size was 20 nm. Hence, tiny particles are generally formed.

4.2.1.4 Dynamic Light Scattering (DLS)

Dynamic light scattering is an analytical technique to investigate the size distribution profile and hydrodynamic average diameter of CQDs. DLS technique observes the Brownian motion of particles in a fluid medium. It generates information by scattering the light at different intensities that provide information on the size distribution of CQDs (Larsson et al., 2022).

An investigation by Rojas-Valencia et al. (2021) demonstrated the distribution of dynamic diameter of CQDs, synthesized from *Hibiscus sabdariffa* flower as a carbon source at different carbonization temperatures of 200°C (A1), 300°C (B1), and 400°C (C1), wherein the average diameter from the analysis obtained was 137, 30, and 50 nm, respectively as illustrated in Figure 4.8.

In a study conducted by Dager et al. (2019) using DLS to obtain the size distribution curve of the CQDs synthesized from fennel seeds, the produced CQDs possessed

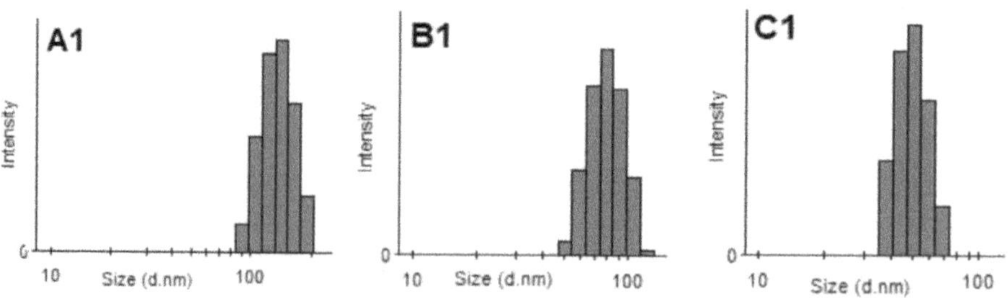

FIGURE 4.8 Average hydrodynamic diameter of the synthesized CQDs from *Hibiscus sabdariffa* flower (Rojas-Valencia et al., 2021).

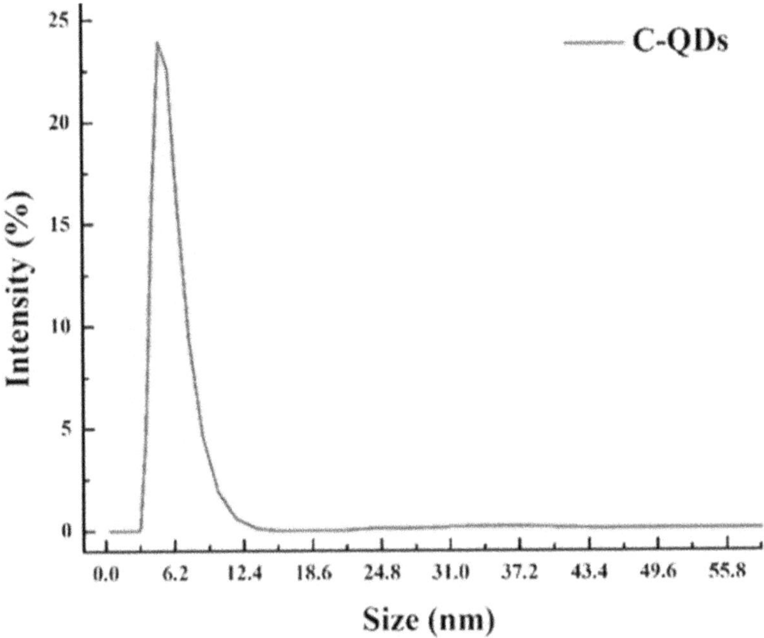

FIGURE 4.9 DLS study of CQDs synthesized from fennel seeds (Dager et al., 2019).

an average size of 6.1 nm, as illustrated in Figure 4.9. Hence, the data obtained in DLS can also be represented in different ways, which depends on the ease of the method and is done for straightforward interpretation.

4.3 DIFFRACTION BASED TECHNIQUES

4.3.1 X-ray Diffraction (XRD)

X-ray diffraction (XRD) is utilized to examine the phase purity, crystal structure, particle size, and crystallinity phase of the CQDs. XRD can be used to estimate the crystal spacing internally in the crystalline carbon cores of CQDs. Constructive interference is generated when a monochromatic X-ray interacts with a CQD. X-rays cause the electrons to be excited, forming a diffraction pattern contributing to a regular spatial arrangement. XRD is an essential analytical technique for investigating the crystallite structure and critical features of CQDs; it is not suitable for the analysis of amorphous CQDs.

When X-rays interact with carbon quantum dots, they interfere constructively, creating a diffraction pattern. The structure and phases of CQDs are attributed to signal processing, the brilliant fringe diffracted X-rays, and counting them with the detector's X-ray counter. A non-destructive characterization method used to identify the crystalline regime and phases of PCQDs (photoluminescent carbon dots) is XRD. Using an X-ray diffractogram, the average crystallite size can be calculated using the Scherer formula (4.1) from the recorded XRD peaks line broadening. Based on this formula, the broad peak generated in the XRD pattern has revealed the formation of CQDs with smaller sizes (Jing et al., 2023; Sachdev & Gopinath, 2015).

$$D = \frac{k\lambda}{\beta \cos\theta} \cdots \qquad (4.1)$$

where
    D = the average size of the crystalline domains (nm),
    K = followed by crystallite shape (~0.9)
    λ = X-ray wavelength (nm/Å)
    β = Full width of the diffraction peak's half maxima (radians)
    Θ = Bragg's angle of the plane (degree/ radians) calculated using Bragg's equation (4.2), and the d-spacing value can be calculated for the synthesized CQDs.

$$n\lambda = 2\text{d}\sin\theta \qquad (4.2)$$

$$\text{d} = \frac{n\lambda}{2\sin\theta}$$

where
    n = the positive integer (4.1)
    λ = the wavelength of incident X-rays
    θ = the incident angle

The study was carried out by Arul and Sethuraman (2018), which exhibited the XRD pattern of nitrogen-doped carbon dots utilizing *Actinidia deliciosa* as a carbon source, as shown in Figure 4.10, wherein the obtained CQDs revealed a weak peak $2\theta = 40.3°$ and an intense broad peak *of* $2\theta = 28.5°$ correlated to (001) and (002) diffraction patterns of the graphitic carbon.

In another study by Rojas-Valencia et al. (2021) on the production of CQDs from the *Hibiscus sabdariffa* flower, the XRD patterns (Figure 4.11) were created at the higher and lower ambiance of synthesis. The sample was produced at 400°C, kept for 4 hours, and had a crystalline diffractogram, which possessed a characteristic reflection at 26.6°, 42.46°, 43.01°, 44.67°, 47.30°, and 50.83° that could be correlated with carbon having a hexagonal crystal system, following a space group P63mc (186), with lattice parameters of a=b=2.4560Å and c=13.392Å and angles of $\alpha = \beta = 90°$ and $\Upsilon = 120°$, could be observed in the 26–1080 diffraction card. For the case with 200°C for 1 hour, semicrystalline composition was observed, and the XRD pattern reflections were observed at $2\theta = 26.61°$, 43.45°, 46.32°, 54.81°, and 63.67°. The primary peak of the CQDs was marked at 26.611° with hkl = (111), where a rhombohedral crystal structure is described, R-3m (166) space group, and lattice parameters a=b=c=3.635Å with angles $\alpha=\beta=\Upsilon=39.49°$. The calcium oxalate hydrate was responsible for the remaining peaks, according to the 03–0087 XRD card. Hence, a detailed analysis of the crystallite structure of the CQDs is possible using XRD (Table 4.3).

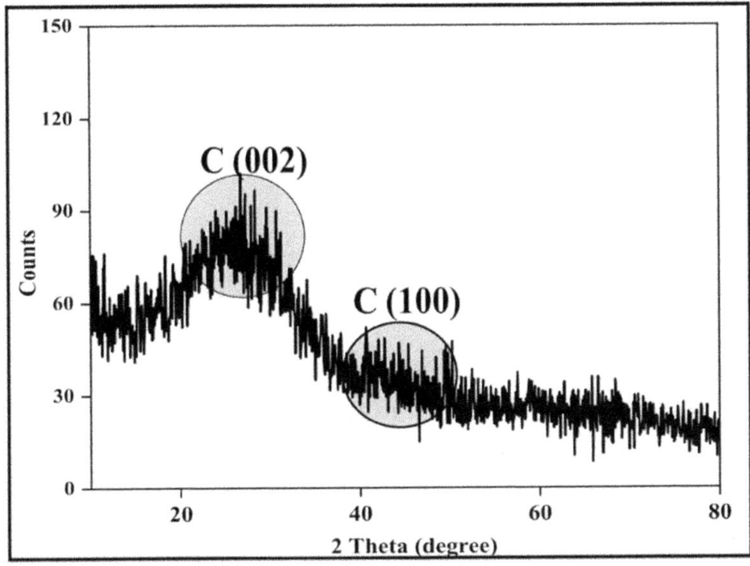

FIGURE 4.10 XRD results of the obtained nitrogen-doped carbon dots utilizing *Actinidia deliciosa* as a carbon source (Arul & Sethuraman, 2018).

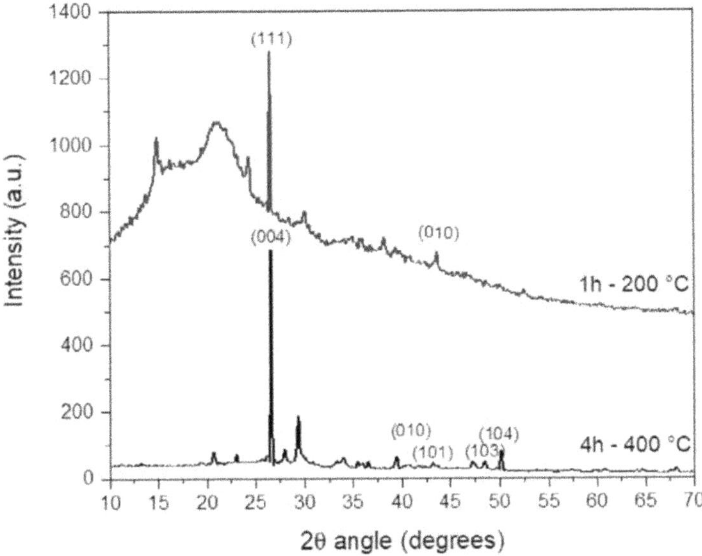

FIGURE 4.11 XRD pattern of the synthesized CQDs attained at higher and lower synthesis levels (Rojas-Valencia et al., 2021).

TABLE 4.3

XRD Pattern (Bragg's reflection, two θ) of Various CQDs from Different Sources

Source of Carbon	Bragg's Reflection 2 θ (°)	References
Flour	27.8	Zhang et al. (2015)
Algal blooms	24.1	Ramanan et al. (2016)
Grass	28	Khalid et al. (2022)

4.4 SPECTROSCOPIC ANALYSIS AND LUMINESCENT OPTICAL PROPERTIES-BASED TECHNIQUES

There are various spectroscopic analyses used for the study of carbon dots, such as UV-visible spectroscopy, photoluminescence spectroscopy, FTIR, X-ray photoelectron spectroscopy (XPS), Raman spectroscopy, nuclear magnetic resonance (NMR), and energy dispersive spectroscopy (EDS).

4.4.1 SPECTROSCOPY AND PHOTO-LUMINESCENT TECHNIQUES

4.4.1.1 UV-Visible Spectroscopy

UV-visible spectroscopy is utilized to determine the optical characteristics, including the absorption and emission behavior of CQDs under ultraviolet and visible regions. The principle involved in the UV-Vis spectrometer is based on the absorption of UV light/visible light from chemical compounds, leading to the generation of distinctive spectra. When the CQDs absorb light, it undergoes excitation and de-excitation phases, leading to spectrum development. The energy difference between the excited and ground state is observed when the matter absorbs a particular wavelength of light. The absorption of a specific light intensity decreases the transmittance of light at a particular wavelength by the sample matter. Hence, spectroscopy depicts results according to the interaction between matter and light. CQDs procured through different techniques demonstrate strong UV absorption, resulting in the variation of absorption peaks (Singh et al., 2018).

The UV-Vis spectrophotometer provides essential information about the CQDs, such as absorption peaks, bandgap energy, and optical properties. CQDs possess excellent optical absorption in the range of the UV zone between 260 and 320 nm, with the tail reaching the area of the visible region. Pure CQDs mainly exhibit two absorption peaks: (a) π-π* transition containing aromatic sp^2 domains and (b) n-π* transition of surface functional moieties consisting of hydroxyl, carboxyl, carbonyl, and ester groups. However, the position of absorption peaks chiefly depends on the nature of surface functional groups and the synthetic production method available for CQDs. From the literature, the characterization of carbon dots through UV-Vis spectroscopy demonstrates that all types of CQDs are active in the electromagnetic spectrum in the UV-Vis region, and carbon dot fluorescence radiation displays λ_{ex} as a dependent behavior (Dong et al., 2013). Moreover, UV-Vis spectroscopy can

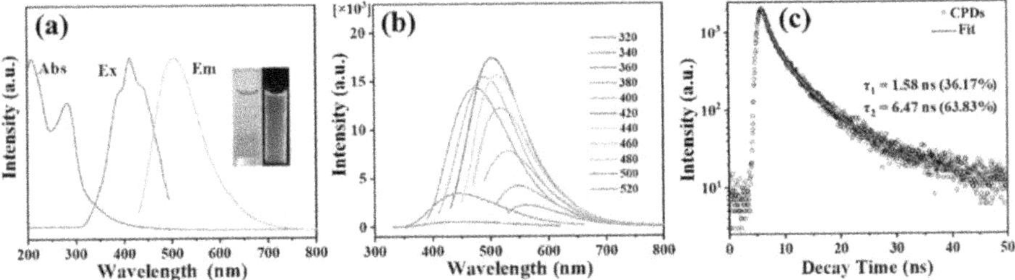

FIGURE 4.12 (a) UV-vis absorbance, fluorescence emission, and excitation of the spectrum of carbon dots prepared from *Allium fistulosum*, (b) *Allium fistulosum*-based carbon dots fluorescence emission spectra in an aqueous solution, from 320 nm on the left to 520 nm on the right, using increasingly longer excitation wavelengths, (c) the CQD aqueous solution's photoluminescence decayed at 501 nm under 420 nm excitation (Wei et al., 2019).

be utilized to investigate the photoluminescence (PL) emission of the CQDs. The PL emission property of the CQDs can be applied in optoelectronic devices and bioimaging.

The study reported by Wei et al. (2019) experimented on the synthesis of CQDs *Allium fistulosum*, as shown in Figure 4.12, which exhibits various absorption peaks at 282 nm (blue line). These possess an aromatic C=C (π-π*) bond. CQDs' fluoroluminance excitation spectrum (green line) was plotted during a study, with FL intensity (503 nm) versus the excitation wavelength, which acquired a broad peak with a maximal of 412 nm. When excited at 412 nm, the CQDs reveal high fluoroluminance (FL) between 400 and 700 nm with a maximal value near 503 nm (yellow line). Figure. 4.12(b) reveals the FL emission spectra of CQDs acquired from increasing the wavelength from 320 to 520 nm at a difference of 20 nm.

4.4.1.2 Photo-luminescence Spectroscopy

The analytical instrument used for the investigation of the photoluminescence of carbon dots is carried out using photoluminescence (PL) spectroscopy (Table 4.4). The photoluminescence effect can be witnessed in the carbon dots when the nanoparticles are lesser than excitons, and the charge present there becomes spatially confined between the nanoparticles; this phenomenon is known as the quantum confinement effect. CQDs possess the quantum confinement effect, which depends on the

TABLE 4.4

Photoluminescence Activity of Carbon Quantum Dots (H. Li et al., 2010)

Size of CQDs (nm)	Radiation Emitted
1.2 (small-sized CQDs)	Ultraviolet spectrum
1.5-3 (medium-sized CQDs)	Visible spectrum
>3.8 (Large-sized CQDs)	Near-infrared range

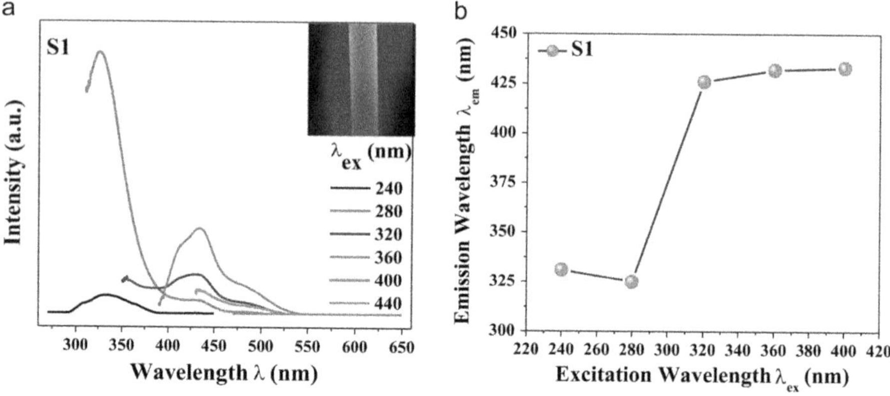

FIGURE 4.13 (a) Variation of photoluminance spectra of hydrothermally synthesized CQDs and (b) excitation wavelength vs. emission wavelength of the sample (Sarkar et al., 2016).

intensities and emission wavelengths upon absorption (λ_{ex}). Consequently, carbon dots carry the emission spectrum as it may be altered over the visible spectrum by alternating the synthesis characteristics and chemical reagents (H. Wang et al., 2017).

In a study by Sarkar et al. (2016), the CQDs were synthesized from hydrothermal treatment as illustrated in Figure 4.13 (S1 = sample synthesized by heating in an autoclave for 120 min at 120°C). It is observed that the increment of the excitation wavelengths from 240 to 440 nm with a gradual increase of 40 nm led to the modification of photoluminance characteristics. Moreover, the highest intensity of the sample was determined when the sample was excited at 280 nm. Figure 4.13(b) reveals the variation in the emission wavelength (λ_{em}) corresponding to the excitation wavelength (λ_{ex}).

4.4.2 Optical Properties of Carbon Quantum Dots

4.4.2.1 Fluorescence and Photoluminescence (PL)

Fluorescence is one of the optical properties of the CQDs significant in the fundamental and application sectors. Photoluminescence is one of the fascinating features of CQDs; it depends on excitation and is also named excitation-dependent fluorescence emission. The photoluminescence characteristics of λ_{ex} depend on the intensity and wavelength of emission of CQDs. According to the study by Zhang et al. (2017), the excitation-dependent PL property of CQDs is analogous to luminescent carbon nanoparticles (Jelinek, 2017).

The study by H. Li et al. (2010) reported on the optical/photoluminance characterization of the CQDs, as illustrated in Figure 4.14. Figure 4.14(a) shows the visual images of CQDs varying at four different size distributions; CQDs were illuminated on the left with a white/daylight lamp, and the right was illuminated under UV light. The naked eye can easily witness CQDs' bright red, yellow, green, and blue PL. Figure 4.14(b) shows the PL spectra for red, yellow, green, and blue CQDs.

An experiment by Thambiraj et al. (2016) produced highly fluorescent CQDs synthesized from sugarcane bagasse pulp as a carbon source, as shown in Figure 4.15.

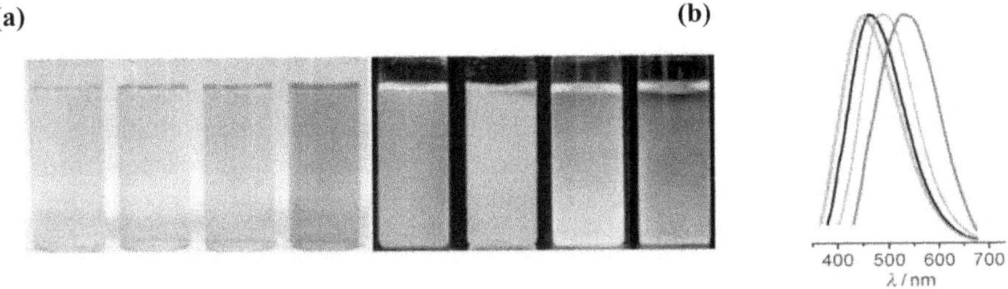

FIGURE 4.14 (a) Optical images of CQDs (left: Illuminated under white/daylight lamp, suitable: Illuminated under UV light-365 nm). (b) Photoluminance (PL) spectra of CQDs – blue, green, black, and red lines are the PL spectra for red, yellow, green, and blue CQDs, respectively (Li et al., 2010).

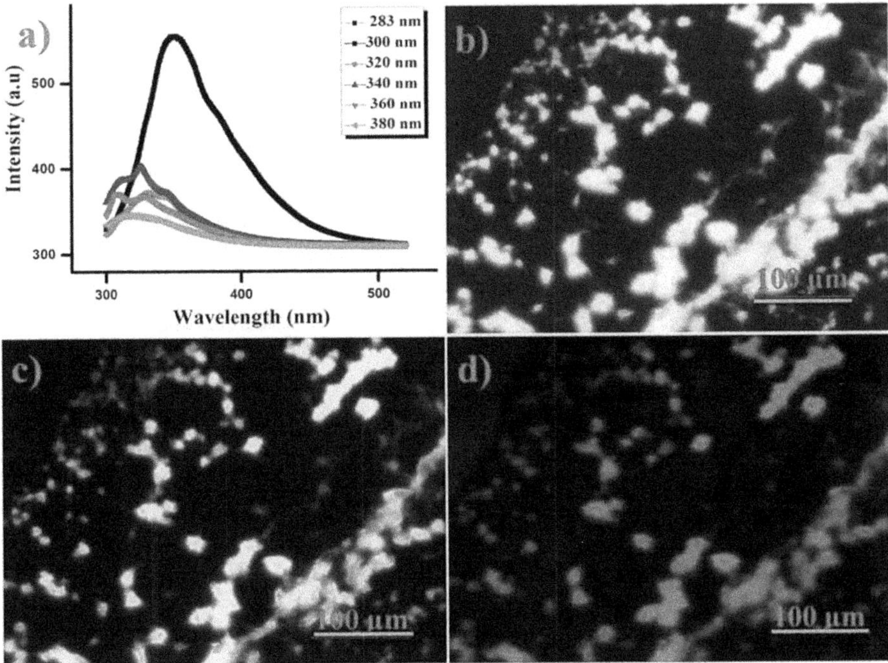

FIGURE 4.15 Fluorescence properties of CQDs synthesized from sugarcane bagasse pulp. (a) Fluorescence spectra of CQDs examined at different wavelengths viz., λ_{em} = 300, 320, 340, 360, and 380 nm and λ_{ex} = 283, (b) fluorescence microscopy images of CQDs investigated under a UV filter, (c) red filter, and (d) green filter (Thambiraj et al., 2016).

Fluorescence microscopic experiments reveal the high fluorescence nature of CQDs with multiple bandwidths. The particle emissions were observed blue under a UV filter (Figure 4.15(b)), green under a red filter (Figure 4.15(c)), and red under a green filter (Figure 4.15(d)). The findings imply that the current CQDs are a suitable replacement for conventional dyes in fluorescent labeling, bioimaging, and biosensing applications.

4.4.2.2 Electrochemical Luminescence (ECL)

Electrochemical luminescence (ECL) is a characteristic property exploited to investigate carbon quantum dots' composition, surface structure, and morphology (Farshbaf et al., 2018) (Farshbaf et al., 2018). ECL is acquired during the excitation of electrons in the target carbon dots. This exerts the relaxation of carbon dots from the excitation state to the ground state simultaneously after the emission of light (Jelinek, 2017). Most CQDs produced are highly oxidized; oxidation does not accelerate the emission, but CQD reduction can increase luminescence (Zheng et al., 2011).

The research carried out by Xu et al. (2013) investigated the photoluminescence and electrochemiluminescence (PL and ECL) for selected applications. Reduced CQDs (r-CQDs) are carbon dots that have undergone a carbonization-extraction process and have a low oxidation level. Oxidized carbon dots (o-CQDs) refer to the highly oxidized carbon dots produced by a carbonization-oxidation process. The PL mechanism of CQDs is presented in Figure 4.16(a). The electrons in the core are stimulated by photons, passing from the valence band (VB) to the conduction band

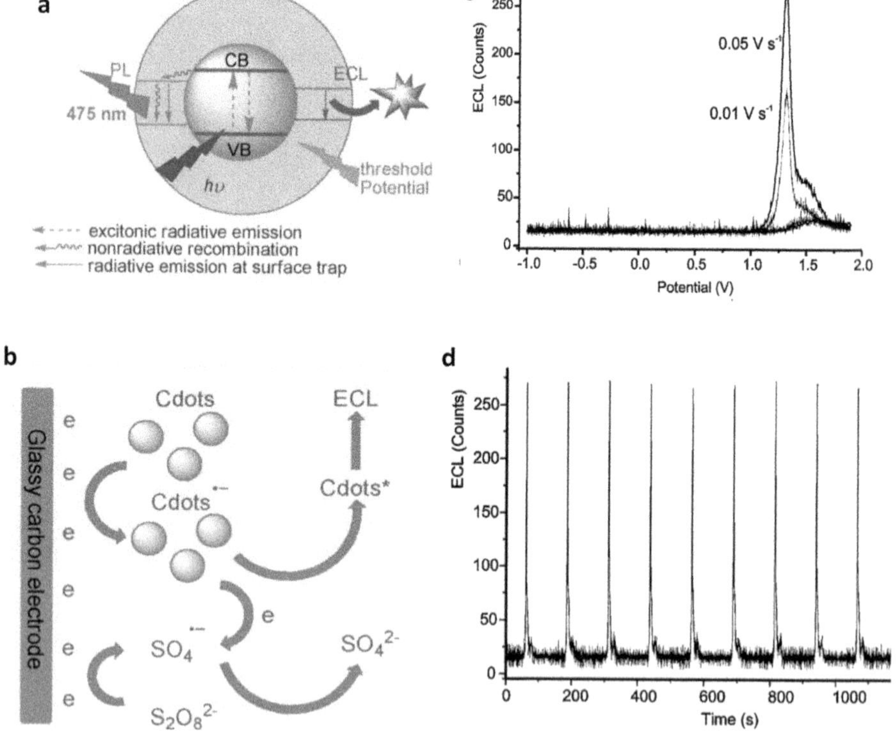

FIGURE 4.16 Illustrative representation of (a) photoluminance and electrochemical luminescence of CQDs, (b) the mechanism of ECL in the oxidized-CQDs/$K_2S_2O_8$ structure, (c) ECL profiles of oxidized-CQDs at a scan rate of 0.01 and 0.05 V s^{-1}, (d) the reproducibility of ECL in a continuous scan mode (Wang and Hu 2014).

(CB), and the generation of PL and ECL occurs because of the energy difference. The cathodic ECL of the o-CQDs/$K_2S_2O_8$ arrangement is shown in Figure 4.16(b), and the results indicated that o-CQD diffusion onto the electrode surface was responsible for controlling the electrochemical response. The electro-generation of o-CQDs radicals is facilitated by the "loose shell" of oxygen-containing groups on the o-CQDs. The anionic o-CQDs absorb an electron from the potent oxidizing agent, the SO_4^- radical, which is released during the reduction of $S_2O_8^{2-}$ to create the emitters for ECL emission. The low ECL emission of r-CQDs reveals that the ECL is connected to the direct oxidization state of the surface. The ECL wave initiated at 1.10 V gains its peak value at 1.30 V, comparable to the oxidation peak in the cyclic voltammograms (CVs) as shown in Figure 4.16(c). From Figure 4.16(d), it can be observed that the ECL undergoes continuous, highly reproducible cyclic scanning.

4.4.2.3 Phosphorescence

Phosphorescence in carbon dots reveals strong fluorescence effects with a minimum at room temperature. The phosphorescence characteristics of CQDs are applied in the field of fluorescence sensors for the detection of ions, bioimaging, and biomedical areas as they possess a high signal-to-noise ratio, large stokes, and enduring luminescence properties (Li et al., 2018). The phosphorescent CQDs exhibit good potential for room temperature phosphorescence (RTP). They can be used to replace common RTP substances, such as sulfides, rare earth fluorescent substances, and oxides, which are expensive, toxic, and difficult to employ (Y. Wang & Hu, 2014).

4.4.2.4 Chemical Luminescence (CL)

Chemical luminescence (CL) of carbon dots is noticed when the CQDs coexist with classical oxidants such as potassium permanganate ($KMnO_4$) and cerium (IV). The principle behind this mechanism is the production of electrons and holes in the CQDs from the oxidants, which result in the liberation of energy in the form of chemical luminescence emission. The ensuing fluorescence is visible after the injection of electrons during the electronic transition from the higher/excited energy level to a lower level. The concentration of CQDs, the yield, temperature, and incidence of the redox events responsible for the hole or electron transfer, and the effectiveness of coupling between these reactions together, affect the degree of CL emission. The electron distribution due to thermal equilibrium is shown in Figure 4.17 (Jelinek, 2017, n; Wang & Hu, 2014). The CL in CQDs is employed in studies on reductive material and to analyze the dual characteristics of CQDs as an electron acceptor and donor, which could be further exploited as a good opportunity in catalysis and optronics (Y. Wang & Hu, 2014).

4.4.2.5 Up-conversion photoluminescence (UCPL)

Up-conversion photoluminescence (UCPL) characteristics of the CQDs have been observed as a multiphoton activation process, wherein emission and absorption of two or more photons take place simultaneously, initiating the emission of light with a shorter wavelength range as compared to the excitation wavelength, i.e., anti-stoke emission. The UCPL of CQDs delivers a novel application in cell imaging with

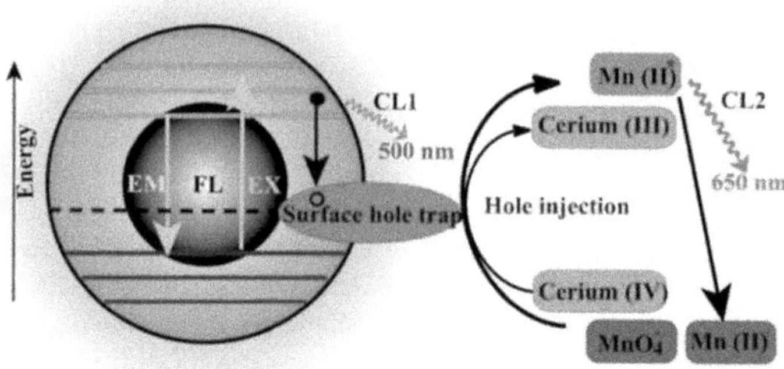

FIGURE 4.17   Fluorescence and chemical luminescence (CL) mechanism in $KMnO_4$ and cerium $_{(IV)}$ CQD system. CL1 and CL2 are two CL routes in the system (Lin et al., 2012)

support from two-photon luminescence microscopy and catalyst design utilized in energy and bioscience technology.

A study was performed by Aghamali et al. (2018) on the UCPL characteristics of the nitrogen-CQDs synthesized from citric acid (CA) as a carbon source and diethylenetriamine (DETA) as surface passivation by employing hydrothermal method as illustrated in Figure 4.18. As the excitation wavelength varied from 600 to 790 nm, the UCPL spectra consisted of a uniform emission band at approximately 431 nm. As the excitation wavelength increased, the intensity of the peaks initially increased and then decreased. The peaks of wavelengths from 680 to 760 nm were higher than other regions. These results predicted that the absorption of N-CQDs was quite potent in the region from UV to red/blue spectral region.

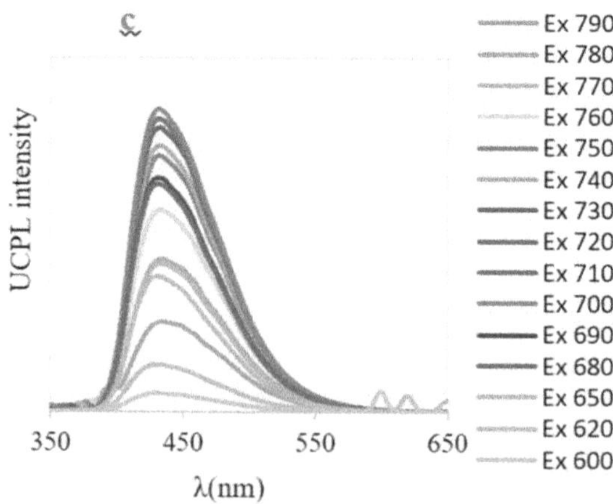

FIGURE 4.18   UCPL characteristics of the N-CQDs synthesized from citric acid as a carbon source (Aghamali et al., 2018).

4.5 SPECTROSCOPY TECHNIQUES

4.5.1 FTIR SPECTROSCOPY

FTIR spectroscopy is a prime technique utilized to investigate functional groups that are available on the surface of CQDs – carbon, oxygen, and hydrogen are mainly available in CQDs. The basic principle of FTIR spectroscopy is stretching vibrations of cluster/individual bonds and functional groups. This technique is established on the absorption of electromagnetic radiation in the wavelengths between the infrared spectrum, i.e., 4000–400 cm^{-1}. The light utilizes an infrared spectrometer, which helps to generate an output in an infrared region. CQDs are developed by the partial oxidation of carboxylic acid (–COOH), carbonyl (–C=O), ether, aldehyde (–CHO), ketone (–CO–), and hydroxyl (–OH) groups, as these functional groups are abundant on the surface of carbon dots. Consequently, investigating these functional groups is significant for characterization (Jing et al., 2023; Sharma & Chowdhury, 2023) and enhances the analytical performance of the carbon dots, which can be conveniently done using FTIR spectroscopy. Carbon dots are further altered in the structure to enhance analytical performance through elemental doping and composite creation, resulting in a high quantum yield, stable PL emission intensity, and exceptional electrical characteristics. The FTIR technique for the characterization of CQDs is easy to operate with ease in preparing samples, a rapid and affordable method. Furthermore, as infrared radiation cannot offer sufficient structural information on CQDs, doping with metal heteroatoms on CQDs can be efficacious. The heteroatom doping of alkyl sulfide (C–S), amines/amides (–NH2, –CN), thiols (–SH), phosphates (P=O and P–OR), and organosiloxane (Si–OSi/Si–O–C) has been utilized for the characterization of carbon dots (Z. Zhang et al., 2015).

A study carried by Ramanan et al. (2016) analyzed the FTIR spectrum of CQDs synthesized from the eutrophic algal blooms as illustrated in Figure 4.19, to determine

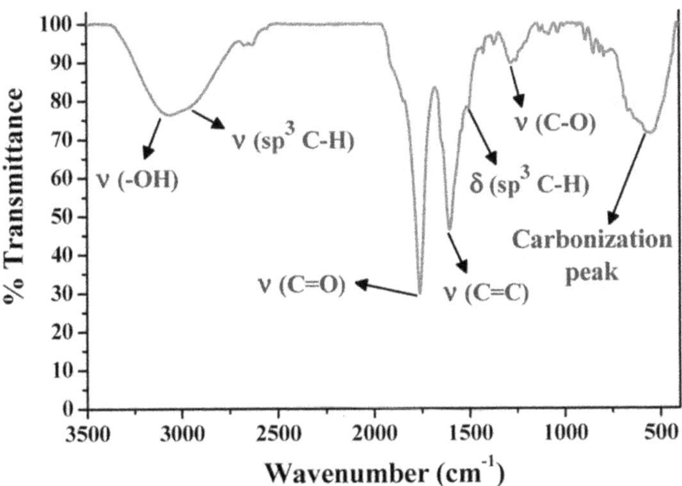

FIGURE 4.19 FTIR spectrum of CQDs synthesized from eutrophic algal blooms (Ramanan et al., 2016).

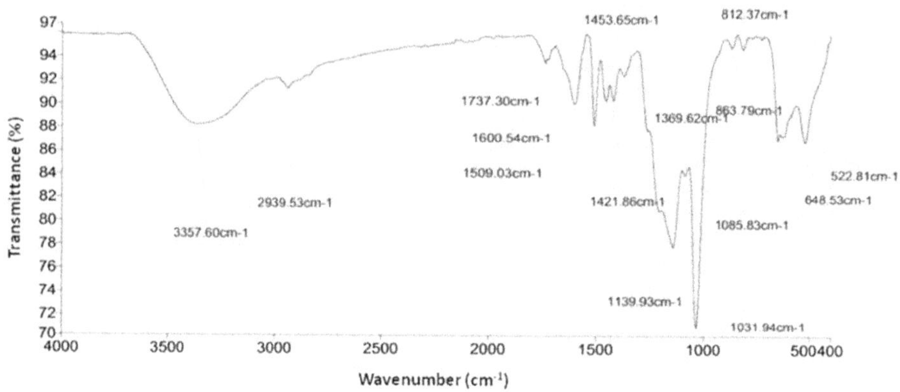

FIGURE 4.20   FTIR spectrum of carbon dots using lignin as a carbon source (Rai et al., 2017).

the surface functions of the CQDs. The broad absorption was observed in the range from 3360 to 2550 cm⁻¹, which was centered at 3050 cm⁻¹, the sharp and strong absorption at 1763 cm⁻¹ and the weak absorption at 1279 cm⁻¹ are all caused by the O-H, C=O, and C-O stretching vibrations of the carboxylic acid functionality. Absorption at 1763 cm⁻¹ demonstrates the unconjugated characteristic of the surface carboxylic groups. Two absorptions at 2670 and 2630 cm⁻¹ resulting from the intramolecular hydrogen bonding (O-H) of the carboxyl functional group revealed the closeness of the surface carboxyl groups. They suggested that the surface carboxyl group density was higher in CQDs. The carbon core of CQDs is thought to be composed of well-conjugated and/or aromatic C=C molecules based on the strong absorption at 1590 cm⁻¹. Peaks at 2960 and 1495 cm⁻¹ were attributed to the in-plane bending and sp³ C-H stretching vibrations of surface methyl/methylene groups, respectively. At about 570 cm⁻¹, the carbonization peak finally emerged.

In another study done by Rai et al. (2017), as shown in Figure 4.20, in the case of CQDs, the characteristic absorption band at 3357 cm⁻¹ was exhibited by lignin, which was attributed to the O-H stretching vibrations. The functional group C-H stretching, C-O, and -COOH were represented by the absorption bands at 2939, 1737, and 1600 cm⁻¹, respectively. Additionally, extending vibration bands to a length of 1509 cm⁻¹ demonstrated the presence of aromatic ring stretch. The sulfur-containing functional groups corresponded to the absorption band at 1139 and 1031 cm⁻¹. Thus, FTIR spectroscopy has been identified as an essential tool for the characterization of CQDs.

4.5.2   X-ray Photoelectron Spectroscopy (XPS)

XPS is an analytical technique beneficial for the investigation of surface chemicals/surface functionalization, functional moieties, elemental composition, and nanoscale structure and components present in CQDs. This technique is based on the photoelectric effect that can be applied to perceive the carbon dots' knowledge

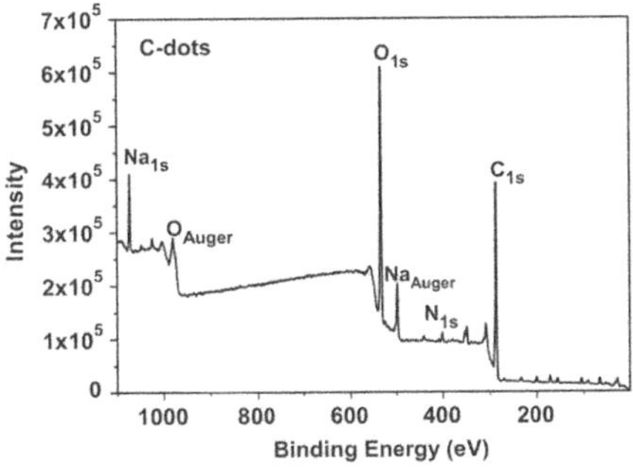
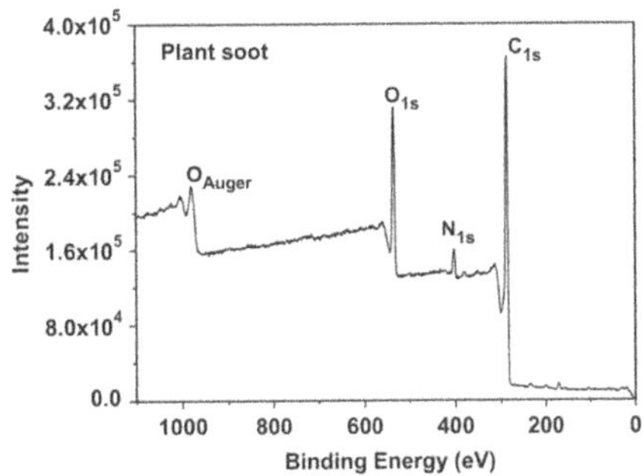

FIGURE 4.21 XPS spectra of carbon dots obtained from the plant soot as a carbon source (Tan et al., 2013).

about elemental composition, oxidation states, and electronic structure (Sharma & Chowdhury, 2023). The ejected (1s, 2s) electrons from the shell contribute to the XPS spectral lines. The elemental functional groups, elemental composition, and doping of CQDs utilizing heteroatoms with metallic/non-metalloid nature, such as N, P, S, B, and Si, can be accurately investigated via the XPS technique synergistically with FTIR spectroscopy (Dong et al., 2013; Saha et al., 2015). The utility of the XPS technique is to surmise the structural state of carbon dots when metallic heteroatoms (Mg, Ni., etc.) are doped in that.

In the XPS analysis done by Tan et al. (2013) on CQDs synthesized from the plant soot (Figure 4.21), two peaks were observed at 498.0 and 1072 eV for Na_{Auger} and Na_{1s} CQDs, respectively. Another peak at 979.7 eV corresponding to O_{Auger} was also observed. In the XPS spectrum of plant soot, the primary graph included a C_{1s} peak at ca. 284 eV, an O_{1s} peak at ca. 532 eV, and a N_{1s} peak at ca. 400 eV. Hence, it was concluded that the plant soot possessed carbon, oxygen, and nitrogen in a weight ratio of 79.54:16.46:4.00.

In a different study reported by Arul and Sethuraman (2018), N-doped carbon dots from *Actinidia deliciosa* were obtained. In his research, the XPS spectrum of the developed carbon dots, as illustrated in Figure 4.22 revealed high-resolution XPS spectra that constituted three elements including carbon (C): 1s, nitrogen (N): (1s), and oxygen (O): (1s). The peak positions of C, N, and O were at 285, 400, and 532 eV, respectively.

Bano et al. (2018) reported the XPS spectrum of CQDs synthesized from *Tamarindus indica* leaves. As illustrated in Figure 4.23, the produced CQDs possessed a wide range of XPS spectra, peaks at 284.6 eV, 400 eV, and 531 eV, confirming that C (51.1%), N (14.2%), and O (34.7%) are the main components. In the figure, four peaks can be observed in the C 1s spectrum and they are located at peaks of 284.6 eV, 285.7 eV, 286.6 eV, and 287.8 eV, which correspond to the availability of C-C, C=C, C-O/C-N chemical bonds, respectively. The N 1s spectra included three peaks at 399.3 eV, 400.7 eV, and 401.6 eV, which revealed the presence of the C-N-C, N-C_3, and N-H bonds, respectively. Two peaks at 531.6 eV and 533.0 eV were attributed to C=O and C-OH/C-O-C, respectively, and were reported in the O 1s spectra as illustrated in Figure 4.20.

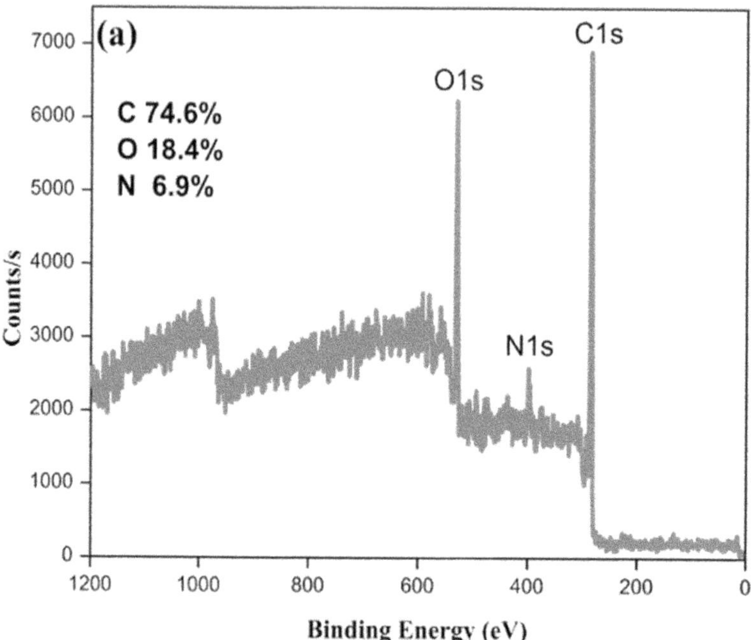

FIGURE 4.22   XPS spectrum of the synthesized carbon dots (Arul & Sethuraman, 2018).

4.5.3 RAMAN SPECTROSCOPY

Raman spectroscopy is a non-destructive spectroscopy process, which provides details about the carbon state in carbon dots. The Raman spectrum of CQDs reveals two bands, the intensity, and position of the D-band (disorder-induced band) and G-band (graphitic band). The vibrations of disordered carbon atoms with dangling bonds in the final plane of graphitic carbon are connected with the D-band, indicating the existence of defects with primarily sp^3 orbital alloying (M. Wu et al., 2017). G-band is connected to the vibration of sp^2-bonded carbon atoms in a planar (two-dimensional) hexagonal lattice with a higher degree of the crystalline regime. The intensity ratio of the D band (containing faults, the higher degree of disorder) to the G band (ID/IG) indicates the degree of graphitization of C-dots. Before, CQDs with greater (ID/IG) ratio values had more flaws, which led one to surmise that carbon was amorphous. A higher level of graphitization is observed with the volte-face scenario (ID/IG), which meant that C-dots are primarily crystalline. Moreover, the intensity ratio of (ID/IG) less than 1 indicated the less defective carbon structures (W. Wu et al., 2015).

In a different study done by Ramanan et al. (2016), as in Figure 4.24, the Raman spectrum of the CQDs prepared from eutrophic algal blooms indicated two peaks at 1564 and 1352 cm^{-1} corresponding to the G and D bands of carbon subsequently. The ratio ID/IG revealed the ratio of sp^3/ sp^2 and the disorder of carbon, indicating that there is an adequacy of structural defects in the synthesized CQDs.

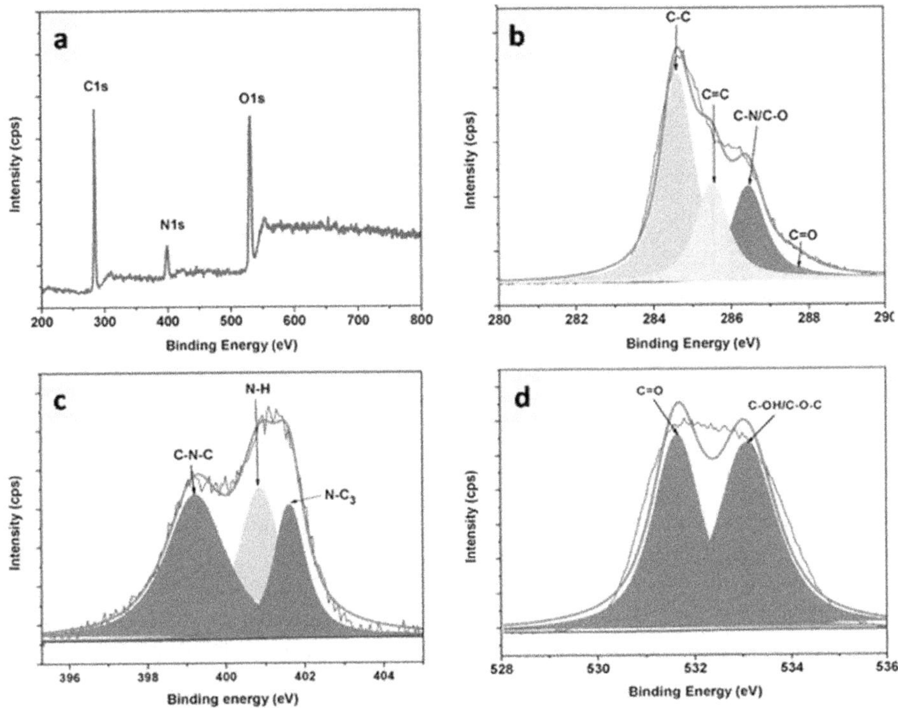

FIGURE 4.23 XPS spectrum of CQDs produced from *Tamarindus indica* leaves. (a) Full scan XPS spectra (b) C 1s spectrum (c) N 1s spectrum (d) O 1s spectrum of the synthesized CQDs. (Bano et al., 2018).

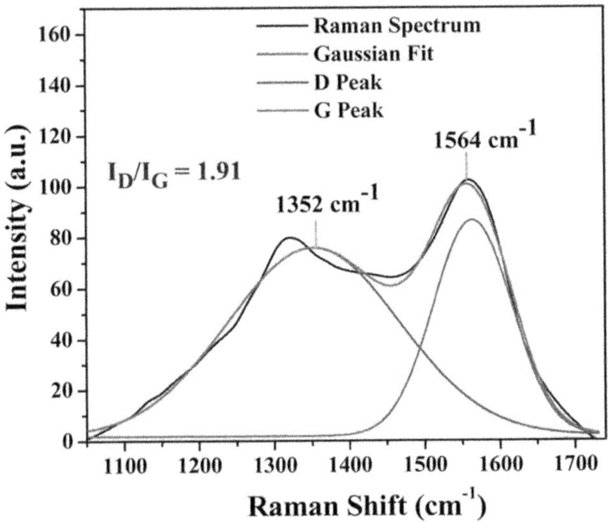

FIGURE 4.24 Raman spectrum of carbon dots synthesized from eutrophic algal blooms as a carbon source (Ramanan et al., 2016).

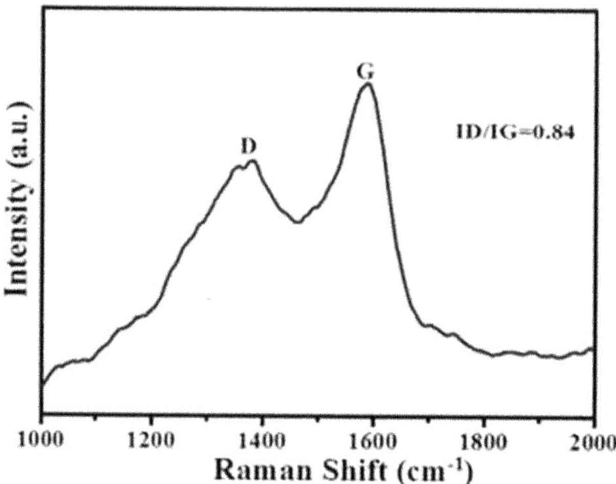

FIGURE 4.25   Raman spectrum of the CQDs prepared from potato starch (Qiang et al., 2019).

Another study carried out by Qiang et al. (2019) reported on the CQDs synthesized from potato starch. The D band at 1368 cm⁻¹ and the G band at 1582 cm⁻¹ as characteristic peaks, and an ID/IG ratio of 0.84 are illustrated in Figure 4.25.

4.5.4   Nuclear Magnetic Resonance (NMR) Spectroscopy

NMR technique is applied to investigate the molecular structural parameters, surface functional groups, impurities, validate elements (such as C, N, and P), and their bond interaction in the CQDs at the atomic level. It is based on the principle of nuclear magnetic resonance- when definite atomic nuclei possess a non-zero magnetic moment (nuclear spin) while arranged in the magnetic field. It is applied to investigate the quantitative (concentration of various components), dynamic (molecular rotations and conformational changes), and intermolecular interaction studies in CQDs. Hybrid/modified carbon atoms in the binding mode and crystalline network present in the carbon atoms are observed through NMR (Singh et al., n.d.). The two most common types of NMR techniques used for the characterization of CQDs are ^{1}H NMR and ^{13}C NMR. As the name reflects the ^{1}H NMR is used to investigate the number and types of hydrogen atoms available in the water molecule and ^{13}C NMR is utilized to investigate the types and number of carbon atoms in a molecule. Basically, ^{1}H NMR and ^{13}C NMR are the studies of spin changes that occur in proton and carbon nuclei respectively (Holzgrabe, 2010).

F. Li et al. (2017) studied the NMR spectroscopy of Selenium (Se) doped CQDs for structural analysis (Figure 4.26). In the ^{13}C NMR spectra of Se-CQDs, the range of signals between 100–180 and 25–70 ppm was observed, which is correlated with sp² hybridized carbon atoms and sp³ (aliphatic) carbon atoms. Readings between 160 and 180 ppm belong to amide/carboxyl groups, which indicated the availability of amino acid traces on the surface of procured Se-CQDs. In the ^{1}H NMR spectra,

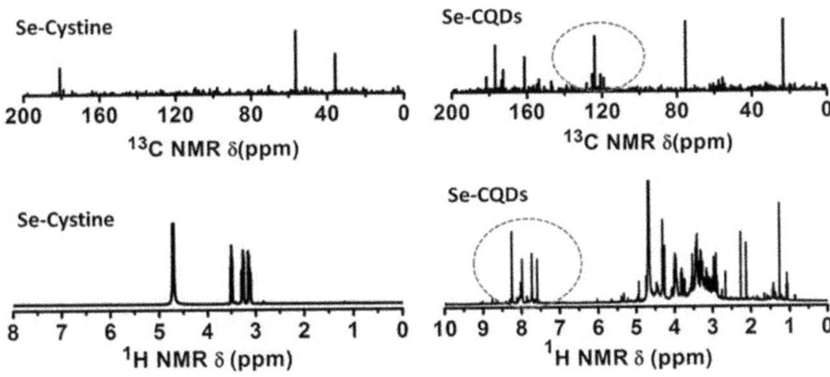

FIGURE 4.26   Structural analysis of selenium (se)-based CQDs by NMR spectroscopy (F. Li et al., 2017).

signals between 7 and 9 ppm correspond to the aromatic structure i.e., sp^2 hybridized carbon atoms.

Das et al. (2017) developed CQDs from the roasted grams shells as a green approach as illustrated in Figures 4.27 and 4.28. The ^1H NMR spectroscopy of gram shell carbon dots contributed toward evaluation in a different chemical environment. It was evaluated in D_2O, which exhibited a signal in three chemical environments. Peaks in the region 6 to 8 ppm corresponded to the sp^2 protons/aromatic group, in the range of 3 to 6 ppm to the ether groups and at 1 to 3 ppm correlated to sp^3 C-H

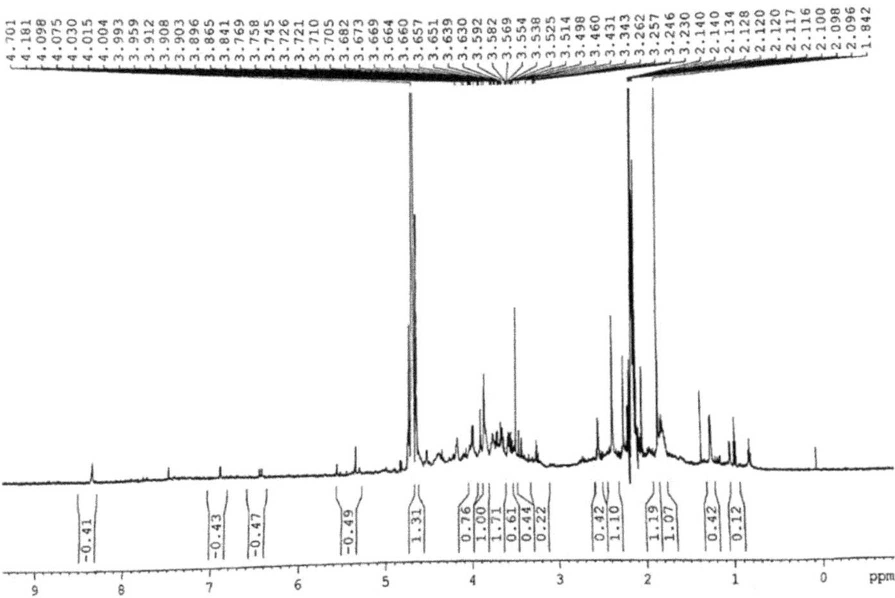

FIGURE 4.27 ^1H NMR spectroscopy of CQDs synthesized from gram shells (Das et al., 2017).

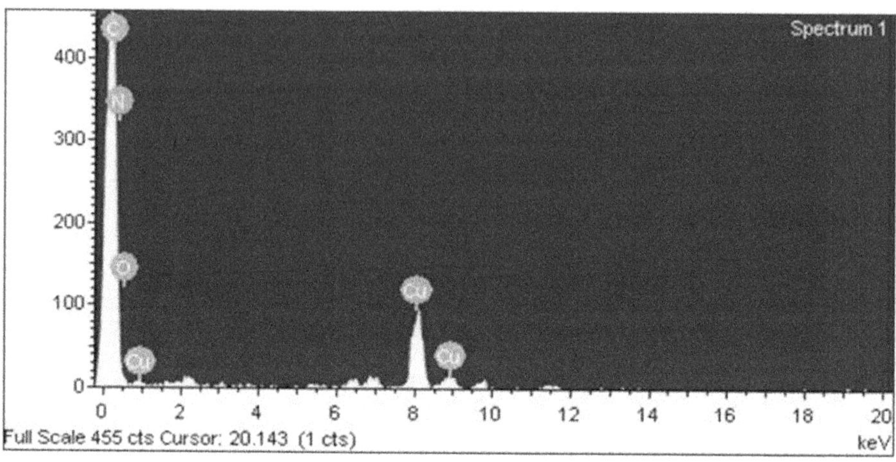

FIGURE 4.28   Energy dispersive spectroscopy (EDS) of CQDs prepared from *Actinidia deliciosa* (Arul & Sethuraman, 2018).

protons and protons adhering to the ether, hydroxyl, and carbonyl groups present on the surface of the synthesized CQDs.

4.5.5   ENERGY DISPERSIVE SPECTROSCOPY (EDS)

EDS is an analytical instrument utilized for the elemental investigation of carbon dots. In this, the high-intensity beam of X-ray is projected into the carbon dots, and an energy-dispersive graded spectrometer is used to determine the energy and quantity of emitted X-rays from carbon dots using the resulting X-ray spectrum. According to the lines drawn from the X-ray spectra, the peak energy provides qualitative information, while the peak intensity foretells the quantitative component. EDS can be used to analyze elemental components, including carbon (C), oxygen (O), phosphorus (P), and silicon (Si). The carbon, oxygen, nitrogen, and silicon, from the carbon quantum dots, are all easily discernible, and additional signals for bromide and potassium from the salt crystals are also visible (Boruah et al., 2020).

In a study, Arul & Sethuraman (2018) investigated the EDS of the procured CQDs from *Actinidia deliciosa* consisting of elements such as Carbon (74.59) %, Nitrogen (6.88%), and Oxygen (18.53%) as illustrated in Figure 4.29. In a different study, Kim et al. (2014) reported on the CQDs prepared from the ionic salt crystals. The fingerprints of silicon, carbon, oxygen, and carbon from the CQDs, as well as the availability of potassium and bromide from the salt crystals, were recorded as illustrated in Figure 4.29.

4.6   THERMOGRAVIMETRIC ANALYSIS

Thermogravimetric analysis is an analytical tool used to investigate the thermal behavior such as thermal stability, phase transition, thermal decomposition, residual impurities, and various thermal phenomena (decomposition, volatilization, oxidation,

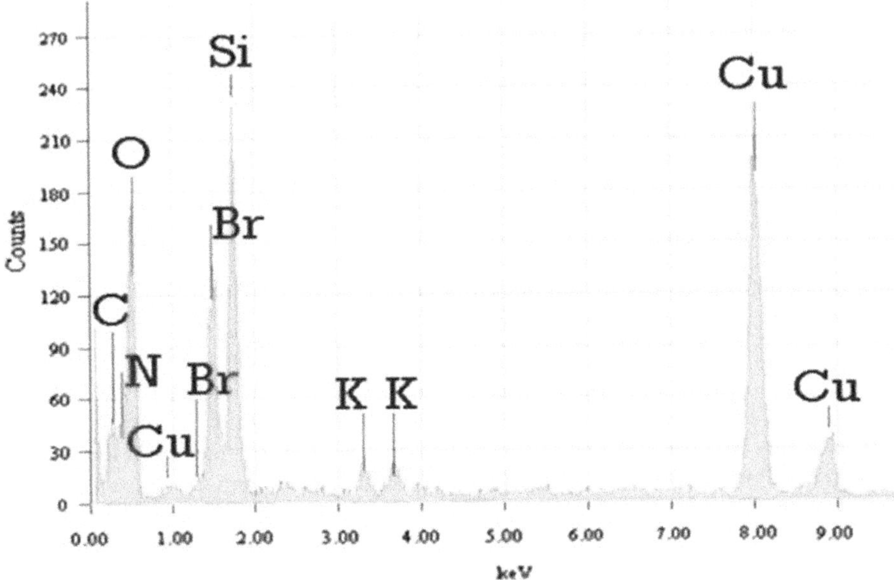

FIGURE 4.29   EDS of CQDs from ionic salt crystals (Kim et al., 2014).

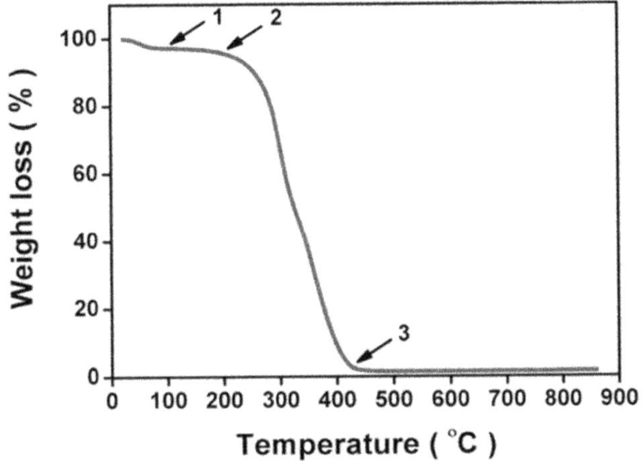

FIGURE 4.30   Thermogravimetric analysis of carbon dots obtained from coriander leaves (Sachdev & Gopinath, 2015).

and desorption) of CQDs. It allows the measurement of weight changes of the CQDs at a maintained temperature (heating/cooling) under reactive/inert atmospheric conditions over a period. The obtained data of CQDs are represented graphically as a thermogravimetric curve, where the gain and loss of weight of the sample are plotted corresponding to time or temperature (Yang, Hu, Liu, & Zhang, 2019).

In a study (Sachdev & Gopinath, 2015), as depicted in Figure 4.30, thermal stability of CQDs was obtained for coriander leaves. In the TGA curve (Figure 4.30), the thermogram revealed a three-step degradation pattern, and an initial weight loss of 3% was observed at 100°C, which was attributed to the loss of water molecules associated with CQDs. In the second phase, the water molecules were lost by 7% at temperatures between 100°C and 200°C. In the final degradation phase, majority of the moisture loss (93%) was observed in between 200°C and 435°C, beyond that phase the curve levelled off.

4.7   ZETA POTENTIAL

Zeta potential is an important characteristic to be evaluated in the CQDs as it informs about the effective electric charge present on the surface of CQDs and its quantification (Selvamani, 2019). The analysis of zeta potential provides stability assessment, surface functionalization, surface charge characterization, and dispersion behavior of the CQDs. The zeta potential is calculated through the potential difference between the stationary layer and the dispersion medium of the fluid attached to the particle layer. The higher value of the zeta potential illustrates the system's stability; however, the negative and positive signs of zeta potential indicate the surface charge of carbon dots, whereas carbon dots with lower zeta potential values aggregate (Sivasankaran et al., 2017).

In a study done by Sachdev and Gopinath (2015), the zeta potential of the coriander carbon dots was observed as −24.9 mV (negative value), attributed to the availability of carboxylic and hydroxyl groups on the surface as depicted in Figure 4.31. In another study by Dager et al. (2019), the zeta potential of the fennel seeds was obtained (Figure 4.32). The fennel seeds' CQDs exhibited a negative single peak at −23 mV and a peak width of 10.01 mV. The negative value of the zeta potential represented the negative charge moieties present on the surface of the CQDs, and these

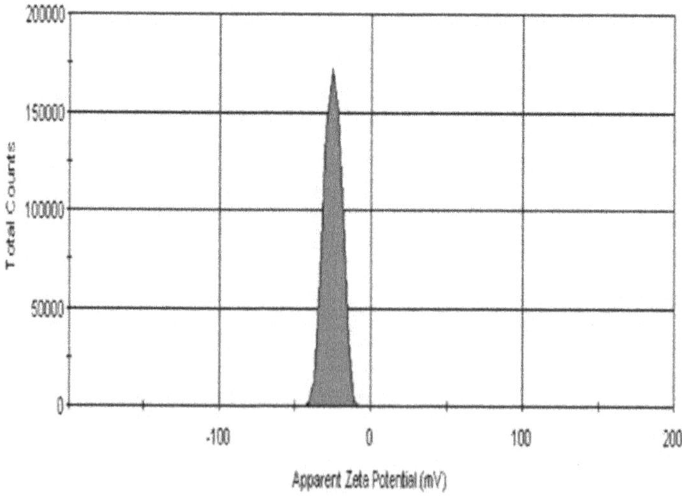

FIGURE 4.31   Zeta potential of CQDs obtained from coriander leaves (Sachdev & Gopinath, 2015).

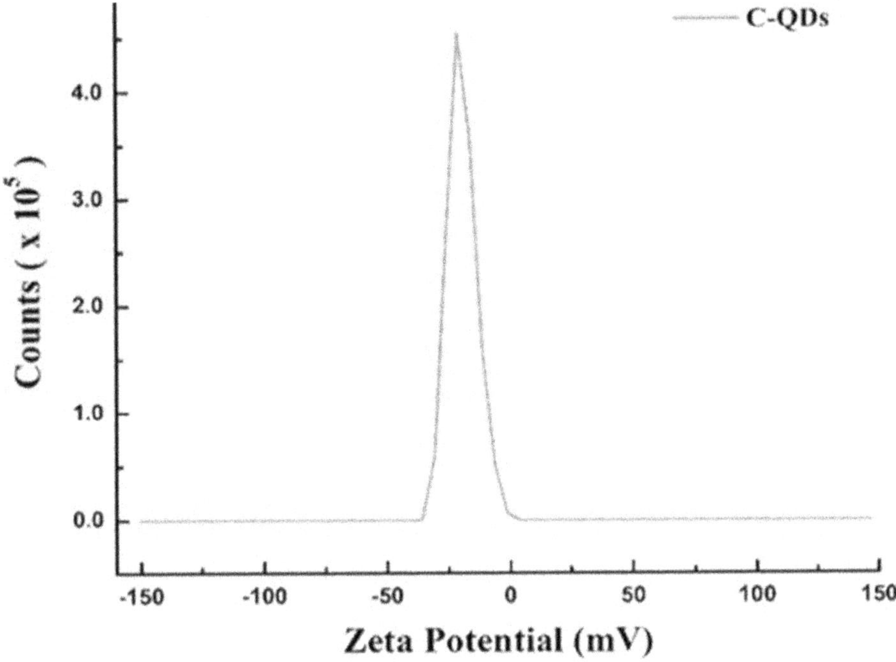

FIGURE 4.32 Zeta potential of CQDs produced from fennel seeds as a carbon source (Dager et al., 2019).

moieties contribute significantly to the characteristic of CQDs in attaining good dispersion in a water-based solvent. Hence, these specific observations are possible through the application of TGA which contributes toward the better utilization of CQDs in the development of thermally stable or controlled materials.

4.8 COLLOIDAL STABILITY

Dager et al. (2019) also studied on the colloidal stability of the synthesized CQDs investigated at room temperature. The storage of the CQDs after 15 months exhibited no significant differences in turbidity and demonstrated that the colloidal stability of the synthesized CQDs is very high and can be used over a certain period of time as shown in Figure 4.33.

4.9 THIN LAYER CHROMATOGRAPHY (TLC)

Thin-layer chromatography is an analytic technique for the characterization of CQDs to assess the purity, identify components, and contribute to the qualitative information about the sample. Dager et al. (2019) studied the TLC of the produced CQDs from the fennel seeds after dialysis, which contained a single fraction and revealed that the produced CQDs possessed a high purity (Figure 4.34). In these cases, TLCs have been found to be extremely useful and conclusive.

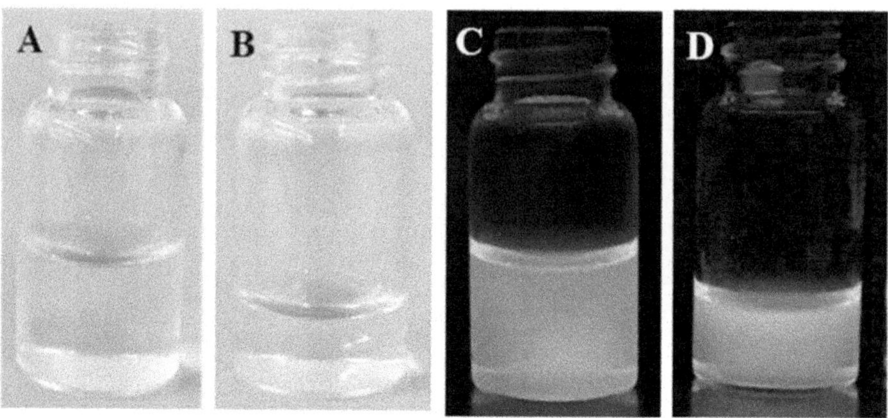

FIGURE 4.33 CQDs reveal no sign of turbidity for a storage period of 15 months under ambient conditions (Dager et al., 2019). (a) Optical image of freshly produced CQDs under daylight exposure when dispersed in water, b) optical image of CQDs under daylight exposure when dispersed in water after 15 months of storage, (c) optical image of freshly produced CQDs under UV exposure when dispersed in water, (d) optical image of CQDs under UV exposure when dispersed in water after 15 months of storage.

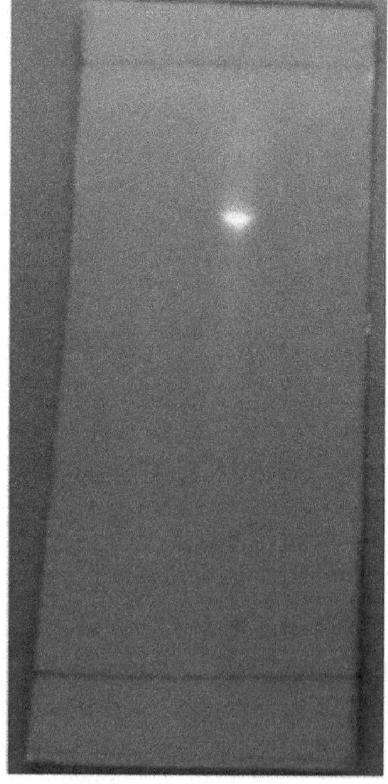

FIGURE 4.34 Thin layer chromatography of CQDs produced from fennel seeds, which exhibits a single luminescent band (Dager et al., 2019).

4.10 QUANTUM YIELD ANALYSIS

The luminescence/fluorescence quantum yield (QY) is an essential photophysical characteristic that enables analyses of the emission performance of CQDs. It refers to the ability to convert absorbed light into emitted light, generally in the form of fluorescence (Sadjadi, 2021). The QY is the ratio of the number of emitted fluorescence photons to the number of absorbed excitation photons.

Lin et al. (2012) studied the absolute quantum yield of various colored CQDs from the Edinburg Instrument (modular-based spectroscope for the detection of luminance). The absolute quantum yield values for GCQD-NBS (green carbon quantum dots-N-bromosuccinimide), GCQD-PCS (p-chloromethylstyrene), GCQD-NBC (4-nitro benzyl chloride), and GCQD-DAB (4-dimethylaminobenzaldehyde) were reported as 21.53%, 21.23%, 54.98%, and 26.19%, respectively. The normalized emission spectra of the synthesized CQDs are illustrated in Figure 4.35. (a). The CIE coordinates for M-CQDs and GCQDs were determined from the corresponding emission spectra, and the outcomes are shown in Figure 4.35. (b). It was reported that the CIE coordinates for GCQD-NBS, GCQD-PCS, GCQD-NBC, and GCQD-DAB were converted from green (GCQDs) to pure green, to yellow-green, then to orange, and finally to the red region.

Qiang et al. (2019) mentioned about the determination of the photoluminescence quantum yield of the CQDs from Rhodamine B in water employed as a reference dye as mentioned in Equation 4.4.3.

$$\eta = \eta_r \frac{I_s \alpha_r \kappa_s^2}{I_r \alpha_s \kappa_r^2} \tag{4.3}$$

ŋ = Quantum yield
I = Photoluminance emission intensity
α = excitation coefficient at a mentioned excitation wavelength
κ = refractive index of the solvent

The subscripts *s* and *r* refer to the sample and reference, respectively.

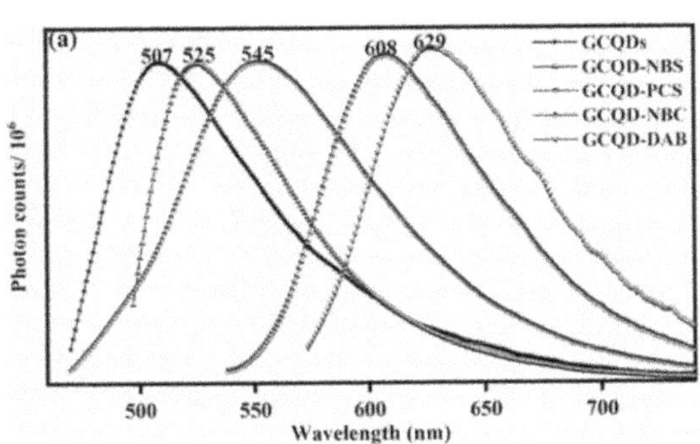
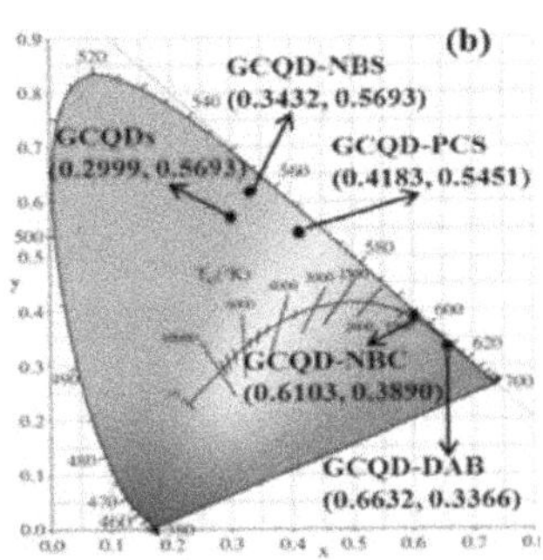

FIGURE 4.35　(a) The normalized emission spectra of GCQDs, GCQD-NBS, GCQD-PCS, GCQD-NBC, and GCQD-DAB. (b) The CIE color coordinates for the M-CQDs (Lin et al., 2012).

4.10.1 Quantum Yield (QY) Measurement

Quantum yield analysis is used to determine the photoluminescence efficiency, surface passivation effects, and optical properties of CQDs. Generally, the QY of carbon dots can be observed by a relative method by using quinine sulfate in 0.10 M of H_2SO_4 solution/fluorescein in the reference standard (0.10 mol/L NaOH).

In a study conducted by Aghamali et al. (2018), nitrogen-doped CQDs (N-CQDs) were synthesized using citric acid (CA) as a carbon source and diethylenetriamine (DETA) for surface passivation employing hydrothermal method. The study presented analysis of quantum yield as illustrated in Figure 4.6 using quinine sulfate, having a refractive index (η) of 1.33 in 0.1 M H_2SO_4, considering quantum yield of 0.54 under 350 nm excitation level (Kwon & Rhee, 2012). The produced N-CQDs were dissolved in pure water (η=1.33) in five different concentrations. Each concentration was tested under 350 nm with less than 0.1 absorbance values. A UV-Vis spectrophotometer was used to determine the absorption values of the different concentrates of solution at an excitation wavelength of 350 nm and the fluorescence spectrometer was utilized to measure the photoluminescence (PL) emission spectrum of the solution at 350 nm excitation wavelength. The quantum yield (QY) was determined by using Equation 4.4.

$$QY_{CQDs} = 0.54 \frac{m_{CQDs}}{m_{QS}} \times \frac{\eta^2_{CQDs}}{\eta^2_{QS}} \tag{4.4}$$

QY = Fluorescence quantum yield
m = slope calculated from the graph (fluorescence intensity vs absorbance)
η = refractive index of the sample (CQDs) and the reference solution (quinine sulfate (QS))

As shown in Figure 4.36, the produced N-CQDs were diluted in an aqueous solution. In visible light and daylight (Figure a and c), the solution was colorless. Under

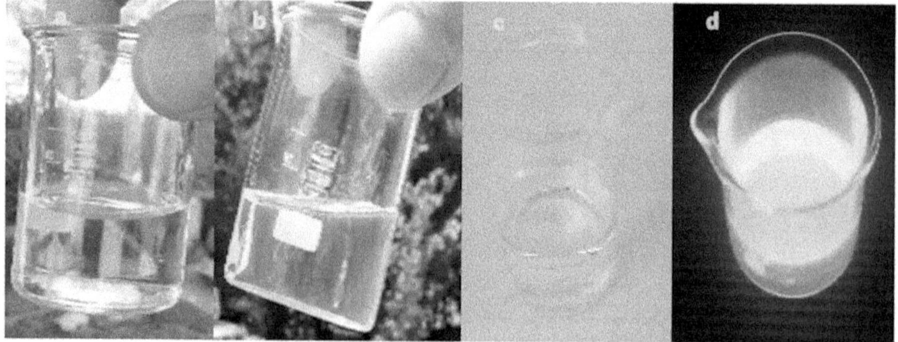

FIGURE 4.36 An aqueous solution with the diluted N-CQDs; (a and c): under visible and daylight (colorless), (b and d): under direct sunlight and 365 nm UV light (intense blue fluorescence) (Aghamali et al., 2018).

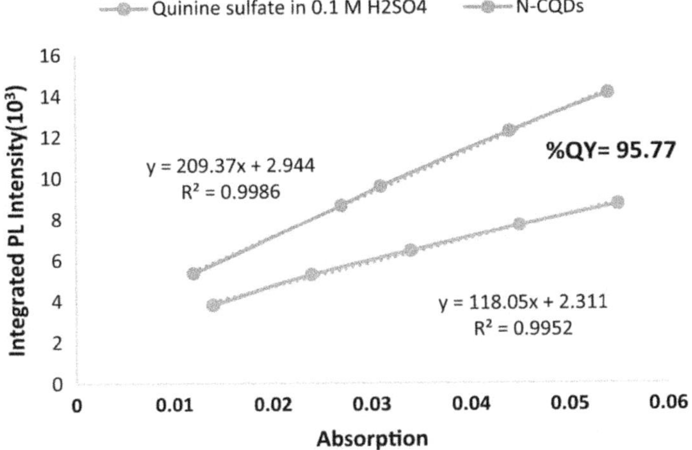

FIGURE 4.37 Quantum yield measurement of N-CQDs employing quinine sulfate (QS) as a reference (Aghamali et al., 2018).

direct sunlight and 365 nm UV light (Figure b and d), an intense blue fluorescence color was observed.

As observed in Figure 4.37, the synthesized N-CQDs exhibited a high QY of about 95% by utilizing quinine sulfate as a reference (Aghamali et al., 2018).

4.11 RADICAL SCAVENGING ACTIVITY

Analyses of radical scavenging activity are used to examine the antioxidant potential of the CQDs. Various common methods have been employed for the assessment of CQDs' antioxidant activities, including DPPH (2,2-diphenyl-1-picrylhydrazyl) radical scavenging assay, ABTS (2,2'-azino-bis (benzoathiazoline-6-sulfonic acid)) radical scavenging assay, FRAP (ferric reducing antioxidant power), and ORAC (oxygen radical absorbance capacity) assay.

A study on CQDs from garlic was carried out wherein the free radical scavenging activity of the synthesized CQDs through a DPPH free radical was analyzed using methanol solutions. In the tests, 2 mL of DPPH (100 µM) solution and 10 µL of aqueous CQDs were combined and decreased values in absorption at 515 nm were observed. The DPPH radical scavenging activity was determined using the following Equation 4.5:

$$\text{Inhibition}\left(\%\right) = \frac{A_c - A_s}{A_C} \times 100 \tag{4.5}$$

where A_s and A_c are the absorbances of DPPH at 515 nm in the presence and absence of the CQDs, respectively.

The experimental solution changes from deep violet to light yellow color when DPPH accepts a hydrogen radical and forms a stable DPPH-H complex. As shown in

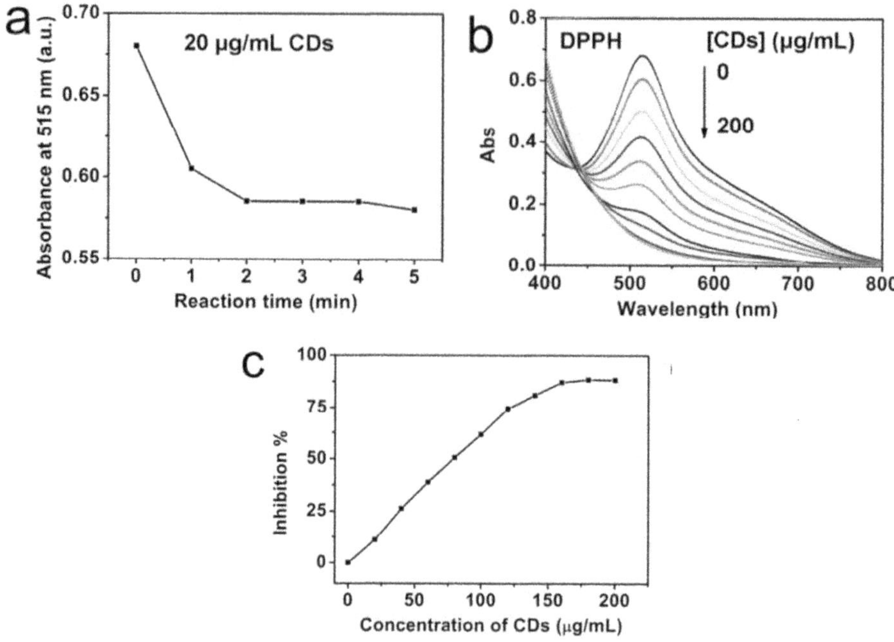

FIGURE 4.38 DPPH radical scavenging. (a) DPPH radical scavenging as a function of time in the availability of 20 µg/mL of the CQDs. (b) Absorbance titration of the spectra of DPPH upon increasing the CQDs from 0 to 200 µg/mL. (c) CQD concentration (Zhao et al., n.d.).

Figure 4.38 (a), it was reported that the absorbance of the DPPH methanol solution at 515 nm was reduced and equilibrated after 2 minutes of addition of 20 µg/mL CQDs. In Figure 4.38 (b), the work on the dose-dependent scavenging activity of the DPPH radical by CQDs at concentrations ranging from 0 to 200 µg/mL has been reported. The absorbance of DPPH decreased as the CQD concentration increased until it reached saturation at 160 µg/mL. Figure 4.38 (c) is a plot between the concentration of CQDs and the inhibition value.

4.12 CYTOTOXICITY

The potential of a certain chemical/mediator to demolish living cells is known as cytotoxicity. Cytotoxicity is analyzed using rat mesangial cells (RMC). Characterization of cytotoxicity by RMC involves assessing the toxic effects of CQDs on the cells in vitro. For determining the cytotoxicity, assays and experiments were conducted considering cell viability, cell death, and other cellular responses. Various methods have been used for the cytotoxicity characterization with RMCs such as cell viability assays, lactate dehydrogenase (LDH) release assay, cell morphological examination, cell cycle analysis, reactive oxygen species (ROS) measurement, etc. One or more assays can be utilized for the validation of the cytotoxic effects of the CQDs on RMCs. These characterization techniques deliver significant information related to the mechanism of cytotoxicity and assist in the development of potential CQDs and recognition of harmful substances.

4.12.1 Characterization of the Cytotoxicity of CQDs using RMC Method

During a study (Zhang et al., 2015), the cytotoxicity of the synthesized CQDs from the flour was considered and compared with the CQDs produced from $Cd2^+$ and NaHTe solution (CdTe quantum dots). The RMC was utilized to estimate the cytotoxicity of the test samples. RMC line was cultured in Dulbecco minimum essential media (DMEM) and 5.5 mM D-glucose, and supplemented with 10 % FBS (Fetal bovine serum), 100 units/mL of penicillin, and 100 mg/mL of streptomycin. Then MTT assay was assessed in terms of cell viability (Figures 4.39 and 4.40).

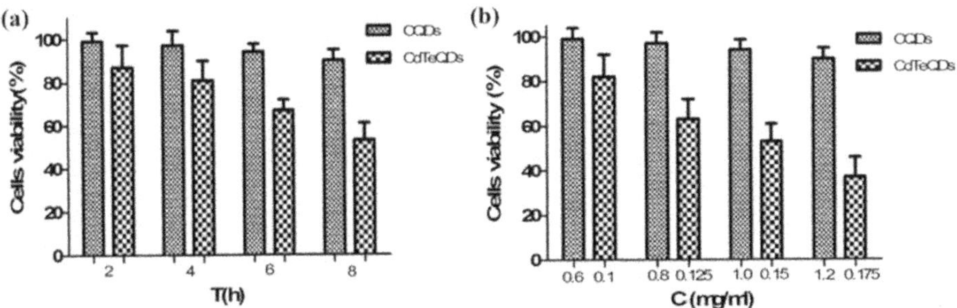

FIGURE 4.39   (a) The cell viability of RMCs co-incubated with the synthesized CQDs from flour and CdTe quantum dots at different concentrations for 8 hours; (b) the cell viability of RMCs co-incubated with the synthesized CQDs and CdTe quantum dots at concentrations of 0.8 mg/mL and 0.15 mg/mL, respectively at different time intervals (Zhang et al., 2015).

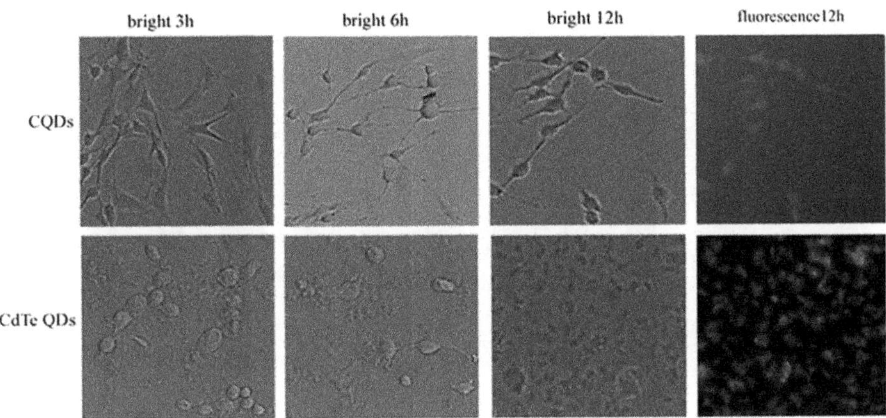

FIGURE 4.40   Image of RMCs co-incubated with CQDs and CdTe quantum dots at concentrations of 0.8 mg/mL and 0.15 mg/mL, respectively, at different time intervals (Zhang et al., 2015).

4.12.2 In Vitro Cytotoxicity Assay

The CQDs synthesized from the essential oil of *Thymus vulgaris* L. as a carbon source were reported by Bayat et al. (2019). The study demonstrated the investigation of cell viability utilizing a calorimetric assay agent. During the procedure, MTT, a light yellow tetrazole, was converted to violet formazan crystals by the action of the mitochondrial enzyme 3-(4,5-dimethylthiazol-2-yl)-2,5-diphenyltetrazolium bromide (MTT). For an additional 24-hour incubation, different CQDs concentrations (0–1400 mg/L) of the as-prepared CQDs were added. The fresh culture media containing MTT (20 μL, 5 mg/mL) was then added to 100 μL of the mixture. Cells were then incubated for 4 hours while mitochondrial enzymes worked to create formazan crystals. In place of the growth media, 150 μL of dimethyl sulfoxide (DMSO) was added to the CQD-conjugated cells. A Bio-Rad ELISA reader measured dye absorbance at a wavelength of 570 nm. Equation 4.6 was used to calculate the cell viability:

$$\text{Cell viability}\left(\%\right) = \frac{A_{Treated}}{A_{Control}} \times 100 \tag{4.6}$$

where $A_{Treated}$ and $A_{Control}$ were obtained in the presence and absence of CQDs, respectively.

CQDs are biocompatible with cells and safe for biomedical applications based on cell viability results. The cytotoxicity of the CQDs obtained from *Thymus vulgaris* L was low at 1400 mg/L, and the viability of the cells was about 76% (Figure 4.41). In a different study, Xue et al. (2019) developed CQDs from lignin and investigated the

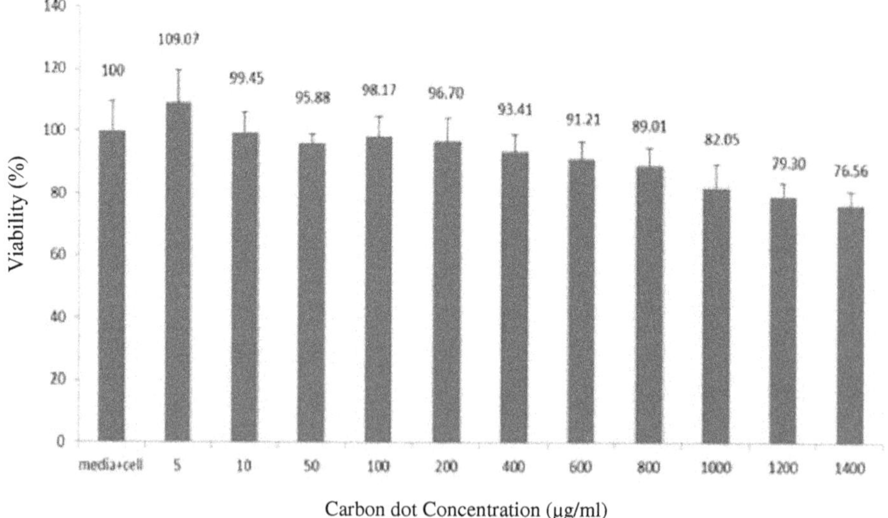

FIGURE 4.41 Cytotoxicity effects of carbon dots at different concentrations of carbon dots on SKOV3 cells (Bayat et al., 2019).

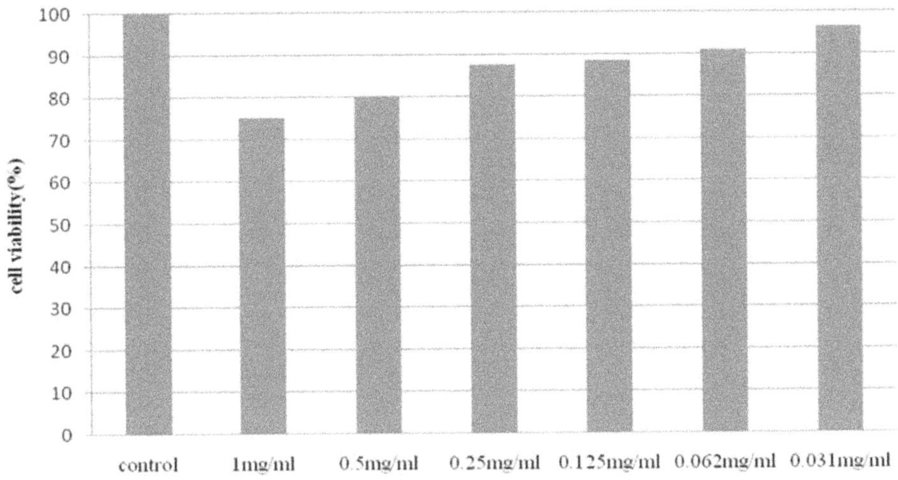

FIGURE 4.42   Cell viability results (%) evaluated by MTT assay (Xue et al., 2019).

cytotoxicity of the produced CQDs in HeLa cells using the MTT assays. A 96-well plate was loaded with raw HeLa cells (6×10^3 cells per well), which were then incubated for 24 hours at 37 °C in a 5% CO_2 condition. The cells were then exposed to L-CQDs at various doses (0–1 mg/mL), and they were then incubated for a further 24 hours at 37 °C with 5% CO_2. The cells were then treated with MTT solution (20 µL, 5 mg/mL) and washed with phosphate-buffered saline (PBS) (pH = 7.4) before being further cultured for 4 hours. To determine the cell viability, the optical absorbance at 570 nm of each well was measured using a microplate reader (Bio-Rad). The study revealed that the cell viability values increased progressively as the CQD concentration decreased, as illustrated in Figure 4.42. After 24 hours of incubation, the cell viabilities at 0.062 mg/mL and 0.031 mg/mL concentrations were both greater than 90%. Even after increasing the CQD concentration from 0.125 mg/mL to 0.5 mg/mL, their cell viability remained greater than 80%. According to the results, the CQDs showed high biocompatibility and minimal cytotoxicity toward HeLa cells, which was presumably attributed to CQDs' low toxicity.

4.13   CONCLUSION

The characterization techniques discussed in this chapter serve as a fundamental approach to understanding these properties and relate to their intended applications. Furthermore, broader knowledge in nanomaterials science and technology can be obtained through the characterization of CQDs. Advanced techniques and methodologies are utilized to understand the unique properties of carbon quantum dots in the nanoscale, emphasizing the importance of analytical techniques for effective characterization of the CQDs. Primary characterization techniques, including microscopic, diffraction, spectroscopic, optical, structural, surface functionalities, quantum yield, antioxidant, and cytotoxicity of the CQDs, are in continuous use; however, they need regular updates and scientific innovation as data available on this material is still sparse as compared to others. Hence in the future, with further advancement and data availability, the understanding and application of carbon dots will be much more precise and widespread.

REFERENCES

Aghamali, A., Khosravi, M., Hamishehkar, H., Modirshahla, N., & Behnajady, M. A. (2018). Synthesis and characterization of high efficient photoluminescent sunlight driven photocatalyst of N-Carbon Quantum Dots. *Journal of Luminescence*, 201, 265–274. Retrieved from https://doi.org/10.1016/j.jlumin.2018.04.061

Arul, V., & Sethuraman, M. G. (2018). Facile green synthesis of fluorescent N-doped carbon dots from *Actinidia deliciosa* and their catalytic activity and cytotoxicity applications. *Optical Materials*, 78, 181–190. Retrieved from https://doi.org/10.1016/j.optmat.2018.02.029

Bano, D., Kumar, V., Singh, V. K., & Hasan, S. H. (2018). Green synthesis of fluorescent carbon quantum dots for the detection of mercury (<scp>ii</scp>) and glutathione. *New Journal of Chemistry*, 42(8), 5814–5821. Retrieved from https://doi.org/10.1039/C8NJ00432C

Bayat, A., Masoum, S., & Hosseini, E. S. (2019). Natural plant precursor for the facile and eco-friendly synthesis of carbon nanodots with multifunctional aspects. *Journal of Molecular Liquids*, 281, 134–140. Retrieved from https://doi.org/10.1016/j.molliq.2019.02.074

Boruah, A., Saikia, M., Das, T., Goswamee, R. L., & Saikia, B. K. (2020). Blue-emitting fluorescent carbon quantum dots from waste biomass sources and their application in fluoride ion detection in water. *Journal of Photochemistry and Photobiology B: Biology*, 209. Retrieved from https://doi.org/10.1016/j.jphotobiol.2020.111940

Dager, A., Uchida, T., Maekawa, T., & Tachibana, M. (2019). Synthesis and characterization of mono-disperse carbon quantum dots from fennel seeds: Photoluminescence analysis using Machine Learning. *Scientific Reports*, 9(1). Retrieved from https://doi.org/10.1038/s41598-019-50397-5

Das, P., Bose, M., Ganguly, S., Mondal, S., Das, A. K., Banerjee, S., & Das, N. C. (2017). Green approach to photoluminescent carbon dots for imaging of gram-negative bacteria *Escherichia coli*. *Nanotechnology*, 28(19), 195501. Retrieved from https://doi.org/10.1088/1361-6528/aa6714

Dong, Y., Pang, H., Yang, H. Bin, Guo, C., Shao, J., Chi, Y., … Yu, T. (2013). Carbon-based dots co-doped with nitrogen and sulfur for high quantum yield and excitation-independent emission. *Angewandte Chemie International Edition*, 52(30), 7800–7804. Retrieved from https://doi.org/10.1002/anie.201301114

Farshbaf, M., Davaran, S., Rahimi, F., Annabi, N., Salehi, R., & Akbarzadeh, A. (2018). Carbon quantum dots: Recent progresses on synthesis, surface modification and applications. *Artificial Cells, Nanomedicine, and Biotechnology*, 46(7), 1331–1348. Retrieved from https://doi.org/10.1080/21691401.2017.1377725

Gu, D., Shang, S., Yu, Q., & Shen, J. (2016). Green synthesis of nitrogen-doped carbon dots from lotus root for Hg(II) ions detection and cell imaging. *Applied Surface Science*, 390, 38–42. Retrieved from https://doi.org/10.1016/j.apsusc.2016.08.012

Li, H., He, X., Kang, Z., Huang, H., Liu, Y., Liu, J., … Lee, S. T. (2010). Water-soluble fluorescent carbon quantum dots and photocatalyst design. *Angewandte Chemie - International Edition*, 49(26), 4430–4434. Retrieved from https://doi.org/10.1002/anie.200906154

Holzgrabe, U. (2010, August). Quantitative NMR spectroscopy in pharmaceutical applications. *Progress in Nuclear Magnetic Resonance Spectroscopy*. Retrieved from https://doi.org/10.1016/j.pnmrs.2010.05.001

Jing, H. H., Bardakci, F., Akgöl, S., Kusat, K., Adnan, M., Alam, M. J., … Sasidharan, S. (2023, January 1). Green carbon dots: Synthesis, characterization, properties and biomedical applications. *Journal of Functional Biomaterials*. MDPI. Retrieved from https://doi.org/10.3390/jfb14010027

Karatutlu, A., Patil, B., Seker, I., Istengir, S., Bolat, A., Yildirim, O., … Sapelkin, A. (2018). Structural, optical, electrical and electrocatalytic activity properties of luminescent organic carbon quantum dots. *ChemistrySelect*, 3(17), 4730–4737. Retrieved from https://doi.org/10.1002/slct.201800714

Khalid, H., Khan, M. F., Ahmad, B., Ismail, M., Zahid, M., & Ismail, A. (2022). Grass-derived carbon nanodots as a fluorescent-sensing platform for label-free detection of Cu (II) ions. *Journal of Materials Science: Materials in Electronics*, 33(8), 5626–5634. Retrieved from https://doi.org/10.1007/s10854-022-07749-1

Kim, T. H., Wang, F., McCormick, P., Wang, L., Brown, C., & Li, Q. (2014). Salt-embedded carbon nanodots as a UV and thermal stable fluorophore for light-emitting diodes. *Journal of Luminescence*, 154, 1–7. Retrieved 29 August 2023 from https://doi.org/10.1016/J.JLUMIN.2014.04.002

Kwon, W., & Rhee, S. W. (2012). Facile synthesis of graphitic carbon quantum dots with size tunability and uniformity using reverse micelles. *Chemical Communications*, 48(43), 5256–5258. Retrieved 1 September 2023 from https://doi.org/10.1039/C2CC31687K

Larsson, M. A., Ramachandran, P., Jarujamrus, P., & Lee, H. L. (2022). Microwave synthesis of blue emissive N-Doped carbon quantum dots as a fluorescent probe for free chlorine detection. *Sains Malaysiana*, 51(4), 1197–1212. Retrieved from https://doi.org/10.17576/jsm-2022-5104-20

Li, F., Li, T., Sun, C., Xia, J., Jiao, Y., & Xu, H. (2017). Selenium-doped carbon quantum dots for free-radical scavenging. *Angewandte Chemie*, 129(33), 10042–10046. Retrieved from https://doi.org/10.1002/ange.201705989

Li, Q., Zhou, M., Yang, M., Yang, Q., Zhang, Z., & Shi, J. (2018). Induction of long-lived room temperature phosphorescence of carbon dots by water in hydrogen-bonded matrices. *Nature Communications*, 9(1). Retrieved from https://doi.org/10.1038/s41467-018-03144-9

Lin, Z., Xue, W., Chen, H., & Lin, J. M. (2012). Classical oxidant induced chemiluminescence of fluorescent carbon dots. *Chemical Communications*, 48(7), 1051–1053. Retrieved from https://doi.org/10.1039/c1cc15290d

Liu, H., Ye, T., & Mao, C. (2007). Fluorescent carbon nanoparticles derived from candle soot. *Angewandte Chemie*, 119(34), 6593–6595. Retrieved from https://doi.org/10.1002/ange.200701271

Murru, C., Badía-Laíño, R., & Díaz-García, M. E. (2020). Synthesis and characterization of green carbon dots for scavenging radical oxygen species in aqueous and oil samples. *Antioxidants*, 9(11), 1–18. Retrieved from https://doi.org/10.3390/antiox9111147

Qiang, R., Yang, S., Hou, K., & Wang, J. (2019). Synthesis of carbon quantum dots with green luminescence from potato starch. *New Journal of Chemistry*, 43(27), 10826–10833. Retrieved from https://doi.org/10.1039/C9NJ02291K

R Jelinek - quantum dots. Springer International Publishing, & 2017, undefined. Carbon quantum dots. *Quantum Dots. Springer International Publishing, Cham, 2017•Springer*. Retrieved 25 July 2023 from https://link.springer.com/content/pdf/10.1007/978-3-319-43911-2.pdf

Rai, S., Singh, B. K., Bhartiya, P., Singh, A., Kumar, H., Dutta, P. K., & Mehrotra, G. K. (2017). Lignin derived reduced fluorescence carbon dots with theranostic approaches: Nano-drug-carrier and bioimaging. *Journal of Luminescence*, 190, 492–503. Retrieved from https://doi.org/10.1016/j.jlumin.2017.06.008

Ramanan, V., Thiyagarajan, S. K., Raji, K., Suresh, R., Sekar, R., & Ramamurthy, P. (2016). Outright green synthesis of fluorescent carbon dots from eutrophic algal blooms for in vitro imaging. *ACS Sustainable Chemistry and Engineering*, 4(9), 4724–4731. Retrieved from https://doi.org/10.1021/acssuschemeng.6b00935

Rojas-Valencia, O. G., Regules-Carrasco, M., Hernández-Fuentes, J., Germán, C. M. R. S., Estrada-Flores, M., & Villagarcía-Chávez, E. (2021). Synthesis of blue emissive carbon quantum dots from Hibiscus Sabdariffa flower: Surface functionalization analysis by FT-IR spectroscopy. *Materialia*, 19. Retrieved from https://doi.org/10.1016/j.mtla.2021.101182

Sabet, M., & Mahdavi, K. (2019). Green synthesis of high photoluminescence nitrogen-doped carbon quantum dots from grass via a simple hydrothermal method for removing organic and inorganic water pollutions. *Applied Surface Science*, 463, 283–291. Retrieved from https://doi.org/10.1016/j.apsusc.2018.08.223

Sachdev, A., & Gopinath, P. (2015). Green synthesis of multifunctional carbon dots from coriander leaves and their potential application as antioxidants, sensors and bioimaging agents. *Analyst*, 140(12), 4260–4269. Retrieved from https://doi.org/10.1039/c5an00454c

Sadjadi, S. (2021). The utility of carbon dots for photocatalysis. In *Emerging Carbon Materials for Catalysis* (pp. 123–160). Elsevier. Retrieved from https://doi.org/10.1016/B978-0-12-817561-3.00004-4

Saha, S., Das, S., Ghorai, U. K., Mazumder, N., Ganguly, D., & Chattopadhyay, K. K. (2015). Controlling nonradiative transition centers in Eu^{3+} activated $CaSnO_3$ nanophosphors through Na^+ Co-Doping: Realization of ultrabright red emission along with higher thermal stability. *The Journal of Physical Chemistry C*, 119(29), 16824–16835. Retrieved from https://doi.org/10.1021/acs.jpcc.5b03500

Sarkar, S., Banerjee, D., Ghorai, U. K., Das, N. S., & Chattopadhyay, K. K. (2016). Size dependent photoluminescence property of hydrothermally synthesized crystalline carbon quantum dots. *Journal of Luminescence*, 178, 314–323. Retrieved from https://doi.org/10.1016/j.jlumin.2016.05.033

Selvamani, V. (2019). Stability studies on nanomaterials used in drugs. In *Characterization and Biology of Nanomaterials for Drug Delivery* (pp. 425–444). Elsevier. Retrieved from https://doi.org/10.1016/B978-0-12-814031-4.00015-5

Sharma, S., & Chowdhury, P. (2023). Fluorescence signal from carbon quantum dots synthesized from natural resources. *Materials Today: Proceedings*. Retrieved from https://doi.org/10.1016/j.matpr.2023.05.676

Singh, I., Arora, R., Dhiman, H., & Pahwa, R. (n.d.). *Carbon Quantum Dots: Synthesis, Characterization and Biomedical Applications*.

Sivasankaran, U., Jesny, S., Jose, A. R., & Girish Kumar, K. (2017). Fluorescence determination of glutathione using tissue paper-derived carbon dots as fluorophores. *Analytical Sciences*, 33(3), 281–285. Retrieved from https://doi.org/10.2116/analsci.33.281

Tan, M., Zhang, L., Tang, R., Song, X., Li, Y., Wu, H., Ma, X. (2013). Enhanced photoluminescence and characterization of multicolor carbon dots using plant soot as a carbon source. *Talanta*, 115, 950–956. Retrieved from https://doi.org/10.1016/j.talanta.2013.06.061

Thimbiraj, S., & Shankaran, R. (2016). Green synthesis of highly fluorescent carbon quantum dots from sugarcane bagasse pulp. *Applied Surface Science*, 390, 435–443. Retrieved from https://doi.org/10.1016/j.apsusc.2016.08.106

Wang, H., Sun, C., Chen, X., Zhang, Y., Colvin, V. L., Rice, Q., Yu, W. W. (2017). Excitation wavelength independent visible color emission of carbon dots. *Nanoscale*, 9(5), 1909–1915. Retrieved from https://doi.org/10.1039/c6nr09200d

Wang, Y., & Hu, A. (2014). Carbon quantum dots: Synthesis, properties, and applications. *Journal of Materials Chemistry C*, 2(34), 6921–6939. Retrieved from https://doi.org/10.1039/c4tc00988f

Wei, Z., Wang, B., Liu, Y., Liu, Z., Zhang, H., Zhang, S., … Lu, S. (2019). Green synthesis of nitrogen and sulfur co-doped carbon dots from Allium fistulosum for cell imaging. *New Journal of Chemistry*, 43(2), 718–723. Retrieved from https://doi.org/10.1039/c8nj05783d

Wu, M., Zhan, J., Geng, B., He, P., Wu, K., Wang, L., … Pan, D. (2017). Scalable synthesis of organic-soluble carbon quantum dots: superior optical properties in solvents, solids, and LEDs. *Nanoscale*, 9(35), 13195–13202. Retrieved from https://doi.org/10.1039/C7NR04718E

Wu, W., Zhan, L., Ohkubo, K., Yamada, Y., Wu, M., & Fukuzumi, S. (2015). Photocatalytic H2 evolution from NADH with carbon quantum dots/Pt and 2-phenyl-4-(1-naphthyl) quinolinium ion. *Journal of Photochemistry and Photobiology B: Biology*, 152, 63–70. Retrieved from https://doi.org/10.1016/j.jphotobiol.2014.10.018

Xu, Y., Wu, M., Feng, X. Z., Yin, X. B., He, X. W., & Zhang, Y. K. (2013). Reduced carbon dots versus oxidized carbon dots: Photo- and electrochemiluminescence investigations for selected applications. *Chemistry - A European Journal*, 19(20), 6282–6288. Retrieved from https://doi.org/10.1002/chem.201204372

Xue, B., Yang, Y., Sun, Y., Fan, J., Li, X., & Zhang, Z. (2019). Photoluminescent lignin hybridized carbon quantum dots composites for bioimaging applications. *International Journal of Biological Macromolecules*, 122, 954–961. Retrieved from https://doi.org/10.1016/j.ijbiomac.2018.11.018

Yang, J.-M., Hu, X.-W., Liu, Y.-X., & Zhang, W. (2019). Fabrication of a carbon quantum dots-immobilized zirconium-based metal-organic framework composite fluorescence sensor for highly sensitive detection of 4-nitrophenol. *Microporous and Mesoporous Materials*, 274, 149–154. Retrieved from https://doi.org/10.1016/j.micromeso.2018.07.042

Zainal Abidin, N. H., Shafie, S. N. A., Suhaimi, H., Sambudi, N. S., & Sapiaa Md Nordin, N. A. H. (2021). Incorporation of carboxyl and amino functionalized carbon quantum dots in thin film membrane for nanofiltration. *Polymer Testing*, 100, 107270. Retrieved from https://doi.org/10.1016/j.polymertesting.2021.107270

Zhang, Q., Sun, X., Ruan, H., Yin, K., & Li, H. (2017). Production of yellow-emitting carbon quantum dots from fullerene carbon soot. *Science China Materials*, 60(2), 141–150. Retrieved from https://doi.org/10.1007/s40843-016-5160-9

Zhang, Z., Duan, Y., Yu, Y., Yan, Z., & Chen, J. (2015). Carbon quantum dots: synthesis, characterization, and assessment of cytocompatibility. *Journal of Materials Science: Materials in Medicine*, 26(7). Retrieved from https://doi.org/10.1007/s10856-015-5536-x

Zhao, S., Lan, M., Zhu, X., Xue, H., Ng, T.-W., Meng, X., … Zhang, W. (n.d.). *Green Synthesis of Bifunctional Fluorescent Carbon Dots from Garlic for Cellular Imaging and Free Radicals Scavenging*.

Zheng, H., Wang, Q., Long, Y., Zhang, H., Huang, X., & Zhu, R. (2011). Enhancing the luminescence of carbon dots with a reduction pathway. *Chemical Communications*, 47(38), 10650. Retrieved from https://doi.org/10.1039/c1cc14741b

Zuo, P., Lu, X., Sun, Z., Guo, Y., & He, H. (2016, February 1). A review on syntheses, properties, characterization and bioanalytical applications of fluorescent carbon dots. *Microchimica Acta*. Springer-Verlag Wien. Retrieved from https://doi.org/10.1007/s00604-015-1705-3

5 Antimicrobial Mechanisms Exhibited by Carbon Quantum Dots

*Jeyakumar Saranya Packialakshmi
and Jun Tae Kim*

5.1 INTRODUCTION

Modern society relies on the use of antibiotics to eliminate pathogenic bacteria which causes several illnesses. Initially discovered for utilization in human medicine, the use of antibiotics is extended to various fields like farming, aquaculture, food preservation, and food packaging. The antibiotic drugs prescribed are fast-acting, easy to use, slow the growth of bacteria, and kill them. As irreplaceable as they are in the medical field, it is observed that at recent times many clinical pathogens are developing resistance to most antibiotics. Though naturally occurring, antibiotic resistance is aggravated by inappropriate and overuse of antibiotics. Being one of the biggest public health threats, 700,000 deaths are reported in association with antibiotic-resistant bacteria every year (Tarín-Pelló et al., 2022). Bacteria, viruses, fungi, and parasites develop resistance and do not respond to antibiotic drugs, whose dosages are standardized to treat infection. When pathogens develop resistance and refrain from responding to antibiotics, deaths occur, especially in immune-compromised groups of individuals such as newborn babies, the elderly population, those undergoing cancer therapies, surgeries, etc. Responsible intake of antibiotics, reduction of unnecessary prescriptions, and abstaining from the availability of antibiotic drugs over the counter successfully reduced the resistance-selective pressure among the bacteria. Despite the efforts, combating already developed multidrug-resistant bacteria, developing resistance and emergence of resistance pertaining to various geographic regions remains a challenge. Addressing these issues, developing novel, effective antimicrobials with special attention to multidrug-resistant and community-developed pathogens is necessary.

Antimicrobial agents can be microbiostatic or microbicidal. These antimicrobial agents belong to various broad-spectrum chemical classes. The widespread list of pathogens and the development of antimicrobial resistance all over the world demanded the requirement of novel and powerful molecules for control. Phytoextracts, secondary metabolites, bacteriocins, antimicrobial peptides, pigments, nanomaterials,

DOI: 10.1201/9781003437857-6

etc. were novel classes of molecules used for the control of pathogens (Amaning Danquah et al., 2022; Stan et al., 2021). Slow progress in antibiotic discovery, redundancy of the compounds identified, and development of multidrug-resistant antibiotics exacerbate the requirements. Accordingly, new-age chemical molecules emerge. One such nanomaterial recently been discovered is the CQDs. The CQDs are zero-dimensional fluorescent materials with a size lesser than 10 nm and that carry some form of surface passivation (Alshammari et al., 2023; Xu et al., 2004). Initially, CQDs were exploited for applications like photocatalysis, absorption, metal ion sensing, bio-imaging, drug delivery, etc. The microbial activities of the CQDs have gained attention in recent times owing to their versatile functionalities.

Unlike conventional antibiotics, the CQDs inherit a multidimensional approach to battle microbial pathogens. A combination of physical, chemical, and biological interactions directs the antimicrobial mechanisms of the CQDs. The major antimicrobial mechanisms of CQDs are associated with the destruction of the cell wall/membranes, cessation of membrane transport, interference with gene expression, generation of free radicals, etc. The antimicrobial activities of the CQDs are widely studied but with less focus on the mechanisms of antibiosis.

This review is focused on possible antimicrobial mechanisms imposed by the CQDs. A trivial section explores the factors that influence the antimicrobial activities of the CQDs. In conclusion, carbon quantum dots represent a novel and multifaceted approach to addressing the pressing issue of antibiotic resistance and bacterial infections. This review paper aims to comprehensively elucidate the antimicrobial and antibiofilm mechanisms of CQDs, inspiring further research to unlock their full potential as an innovative solution in the fight against bacterial pathogens.

5.2 ANTIBACTERIAL MECHANISMS OF CQDs

Bacterial pathogens and infections caused by them are the second leading cause of human and animal mortality worldwide. Bacterial infections cause 7.7 million deaths which accounts for almost 13.6%. Carbon quantum dots (CQDs) are now emerging as antibacterial compounds with remarkable multifaceted and innovative antibacterial mechanisms against bacterial pathogens and antibiotic-resistant bacterial strains (Ghirardello et al., 2021). The following section focuses on divulging the intricate mechanisms by which the CQDs achieve pronounced antibacterial effects. Unlike the antibiotics that have specific targets, CQDs unveil a range of interactions with the bacterial cell to inactivate them and reduce the number of viable cells. By examining the multifaceted antibacterial mechanisms of CQDs, we aim to provide a comprehensive insight into the potential of these nanomaterials as a promising solution to address the growing concerns of antibiotic resistance and bacterial infections.

5.3 PHYSICAL DAMAGE TO BACTERIAL CELL STRUCTURES

The CQDs encompass a series of multifaceted antibacterial mechanisms, the pivotal being their ability to induce physical damage to the structural components of the bacterial cells. Bacterial membranes composed mainly of lipids and proteins play a pivotal role in the maintenance of cellular structure and regulation of membrane transport

(Strahl & Errington, 2017). Operating at the nanoscale, the CQDs interact with the bacterial cell wall and membranes, making them irregular, causing the disintegration of the native bacterial cell structure, and resulting in intercellular leak (Hao et al., 2021). The diminutive size and versatile surface properties enable the CQDs to infiltrate the membranes, destabilizing and rupturing them. The damage heightens the membrane permeability compromising the ability of the bacterium to withhold the osmatic pressure making the cell vulnerable to external stress. The intercellular components are released into the environment following impediments to the functionality of the bacteria. The onset of membrane damage and loss of cell viability are directly proportional. This loss of cell viability corresponds to the exponential phase of the bacterial growth cycle (Pagán & Mackey, 2000). The damage to the bacterial cell wall and cell membranes results in the release of critical intracellular components of the bacterial cell. Thus, bacterial interaction with the CQDs causes physical damage, and this cell wall damaging ability underpins them as novel antibacterial agents offering a distinct approach to combating bacterial pathogens compared to traditional antibiotics.

5.3.1 IMPACT OF POSITIVE SURFACE CHARGES

Positive surface charges are an eccentric attribute that pronounces CQDs as antibacterial agents that instigate damage to bacterial cell structures. The surface charges are the prime factor that significantly influences the CQD's interaction with the bacterial cell surfaces (Travlou et al., 2018). Positive charges on CQDs which are acquired through surface functionalization play a key role in the antibacterial efficiency of the CQDs. The bacterial cell membranes are negatively charged as they are primarily made of phospholipids. Additionally, teichoic acids, found in the cell wall of Gram-positive bacteria, also contribute to the negative charge due to their phosphate residues (Wu et al., 2021). The positively charged CQDs interact with the negatively charged bacterial membrane through electrostatic forces. The electrostatic interaction promotes the adhesion and binding of the CQDs to the bacterial cell surface.

The electrostatic interactions bring about twofold manifestations. Initially, the proximity and close association of the CQDs with the bacterial surface escalates the chances of penetration into the membrane (Li et al., 2022). Secondly, there occurs a localized increase in the cumulative positive charge disrupting the electrochemical balance of the bacterial membrane leading to an imbalance (Hao et al., 2021). This imbalance leads to disturbances in the membrane integrity increasing the permeability causing structural damage on bacterial surfaces. Knowledge of the effect of positive surface charge of CQD is important to harness their antibacterial potential. By exploring the interaction between surface charge, electrostatic attraction, and membrane disruption, researchers aim to refine CQD-based antibacterial strategies, potentially mitigating the challenges posed by drug-resistant bacterial strains (Saadh et al., 2024).

5.4 INFLUENCE OF HYDROPHOBIC INTERACTIONS

Several complex antibacterial mechanisms of CQDs prevail among which hydrophobic interactions are one pivotal mechanism. The hydrophobic interactions are crucial for the effective antibacterial activity causing physical damage to the cell structures of the bacteria. The CQDs possess inherent hydrophobic properties, which favors non-polar conditions (Varisco et al., 2017). The bacterial membranes primarily being composed of lipid bilayer, they have hydrophobic tails. This inherent contrast between the hydrophobic nature of CQDs and the lipid composition of bacterial membranes plays a vital role in their antibacterial activity (Varghese & Balachandran, 2021).

The hydrophobic CQDs readily interact with the hydrophobic tails of lipids that lie within the bacterial cell membranes. This interaction leads to the embedding themselves to the lipid bilayer inducing compact anchoring. Following the embedding, the integration of CQDs into the hydrophobic core of the membrane disrupts the orderly arrangement of the lipid molecules (Ljungh et al., 2006). There are two critical outcomes to this disturbance caused: firstly, there occurs an augmentation in the cell membrane permeability enabling the unrestricted flow of ions and molecules across the membrane. Secondly, there occurs a compromise to the structural integrity of the lipid bilayer, leading to a weakened and compromised cell membrane and ultimately resulting in leakage and rupture causing substantial physical damage to the bacterial cell (Alavi et al., 2021). A deeper understanding of the effect of the hydrophobic interaction of CQDs with bacterial cells as antibacterial mechanisms is important for harnessing their complete potential to be used as novel antibacterial agents.

5.5 IMPACT OF PARTICLE SHAPE AND SIZE

The particle morphology and size of the CQDs are crucially significant parameters that determine the antibacterial activity of the CQDs. Their size and morphology influence the CQD's ability to impose physical damage to the bacterial structures. These characteristics are not mere attributes but essential components that dictate the interactions of CQDs with bacterial cell membranes (Sun et al., 2021). CQDs come in a wide array of sizes and morphologies including spherical, quasi-spherical, or irregular shapes. The sizes determine the ability of the CQDs to penetrate the bacterial cell membranes. The smaller the size of the CQDs the higher the chances that the minute-dimensioned CQDs possess an increased ability to infiltrate the cell membranes (Han et al., 2019). Their diminutive size allows them to navigate the lipid bilayer more readily, increasing the likelihood of embedding themselves within the membrane and subsequently causing structural disruption. In addition to the size, the morphology of the CQDs is significant for their interaction with the bacterial cells (Alavi et al., 2021). The counter effect of the size and surface area counter affects the bactericidal activity. Irregularly shaped CQDs often possess a larger surface area and varied surface properties when compared to their spherical counterparts. The irregular morphology and structural diversity allow greater interaction of the particles with the bacterial membranes, potentially leading to more effective membrane disruption (Li et al., 2020). Unraveling the complicated interactions between particle morphology, size, and CQDs' antibacterial effectiveness holds immense promise. Researchers seek to harness this understanding to tailor CQDs with specific structural attributes that enhance their capacity to inflict physical damage on bacterial cell structures. By fine-tuning CQDs to exploit the nuances of size and morphology, researchers are poised to develop more precise and efficient antibacterial agents, offering a potential solution to the challenges of antibiotic resistance and bacterial infections. This section delves into the pivotal role that particle morphology and size play in shaping CQDs' antibacterial mechanisms, elucidating their intricate interplay in the quest for innovative antibacterial solutions.

5.6 OXIDATIVE DAMAGE

Exploring the multifaceted antibacterial mechanisms of the CQDs, oxidative injury emerges as a critical facet with potential implications for their ability to combat bacterial pathogens. The oxidative stress leads to the disruption and elimination of the microorganisms. The CQDs possess inherent potential to generate reactive oxygen species (ROS), including singlet oxygen, superoxide anions, and hydroxyl radicals within the bacterial cells (Levy et al., 2019). The ROS are highly reactive and can disrupt the macromolecular cellular components including proteins, lipids, and DNA resulting in detrimental effects on the bacterial cells. ROS attacks and damage critical cellular structures, leading to protein denaturation, lipid peroxidation, and DNA fragmentation (Zhao & Drlica, 2014). This multifaceted damage causes a breakdown in essential cellular functions, ultimately culminating in bacterial cell death.

Comprehensive understanding of the oxidative damage mechanism is integral to comprehending CQDs' antibacterial effectiveness. Researchers are deeply studying paths to fine-tune CQDs to promote their ROS generation, thereby improving their capacity of the bacterial cells to induce oxidative stress. By delving into the intricate details of the oxidative damage mechanism, CQDs are poised to provide a promising avenue in addressing antibiotic resistance and tackling bacterial infections.

5.7 PHOTOTHERMAL IMPACT

In the recent years, the photothermal effect is emerging as one remarkable mechanism that CQDs employ to eliminate bacterial pathogens. This mechanism is revolutionizing as it involves the ability of CQDs to harness light and convert them to thermal energy (Zhai et al., 2023), exerting precise, directed, and localized destruction to the bacterial cells. The CQD photothermal effect can be strongly dedicated to their notable optical properties primarily their strong photoluminescence. When exposed to specific wavelengths of light, the CQDs absorb photons and generate copious amount of heat energy (Anwar et al., 2019; Rawat et al., 2023). This photothermal conversion allows the CQDs to eliminate bacterial cells by selectively increasing the temperature that affects only the cells rather than the surrounding healthy tissues/environment. The elevated temperature has a profound effect on the bacterial cells like disruption of the integrity of the cell membrane, denaturation of vital proteins, and interference with cellular metabolic processes (Yu et al., 2023). These structural and functional damages impair bacterial growth and ultimately results in bacterial cell death. Compared to other methods, the photothermal effect has high level of precision and specificity, which is highly advantageous. Modulation of the wavelengths of the lights used and fine tuning the properties of CQDs enables the researchers to optimize the photothermal activity for efficient bacterial cell damage (Han et al., 2021). The photothermal potential of the CQDs should further be explored for its role in targeted fight against antibiotic resistance and bacterial infections.

5.8　DISRUPTION OF BACTERIAL CELLULAR AND *DNA/RNA STRUCTURE AND FUNCTION*

Bacterial cellular activities encompass a complex array of functions, from DNA replication and protein synthesis to cellular respiration and membrane integrity. CQDs, with their unique structural and chemical attributes, have shown a remarkable ability to intervene with and perturb these fundamental processes. This interference may lead to a cascade of disruptions that ultimately affect bacterial multiplication and survival. As discussed earlier, the CQDs interfere with the bacterial membrane which is the first line of defense in a bacterial cell. Once gaining entry into the bacterial cell, the CQDs affect the genetic components (DNA/RNA) of the cell (Rajendiran et al., 2019). Because of their nanoscale size and adaptable surface chemistry, CQDs have a variety of interactions with nucleic acids. For bacterial cells, this interaction may have a number of negative effects. Significantly, it has been noted that CQDs can cause oxidative stress and base pairing disruption, which can lead to damage to DNA and RNA. Lesions in the genetic material can result from the oxidation of DNA and RNA bases due to oxidative stress caused by CQDs. Furthermore, CQDs have the ability to obstruct transcription and DNA replication, the two critical processes that result in the disruption of the synthesis of the crucial genetic material (Zhang et al., 2015).

The effect of CQDs' actions on DNA and RNA is profound, as they disintegrate the genetic integrity and transcriptional processes essential for the bacterial survival and growth. This disturbance ultimately impairs the bacterial cell's ability to proliferate and function effectively. Understanding how CQDs affect the structure and functions of DNA and RNA is essential in the quest for innovative antibacterial solutions. Researchers are actively investigating these mechanisms to harness CQDs as agents that can specifically target the genetic material of bacterial cells, offering a potential approach to tackling bacterial infections and antibiotic resistance.

5.9　EFFECT ON PROTEIN ACTIVITY

One important aspect of the investigation into the complex antibacterial processes of Carbon Quantum Dots (CQDs) and how they affect bacterial cellular life activities is how much of an impact they have on bacterial protein activity. Bacterial cells store proteins, which control a number of vital processes. Because of their special characteristics, CQDs have been shown to obstruct these processes (Typas & Sourjik, 2015).

CQDs can disrupt protein activity through multiple mechanisms. One notable pathway is the denaturation of proteins induced by oxidative stress generated by CQDs. Oxidative stress can lead to the alteration of protein structures and loss of their biological activity. Additionally, CQDs can interfere with protein synthesis, hampering the production of critical bacterial proteins. This interference can result from disruptions in cellular processes, such as transcription and translation, all of which are essential for protein synthesis (Czarnecka et al., 2021). The impact of CQDs on protein activity has far-reaching consequences for bacterial cells. It can lead to dysfunction in key metabolic pathways, enzymatic processes, and regulatory functions. As a result, bacterial cells may experience impaired growth and survival.

Understanding the mechanisms through which CQDs influence protein activity is pivotal for developing innovative antibacterial strategies. Researchers are actively exploring these mechanisms to fine-tune CQDs as agents that can selectively target bacterial proteins, offering a promising approach to combat bacterial infections and tackle antibiotic resistance.

5.10   PERTURBATION OF CELL METABOLISM

The CQDs influence the bacterial cellular activities that dictate bacterial life, especially bacterial cell metabolism. Bacterial metabolism encompasses a complex network of biochemical reactions that are essential for energy production, growth, and overall cellular function. CQDs, with their exceptional properties, have been found to interfere with these metabolic processes, significantly affecting bacterial survival and proliferation (Zhao et al., 2022). CQDs employ several mechanisms to disrupt the bacterial cell mechanism. One primary pathway involves oxidative stress induced by CQDs, leading to the oxidation of key metabolites and enzymes critical for metabolic pathways. A reduction in energy production and metabolic malfunction may arise from this oxidative damage. Furthermore, CQDs have the ability to obstruct regulatory systems that govern bacterial metabolism and interfere with enzymatic activities. The impact of CQDs on cell metabolism has significant ramifications. A decrease in energy production and essential cellular building blocks caused by impaired metabolism can impede bacterial growth and general cell activity (Sun et al., 2022). CQDs have a substantial effect on the ability of bacterial cells to multiply and survive by interfering with metabolic pathways.

A deeper understanding of the pathways with which CQDs affect bacterial cell metabolism is instrumental in developing novel antibacterial strategies. Research studies are actively carried out to harness the potential of CQDs as antibacterial agents specifically targeting and offering a promising avenue to combat bacterial infections and address antibiotic resistance.

5.11   PROGRAMMED CELL DEATH

CQDs have the capability to induce programmed cell death in bacterial populations. Programmed cell death, or apoptosis, is a controlled and orchestrated process that leads to the demise of individual bacterial cells, thereby inhibiting bacterial growth and colonization (Li et al., 2022). The CQDs display the ability to induce programmed cell death in bacterial cells through a combined effect of oxidative stress and disruption of essential cellular functions (Singh et al., 2012). The oxidative stress generated by CQDs can trigger signaling pathways within the bacterial cells that initiate the process of apoptosis. This activates the apoptotic genes and releases enzymes that lead to the breakdown of cellular components. Furthermore, CQDs can interfere with crucial bacterial processes, such as DNA replication and protein synthesis, ultimately disrupting the bacterial life cycle. This interference contributes to the initiation of programmed cell death in bacterial populations. The induction of programmed cell death in bacterial cells is a significant antibacterial mechanism, as it effectively reduces bacterial growth and the risk of infection.

5.12 ANTIFUNGAL MECHANISMS OF CQDs

Carbon quantum dots exhibit promising antifungal properties through multifaceted mechanisms. The antifungal ability can be attributed to their unique physiochemical characteristics. The CQDs possess inherent photodynamic activity and generate ROS, which effectively damages the fungal cell wall. The CQDs affect the fungal cell wall structure causing the fungal cells to lose their fibrous structure causing membrane detachment. In a study by Zhao et al. (2021), CQDs generated from *Forsythia* were tested for their antifungal activity against wood rot fungi *Coriolus versicolor* and *Gloeophyllum trabeum*. The *in vivo* results indicate that the CQDs effectively inhibited *Gloeophyllum trabeum* than *Coriolus versicolor*. Disintegration of the chitinaceous cell wall occurs, displaying excellent antifungal activity, which is due to the amino groups present in the CQDs with positive charges, and the fungal cell wall is negatively charged, which effectively explains increased interaction. CQDs possess inherent photodynamic activity, generating reactive oxygen species (ROS) upon exposure to light, which effectively damages fungal cell membranes and biomolecules. CQDs can disrupt fungal cell walls through electrostatic interactions and induce apoptosis by triggering intracellular oxidative stress pathways. Moreover, CQDs can interfere with vital fungal metabolic processes, such as energy production and enzyme function, through interactions with cellular components (Le et al., 2022). These mechanisms collectively contribute to the antifungal efficacy of CQDs, making them promising candidates for combating fungal infections. N-doped CQDs derived from *Moringa oleifera* roots were tested for their antifungal and antioomycete activity. The test results revealed that the N-doped CQDs had a broad spectrum of antifungicidal activity against two phytopathogens, *Corynespora cassiicola* and *Phytophthora nicotianae*; the inhibitory rates were 82.8% and 75.3%, respectively, at 11 µL/mL N-CQDs. Similarly, an inhibitory efficiency of almost 100% was identified at 22 µL/mL (Wang et al., 2021). There are several studies on antifungal activity, but there is very little effort directed toward decoding the antifungal mechanisms. Fewer proven mechanisms are discussed (Figure 5.1).

5.13 ANTIVIRAL ACTIVITY OF CQDs

Infection of virus to living cells occurs in four stages: attachment, penetration, replication, and budding. CQDs combat viral infection by impeding attachment of the virus to the host, hampering virus penetration, hindering viral replication, and intercepting viral budding (Chen & Liang, 2020). Firstly, CQDs exhibit strong binding affinity toward viral particles, effectively preventing their attachment to host cells, thus inhibiting viral entry. CQDs derived from polyamine inhibit the white spot syndrome virus envelope (Huang et al., 2020). Furthermore, CQDs possess inherent photodynamic properties, allowing them to generate reactive oxygen species (ROS)

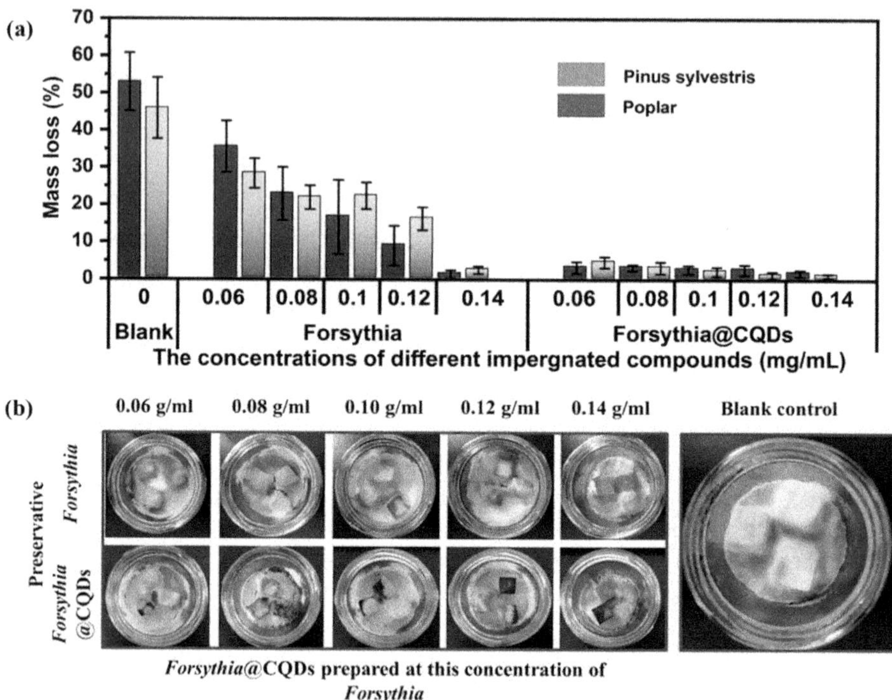

FIGURE 5.1 Forsythia wood blocks infected with *Gloeophyllum trabeum* and challenge with Forsythia CQDs with antifungal activity. (a) Weight loss rate of wood blocks of *Forsythia* and *Forsythia* @CQDs with different impregnation concentrations. (b) Digital photo of wood after 12 weeks of corrosion resistance test inoculated with *Gloeophyllum trabeum*.

upon exposure to light. These ROS can induce damage to viral capsids or envelopes, making the viruses non-infectious. Additionally, CQDs have been reported to modulate host immune responses by stimulating the production of antiviral cytokines and enhancing the activity of immune cells such as macrophages and natural killer cells, thereby bolstering the host's defense against viral infections. Moreover, the versatile surface chemistry of CQDs enables functionalization with antiviral agents or targeting ligands, further enhancing their efficacy and specificity against specific viral strains. Overall, the multifunctional antiviral mechanisms of CQDs make them promising candidates for the development of novel antiviral therapeutics with broad-spectrum activity and potential applications in combating viral outbreaks and pandemics.

5.14 ANTIBIOFILM ACTIVITY OF CQDs

Biofilms are a complex community of bacterial populations that adhere to each other and to biotic and abiotic surfaces by the self-produced matrix of extracellular polysaccharides (Zhang et al., 2020). The biofilms are more prevalent in environment, industries, hospitals, etc. The biofilm formation causes significant problems in water supply lines, food processing plants, food packaging industries, healthcare systems, manufacturing units, marine industries, and sanitation industries. Each industry suffers severe economic losses owing to the strenuous removal of the biofilms (Shineh et al., 2023). The waste water treatment plants suffer the most in terms of the cost involved. In medical and food industry, the biofilms cause severe morbidity and mortality. The biofilms are much resistant than their planktonic counterparts and are hard to remove. Removal of biofilms are highly challenging as the involvement of antibiotics and other chemicals leads to the development of antibiotic resistance (Gebreyohannes et al., 2019). Hence, novel materials are being developed and tested for their antibiofilm properties. CQDs are one addition to the extended list of choices for the eradication of the biofilms. CQDs stand as a beacon of hope, holding the potential to disrupt and inhibit the initial stages of biofilm development (Pabbati et al., 2021). CQDs, with their unique properties, introduce innovative strategies to combat this resilience. They act as disruptors at the very foundation of biofilm formation. This section discusses the antibiofilm mechanisms exerted by the CQDs.

5.15 INHIBITION OF BIOFILM FORMATION

The CQDs primarily inhibit biofilm formation by thwarting bacterial adhesion. The CQDs effectively compete for the surface to which the biofilm-forming bacteria is adhered, thus reducing the availability of spaces for bacterial adhesion. Biofilm formation involves five stages which are initial reversible attachment, microcolony formation, irreversible attachment, maturation, and dispersion (Alotaibi, 2021). The CQDs have the ability to hinder the initial reversible attachment. Bacterial adhesion followed by initial attachment is an important step as the biofilm build on the surfaces to which they firmly attach. CQDs with their distinctive attributes play a significant role in disrupting this process and preventing the establishment of biofilms. CQDs curtail the initial adhesion of bacteria, thereby impeding the foundation of biofilm formation. The competitive inhibition of the attachment surface by the CQDs reduces the availability of locations for bacterial aggregation (Desmau et al., 2020). Additionally, the CQDs have the ability to modify the surface characteristics of the substrates, making them less favorable for bacterial attachment. They modify the physicochemical properties of surfaces altering the surface charge and hydrophobicity of substrates, making them less favorable for bacterial adhesion. This alteration creates a less hospitable environment for bacteria, further hindering their attachment (Rani et al., 2020). CQDs show a profound impact against biofilms by quorum quenching, a molecular mechanism that inhibits quorum sensing, the signaling mechanism by which biofilms are formed (Singh et al., 2017). The inhibition of biofilm formation by CQDs holds wide promise in mitigating the consequences of biofilm-related issues. This approach, by impeding the foundational steps of biofilm development, provides an innovative strategy to tackle biofilms' adverse effects in diverse sectors. It not only offers potential solutions for healthcare-associated infections but also addresses challenges in the preservation of industrial equipment and water management systems. The CQDs exert antibiofilm activity at every stage of biofilm formation right from initial attachment to maturation.

5.16   INTERRUPTION OF QUORUM SENSING

Quorum sensing is the cell-population density-dependent bacterial gene regulation which corresponds to physiological expression. Biofilm formation occurs by quorum sensing. The bacterial cells produce and secrete extracellular signaling molecules called autoinducers. Once the autoinducers reach a threshold level, it induces the genes responsible for biofilm formation. This quorum sensing mechanism is pivotal for biofilm formation. Chemical or enzymatic degradation of the signals, the autoinducers is quorum quenching (Jeyakumar et al., 2024). CQDs with their unique physical, optical, and chemical properties are recently emerging as potent inhibitors of quorum sensing, quorum quenchers. They have the capacity to impede the signaling molecules significant to this communication process, thus impeding bacteria's ability to sense and respond to population density effectively. This results in faltering of bacterial coordination, rendering significantly less aggregation which leads to cohesive biofilm structures that pose significant challenges in various fields. The quorum quenching ability of the CQDs serves as a promising strategy for mitigation of the biofilms and biofilm-related issues (Cui et al., 2022).

5.17   ELIMINATION OF CONVENTIONAL BIOFILM

Bacterial cells that form biofilms undergo five typical stages of formation. When the final stage is achieved, a matured biofilm gets itself established in the conducive environment. Once the biofilm reaches the final stage, they become resilient and difficult to eradicate. CQDs with antibacterial activity kill the bacterial cells by various mechanisms, thus preventing the biofilm formation. By inducing bacterial cell death, CQDs thwart the growth and maturation of biofilm structures, preventing their establishment (Wang et al., 2019). CQDs' impact on biofilms is inherently mechanical. When CQDs are introduced into the biofilm matrix, mechanical destabilization of the matrix occurs. The infiltration creates fractures, breaking the intercellular bonds and weakening the structural integrity of the biofilm. This mechanical stress renders the biofilm more vulnerable to disintegration and removal (Shaikh et al., 2019). The CQDs generate ROS including singlet oxygen, superoxide anions, and hydroxyl radicals. These CQDs are highly reactive and they have the ability to infiltrate into the biofilm matrix by penetration. This oxidative stress damages the structural components of the biofilm and the resident bacterial cells (Li et al., 2023). The ROS generated by CQDs acts against mature microbial communities. CQDs affect the biofilm's integrity, disrupting the biofilm matrix and inflicting oxidative damage upon the embedded planktonic bacterial cells. This oxidative assault weakens the biofilm's defenses, rendering it susceptible to disintegration. The use of ROS for biofilm removal by CQDs introduces a potent and selective approach in the ongoing battle against well-established biofilms.

The CQDs obstruct the self-assembly of amyloid proteins within the biofilm matrix. Amyloid proteins are prime components of the extracellular matrix in certain biofilms, contributing to their structural integrity. CQDs, with their unique properties, introduce an innovative strategy to disrupt this self-assembly process and weaken the biofilm's structural stability. CQDs have been observed to interact with amyloid proteins, hindering their aggregation and self-assembly (Wang et al., 2019). While biofilm inhibition is critical, the eradication of pre-existing biofilms represents a more formidable challenge. CQDs, with their unique properties and multifaceted strategies, offer a glimmer of hope in this endeavor. This exploration delves into the intricate mechanisms CQDs employ to dismantle well-established biofilms, offering insights into how they may revolutionize biofilm management.

5.18 SUMMARY AND FUTURE PERSPECTIVES

In this comprehensive exploration of Carbon Quantum Dots' (CQDs) antimicrobial mechanisms, we have delved into their multifaceted roles in combating microbial challenges. CQDs, with their notable properties and versatility, offer innovative strategies in the realms of microbial infection control and biofilm management. Firstly, in the antibacterial domain, CQDs exhibit a remarkable array of mechanisms. They cause physical damage to bacterial structures, affecting cellular membranes and morphology. The positive surface charges, hydrophobic interactions, and particle size and morphology of CQDs play pivotal roles in these interactions. Furthermore, CQDs induce oxidative damage, disrupt bacterial cellular life activities, and stimulate programmed cell death, offering a diverse toolkit for combatting bacterial pathogens. They also demonstrate the capability of retaining the active structures of drug molecules, potentially revolutionizing drug delivery systems.

Carbon quantum dots (CQDs) possess antifungal properties by disrupting fungal cell membranes, inhibiting growth. Additionally, they exhibit antiviral activity by interfering with viral entry, replication, and release, primarily through interactions with viral surface proteins and nucleic acids. The small size of CQDs allows for efficient penetration into microbial cells, enhancing their efficacy as broad-spectrum antimicrobial agents. Their multifaceted mechanisms make CQDs promising candidates for combating fungal and viral infections, offering potential solutions in biomedical and environmental applications. In the context of antibiofilm mechanisms, CQDs tackle the resilient world of biofilms in several ways. They inhibit biofilm formation by hampering bacterial adhesion and interfering with quorum sensing. CQDs also contribute to the eradication of mature biofilms through physical action, the generation of reactive oxygen species (ROS), and the disruption of amyloid protein self-assembly.

5.19 CONCLUSION

In summary, carbon quantum dots emerge as potent and versatile agents in the ongoing battle against bacterial infections and biofilm-related challenges. Their multifaceted mechanisms offer a diverse range of strategies to address these issues. With continued research and innovation, the future holds exciting prospects for the use of CQDs in antibacterial and antibiofilm applications, paving the way for more effective, sustainable, and targeted solutions in the healthcare industry and beyond.

REFERENCES

Alavi, M., Jabari, E., & Jabbari, E. (2021). Functionalized carbon-based nanomaterials and quantum dots with antibacterial activity: A review. *Expert Review of Anti-Infective Therapy*, *19*(1), 35–44. https://doi.org/10.1080/14787210.2020.1810569

Alotaibi, G. F. (2021). Factors influencing bacterial biofilm formation and development. *American Journal of Biomedical Science & Research*, *12*(6), 617–626. https://doi.org/10.34297/AJBSR.2021.12.001820

Alshammari, G. M., Al-Ayed, M. S., Abdelhalim, M. A., Al-Harbi, L. N., Qasem, A. A., & Abdo Yahya, M. (2023). Development of luminescence carbon quantum dots for metal ions detection and photocatalytic degradation of organic dyes from aqueous media. *Environmental Research*, *226*, 115661. https://doi.org/10.1016/j.envres.2023.115661

Amaning Danquah, C., Minkah, P. A. B., Osei Duah Junior, I., Amankwah, K. B., & Somuah, S. O. (2022). Antimicrobial compounds from microorganisms. *Antibiotics*, *11*(3), 285. https://doi.org/10.3390/antibiotics11030285

Anwar, S., Ding, H., Xu, M., Hu, X., Li, Z., Wang, J., Liu, L., Jiang, L., Wang, D., Dong, C., Yan, M., Wang, Q., & Bi, H. (2019). Recent advances in synthesis, optical properties, and biomedical applications of carbon dots. *ACS Applied Bio Materials*, *2*(6), 2317–2338. https://doi.org/10.1021/acsabm.9b00112

Chen, L., & Liang, J. (2020). An overview of functional nanoparticles as novel emerging antiviral therapeutic agents. *Materials Science and Engineering: C*, *112*, 110924. https://doi.org/10.1016/j.msec.2020.110924

Cui, F., Li, T., Wang, D., Yi, S., Li, J., & Li, X. (2022). Recent advances in carbon-based nanomaterials for combating bacterial biofilm-associated infections. *Journal of Hazardous Materials*, *431*, 128597. https://doi.org/10.1016/j.jhazmat.2022.128597

Czarnecka, J., Kwiatkowski, M., Wiśniewski, M., & Roszek, K. (2021). Protein corona hinders N-CQDs oxidative potential and favors their application as nanobiocatalytic system. *International Journal of Molecular Sciences*, *22*(15), 8136. https://doi.org/10.3390/ijms22158136

Desmau, M., Levard, C., Vidal, V., Ona-Nguema, G., Charron, G., Benedetti, M. F., & Gélabert, A. (2020). How microbial biofilms impact the interactions of Quantum Dots with mineral surfaces? *NanoImpact*, *19*, 100247. https://doi.org/10.1016/j.impact.2020.100247

Gebreyohannes, G., Nyerere, A., Bii, C., & Sbhatu, D. B. (2019). Challenges of intervention, treatment, and antibiotic resistance of biofilm-forming microorganisms. *Heliyon*, *5*(8), e02192. https://doi.org/10.1016/j.heliyon.2019.e02192

Ghirardello, M., Ramos-Soriano, J., & Galan, M. C. (2021). Carbon dots as an emergent class of antimicrobial agents. *Nanomaterials*, *11*(8), 1877. https://doi.org/10.3390/nano11081877

Han, G., Zhao, J., Zhang, R., Tian, X., Liu, Z., Wang, A., Liu, R., Liu, B., Han, M., Gao, X., & Zhang, Z. (2019). Membrane-Penetrating carbon quantum dots for imaging nucleic acid structures in live organisms. *Angewandte Chemie*, *131*(21), 7161–7165. https://doi.org/10.1002/ange.201903005

Han, Q., Lau, J. W., Do, T. C., Zhang, Z., & Xing, B. (2021). Near-Infrared light brightens bacterial disinfection: recent progress and perspectives. *ACS Applied Bio Materials*, *4*(5), 3937–3961. https://doi.org/10.1021/acsabm.0c01341

Hao, X., Huang, L., Zhao, C., Chen, S., Lin, W., Lin, Y., Zhang, L., Sun, A., Miao, C., Lin, X., Chen, M., & Weng, S. (2021a). Antibacterial activity of positively charged carbon quantum dots without detectable resistance for wound healing with mixed bacteria infection. *Materials Science and Engineering: C*, *123*, 111971. https://doi.org/10.1016/j.msec.2021.111971

Hao, X., Huang, L., Zhao, C., Chen, S., Lin, W., Lin, Y., Zhang, L., Sun, A., Miao, C., Lin, X., Chen, M., & Weng, S. (2021b). Antibacterial activity of positively charged carbon quantum dots without detectable resistance for wound healing with mixed bacteria infection. *Materials Science and Engineering: C*, *123*, 111971. https://doi.org/10.1016/j.msec.2021.111971

Huang, H.-T., Lin, H.-J., Huang, H.-J., Huang, C.-C., Lin, J. H.-Y., & Chen, L.-L. (2020). Synthesis and evaluation of polyamine carbon quantum dots (CQDs) in *Litopenaeus vannamei* as a therapeutic agent against WSSV. *Scientific Reports, 10*(1), 7343. https://doi.org/10.1038/s41598-020-64325-5

Jeyakumar, S. P., Tamilvendan, K., Kumar, M. K. P., Reddy, Y. N., Earanna, N., & Biplab, D. (2024). Stopping not till the rot rots: Quorum quenching as a biocontrol method for soft rot control in agriculture. *Biocatalysis and Agricultural Biotechnology, 57*, 103098. https://doi.org/10.1016/j.bcab.2024.103098

Le, N., Zhang, M., & Kim, K. (2022). Quantum dots and their interaction with biological systems. *International Journal of Molecular Sciences, 23*(18), 10763. https://doi.org/10.3390/ijms231810763

Levy, M., Chowdhury, P. P., & Nagpal, P. (2019). Quantum dot therapeutics: A new class of radical therapies. *Journal of Biological Engineering, 13*(1), 48. https://doi.org/10.1186/s13036-019-0173-4

Li, J., Mao, X., Lu, X., & Feng, J. (2022a). Bacterial programmed cell death. In *Stress Responses of Foodborne Pathogens* (pp. 537–547). Springer International Publishing. https://doi.org/10.1007/978-3-030-90578-1_19

Li, P., Yang, X., Zhang, X., Pan, J., Tang, W., Cao, W., Zhou, J., Gong, X., & Xing, X. (2020). Surface chemistry-dependent antibacterial and antibiofilm activities of polyamine-functionalized carbon quantum dots. *Journal of Materials Science, 55*(35), 16744–16757. https://doi.org/10.1007/s10853-020-05262-6

Li, P., Yu, M., Ke, X., Gong, X., Li, Z., & Xing, X. (2022b). Cytocompatible amphipathic carbon quantum dots as potent membrane-active antibacterial agents with low drug resistance and effective inhibition of biofilm formation. *ACS Applied Bio Materials, 5*(7), 3290–3299. https://doi.org/10.1021/acsabm.2c00292

Li, Q., Shen, X., & Xing, D. (2023). Carbon quantum dots as ROS-generator and -scavenger: A comprehensive review. *Dyes and Pigments, 208*, 110784. https://doi.org/10.1016/j.dyepig.2022.110784

Ljungh, Å., Yanagisawa, N., & Wadström, T. (2006). Using the principle of hydrophobic interaction to bind and remove wound bacteria. *Journal of Wound Care, 15*(4), 175–180. https://doi.org/10.12968/jowc.2006.15.4.26901

Pabbati, R., Aerupula, M., Shaik, F., & Kondakindi, V. R. (2021). *Nanoparticles for Biofilm Control* (pp. 227–247). https://doi.org/10.1007/978-981-15-9916-3_9

Pagán, R., & Mackey, B. (2000). Relationship between membrane damage and cell death in pressure-treated *Escherichia coli* cells: Differences between exponential- and stationary-phase cells and variation among strains. *Applied and Environmental Microbiology, 66*(7), 2829–2834. https://doi.org/10.1128/AEM.66.7.2829-2834.2000

Rajendiran, K., Zhao, Z., Pei, D.-S., & Fu, A. (2019). Antimicrobial activity and mechanism of functionalized quantum dots. *Polymers, 11*(10), 1670. https://doi.org/10.3390/polym11101670

Rani, U. A., Ng, L. Y., Ng, C. Y., & Mahmoudi, E. (2020). A review of carbon quantum dots and their applications in wastewater treatment. *Advances in Colloid and Interface Science, 278*, 102124. https://doi.org/10.1016/j.cis.2020.102124

Rawat, P., Nain, P., Sharma, S., Sharma, P. K., Malik, V., Majumder, S., Verma, V. P., Rawat, V., & Rhyee, J. S. (2023). An overview of synthetic methods and applications of photoluminescence properties of carbon quantum dots. *Luminescence, 38*(7), 845–866. https://doi.org/10.1002/bio.4255

Saadh, M. J., Al-dolaimy, F., Alamir, H. T. A., Kadhim, O., Al-Abdeen, S. H. Z., Sattar, R., Jabbar, A. Mhussan, Kadhem Abid, M., Jetti, R., Alawadi, A., & Alsalamy, A. (2024). Emerging pathways in environmentally friendly synthesis of carbon-based quantum dots for exploring antibacterial resistance. *Inorganic Chemistry Communications, 161*, 112012. https://doi.org/10.1016/j.inoche.2023.112012

Shaikh, A. F., Tamboli, M. S., Patil, R. H., Bhan, A., Ambekar, J. D., & Kale, B. B. (2019). Bioinspired carbon quantum dots: An antibiofilm agents. *Journal of Nanoscience and Nanotechnology*, *19*(4), 2339–2345. https://doi.org/10.1166/jnn.2019.16537

Shineh, G., Mobaraki, M., Perves Bappy, M. J., & Mills, D. K. (2023). Biofilm formation, and related impacts on healthcare, food processing and packaging, industrial manufacturing, marine industries, and sanitation–A review. *Applied Microbiology*, *3*(3), 629–665. https://doi.org/10.3390/applmicrobiol3030044

Singh, A. K., Prakash, P., Singh, R., Nandy, N., Firdaus, Z., Bansal, M., Singh, R. K., Srivastava, A., Roy, J. K., Mishra, B., & Singh, R. K. (2017). Curcumin quantum dots mediated degradation of bacterial biofilms. *Frontiers in Microbiology*, *8*. https://doi.org/10.3389/fmicb.2017.01517

Singh, B. R., Singh, B. N., Khan, W., Singh, H. B., & Naqvi, A. H. (2012). ROS-mediated apoptotic cell death in prostate cancer LNCaP cells induced by biosurfactant stabilized CdS quantum dots. *Biomaterials*, *33*(23), 5753–5767. https://doi.org/10.1016/j.biomaterials.2012.04.045

Stan, D., Enciu, A.-M., Mateescu, A. L., Ion, A. C., Brezeanu, A. C., Stan, D., & Tanase, C. (2021). Natural compounds with antimicrobial and antiviral effect and nanocarriers used for their transportation. *Frontiers in Pharmacology*, *12*. https://doi.org/10.3389/fphar.2021.723233

Strahl, H., & Errington, J. (2017). Bacterial membranes: Structure, domains, and function. *Annual Review of Microbiology*, *71*(1), 519–538. https://doi.org/10.1146/annurev-micro-102215-095630

Sun, B., Wu, F., Zhang, Q., Chu, X., Wang, Z., Huang, X., Li, J., Yao, C., Zhou, N., & Shen, J. (2021). Insight into the effect of particle size distribution differences on the antibacterial activity of carbon dots. *Journal of Colloid and Interface Science*, *584*, 505–519. https://doi.org/10.1016/j.jcis.2020.10.015

Sun, Y., Zhang, M., Bhandari, B., & Yang, C. (2022). Recent development of carbon quantum dots: biological toxicity, antibacterial properties and application in foods. *Food Reviews International*, *38*(7), 1513–1532. https://doi.org/10.1080/87559129.2020.1818255

Tarín-Pelló, A., Suay-García, B., & Pérez-Gracia, M.-T. (2022). Antibiotic resistant bacteria: current situation and treatment options to accelerate the development of a new antimicrobial arsenal. *Expert Review of Anti-Infective Therapy*, *20*(8), 1095–1108. https://doi.org/10.1080/14787210.2022.2078308

Travlou, N. A., Giannakoudakis, D. A., Algarra, M., Labella, A. M., Rodríguez-Castellón, E., & Bandosz, T. J. (2018). S- and N-doped carbon quantum dots: Surface chemistry dependent antibacterial activity. *Carbon*, *135*, 104–111. https://doi.org/10.1016/j.carbon.2018.04.018

Typas, A., & Sourjik, V. (2015). Bacterial protein networks: properties and functions. *Nature Reviews Microbiology*, *13*(9), 559–572. https://doi.org/10.1038/nrmicro3508

Varghese, M., & Balachandran, M. (2021). Antibacterial efficiency of carbon dots against Gram-positive and Gram-negative bacteria: A review. *Journal of Environmental Chemical Engineering*, *9*(6), 106821. https://doi.org/10.1016/j.jece.2021.106821

Varisco, M., Zufferey, D., Ruggi, A., Zhang, Y., Erni, R., & Mamula, O. (2017). Synthesis of hydrophilic and hydrophobic carbon quantum dots from waste of wine fermentation. *Royal Society Open Science*, *4*(12), 170900. https://doi.org/10.1098/rsos.170900

Wang, H., Song, Z., Gu, J., Li, S., Wu, Y., & Han, H. (2019b). Nitrogen-Doped carbon quantum dots for preventing biofilm formation and eradicating drug-resistant bacteria infection. *ACS Biomaterials Science & Engineering*, *5*(9), 4739–4749. https://doi.org/10.1021/acsbiomaterials.9b00583

Wang, Y., Kadiyala, U., Qu, Z., Elvati, P., Altheim, C., Kotov, N. A., Violi, A., & VanEpps, J. S. (2019a). Anti-Biofilm activity of graphene quantum dots *via* self-assembly with bacterial amyloid proteins. *ACS Nano*, *13*(4), 4278–4289. https://doi.org/10.1021/acsnano.8b09403

Wang, Z., Liu, Q., Leng, J., Liu, H., Zhang, Y., Wang, C., An, W., Bao, C., & Lei, H. (2021). The green synthesis of carbon quantum dots and applications for sulcotrione detection and anti-pathogen activities. *Journal of Saudi Chemical Society*, *25*(12), 101373. https://doi.org/10.1016/j.jscs.2021.101373

Wu, X., Han, J., Gong, G., Koffas, M. A. G., & Zha, J. (2021). Wall teichoic acids: physiology and applications. *FEMS Microbiology Reviews*, *45*(4). https://doi.org/10.1093/femsre/fuaa064

Xu, X., Ray, R., Gu, Y., Ploehn, H. J., Gearheart, L., Raker, K., & Scrivens, W. A. (2004). Electrophoretic analysis and purification of fluorescent single-walled carbon nanotube fragments. *Journal of the American Chemical Society*, *126*(40), 12736–12737. https://doi.org/10.1021/ja040082h

Yu, M., Li, P., Huang, R., Xu, C., Zhang, S., Wang, Y., Gong, X., & Xing, X. (2023). Antibacterial and antibiofilm mechanisms of carbon dots: a review. *Journal of Materials Chemistry B*, *11*(4), 734–754. https://doi.org/10.1039/D2TB01977A

Zhai, Z., Dong, X., Qi, H., Tao, R., & Zhang, P. (2023). Carbon quantum dots with high photothermal conversion efficiency and their application in photothermal modulated reversible deformation of Poly(*N* -isopropylacrylamide) hydrogel. *ACS Applied Bio Materials*, *6*(9), 3395–3405. https://doi.org/10.1021/acsabm.3c00046

Zhang, K., Li, X., Yu, C., & Wang, Y. (2020). Promising therapeutic strategies against microbial biofilm challenges. *Frontiers in Cellular and Infection Microbiology*, *10*. https://doi.org/10.3389/fcimb.2020.00359

Zhang, T., Wang, Y., Kong, L., Xue, Y., & Tang, M. (2015). Threshold dose of three types of quantum dots (QDs) induces oxidative stress triggers DNA damage and apoptosis in mouse fibroblast L929 cells. *International Journal of Environmental Research and Public Health*, *12*(10), 13435–13454. https://doi.org/10.3390/ijerph121013435

Zhao, C., Wang, X., Yu, L., Wu, L., Hao, X., Liu, Q., Lin, L., Huang, Z., Ruan, Z., Weng, S., Liu, A., & Lin, X. (2022). Quaternized carbon quantum dots with broad-spectrum antibacterial activity for the treatment of wounds infected with mixed bacteria. *Acta Biomaterialia*, *138*, 528–544. https://doi.org/10.1016/j.actbio.2021.11.010

Zhao, X., & Drlica, K. (2014). Reactive oxygen species and the bacterial response to lethal stress. *Current Opinion in Microbiology*, *21*, 1–6. https://doi.org/10.1016/j.mib.2014.06.008

Zhao, X., Wang, L., Ren, S., Hu, Z., & Wang, Y. (2021). One-pot synthesis of Forsythia@carbon quantum dots with natural anti-wood rot fungus activity. *Materials & Design*, *206*, 109800. https://doi.org/10.1016/j.matdes.2021.109800

Section II

Applications

6 Antioxidant Properties and UV-blocking of Carbon Quantum Dots in Food Packaging Applications

Zohreh Riahi, Alireza Kaviani, Ajahar Khan,
Gholamreza Pircheraghi and Jun Tae Kim

6.1 INTRODUCTION

Each year, a substantial quantity of food is lost within the supply chain. The reports indicate that approximately 60% of this loss could be avoided. The primary factors contributing to food spoilage are oxidation, microbial contamination, exposure to light, undesirable moisture levels, excessive ethylene presence, and inadequate temperature control (Riahi, Hong, Rhim, Shin, & Kim, 2023a). Effective food packaging is crucial for reducing food wastage throughout storage and distribution processes (Jung et al., 2020). Active packaging involves the deliberate incorporation of active constituents with the capacity to absorb or release substances within the packaged food or its surrounding environment. This process aims to uphold the quality, sensory properties, and safety of the food product (Ahmed et al., 2022). For example, the active component may serve as a scavenger to absorb residual oxygen, water vapor, and ethylene or alternatively act as an emitter to release carbon dioxide/ethanol or provide UV-shielding and gas barrier capabilities. Hence, active packaging systems significantly contribute to mitigating food wastage (Roopa et al., 2023). Various active compounds, encompassing natural plant extracts, food-derived sources, essential oils, and nanomaterials, are utilized in the fabrication of such active packaging systems (Riahi, Khan, Rhim, Shin, & Kim, 2023b). At present, nanocomposite food packaging technology utilizing nanomaterials stands as one of the forefront areas within the food industry (Garcia, Shin, & Kim, 2018). In the last few years, carbon dots (CDs) have emerged as active additives for packaging films, addressing the requirements of food safety applications (Khan, Riahi, Tae Kim, & Rhim, 2024). These particles exhibit distinctive characteristics, including photoinduced electron transfer, pronounced absorption within the blue and UV spectra, adjustable photoluminescence, fluorescence sensing capabilities, photocatalytic activity, biocompatibility, notable chemical stability, straightforward functionalization, and antioxidant as well as antimicrobial attributes (Khan, Ezati, Kim, & Rhim, 2023a). CDs have demonstrated the ability to scavenge reactive oxygen species (ROS), including hydroxyl radicals, superoxide anions, nitric oxide, and peroxynitrite, in both extracellular and intracellular environments through mechanisms involving adduct formation, hydrogen donation, and electron transfer (Moradi, Molaei, Kousheh, T. Guimarães, & McClements, 2023). Furthermore, CDs have garnered significant interest as ultraviolet (UV) absorbers due to their exceptional UV absorption capabilities and high visible transmittance rates, stemming from their particle sizes being less than 10 nm. These characteristics are anticipated to revolutionize traditional UV absorbers (Hu et al., 2019). The antioxidative and UV-blocking efficacy of carbon dots in packaging materials has been documented in several investigations (Ezati, Priyadarshi, & Rhim, 2022; Kousheh, Moradi, Tajik, & Molaei, 2020; Linlin Zhao, Zhang, Mujumdar, & Wang, 2023). This chapter presents insights into the antioxidative and UV-blocking characteristics of carbon dots, elucidating their mechanisms of action, followed by an overview of their application in food packaging technology. In the end, the challenges and future recommendations of carbon dots as an active filler of packaging materials are briefly discussed.

6.2 ANTIOXIDANT ACTIVITY OF CARBON DOTS

Free radicals are molecules characterized by a highly reactive nature due to the presence of unpaired electrons (Gómez-Estaca, López-de-Dicastillo, Hernández-Muñoz, Catalá, & Gavara, 2014). In the realm of food, the generation of free radicals can occur through different processes, including exposure to oxygen, light, heat, metal ions, as well as during food processing and storage (Meitha, Pramesti, & Suhandono, 2020). It is recognized that reactive oxygen species (ROS), encompassing singlet oxygen ($^1O_2$) and various free radicals (such as hydrogen peroxide ($HO_2^{\cdot}$), hydroxyl ($^{\cdot}OH$), and superoxide ($O_2^{\cdot-}$) radicals), exert a significant influence on food spoilage, degradation of polymers and chemical products, and deterioration of biological structures (Linlin Zhao et al., 2023).

The initiation stage of food oxidation commences with the abstraction of hydrogen atoms by free radicals from vulnerable compounds within foods, such as unsaturated fatty acids, resulting in the generation of lipid radicals. Following the formation of lipid radicals, they undergo reaction with oxygen to generate peroxy radicals. These peroxy radicals can subsequently initiate a cascade of lipid oxidation by further attacking other unsaturated fatty acids. Throughout the propagation stage, lipid oxidation reactions generate a range of secondary products, including hydroperoxides, which have the potential to decompose into volatile compounds, contributing to undesirable flavors and odors in food products (Shahidi & Zhong, 2010). Lipid oxidation has the potential to degrade food quality, causing alterations in attributes such as color, flavor, texture, and nutritional composition and rendering the product unsuitable for human consumption. The odors and rancid flavors are correlated with the existence of volatile oxidation by-products produced during the process of lipid oxidation. This phenomenon is evident in nuts, vegetable and fish oils, as well as meat or fish products that are treated or processed with preservation techniques aimed at minimizing microbial proliferation (Gómez-Estaca et al., 2014). The lipid oxidation process persists until it is halted by either the elimination of free radicals or the consumption of antioxidants (Othón-Díaz et al., 2023). Therefore, free radical scavengers or antioxidants play a crucial role in various domains, such as cosmetics, health, food science, packaging, and other related fields (Jia, Wu, & Kang, 2023). Specifically, food items containing high levels of lipids, particularly those with a high degree of unsaturation, are prone to degradation via this mechanism. Currently, the consumer demand for food products that are healthier and safer has stimulated research into innovative preservation methods.

Various strategies have been implemented to mitigate lipid oxidation, including the direct incorporation of antioxidants into food matrices or the development of appropriate packaging technologies. The direct incorporation of antioxidants into food products is the most commonly employed approach currently due to its cost-effectiveness and practicality. However, two limitations exist with this strategy: firstly, antioxidants may experience diminished or inhibited activity as a result of interactions with food constituents during processing, and secondly, the quality of the food may deteriorate rapidly following the consumption of active compounds within the food (Mastromatteo, Mastromatteo, Conte, & Nobile, 2010). Regarding the packaging strategy, the combination of vacuum or modified-atmosphere packaging with high-barrier materials can restrict the ingress of oxygen. However, complete and efficient elimination is not always achieved due to residual oxygen present during packaging or its penetration from the external environment through the packaging material (Lopez-de-Dicastillo, Alonso, Catala, Gavara, & Hernandez-Munoz, 2010). Furthermore, certain food items like fresh red meat or specific fish products necessitate packaging with the presence of oxygen (Mastromatteo, Mastromatteo, Conte, & Del Nobile, 2010). To address these shortcomings, scientists have proposed active antioxidant packaging systems. This innovative approach in packaging technology involves integrating antioxidant agents into the packaging material to enhance the stability of food products susceptible to oxidation (Kuai et al., 2021).

Typical antioxidants employed in active packaging encompass natural compounds like tocopherols (vitamin E), ascorbic acid (vitamin C), polyphenols (derived from sources like green tea, grape seed extract, etc.), as well as synthetic antioxidants including butylated hydroxyanisole (BHA), butylated hydroxytoluene (BHT), and tertiary butylhydroquinone (TBHQ) (López-Pedrouso, Lorenzo, & Franco, 2022). Traditionally, synthetic food additive antioxidants like polyphenols, organophosphates, and thioester compounds have been utilized. However, concerns regarding their potential toxicity resulting from migration into food products have raised doubts about their continued application (Gómez-Estaca et al., 2014).

Recently, a range of carbon nanodots, including graphene quantum dots (GQDs), nitrogen-doped carbon dots, selenium-doped CDs, chlorine-doped GQDs, and nitrogen/sulfur co-doped CDs, have emerged as potential antioxidants for the elimination of ROS (Linlin Zhao et al., 2023). The researchers suggested that CDs derived from green sources have the potential to serve as antioxidants in applications such as cosmetics or food packaging in forthcoming endeavors. Plant-derived CDs by a hydrothermal synthesis method are commonly employed for the preparation of such sustainable antioxidant materials for food packaging purposes (Moradi et al., 2023).

Chunduri et al. (2016) fabricated CDs utilizing coconut shells as the carbon source through a hydrothermal approach. The DPPH (2,2-diphenyl-1-picrylhydrazyl) assay demonstrated the effective scavenging capability of the prepared CQDs against free radicals.

F. Li et al. (F. Li et al., 2017) prepared selenium-doped carbon quantum dots (Se-CQDs) via a hydrothermal method employing citric acid and selenocysteine. They demonstrated that Se-CQDs exhibited remarkable in vitro scavenging capacity against H_2O_2 and hydroxyl radicals ($\cdot$OH). Lin et al. (2019) fabricated CDs incorporating P^{3+} and Mn^{2+} via a microwave-assisted pyrolysis technique in an aqueous medium. The CDs exhibited antioxidant properties similar to ascorbic acid against DPPH, hydroxyl radicals, and superoxide anion radicals (Lin, Tsai, Dehvari, Huang, & Chang, 2019).

Plant waste (grapes and tea)-derived CDs are synthesized, and their antioxidant capacity was assessed in an aqueous environment using the DPPH assay and Folin-Coicalteau method (Murru, Badía-Laíño, & Díaz-García, 2020). Additionally, the peroxide value measurements illustrated that the incorporation of CDs derived from tea waste into mineral oil as an eco-friendly antioxidant agent resulted in enhanced oxidation stability.

Typically, various mechanisms operate independently or synergistically to facilitate radical scavenging: (i) Transfer of hydrogen from functional moieties. (ii) Electron transfer mechanism (ETM). ETM can be described using a donor-acceptor map, which shows the electron-donating and electron-accepting capabilities of molecules. (iii) Formation of radical adducts at sp^2 carbon sites. The abundance of sp^2-rich regions promotes the formation of adducts with radical species. These regions facilitate electron delocalization within the conjugated, graphene-like areas and neutralize radicals by creating a secondary adduct (Innocenzi & Stagi, 2023). Therefore, the antioxidant activity is influenced by factors such as the sp^2 hybrid carbon domain, electron transport, unpaired electrons produced by defects and vacancies, hydrogen donor action, charge transfer capacity, doping element type, and surface functional groups (Linlin Zhao et al., 2023). For example, Lin Zhao, Wang, and Li (2019) demonstrated that carbon dots synthesized under NaOH electrolysis conditions exhibited an increased abundance of active oxygen-containing groups, including carbonyl and hydroxyl groups. These functional groups can act as hydrogen donors for scavenging free radicals, thereby enhancing the antioxidant capacity of the carbon dots. Simultaneously, the defect states and charge transfer capacity of CDs were augmented, contributing to their amplified antioxidant potential. Besides, recent investigations have indicated that carboxyl groups and amino groups facilitate the removal of ROS from CDs, increasing their antioxidant ability (Kou et al., 2021). Ruiz et al. (2017) also demonstrated that CDs with a significant quantity of sp^2 hybrid carbon domains and robust hydrogen donor action exhibited enhanced efficacy in scavenging free radicals. The antioxidant efficiency of CDs was also correlated with the antioxidant ability of their precursors. Precursors possessing antioxidant capacity were more inclined to yield CDs with the ability to scavenge free radicals. Y. Li et al. (2021) documented that *Salvia miltiorrhiza* has been extensively investigated for its antioxidant properties. They showed the *Salvia miltiorrhiza*-derived CDs illustrated good antioxidant activity compared to the normal *Salvia miltiorrhiza* extract (M. Li, Feng, Liu, Wu, & Wang, 2021). Son, Park, and Jung (2021) devised

CDs utilizing tannic acid as a precursor. Their anti-aging and antioxidant efficacy was more than the strong antioxidant positive control materials (such as surpassed that of quercetin, L-ascorbic acid, and tannic acid).

In addition, the type of radicals [reactive nitrogen species (NO· and NO$_2$), hydroxyl radicals (·OH), and superoxide radical anions (O$_2$·)] is an important factor affecting the antioxidant capacity of CDs (Innocenzi & Stagi, 2023). Various carbon nanomaterials presented reactive nitrogen species (RNS) scavenging ability (Ferreira, Ni, Rosenkrans, & Cai, 2018). The scavenging activity is assessed by quantifying the radical concentration in solutions containing dots compared to a control lacking them. The standard molecule utilized for this objective is 1,1-Diphenyl-2-picrylhydrazyl radical (DPPH·). It is a stable, nitrogen-centered free radical wherein three benzene rings surround the nitrogen atom and possess two lone-pair electrons. Due to its electronic configuration, DPPH readily accepts a hydrogen radical (H·) to generate a stable DPPH-H complex (Ionita, 2021). The radical scavenging efficiency of DPPH is evaluated by quantifying the reduction in the Electronic Spin Resonance (ESR) signal produced by a free radical in the existence of the CDs or by using a simple detection method relying on UV-vis spectroscopy. UV-vis spectroscopy is a commonly used technique for evaluating the radical scavenging ability of CDs. In methanolic solution, DPPH· absorbs light in the visible spectrum, with a peak maximum of around 517 nm. As the concentration of CDs increases, the purple color of the DPPH solution gradually shifts to yellow, resulting in a decrease in the absorption band at 517 nm. This change is used to quantify the scavenging activity (Ionita, 2021). Scavenging activity against RNS has been documented for CDs synthesized from various sources, including *Thymus vulgaris*, date molasses (B. Das et al., 2014), natural extracts such as coriander leaves (Sachdev & Gopinath, 2015), green tea leaves (Murru et al., 2020), lutein (Yang et al., 2020), and grape pomace (Murru et al., 2020). The results confirmed a concentration-dependent behavior of CDs for radical neutralization. However, many of these studies lack the experimental details necessary for ensuring reproducibility and comprehensive characterization of the material. Moreover, the published research didn't provide sufficient insights for a comprehensive understanding of the process. The mechanism proposed for the potential radical scavenging activity involves hydrogen transfer from the surface groups of CDs to DPPH (Figure 6.1a). The presence of functional moieties such as carboxyls (-COOH), hydroxyls (-OH), and amines (-NH$_2$, -NH) facilitates the hydrogen transfer, leading to the reduction of DPPH· to DPPH-H. The unpaired electrons present on the surface of CDs can undergo delocalization through resonance within the aromatic domains or via rearrangement of chemical bonds (Figure 6.1b) (Innocenzi & Stagi, 2023).

CDs have demonstrated the ability to scavenge hydroxyl and superoxide radicals as well. OH radicals are potent oxidizing agents capable of rapidly deteriorating various organic molecules, leading to oxidative damage to DNA, lipids, and proteins. Hydroxyl radicals are recognized as primary contributors to oxidative stress within biological systems. The radical scavenging efficiency of CDs is assessed by measuring their capacity to mitigate the produced OH· in solution (Nimse & Pal, 2015). The OH· scavenging has been documented for numerous CDs with various structures and compositions. However, conducting a comprehensive comparison is challenging due

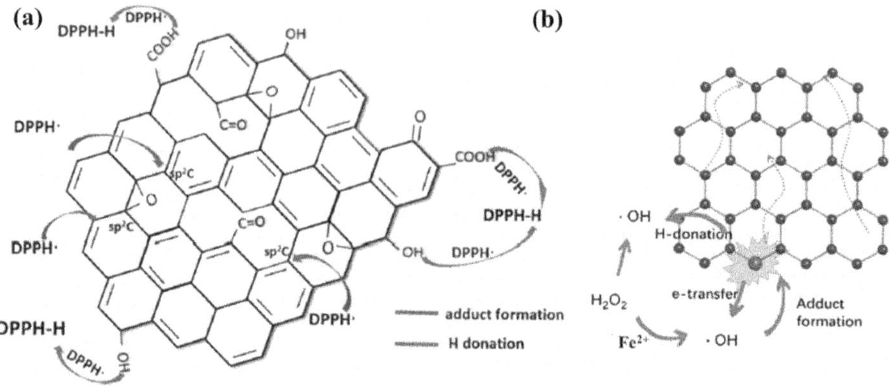

FIGURE 6.1　(a) The suggested mechanism for the interaction between GQDs and the DPPH radical, and (b) proposed pathway for the ·OH scavenging by Se-CDs at the active edge of selenium-doped sp^2-C (Innocenzi & Stagi, 2023).

to the diversity of testing protocols and the considerable variability in CD compositions documented in the literature (Innocenzi & Stagi, 2023).

The carbon dots have also been used to scavenge superoxide radical anions ($O_2^{·-}$), which are generated through the one-electron reduction of oxygen molecules (O_2). The presence of excess superoxide radical anions can expedite aging processes through the mechanism of lipid peroxidation (Innocenzi & Stagi, 2023). The literature regarding the $O_2^{·-}$ scavenging ability of CDs indicates comparatively lower efficacy against $O_2^{·-}$ in contrast to RNS and hydroxyl radicals (Qiu et al., 2014). Overall, they exhibit limited efficacy in reducing $O_2^{·-}$, with only a few exceptions. The $O_2^{·-}$ scavenging performance depends on the electron transfer ability of the system, and a proper design of the system and materials is necessary to reach optimum efficiency (Innocenzi & Stagi, 2023).

6.3　UV-BLOCKING PROPERTIES OF CARBON DOTS

Our daily food is subjected to both natural and artificial light sources throughout the food supply chain, encompassing stages such as harvesting, storage, transportation, processing, retailing, eateries, and consumption (Vijayakumar, Sivaraman, Pavagada Siddappa, & Dandu, 2022). Continuous exposure to light, particularly ultraviolet radiation, deteriorates food quality by photolysis and photooxidation processes. Consequently, the production of active oxygen and free radicals occurs, leading to the generation of undesirable odors and flavors, degradation of nutritional content, discoloration of food, and overall food deterioration (Pandiselvam et al., 2022). Another noteworthy characteristic of UV light, distinguishing it from visible light, is its ability to ionize molecules and instigate chemical reactions. Primarily, oxidation processes take place in food items rich in lipids or proteins, including bakery products, meat, fish, walnuts, almonds, nuts, dairy items, and wines. These types of food facilitate light-triggered autooxidation by augmenting the interfacial area between hydrophilic pro-oxidants and lipids (Skibsted, Risbo, & Andersen, 2010).

Ultraviolet radiation constitutes electromagnetic radiation within the wavelength range of 200–400 nm, possessing a shorter wavelength compared to visible light. Radiations within the ultraviolet spectrum can be categorized based on their wavelengths as UVC (200–280 nm), UVB (280–315 nm), and UVA (315–400 nm) (L. Wang et al., 2022). UV-A and UV-B radiation are deemed hazardous as they can penetrate the Earth's atmosphere, whereas UV-C radiation does not penetrate, rendering it less hazardous. Over recent decades, human-induced activities have contributed to the depletion of the ozone layer, resulting in increased exposure to ultraviolet radiation in the atmosphere (Marabini et al., 2020). At sea level, the substantial flux of UVA radiation ranges from approximately 35 to 50 W m^{-2}. Under these conditions, an exposure duration of approximately 1 hour results in an administered dose of about 200 kJ m^{-2}. Consequently, the production of harmful photoproducts may increase substantially, necessitating the implementation of effective strategies to mitigate losses attributed to UV-A radiation exposure during outdoor activities (Ezati et al., 2023). Figure 6.2a illustrates a schematic delineation of various classifications of ultraviolet radiation (UV-A, UV-B, and UV-C) along with their placement within the electromagnetic spectrum.

Therefore, there has been increasing concern regarding the photooxidation of food products induced by UV radiation. The occurrence of photooxidation in food products is contingent upon factors such as oxygen concentration, optical characteristics of packaging films, temperature, and duration of exposure to UV radiation (Krehula et al., 2017). Hence, the development of novel strategies to mitigate food spoilage is imperative. For this purpose, active food packaging incorporating UV-absorbing agents is employed to safeguard the food during its journey through the supply chain, shielding it from external factors like UV radiation. This approach aims to prolong the shelf life of foods by minimizing alterations in their physico-chemical properties, such as color, flavor, weight, bioavailability, texture, and moisture content (Ezati et al., 2023). Materials like aluminum foil, paper, brown glass bottles, and paperboard are recognized to attenuate UV radiation. However, there has been a significant demand for transparent packaging aimed at enhancing and distinguishing the visual appeal of packaged food products along with UV-blocking ability (Atta et al., 2022). Therefore, the UV protection-active packaging film consisting of a polymer matrix with a UV inhibitor filler is proposed (Channa et al., 2022).

Two types of commercially accessible UV absorbers are present: organic UV absorbers and inorganic UV absorbers (Uthirakumar, Devendiran, Kim, & Lee, 2018). Organic UV absorbers predominantly consist of compounds such as triazine, benzophenone, salicylic acid, benzotriazole, and various other organic compounds. The conjugated π-π* electronic systems are known as common features of these compounds, and most of them are soluble in oil. Two water-soluble commercially available types are 2-hydroxy-4-methoxy benzophenone-5-sulfonic acid (BP-4) and 2-phenylbenzimidazole-5-sulfonic acid (UV-T). This category of UV absorbers exhibits certain drawbacks, including a limited absorption spectrum, toxicity, and high cost. Inorganic UV absorbers primarily consist of metal oxides like zinc oxide, titanium dioxide, and other similar compounds. Additionally, this category of UV shielding agent exhibits limited compatibility with organic substances, posing challenges in its integration into polymer materials (Z. Xu et al., 2023).

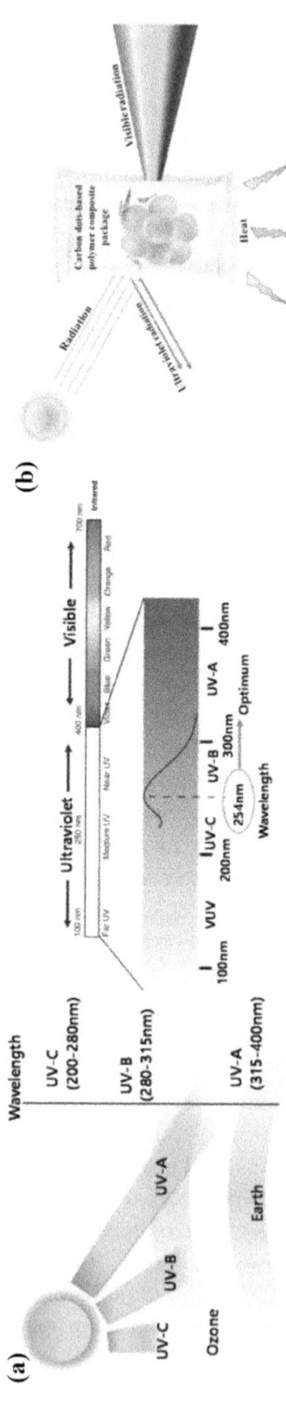

FIGURE 6.2 (a) Different categories of ultraviolet radiations (UV-A, UV-B, and UV-C) and their position in the electromagnetic spectrum (Ezati et al., 2023), and (b) mechanism of UV-barrier action of CDs-based nanocomposite polymeric films (Kumar & Gaikwad, 2023).

Interestingly, CDs have emerged as a notable anti-UV material in food packaging technology over the last couple of years (Tripathi, Kumar, Deshmukh, & Gaikwad, 2023). The straightforward synthesis methods and cost-effectiveness render CDs a promising alternative to conventional commercial UV absorbers (Hu et al., 2019). Although the exact UV-light blocking mechanism of CDs remains incompletely understood, some researchers attribute this property to various functional groups present on the surfaces of the CDs (Moradi et al., 2023). The absorption of UV light by CDs is facilitated by the transition of orbital electrons from n to π^* and/or π to π^* within the CD network. Here, the π and n states stem from the core sp^2 carbons and the functional groups containing lone-pair electrons, respectively (Chung, Kim, & Park, 2020). While CDs exhibit diverse structures, they present similar UV-visible absorption characteristics. Typically, a clear absorption peak observed in the UV region ranged from 260 nm to 320 nm, attributing to the electron transition from the π orbital to C=N bonds. Moreover, the absorption peak observed in the range of 280~350 nm is ascribed to electronic transitions from C–O or C=O bonds to the π^* orbital. The absorption peak wavelength within the range of 350~600 nm is ascribed to electron transitions of the surface functional moieties of CDs, suggesting the contribution of surface chemical moieties groups to the UV–visible absorption. Certain investigations suggest that the absorption peaks of CDs exhibit a red shift following the treatment of surface functional groups or modification of their sizes (Cui, Ren, Sun, Liu, & Xia, 2021). Moreover, certain unique CDs exhibit extended absorption ranges in the long-wavelength spectrum of 600–800 nm, arising from structures containing aromatic rings (Hola et al., 2017). As a result, the modulation of oxygen/nitrogen content, structural defects, and morphology significantly influences the absorption peak positions of CDs. Consequently, factors such as synthesis protocols, precursor selection, and surface modifications, including element doping, exert considerable impact on the light absorption characteristics of CDs (Cui et al., 2021).

Li et al. (2011) dispersed 4.0 g of active carbon in 70 mL of hydrogen peroxide to create a suspension, followed by sonication treatment for 2 hours at 25°C. The spherical fluorescent CDs (diameter: 5 to 10 nm) were collected after the filtration step. Their UV–vis absorption spectrum exhibited a peak in the 250~300 nm region, characteristic of an aromatic pi system. Wang et al. (2011) rapidly poured 0.5 g of anhydrous citric acid into an AEAPMS solution at 240°C under vigorous stirring, maintaining the temperature for 1 minute. Following natural cooling and purification steps, they successfully synthesized highly luminescent (diameter = ~0.9 nm and quantum yield=47%) amorphous carbon nanoparticles. In the UV–vis absorption spectrum of produced CDs, a prominent absorption peak was observed at 360 nm.

Dong et al. (2012) synthesized photoluminescent CDs through the carbonization process of citric acid at 200°C, resulting in nanosheet CDs with a width of approximately 15 nm and a thickness ranging from 0.5nm to 2.0 nm. Their absorption spectrum displayed a UV absorption peak at 362 nm with a narrow peak width, suggesting uniformity in nanoparticle size.

Tang et al. (2012) synthesized CDs with a diameter of 1.65 nm using microwave-assisted pyrolysis of glucose solution. The fluorescence quantum yield was measured to be 7%~10%. UV absorption analysis of the CDs in aqueous solution revealed two distinct peaks positioned at 228 and 282 nm.

Hence, the film consisting of CDs offers UV-blocking capabilities via excited-state intramolecular proton transfer facilitated by tunnels such as O...H...O, O...H...N, alongside extensive conjugated structures (Chung et al., 2020). Studies have also proved that CDs induce robust UV-absorbing properties to packaging film, allowing them to convert light energy by absorbing specific characteristic wavelengths. A conceivable UV barrier mechanism for the UV barrier effect of a polymer film loaded with CDs is depicted in Figure 6.2b. The considerable light reflection and scattering induced by CDs efficiently convert UV photon energy into heat, leading to energy dissipation due to the CDs' robust down-conversion properties.

6.4 APPLICATION OF ANTIOXIDANT AND UV-SHIELDING CHARACTERISTICS OF CARBON DOTS IN FOOD PACKAGING FILMS

In the field of food technology, CDs find predominant applications in detecting and quantifying pathogens, heavy metal ions, additives, antibiotics, pesticide residues, as well as nutritional and functional constituents. The fundamental operational principle of fluorescence sensors involves the interaction between the recognition element and the target analyte, leading to alterations in the fluorescence behavior of CDs. These changes are quantitatively correlated with the concentration or structure of the target analyte (Linlin Zhao et al., 2023). Lately, researchers have initiated investigations into the prospective applications of CDs for food preservation purposes. For this, CDs have been harnessed to pioneer novel technologies aimed at enhancing the freshness or extending the shelf life of food products, devising tools or methodologies for swift on-site analysis, and fabricating eco-friendly and functional food packaging solutions. Herein, we provide recent advancements in utilizing CDs for augmenting food packaging and preservation, focusing particularly on their UV-barrier and antioxidant effects. The outlined contents include (1) utilization in protective food packaging, (2) integration into intelligent packaging systems, (3) incorporation into coatings, and (4) utilization as nanoscale food additives to prolong the shelf life of food samples (Figure 6.3).

CDs can be easily integrated into polymer matrices to fabricate biocompatible packaging films or coatings. Two primary methods utilized for the fabrication of CD-based active films or coatings include solvent casting and absorption/coating methods. Examples of the utilization of carbon dots as active (antioxidant and anti-UV) filler for the development of sustainable active food packaging for shelf-life enhancement of various foods over the recent years are summarized in Table 6.1.

Riahi et al. (2022) synthesized chitosan-based CDs with multifunctional properties using a hydrothermal process. The CDs imparted strong antioxidant activity, showing 100% ABTS and 88% DPPH radical scavenging for the film with 5 wt% CD. Moreover, CMC/CD$^{5\%}$ demonstrated 100% UV-shielding properties. Fan et al. (2019) showed that kelp-derived CDs improved the quality of fresh stored cucumbers at 4°C. The chitosan coating with 4.5% CDs significantly reduced weight loss, prevented peroxidase activity and inhibited the growth of molds and yeasts during storage for 15 days. Das Purkayastha et al. (2014) investigated the impact of packaging rapeseed oil in

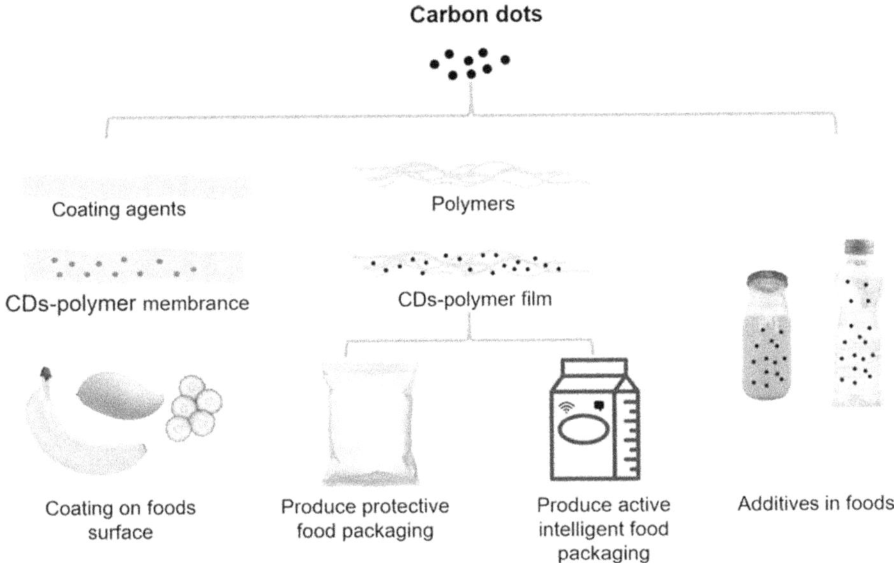

FIGURE 6.3 The utilization methods of carbon dots as an active filler (antioxidant, anti-UV) for food preservation purposes (Linlin Zhao et al., 2023).

composite film bags made from rapeseed protein and CDs on the oil's shelf life. After 28 days of storage, the oil samples in the rapeseed protein-CD bags showed significantly reduced oxidative rancidity compared to those in standard protein bags. The levels of thiobarbituric acid, free fatty acids, and peroxide values decreased to 2, 1.4, and 1.2 times, respectively. These findings demonstrate that composite packaging containing CDs can enhance the oxidative stability of lipid-rich foods during storage.

In another study, Das et al. (2021) found that polypropylene film integrated with nitrogen, phosphorous, and sulfur-doped (NPSC) carbon dots presented antioxidant activity. DPPH, hydroxyl, superoxide anion, and $KMnO_4$ are used to evaluate the radical scavenging capacity of NPSC. The antioxidant effectiveness of the NPSC dots displayed a concentration-dependent response across all free radicals, with the highest efficacy observed in scavenging DPPH radicals at 417 mg/mL NPSC dots, achieving a 74% activity level.

Min et al. (2022) engineered a gelatin/CD film characterized by potent antioxidant activity and UV-barrier capabilities, aiming to mitigate the degradation of food items susceptible to oxidative processes during storage. The film's antioxidant efficacy was contingent upon the concentration of carbon dots, as evidenced by substantial activity observed in both ABTS and DPPH assays. Notably, 100% ABTS and 72% DPPH neutralization were achieved with a concentration of 200 μg/mL of carbon dots derived from potato peels. The films loaded with 2 wt% CDs exhibited complete UV-shielding capability (100%), likely associated with the surface structural characteristics of CDs facilitating the elimination of free radicals. The pristine gelatin film demonstrated 27.4% and 1.8% scavenging activity against ABTS and DPPH assays, respectively, possibly due to the presence of antioxidant peptides inherent in gelatin (Table 6.1).

TABLE 6.1

Summary of Recently Reported Carbon Dot-based Active Packaging Materials for Food Preservation

Biopolymer Film	Functional Fillers	Food Type	Application	References
Carrageenan/sodium alginate	Garlic (Allium sativum) cloves-derived carbon dots	Sliced raw meat	UV-blocking, Antimicrobial, and antioxidant	Khan, Priyadarshi, Bhattacharya, & Rhim (2023c)
Polyvinyl alcohol	Carbon dots derived from banana paste	Banana, jujube, and fried meatballs	Antimicrobial, antioxidant, and UV-blocking	Linlin Zhao, Zhang, Mujumdar, Adhikari, & Wang (2022)
Cellulose nanofiber	Carbon dots and anthocyanins from *Brassica oleracea*	Pork, fish, and shrimp	Antimicrobial, antioxidant, UV barrier, and pH response	Wagh, Khan, Priyadarshi, Ezati, & Rhim (2023)
Cellulose nanofibers	Coffee grounds-based carbon dots	Minced pork	UV barrier, antioxidant, and antibacterial	Sul, Khan, & Rhim (2024)
Carrageenan	Coconut husk-lignin derived carbon dots	Milk	Antioxidant, UV barrier, antimicrobial, and pH response	Sangeetha et al. (2024)
Polyvinyl alcohol	Pseudomonas aeruginosa-derived carbon dots doped with sulfur	Pork meat and sliced apples	Antioxidant and UV shielding	Hong, Riahi, Shin, & Kim (2024)
Fish scale gelatin/ alginate dialdehyde	Carbon dots derived from pomelo peel waste	Strawberry	Antioxidant, UV resistance, and antimicrobial	Y. Li et al. (2023)
Chitosan	Egg-yolk-derived carbon dots	Litchi	Antioxidant, UV resistance, and antimicrobial	Su et al. (2023)
Casein/modified tragacanth gum	Milk permeate-derived carbon dots	Butter	UV barrier and antioxidant	Khoshkalampour, Ahmadi, Ghasempour, Lim, & Ghorbani, (2023a)
Gelatin/ dialdehyde persian gum	Carbon dots from grape leaves	Trout fish	Antioxidant, UV barrier, and antimicrobial	Khoshkalampour, Ghorbani, & Ghasempour, (2023b)
Cellulose nanofibers/ polyvinyl alcohol	Chitosan-derived carbon dots and anthocyanin extracted from the *Lycium ruthenicum* fruit	Shrimp	Antioxidant, UV barrier, antimicrobial, and pH response	Cheng et al., (2023)
Cellulose nanofiber/ pullulan	Zn-doped avocado-derived carbon dots	Breast chicken and tofu	Antioxidant, UV barrier, and antimicrobial,	Riahi, Khan, Rhim, Shin, & Kim (2024)

The incorporation of 2.0% and 4.0% CDs notably enhanced the scavenging capacity of the films to 99.2% and 99.6% in the ABTS assay and 72.8% and 93.6% in the DPPH assay. Based on the aforementioned findings, it is evident that the antioxidant efficacy of the films containing CDs was more pronounced when assessed using the ABTS method in comparison to the DPPH method. This discrepancy could be attributed to the higher swelling capacity of the gelatin film when immersed in an aqueous ABTS solution compared to a methanolic DPPH solution. The observed antioxidant effect of CDs may be attributed to the presence of surface functional moieties with free radicals scavenging ability.

The incorporation of enoki mushroom-derived carbon dots (mCDs) notably augmented the free radical scavenging capability of the gelatin/carrageenan film, thereby enhancing its antioxidant characteristics compared to the pristine gelatin/carrageenan film (Roy, Ezati, & Rhim, 2021). This heightened antioxidant efficacy may be attributed to the presence of surface hydroxyl groups on the mCDs. Furthermore, the film containing 5wt% mCDs exhibited a UV-blocking efficacy of 65%.

Salimi et al. (2021) formulated an optimized nanopaper utilizing bacterial nanocellulose (BNC). The process involved immersing the BNC paper in a solution of CDs at a concentration of 530 g/L for 14 hours at 30°C. This resulted in nanopaper characterized by exceptional UV-blocking capabilities and notable antibacterial efficacy. Analysis of the transmission spectrum revealed that the UV barrier performance of the CD-nanopaper surpassed 99% under the transmission spectrum below 410 nm.

L. Xu et al. (2020) fabricated a composite film comprising blue luminescent carbon quantum dots (CQDs), polyvinyl alcohol (PVA), and nanocellulosic (CNF) materials. This composite exhibited notable UV and infrared light-blocking capabilities, and light attenuation efficacy improved progressively with a higher CQD content. Wongrerkdee and Pimpang (2020) discovered that composite films composed of graphene quantum dots and PVA exhibited superior UV-blocking performance in comparison to both PVA glass and films.

Patil et al. (2020) employed a solvent casting technique to fabricate a luminescent, flexible, and highly transparent composite film consisting of PVA and waste tea residue carbon dots (WTR-CDs). Incorporating 3 mg of WTR-CDs into the polymer film resulted in the blocking of 20%–60% of UV-A (315–400 nm), 100% of UV-B (280–315 nm), and UV-C (230–280 nm). To assess the UV shielding efficacy of the PVA@WTR-CDs film, a fruit storage experiment was conducted. Following a 30-hour exposure to UV light, grapes covered with the PVA@WTR-CDs film remained unaffected, while those covered with conventional PVA film and uncovered grapes exhibited various degrees of shrinkage and color alteration.

N. Xu et al. (2021) synthesized both undoped carbon quantum dots (1-CQDs) and nitrogen-doped carbon quantum dots (2-CQDs) utilizing acorn cups as carbon sources. These dots were integrated with chitosan (CS) to collectively serve as UV absorbers for the functionalization of the PVA film. The resulting PVA/CS/1-CQDs films exhibited a transparency of 79.34% and a UV-A shielding ability of 83.58%. Conversely, the UV-A shielding ability of the PVA/CS/2-CQDs film reached 94.53%. Evidently, the presence of nitrogen-doped CQDs conferred the composite film with enhanced UV barrier performance.

Riahi et al. (2024) dispersed zinc-doped carbon dots derived from the avocado peel (Zn-ACDs) in cellulose nanofibers/pullulan polymer matrix to prepare a packaging film. The polymer film with 5 wt% Zn-ACDs had 100% UV-blocking ability and excellent antioxidant activity (100.0% for ABTS and 68.0% for DPPH). In another study, Khan et al. (2024) proposed carrageenan-based active/intelligent packaging films containing anthocyanin and ZnO-doped CD (Zn-CD) from purple Kohlrabi peels. The films showed excellent UV blocking ability (85.2% of UV-A and 99.4% of UV-B) and a high antioxidant effect (~99% for ABTS and ~ 58.6% for DPPH radical scavenging activity). The active packaging experiments of shrimp demonstrated that the Car/KA@Zn-CD films extended the shelf life and maintained the quality of the packaged shrimp. Khan et al. (2023c) fabricated garlic (*Allium sativum*) cloves-derived carbon dots (CDs) with high-efficiency UV absorbance to fabricate carrageenan/sodium alginate (Car/Alg)-based functional films for UV-barrier food packaging. The Car/Alg-CD$^{4\%}$ film exhibited excellent UV-blocking properties (~85.1% in the UV-A and 99.0% in the UV-B). In addition, CD-incorporated Car/Alg films showed high antioxidant activity as determined by ABTS (98.6%±0.3%) and DPPH (34.2%±0.3%) free radical scavenging methods. When used for UV protection packaging of raw meat, the functional film could preserve the meat color even when directly exposed to UV light for 30 h (Figure 6.4a).

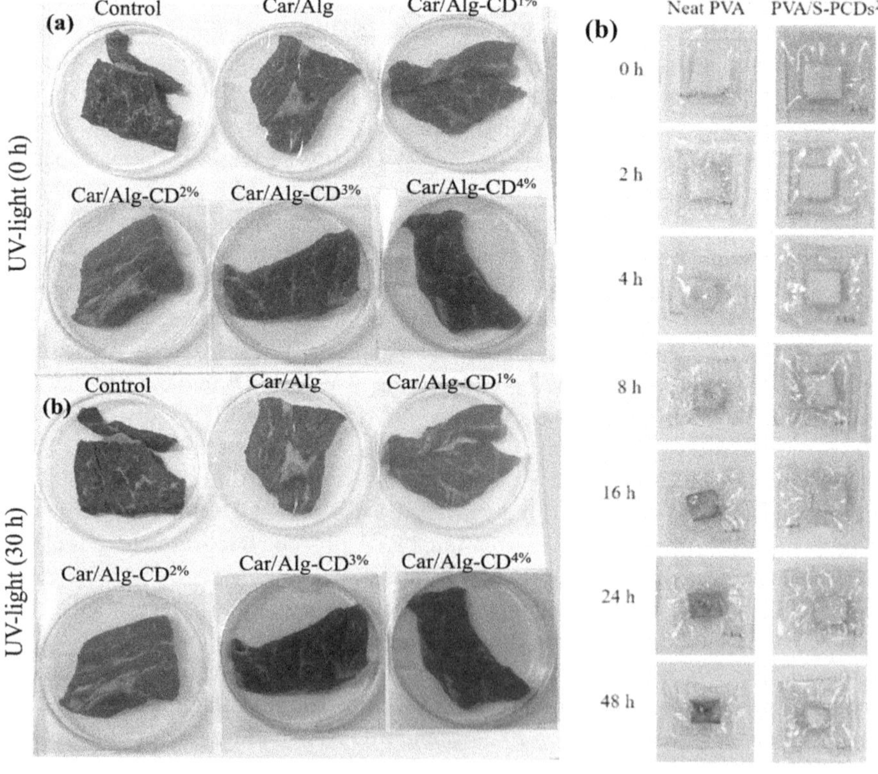

FIGURE 6.4　(a) Digital images of red meat covered with Car/Alg-based films after 30 h exposure to UV-light at 20°C (Khan, Priyadarshi, et al., 2023c), and (b) visual appearance alternation of fresh-cut apple packed with pure PVA and PVA/S-PCDs$^{2\%}$ films sorted for 48 h at room temperature (Hong et al., 2024).

Nitrogen, phosphorus-doped green-tea-derived carbon dots (NP-CDs)-incorporated chitosan/starch (Chi/St)-based multifunctional nanocomposite films were prepared by Khan et al. (2023b). The Chi/St-CD$^{3\%}$ film blocked almost 93.1% of UV-A and ~99.7% of UV-B radiation and exhibited a high antioxidant capacity of about 97.9% for ABTS and 71.4% for DPPH radicals. They stated that the as-prepared films prolonged the storage time of the meat samples due to the high UV-blocking, antioxidant, and antibacterial functionality induced by CDs. Hong et al. (2024) designed *Pseudomonas aeruginosa*-derived carbon dots doped with sulfur (S-PCDs) and further incorporated into the PVA polymer matrix for food preservation purposes. S-PCDs demonstrated exceptional antioxidant activities, achieving 94.98% for ABTS and 83.63% for DPPH radical scavenging. The addition of 2 wt% S-PCDs to the PVA polymer enhanced the UV-shielding action from 22.55 to 97.17%. The PVA/S-PCDs$^{2\%}$ induced 100% ABTS and 61.5% DPPH neutralization, extending the shelf life of pork meat and inhibiting the browning of sliced apples (Figure 6.4b).

The above-mentioned research studies demonstrate the capacity of CDs-doped polymers to be used in protective food packaging.

6.5 CHALLENGES AND FUTURE PERSPECTIVES

Although significant progress has been made in recent years in the study of potential UV protection and antioxidant ability of CDs in active food packaging systems, numerous challenges still remain in this field. A comparative examination of the available literature suggests that CDs can serve dual roles as both radical scavengers and UV absorbers. However, the efficacy of CDs in both roles cannot be universally applied and is contingent upon the source and concentration of the CDs and particular reactive oxygen species (ROS). Therefore, for the future advancement of this research domain, the utilization of "generic" C-dots, whose structure lacks comprehensive description and control, poses a significant concern.

Moreover, the application of CD-based active packaging for real food systems still needs more investigation. A steady release of the desired amount of active compounds onto the surface of food throughout its storage duration is required to prolong the shelf life of food products by active antioxidant packaging. However, the pivotal aspect of active packaging lies in determining the optimal concentration distribution of antioxidants surrounding the food, ensuring that the release kinetics align with the kinetics of food oxidation. The diffusion of active substances from the packaging film into food items is contingent upon various factors, including the compatibility between the incorporated filler and the film, the nature of the food product, the film solubility, and the concentration of the loaded compound (Razavi et al., 2020). Numerous studies have concentrated on employing mathematical models of mass transfer to optimize the active system and elucidate a mechanism for controlled release. Nevertheless, the majority of current research has been conducted using liquid food simulants in containers, which may not adequately predict the release behavior of antioxidants in real food systems. It is imperative to design and conduct well-structured experiments aimed at determining the optimal content released near real food items.

Another challenge lies in the potential release of CDs from packaging film, which could pose safety concerns. The nanoscale dimension of CDs possesses the ability to penetrate the human body via skin contact or inhalation, potentially impacting human health. It is imperative to conduct research to elucidate the migration of CDs into the food systems and assess their potential toxicity.

It is crucial to consider consumers' perspectives regarding the incorporation of CDs in food processing and meals. The utilization of brown-colored CDs (obtained from pyrolysis or thermal approaches) might impose limitations on their widespread applications in various food products. To address this, large-scale synthesis of CDs can be achieved through innovative non-thermal techniques. Additionally, it will be crucial to devise cost-effective methods for the large-scale production of CDs to ensure their commercial viability for food-related applications. Further utilization of CDs as active antioxidants and UV-shielding filler needs more in-depth research to assess the influence of precursor materials, their structure, polymer formulation, and functionalization to achieve optimal enhancement in food packaging efficacy. Then, future endeavors in the advancement of active packaging systems entail focused research on preparation methodologies, incorporation techniques, and concentration optimization.

REFERENCES

Ahmed, M. W., Haque, M. A., Mohibbullah, M., Khan, M. S. I., Islam, M. A., Mondal, M. H. T., & Ahmmed, R. (2022). A review on active packaging for quality and safety of foods: Current trends, applications, prospects and challenges. *Food Packaging and Shelf Life*, *33*, 100913.

Atta, O. M., Manan, S., Shahzad, A., Ul-Islam, M., Ullah, M. W., & Yang, G. (2022). Biobased materials for active food packaging: A review. *Food Hydrocolloids*, *125*, 107419.

Channa, I. A., Ashfaq, J., Gilani, S. J., Shah, A. A., Chandio, A. D., & Jumah, M. N. B. (2022). UV blocking and oxygen barrier coatings based on polyvinyl alcohol and zinc oxide nanoparticles for packaging applications. *Coatings*, *12*(7), 897.

Cheng, X., Zhao, Q., Kang, J., Zhao, X., He, X., & Li, J. (2023). Cellulose nanofiber/poly-vinyl alcohol-based pH-responsive films containing anthocyanin and carbon dots. *ACS Applied Polymer Materials*, *5*(8), 6307–6317.

Chunduri, L. A., Kurdekar, A., Patnaik, S., Dev, B. V., Rattan, T. M., & Kamisetti, V. (2016). Carbon quantum dots from coconut husk: Evaluation for antioxidant and cytotoxic activity. *Materials Focus*, *5*(1), 55–61.

Chung, Y. J., Kim, J., & Park, C. B. (2020). Photonic carbon dots as an emerging nanoagent for biomedical and healthcare applications. *ACS Nano*, *14*(6), 6470–6497.

Cui, L., Ren, X., Sun, M., Liu, H., & Xia, L. (2021). Carbon dots: Synthesis, properties and applications. *Nanomaterials*, *11*(12), 3419.

Das, B., Dadhich, P., Pal, P., Srivas, P. K., Bankoti, K., & Dhara, S. (2014). Carbon nanodots from date molasses: New nanolights for the in vitro scavenging of reactive oxygen species. *Journal of Materials Chemistry B*, *2*(39), 6839–6847.

Das, P., Ganguly, S., Margel, S., & Gedanken, A. (2021). Immobilization of heteroatom-doped carbon dots onto nonpolar plastics for antifogging, antioxidant, and food monitoring applications. *Langmuir*, *37*(11), 3508–3520.

Das Purkayastha, M., Manhar, A. K., Das, V. K., Borah, A., Mandal, M., Thakur, A. J., & Mahanta, C. L. (2014). Antioxidative, hemocompatible, fluorescent carbon nanodots from an "end-of-pipe" agricultural waste: Exploring its new horizon in the food-packaging domain. *Journal of Agricultural and Food Chemistry*, *62*(20), 4509–4520.

Dong, Y., Shao, J., Chen, C., Li, H., Wang, R., Chi, Y., … Chen, G. (2012). Blue luminescent graphene quantum dots and graphene oxide prepared by tuning the carbonization degree of citric acid. *Carbon, 50*(12), 4738–4743.

Ezati, P., Khan, A., Priyadarshi, R., Bhattacharya, T., Tammina, S. K., & Rhim, J.-W. (2023). Biopolymer-based UV protection functional films for food packaging. *Food Hydrocolloids, 142*, 108771. doi:10.1016/j.foodhyd.2023.108771

Ezati, P., Priyadarshi, R., & Rhim, J.-W. (2022). Prospects of sustainable and renewable source-based carbon quantum dots for food packaging applications. *Sustainable Materials and Technologies, 33*, e00494.

Fan, K., Zhang, M., Fan, D., & Jiang, F. (2019). Effect of carbon dots with chitosan coating on microorganisms and storage quality of modified-atmosphere-packaged fresh-cut cucumber. *Journal of the Science of Food and Agriculture, 99*(13), 6032–6041.

Ferreira, C. A., Ni, D., Rosenkrans, Z. T., & Cai, W. (2018). Scavenging of reactive oxygen and nitrogen species with nanomaterials. *Nano Research, 11*, 4955–4984.

Garcia, C. V., Shin, G. H., & Kim, J. T. (2018). Metal oxide-based nanocomposites in food packaging: Applications, migration, and regulations. *Trends in Food Science & Technology, 82*, 21–31.

Gómez-Estaca, J., López-de-Dicastillo, C., Hernández-Muñoz, P., Catalá, R., & Gavara, R. (2014). Advances in antioxidant active food packaging. *Trends in Food Science & Technology, 35*(1), 42–51.

Hola, K., Sudolská, M., Kalytchuk, S., Nachtigallová, D., Rogach, A. L., Otyepka, M., & Zboril, R. (2017). Graphitic nitrogen triggers red fluorescence in carbon dots. *ACS Nano, 11*(12), 12402–12410.

Hong, S. J., Riahi, Z., Shin, G. H., & Kim, J. T. (2024). Pseudomonas aeruginosa-derived carbon dots doped with sulfur as active packaging materials for fresh food preservation. *Food Bioscience, 57*, 103506.

Hu, G., Lei, B., Jiao, X., Wu, S., Zhang, X., Zhuang, J., … Liu, Y. (2019). Synthesis of modified carbon dots with performance of ultraviolet absorption used in sunscreen. *Optics Express, 27*(5), 7629–7641.

Innocenzi, P., & Stagi, L. (2023). Carbon dots as oxidant-antioxidant nanomaterials, understanding the structure-properties relationship: A critical review. *Nano Today, 50*, 101837.

Ionita, P. (2021). The chemistry of DPPH· free radical and congeners. *International Journal of Molecular Sciences, 22*(4), 1545.

Jia, W., Wu, X., & Kang, X. (2023). Integrated the embedding delivery system and targeted oxygen scavenger enhances free radical scavenging capacity. *Food Chemistry: X, 17*, 100558.

Jung, S., Cui, Y., Barnes, M., Satam, C., Zhang, S., Chowdhury, R. A., … Sajadi, S. M. (2020). Multifunctional bio-nanocomposite coatings for perishable fruits. *Advanced Materials, 32*(26), 1908291.

Khan, A., Ezati, P., Kim, J.-T., & Rhim, J.-W. (2023a). Biocompatible carbon quantum dots for intelligent sensing in food safety applications: Opportunities and sustainability. *Materials Today Sustainability, 21*, 100306.

Khan, A., Ezati, P., & Rhim, J.-W. (2023b). Chitosan/Starch-Based active packaging film with N, P-Doped carbon dots for meat packaging. *ACS Applied Bio Materials, 6*(3), 1294–1305.

Khan, A., Priyadarshi, R., Bhattacharya, T., & Rhim, J.-W. (2023c). Carrageenan/Alginate-based functional films incorporated with Allium sativum carbon dots for UV-Barrier food packaging. *Food and Bioprocess Technology*, 1–15.

Khan, A., Riahi, Z., Tae Kim, J., & Rhim, J.-W. (2024). Carrageenan-based multifunctional packaging films containing Zn-carbon dots/anthocyanin derived from Kohlrabi peel for monitoring quality and extending the shelf life of shrimps. *Food Chemistry, 432*, 137215. doi:10.1016/j.foodchem.2023.137215

Khoshkalampour, A., Ahmadi, S., Ghasempour, Z., Lim, L.-T., & Ghorbani, M. (2023a). Development of a novel film based on casein/modified tragacanth gum enriched by carbon quantum dots for shelf-life extension of butter. *Food and Bioprocess Technology*, 1–18.

Khoshkalampour, A., Ghorbani, M., & Ghasempour, Z. (2023b). Cross-linked gelatin film enriched with green carbon quantum dots for bioactive food packaging. *Food Chemistry*, *404*, 134742.

Kou, E., Li, W., Zhang, H., Yang, X., Kang, Y., Zheng, M., … Lei, B. (2021). Nitrogen and sulfur co-doped carbon dots enhance drought resistance in tomato and mung beans. *ACS Applied Bio Materials*, *4*(8), 6093–6102.

Kousheh, S. A., Moradi, M., Tajik, H., & Molaei, R. (2020). Preparation of antimicrobial/ ultraviolet protective bacterial nanocellulose film with carbon dots synthesized from lactic acid bacteria. *International Journal of Biological Macromolecules*, *155*, 216–225.

Krehula, L. K., Papić, A., Krehula, S., Gilja, V., Foglar, L., & Hrnjak-Murgić, Z. (2017). Properties of UV protective films of poly (vinyl-chloride)/TiO 2 nanocomposites for food packaging. *Polymer Bulletin*, *74*, 1387–1404.

Kuai, L., Liu, F., Chiou, B.-S., Avena-Bustillos, R. J., McHugh, T. H., & Zhong, F. (2021). Controlled release of antioxidants from active food packaging: A review. *Food Hydrocolloids*, *120*, 106992.

Kumar, L., & Gaikwad, K. K. (2023). Carbon dots for food packaging applications. *Sustainable Food Technology*, *1*(2), 185–199.

Li, F., Li, T., Sun, C., Xia, J., Jiao, Y., & Xu, H. (2017). Selenium-doped carbon quantum dots for free-radical scavenging. *Angewandte Chemie International Edition*, *56*(33), 9910–9914.

Li, H., He, X., Liu, Y., Yu, H., Kang, Z., & Lee, S.-T. (2011). Synthesis of fluorescent carbon nanoparticles directly from active carbon via a one-step ultrasonic treatment. *Materials Research Bulletin*, *46*(1), 147–151.

Li, M., Feng, Q., Liu, H., Wu, Y., & Wang, Z. (2021). In situ growth of nano-ZnO/GQDs on cellulose paper for dual repelling function against water and bacteria. *Materials Letters*, *283*, 128838.

Li, Y., Yang, J., Sun, L., Liu, B., Li, H., & Peng, L. (2023). Crosslinked fish scale gelatin/alginate dialdehyde functional films incorporated with carbon dots derived from pomelo peel waste for active food packaging. *International Journal of Biological Macromolecules*, *253*, 127290. doi:10.1016/j.ijbiomac.2023.127290

Lin, J.-S., Tsai, Y.-W., Dehvari, K., Huang, C.-C., & Chang, J.-Y. (2019). A carbon dot based theranostic platform for dual-modal imaging and free radical scavenging. *Nanoscale*, *11*(43), 20917–20931.

Lopez-de-Dicastillo, C., Alonso, J. M., Catala, R., Gavara, R., & Hernandez-Munoz, P. (2010). Improving the antioxidant protection of packaged food by incorporating natural flavonoids into ethylene: Vinyl alcohol copolymer (EVOH) films. *Journal of Agricultural and Food Chemistry*, *58*(20), 10958–10964.

López-Pedrouso, M., Lorenzo, J. M., & Franco, D. (2022). Advances in natural antioxidants for food improvement. *Antioxidants*. MDPI.

Marabini, L., Melzi, G., Lolli, F., Dell'Agli, M., Piazza, S., Sangiovanni, E., & Marinovich, M. (2020). Effects of Vitis vinifera L. leaves extract on UV radiation damage in human keratinocytes (HaCaT). *Journal of Photochemistry and Photobiology B: Biology*, *204*, 111810.

Mastromatteo, M., Mastromatteo, M., Conte, A., & Del Nobile, M. A. (2010). Advances in controlled release devices for food packaging applications. *Trends in Food Science & Technology*, *21*(12), 591–598.

Meitha, K., Pramesti, Y., & Suhandono, S. (2020). Reactive oxygen species and antioxidants in postharvest vegetables and fruits. *International Journal of Food Science*, *2020*.

Min, S., Ezati, P., & Rhim, J.-W. (2022). Gelatin-based packaging material incorporated with potato skins carbon dots as functional filler. *Industrial Crops and Products, 181*, 114820.

Moradi, M., Molaei, R., Kousheh, S. A., Guimarães, J.T., & McClements, D. J. (2023). Carbon dots synthesized from microorganisms and food by-products: active and smart food packaging applications. *Critical Reviews in Food Science and Nutrition, 63*(14), 1943–1959.

Murru, C., Badía-Laíño, R., & Díaz-García, M. E. (2020). Synthesis and characterization of green carbon dots for scavenging radical oxygen species in aqueous and oil samples. *Antioxidants, 9*(11), 1147. doi:10.3390/ANTIOX9111147

Nimse, S. B., & Pal, D. (2015). Free radicals, natural antioxidants, and their reaction mechanisms. *RSC Advances, 5*(35), 27986–28006.

Othón-Díaz, E. D., Fimbres-García, J. O., Flores-Sauceda, M., Silva-Espinoza, B. A., López-Martínez, L. X., Bernal-Mercado, A. T., & Ayala-Zavala, J. F. (2023). Antioxidants in oak (Quercus sp.): Potential application to reduce oxidative rancidity in foods. *Antioxidants, 12*(4), 861.

Pandiselvam, R., Barut Gök, S., Yüksel, A. N., Tekgül, Y., Çalişkan Koç, G., & Kothakota, A. (2022). Evaluation of the impact of UV radiation on rheological and textural properties of food. *Journal of Texture Studies, 53*(6), 800–808.

Patil, A. S., Waghmare, R. D., Pawar, S. P., Salunkhe, S. T., Kolekar, G. B., Sohn, D., & Gore, A. H. (2020). Photophysical insights of highly transparent, flexible and re-emissive PVA@ WTR-CDs composite thin films: A next generation food packaging material for UV blocking applications. *Journal of Photochemistry and Photobiology A: Chemistry, 400*, 112647.

Qiu, Y., Wang, Z., Owens, A. C. E., Kulaots, I., Chen, Y., Kane, A. B., & Hurt, R. H. (2014). Antioxidant chemistry of graphene-based materials and its role in oxidation protection technology. *Nanoscale, 6*(20), 11744–11755.

Riahi, Z., Hong, S. J., Rhim, J.-W., Shin, G. H., & Kim, J. T. (2023a). High-performance multifunctional gelatin-based films engineered with metal-organic frameworks for active food packaging applications. *Food Hydrocolloids, 144*, 108984.

Riahi, Z., Khan, A., Rhim, J.-W., Shin, G. H., & Kim, J. T. (2023b). Gelatin/poly (vinyl alcohol)-based dual functional composite films integrated with metal-organic frameworks and anthocyanin for active and intelligent food packaging. *International Journal of Biological Macromolecules*, 126040.

Riahi, Z., Khan, A., Rhim, J.-W., Shin, G. H., & Kim, J. T. (2024). Sustainable packaging film based on cellulose nanofibres/pullulan impregnated with zinc-doped carbon dots derived from avocado peel to extend the shelf life of chicken and tofu. *International Journal of Biological Macromolecules, 258*, 129302. doi:10.1016/j.ijbiomac.2024.129302

Riahi, Z., Rhim, J.-W., Bagheri, R., Pircheraghi, G., & Lotfali, E. (2022). Carboxymethyl cellulose-based functional film integrated with chitosan-based carbon quantum dots for active food packaging applications. *Progress in Organic Coatings, 166*, 106794. doi:10.1016/j.porgcoat.2022.106794

Roopa, H., Panghal, A., Kumari, A., Chhikara, N., Sehgal, E., & Rawat, K. (2023). Active packaging in food industry. *Novel Technologies in Food Science*, 375–404.

Roy, S., Ezati, P., & Rhim, J.-W. (2021). Gelatin/carrageenan-based functional films with carbon dots from enoki mushroom for active food packaging applications. *ACS Applied Polymer Materials, 3*(12), 6437–6445.

Ruiz, V., Yate, L., García, I., Cabanero, G., & Grande, H.-J. (2017). Tuning the antioxidant activity of graphene quantum dots: Protective nanomaterials against dye decoloration. *Carbon, 116*, 366–374.

Sachdev, A., & Gopinath, P. (2015). Green synthesis of multifunctional carbon dots from coriander leaves and their potential application as antioxidants, sensors and bioimaging agents. *Analyst, 140*(12), 4260–4269.

Salimi, F., Moradi, M., Tajik, H., & Molaei, R. (2021). Optimization and characterization of eco-friendly antimicrobial nanocellulose sheet prepared using carbon dots of white mulberry (Morus alba L.). *Journal of the Science of Food and Agriculture, 101*(8), 3439–3447.

Sangeetha, U. K., Sudhakaran, N., Parvathy, P. A., Abraham, M., Das, S., De, S., & Sahoo, S. K. (2024). Coconut husk-lignin derived carbon dots incorporated carrageenan based functional film for intelligent food packaging. *International Journal of Biological Macromolecules, 266*, 131005.

Shahidi, F., & Zhong, Y. (2010). Lipid oxidation and improving the oxidative stability. *Chemical Society Reviews, 39*(11), 4067–4079.

Skibsted, L. H., Risbo, J., & Andersen, M. L. (2010). *Chemical deterioration and physical instability of food and beverages.* Elsevier.

Son, M. H., Park, S. W., & Jung, Y. K. (2021). Antioxidant and anti-aging carbon quantum dots using tannic acid. *Nanotechnology, 32*(41), 415102.

Su, X., Lin, H., Fu, B., Mei, S., Lin, M., Chen, H., … Lin, Y. (2023). Egg-yolk-derived carbon dots@ albumin bio-nanocomposite as multifunctional coating and its application in quality maintenance of fresh litchi fruit during storage. *Food Chemistry, 405*, 134813.

Sul, Y., Khan, A., & Rhim, J.-W. (2024). Effects of coffee bean types on the characteristics of carbon dots and their use for manufacturing cellulose nanofibers-based films for active packaging of meat. *Food Packaging and Shelf Life, 43*, 101282.

Tang, L., Ji, R., Cao, X., Lin, J., Jiang, H., Li, X., … Hao, J. (2012). Deep ultraviolet photoluminescence of water-soluble self-passivated graphene quantum dots. *ACS Nano, 6*(6), 5102–5110.

Tripathi, S., Kumar, L., Deshmukh, R. K., & Gaikwad, K. K. (2023). Ultraviolet blocking films for food packaging applications. *Food and Bioprocess Technology*, 1–20.

Uthirakumar, P., Devendiran, M., Kim, T. H., & Lee, I. H. (2018). A convenient method for isolating carbon quantum dots in high yield as an alternative to the dialysis process and the fabrication of a full-band UV blocking polymer film. *New Journal of Chemistry, 42*(22), 18312–18317. doi:10.1039/C8NJ04615H

Vijayakumar, R., Sivaraman, Y., Pavagada Siddappa, K. M., & Dandu, J. P. R. (2022). Synthesis of lignin nanoparticles employing acid precipitation method and its application to enhance the mechanical, UV-barrier and antioxidant properties of chitosan films. *International Journal of Polymer Analysis and Characterization, 27*(2), 99–110.

Wagh, R. V., Khan, A., Priyadarshi, R., Ezati, P., & Rhim, J.-W. (2023). Cellulose nanofiber-based multifunctional films integrated with carbon dots and anthocyanins from Brassica oleracea for active and intelligent food packaging applications. *International Journal of Biological Macromolecules, 233*, 123567.

Wang, F., Xie, Z., Zhang, H., Liu, C., & Zhang, Y. (2011). Highly luminescent organosilane-functionalized carbon dots. *Advanced Functional Materials, 21*(6), 1027–1031.

Wang, L., Liu, X., Qi, P., Sun, J., Jiang, S., Li, H., … Zhang, S. (2022). Enhancing the thermo-stability, UV shielding and antimicrobial activity of transparent chitosan film by carbon quantum dots containing N/P. *Carbohydrate Polymers, 278*, 118957.

Wongrerkdee, S., & Pimpang, P. (2020). Ultraviolet-shielding and water resistance properties of graphene quantum dots/polyvinyl alcohol composite-based film. *Journal of Metals, Materials and Minerals, 30*(4), 90–96.

Xu, L., Li, Y., Gao, S., Niu, Y., Liu, H., Mei, C., … Xu, C. (2020). Preparation and properties of cyanobacteria-based carbon quantum dots/polyvinyl alcohol/nanocellulose composite. *Polymers, 12*(5), 1143.

Xu, N., Gao, S., Xu, C., Fang, Y., Xu, L., & Zhang, W. (2021). Carbon quantum dots derived from waste acorn cups and its application as an ultraviolet absorbent for polyvinyl alcohol film. *Applied Surface Science, 556*, 149774.

Xu, Z., Huang, W., Chen, C., Ye, W., Guo, B., Qiu, J., … Hu, G. (2023). Preparation of new full UV-absorbing carbon dots from quercetin and their application in UV-absorbing systems for waterborne polyurethane coatings. *Materials Today Chemistry, 27*, 101269.

Yang, D., Li, L., Cao, L., Chang, Z., Mei, Q., Yan, R., … Dong, W.-F. (2020). Green synthesis of lutein-based carbon dots applied for free-radical scavenging within cells. *Materials, 13*(18), 4146.

Zhao, Lin, Wang, Y., & Li, Y. (2019). Antioxidant activity of graphene quantum dots prepared in different electrolyte environments. *Nanomaterials, 9*(12), 1708.

Zhao, Linlin, Zhang, M., Mujumdar, A. S., Adhikari, B., & Wang, H. (2022). Preparation of a novel carbon dot/polyvinyl alcohol composite film and its application in food preservation. *ACS Applied Materials & Interfaces, 14*(33), 37528–37539.

Zhao, Linlin, Zhang, M., Mujumdar, A. S., & Wang, H. (2023). Application of carbon dots in food preservation: a critical review for packaging enhancers and food preservatives. *Critical Reviews in Food Science and Nutrition, 63*(24), 6738–6756.

7 Anti-aging Properties
and Utilization of
Carbon Quantum Dots
in Cosmetics

*Reena Negi, Ashutosh Pandey, Vijay J. Upadhye,
Elyor Berdimurodov, Bhawana Jain
and Sanju Singh*

7.1 INTRODUCTION

Aging eventually occurs in all living things. The human body part that is most obviously affected is the skin. Age-dependent/chronological aging and premature aging/photoaging are two different types of skin aging (Mukherjee, Maity, Nema, & Sarkar, 2011). The second type, which is caused by external sources, showed symptoms like deep furrows, a leathery appearance, and uneven pigmentation (Fisher et al., 2002; Maity, Nema, Abedy, Sarkar, & Mukherjee, 2011). The skin would therefore tend to wrinkle as individuals age naturally. The epidermis, dermis, and subcutaneous tissue are the three layers that make up the skin (Rittié & Fisher, 2002). The outermost layer of the skin is called extracellular matrix (ECM), which made up of proteins like collagen and elastin as well as fibroblasts (Fulop, Khalil, & Larbi, 2012). The ECM offers a structural foundation that is necessary for the skin growth and flexibility and crucial for preservation of physiological processes (Fulop et al., 2012; Kurtz & Oh, 2012). Hyaluronidase, elastase, and collagenase are the three enzymes implicated in skin aging that also has a direct connection with ECM degradation and associated with an increase in activity (Losso, Munene, Bansode, & Bawadi, 2004; Maity et al., 2011; Wary, Thakker, Humtsoe, & Yang, 2003). Collagen, one of the essential elements of the skin's structural makeup, is the major component of the connective tissue, hair, and nails (Mukherjee et al., 2011). The skin structure and flexibility, as well as its ability to retain moisture, are all influenced by hyaluronic acid. Moreover, it speeds up proliferation, regeneration, and repair of tissues (Hsu & Chiang, 2009; Manuskiatti & Maibach, 1996) and improves the interchange of nutrients and waste products. The ECM organization and structural upkeep are likewise handled by this compound (Manuskiatti & Maibach, 1996). When people grow older, their bodies produce less collagen, elastin, and hyaluronic acid, which causes the skin to become less elastic and strong and develop visible wrinkles. In numerous biological

DOI: 10.1201/9781003437857-9

processes, reactive oxygen species (ROS) plays an essential role (K.-H. Wang et al., 2006). Absorption of UV light by skin increases the production of ROS and results in oxidative stress. Protein structure and function could be altered by oxidative damage, which will result in DNA and mitochondrial damage, lipid peroxide production, and protein and gene modification (Irshad & Chaudhuri, 2002). Hyaluronidase, collagenase, and elastase are activated when the ROS level are high, which could accelerate the aging process of the skin (Labat-Robert, Fourtanier, Boyer-Lafargue, Robert, & Biology, 2000; Mukherjee et al., 2011; Rittié & Fisher, 2002). Due to the remarkable UV absorption and visible transmittance rates of quantum dots (QDs), they are anticipated to be a revolutionary advancement over conventional UV absorbers, in recent years. It has received great attention as UV absorbers.

It's interesting to note that graphene and carbon quantum dots (CQDs), both described in recent years (Feng et al., 2017; Hess et al., 2017; Xie, Du, Wu, Hao, & Liu, 2016), provide great anti-UV application effects. In order to prevent nutrition loss, it used in packaging, particularly for CQDs, like polyethylene terephthalate (PET). In addition to comparisons between CQDs and GQDs, CQDs were thought to be the most promising QDs as alternatives to commercial UV absorbers because of their straightforward synthesis procedures and cheap price. As previously indicated, CQDs have a visible light transmittance of above 95% but still have narrow-band absorption and low UV absorption efficiency, which limits their employment in high transparency goods such packing bags, agricultural films, etc. Here, we discuss on CQDs, their anti-aging property, and their use in cosmetics.

7.2 CARBON QUANTUM DOTS (CQDs) AND THEIR SPECIFIC CHARACTERISTICS

In recent years, interest in carbonaceous and carbon-based nanomaterials has increased due to their beneficial characteristics (Atta, El-Mahdy, Al-Lohedan, & Shoueir, 2015; A Mohanty, Baaziz, Lafjah, Da Costa, & Janowska, 2018; Anurag Mohanty & Janowska, 2019; Pirzado et al., 2019). These nanomaterials are less toxic and simple to functionalize (Aljohani et al., 2018; Azizi-Lalabadi, Hashemi, Feng, & Jafari, 2020; Lee, Lo, Lee, Zheng, & Cho, 2019; Trache, Thakur, & Boukherroub, 2020). Due to their special qualities, they exhibit high fluorescence, and fluorescent carbons are more frequently referred to as carbon dots (Thulasi, Kathiravan, & Asha Jhonsi, 2020). Outstanding stability, low hazardous activity, water solubility, and derivatization accessibility set carbon dots apart from other materials. These distinctive characteristics promote their applicability in a variety of areas. Carbon dots, which are mostly composed of heteroatoms (functional groups) connected to a carbonized core, are one of the newest and most promising nanomaterials to be recognized by humans (J. Wang, Wei, Su, & Qiu, 2015). The sp^2 hybrid conjugated carbon core-shell structures between carbon (core) and organic functional groups (shell), such as N-H, -OH, -C = O, COOH, and C-N, or polymer aggregates, would be used to define small (10 nm) nanoparticles (Shi et al., 2019). Outstanding anti-UV application outcomes are seen with CQDs, and they also exhibit good compatibility with polymers. The low UV absorption efficiency and narrow-band absorption constraints of CQDs still prevent their usage in high transparency products like packaging bags, agricultural film, bioimaging, sensing, label free detection, etc.

CQDs are one of the most recent materials with intriguing and distinctive features (Yiqun Zhou, Sharma, Peng, & Leblanc, 2017a). Strong evidence for the chemical components of carbon dots, which included amino groups, oxygen, and polymer chains among other surface function groups, is provided by the amazing properties of these particles. These functions enhance the energy gap and surface energy level while also having a major impact on photoluminescence activity (Tan, Kong, Guan, Wang, & Xu, 2020). Due to their strong tuneable optical properties, lack of toxicity, simplicity, and low cost, these compounds have garnered a lot of interest for application in optical sensors (Meixiu Li, Chen, Gooding, & Liu, 2019). Since biological systems are transparent to these wavelengths and light in this region has a greater tissue-penetrating ability, the ability of carbon dots to emit light in this region is of particular interest (Guo et al., 2018). Because of the n-π^* transition of groups like C-N, C=O, and C-S as well as the π-π^* transition of C = C bonds, CQDs are most successful in capturing photons in the short wavelength area. The visible range expanded into the UV area show a considerable optical absorption. A C = C bond-related π-π^* transition caused absorption in the region between 230 and 270 nm, whereas a C = O bond-related n-π^* transition caused the peak shoulder in the range of 300–390 nm (Iravani & Varma, 2020). Several surface passivation and functionalization techniques could change the absorbance (Gai, Zhao, & Chung, 2019). CQDs seem to be a common choice for surface passivation due to their long wavelengths and declining quantum yield (Tan et al., 2020). The color of the synthesized dots must be either red, green, or blue. Due to the varied chemical compositions, sizes, and increasing heterogeneity of carbon dots, it was not advised for multicolor imaging. These particles have a diverse range of emission spectra.

The usage of carbon dots, notably in bioimaging and cellular imaging, has been greatly influenced by their biocompatibility, one of its most significant properties (M. Zhang et al., 2019). CQDs with a significant number of oxygen groups have demonstrated excellent biocompatibility, low toxicity, and increased radiation performance (X. Yuan et al., 2014; Ya Zhou, Sun, Wang, Ren, & Qu, 2017b). Additionally, they assist in photoluminescence by enhancing the fluorescence brightness and modifying the emission spectra of doped ions, as well as reactive oxygen species (ROS), which was aided by the doped ion capacity to scavenge hydroxyl free radicals (Atabaev, 2018; Kandasamy, 2019; M. Zhang et al., 2019). CQDs open up new opportunities in a variety of devices, including electrical and photonic ones for biological imaging. The abundance and general safety of the material used to create carbon QDs makes them stand out as a potential tool for development in environmentally friendly solar technology (Flores-Pacheco, Álvarez-Ramos, & Ayón, 2020). CQDs were perfect for biological applications since they produce fluorescence in the near-infrared (NIR) spectral region. A wide range of industries, including biomedicine, photocatalysis, light-emitting diodes (LEDs), photosensors, and solar energy conversion, have demonstrated the value of CQDs. Bioimaging, drug administration, DNA delivery, and cancer treatment are examples of therapeutic uses of CQDs (Alaghmandfard et al., 2021; Su et al., 2020). Due to their high biocompatibility, little to no toxicity, and suitability for application in cosmetics, bioimaging, and biosensing, CQDs can be used to create multifunctional sunscreens.

7.3 OPTICAL PROPERTIES

(i)   **Absorption:** CQDs produced utilizing a variety of carbon sources or synthesis techniques always exhibit different absorption tendencies. The absorption bands were attributed to the n-π* transition of the C-O/C-N bond or the π-π* transition of the C-C bond, and they typically did, however, exhibit strong absorption in the ultraviolet (UV) region (200–400 nm), with a tail extending into the visible range (Figure 7.1) (Jiang et al., 2013; Zhu et al., 2013). Moreover, a number of CQDs that emit red or NIR light frequently feature π-conjugated electrons which are connected to the surface groups or polymer chains in sp^2 domains, resulting in the absorption of long wavelengths in the 500–800 nm range (J. Liu et al., 2020a; Qu et al., 2016; F. Yuan et al., 2017). As a result, the absorption properties of CQDs were significantly influenced by the size of π-conjugated domains, the variation in the oxygen/nitrogen concentration of carbon cores, and the types and contents of surface groups.

(ii) **Photoluminescence:** One of the most attractive properties, both theoretically and practically, is photoluminescence (PL). CQDs showed more significant applications in a variety of fields because they have advantages over other fluorescent materials, such as conventional quantum dots (QDs) made of cadmium/lead, rare-earth nanomaterials, and organic dyes. They also have a higher quantum yield, lower toxicity, abundant low-cost sources, and excellent biocompatibility. Quantitatively, the brightness of the PL value is expressed by the quantum yield, which is greatly impacted by the carbon sources, synthesis methods, and post-passivation (Figure 7.2). Although recent research has successfully demonstrated how to produce red and NIR emissive CQDs by altering reaction conditions or carbon sources, CQDs' potential applications in biomedicine are limited because they typically emit blue or green fluorescence (Hui et al., 2020; J. Liu et al., 2020a; Zheng et al., 2016).

(iii) **Phosphorescence:** One of the appealing characteristics of CDs (Figure 7.3) is room-temperature phosphorescence (RTP), which is produced by two

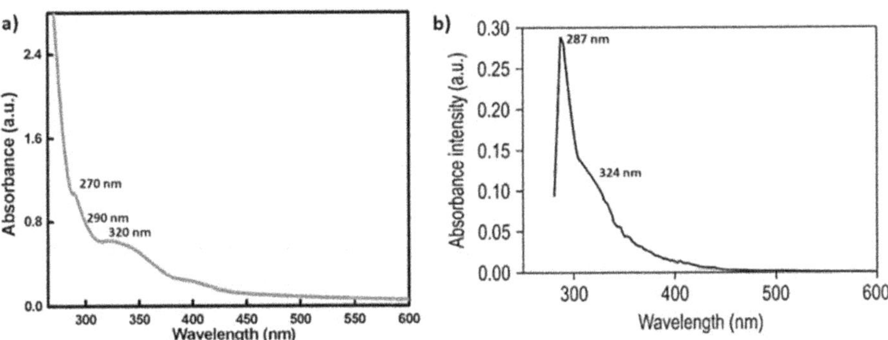

FIGURE 7.1   Based on (a) agarose (Chauhan, Saini, & Chaudhary, 2020) and (b) chondroitin sulfate (Kim, Choi, Kwon, & Kim, 2020) UV-vis absorption spectra of CQDs.

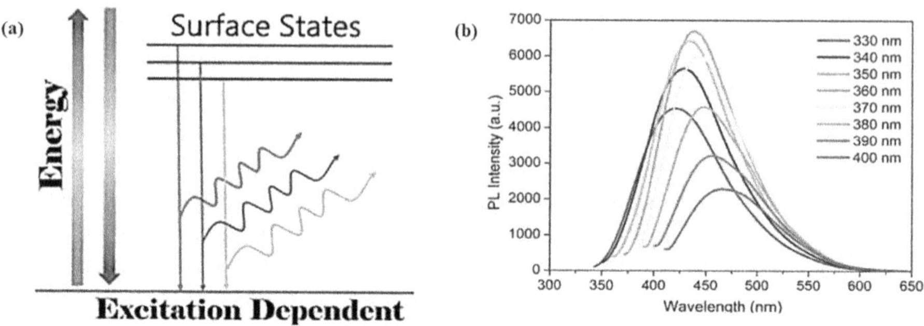

FIGURE 7.2   (a) Different surface energy levels were responsible for the CQDs' multicolored photoluminescence (S. Zhu et al., 2015b); (b) CQD luminescence spectra depend on excitation (X. Wang et al., 2019b).

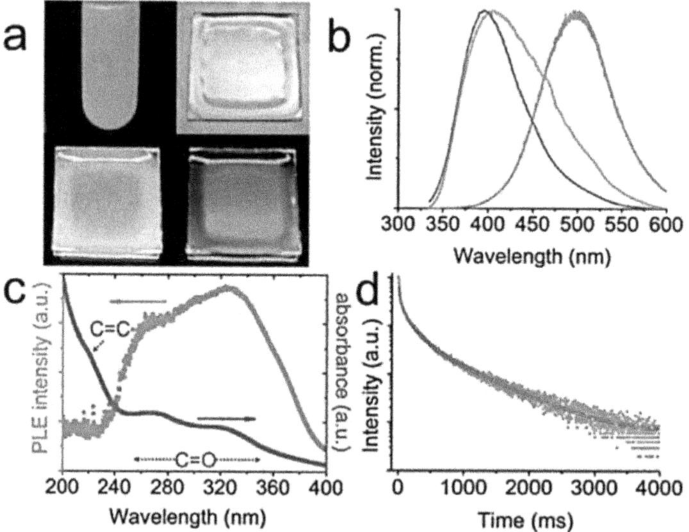

FIGURE 7.3   Digital images of CQDs and their corresponding spectra shown in (a) and (b), respectively. Under UV light (top left; blue line), in a PVA matrix in the presence of daylight (upper right; cyan line), and after UV light had been switched off, CQDs were disseminated in water (a: lower left; b: olive line). The spectra of UV excitation wavelengths were 325 nm and 365 nm, respectively. (c) Phosphorescence excitation spectrum of CQDs dispersed in water (olive dots) and absorption spectrum (blue dots). (d) Time-resolved spectrum of phosphorescence (Youfu Wang & Hu, 2014).

important processes. There are two types of intersystem crossings: (i) the radiative transition from the ground state (S0) to the lowest excited triplet state (T1); and (ii) the transition from the lowest excited singlet state (S1) to a triplet state (Tn) (ISC) (Gan, Shi, An, & Huang, 2018). Moreover, other luminous characteristics of CQDs, including electrochemiluminescence

(Y. Chen, Cao, Ma, & Zhu, 2020b; Jie, Zhou, & Jie, 2019), chemilumines-cence (Molaei, 2019; C. L. Shen et al., 2020), and two- and multiphoton fluorescence (Lan et al., 2017; D.-Y. Zhang et al., 2017), have been gradu-ally exposed and investigated due to their diverse optical characteristics.

7.4 DOPING

In particular, the inclusion of metal ions dramatically improved the photothermal and photodynamic properties of CQDs (Figure 7.4) (Tejwan et al., 2021). After doping, a charge transition between metal ions and the carbon lattice of CQDs forms and alters the charge density because of the empty orbitals in metal ions and their capacity to donate electrons (Lin, Luo, Tsai, Wang, & Chen, 2018). The changed electronic structure of CQDs alters the energy gap between the highest occupied molecular orbital (HOMO) and lowest unoccupied molecular orbital (LUMO), which alters the optical characteristics of the materials. Metal-doped CQDs exhibit a higher quantum yield, a better PL, and improved catalytic and relaxation properties when compared to non-doped CQDs (F. Yuan et al., 2016). Doped CQDs frequently display distinc-tive UV absorption peaks that have been linked to carbon-framework-derived $n - \pi^*$ and $\pi - \pi^*$ transitions (B. B. Chen, Liu, Zou, & Huang, 2016; Lin et al., 2015; M. L. Liu et al., 2017). A metallic dopant increases the absorbance of doped CQDs in the visible region by causing a charge transfer between metallic ions and carbon frameworks (Wu et al., 2015; Q. Zhang et al., 2018). The PL of 365-nm excita-tion wavelength-excited metal-doped CQDs consists of, among other things, ultra-violet (C. Zhu et al., 2015a), blue (B. B. Chen et al., 2016; M. L. Liu et al., 2017;

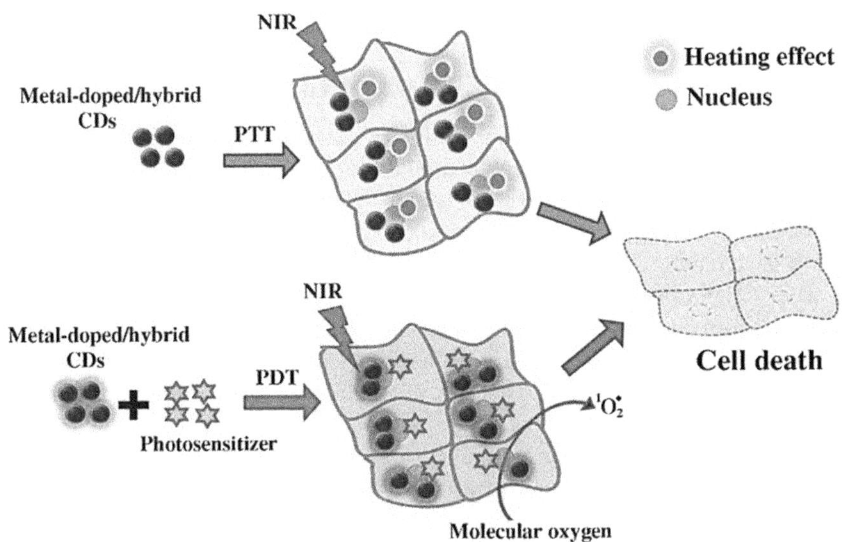

FIGURE 7.4 Metal-doped/hybrid phototherapy induces photodynamic and photothermal therapy (Jovanović et al., 2023).

Ting Liu, Na Li, Jiang Xue Dong, Hong Qun Luo, & Nian Bing Li, 2016a; Q. Zhang et al., 2018), blue-green (Y. H. Yuan et al., 2015), green (Gong et al., 2014), and yellow emissions (Bourlinos et al., 2017; Cheng, Wang, Zhang, Yang, & Chen, 2016). Excitation-dependent photoluminescence is present in the majority of doped CQDs (C. Han et al., 2016; Ting Liu, Na Li, Jiang Xue Dong, Hong Qun Luo, & Nian Bing Li, 2016a). The peak of the PL emission is red-shifted in CQDs that have been doped with metal (Lin et al., 2015). Because of the newly created emission energy traps, electron-hole recombination is encouraged (Yu et al., 2016). The increased PLQY after doping is assumed to be caused by metal nanoparticles having the surface plasmonic resonance (SPR) effect (Sajid et al., 2016). Mn-doped CQDs fluorescence changed when the polarity of the solvent changed (Yu Wang et al., 2016).

The distribution of dopants in CQDs may not be uniform; however, if metals are used as dopants since they have higher radii than carbon (Kou, Jiang, Park, & Meng, 2020). Metal-doped CQD uses in a biological context may be severely hampered by the possible toxicity of metal ions, which is another issue (Ren et al., 2014). Mice receiving intravenously administered Gd-doped CQDs did not experience any pathological tissue damage (Xu, Jia, Yin, He, & Zhang, 2014). HO-8910 cells (C. Han et al., 2016), L929 cells [152], human epidermoid cancer cells (Y. H. Yuan et al., 2015), C6 cells (Gong et al., 2014), and HepG2 cells (Xu et al., 2014) also show little toxicity in response to different metal-doped CQDs. Elements including N, S, P, F, Se, and B are frequently implied when CQDs are doped with non-metals (Huang et al., 2019; Ma et al., 2020). The consistent doping of CQDs illustrates how similar their size is to the size of C. The introduction of new excited energy levels is caused by the dopant alteration of CQD carbon framework surface structure. The photoluminescent characteristics of doped CQDs were significantly influenced by the dopant electronegativity as well.

7.5   REACTIVE OXYGEN SPECIES (ROS) GENERATION VIA CQDs

The main factors influencing the generation of reactive oxygen species (ROS) were functional group type, amount, and spatial distribution. Contrarily, the amount and spatial distribution of aromatic carbon islands, the CD solvent, and the type of polymer used in the creation of nanocomposite materials are the primary determinants of ROS deactivation. The majority of the ROS was created when oxygen electrons and aromatic electrons from CDs came into contact (Dutta et al., 2015). The oxygen molecule's spin changes as a result, increasing internal energy. The pricey family of extremely effective photosensitizers (fullerene, porphyrins, etc.) shares characteristics with CDs (Buglak, Filatov, Hussain, & Sugimoto, 2020; Hamblin, 2018; Yokoi et al., 2021).

The hydroxyl group is one of the most prevalent functional groups on water-soluble CDs. Hurst and Schuster estimated the singlet oxygen-quenching rate constants for various X-Y bonds based on the lifespan of singlet oxygen in various solvents, and they found that the -O-H bond should efficiently quench singlet oxygen (rate constants of 10^3, 10^6, and 10^9 L M^{-1} s^{-1} for some monohydroxy-, dihydroxy-, and trihydroxy-alcohols, respectively). Compared to acetic acid (CH_3COOH), malonic acid $CH_2(COOH)_2$ has a rate constant of 10^3 LM^{-1}s^{-1}, demonstrating the ability of the carboxylic group to quench oxygen (Markovic & Trajkovic, 2008). As a result, we suggest that highly functionalized CDs have extraordinary $_1O^2$ deactivation capacities, and that this remarkable quick increase in singlet oxygen-quenching capacity may also occur as CD functionalization increases.

- Electrochemical cutting of graphite electrodes results in the manufacture of GQDs functionalized with -OH groups on the cathode and -CH groups on the anode (Ristic et al., 2014). Despite the considerable amount of sp2 aromatics, the -OH and -COOH groups effectively quench singlet oxygen in aqueous solutions. The amount of singlet oxygen produced by acetone-soluble GQDs was significantly larger than that of toluene-soluble GQDs.
- Many functional groups in CQDs quench singlet oxygen and they are soluble in aqueous solvents. Some CQD subtypes function admirably as antioxidants (M. H. Son, S. W. Park, & Y. K. Jung, 2021a). Fruits and vegetables considered to be high in antioxidants are frequently used as food sources. Table 7.1 shows the DPPH scavenging activity of several CQDs.
- The ROS production and quenching properties of the CNDs and CQDs are rather comparable (Table 7.2).
- The polymer composition of CPD exhibits both excellent solvent solubility and low singlet oxygen quenching capacity (Lanzilotto et al., 2018). When methyl group-rich hydrophobic copolymers are used as the manufacturing base, quenching would be very small (Nenad K. Stanković et al., 2018a). Singlet oxygen generation is significantly influenced by the size of the π-conjugated domain and the composition of the carbon core.

There were direct and indirect techniques for detecting the singlet oxygen that CQDs emit. At 1270 nm, the singlet oxygen's luminescence was directly measured. EPR, UV-Vis, and visible photoluminescence are the foundations of indirect techniques.

TABLE 7.1

The Advantages of DPPH Scavenging Actions for Specific CQDs

Title	Source Material	Scavenging Activity (%)	References
CQD	Tannic acid	84.5	M. H. Son et al. (2021b)
CQD	Ananas	23.3	Rajamanikandan, Biruntha, & Ramalingam (2022)
Cl-CQD	Citric acid, Urea, NaCl	88	Marković et al. (2020)
CQD	Tomato	63.8	Rodríguez-Varillas et al. (2022)
CQD	Pomelo	56	J. Shen, Shang, Chen, Wang, & Cai (2017)
T-CQD	Thumbai	89	Varsha Raveendran & Renuka (2022)
CQD	Taurine	82.5	Shinoda et al. (2022)
S-CQD	Turmeric and ammonium persulfate	79.5	Ezati, Roy, & Rhim (2022)
CQD	*Citrus clementina* peel	81.4	Šafranko et al. (2021)

TABLE 7.2

Values for Singlet Oxygen Quantum Yields in Different Types of Carbon Quantum Dots

Title	$\Phi\,\Delta$ (%)	Source Material	Measurement Method (Probe)	References
CQD	71	Riboflavin	Visible photoluminescence (SOSG)	Yue et al. (2021)
CQD	27	Polythiophene benzoic acid	UV-Vis (Na-ADPA)	Ge et al. (2016)
Mn/HA-CQD	40	Manganese atoms and hyaluronic acid	UV-Vis (Na-ADPA)	S. Wang et al. (2022)
N,S-co-doped CQDs	8	Polythiophene derivative	UV-Vis (Na-ADMA)	Zhao et al. (2021)
Sn@S-CQD	37	Sodium p-styrene sulfonate and $SnCl_4$	UV-Vis (ABDA)	Q. Luo et al. (2020)
CQD	5.7	Trinitropyrene	Luminescence at 1270 nm	Zhao et al. (2020)
Cu-CQD	36	Poly(acrylic acid) and $Cu(NO_3)_2$	UV-Vis (ABDA)	J. Wang et al. (2019a)
CQD	62	Pheophytin	UV-Vis (DBPF)	Wen et al. (2019)
CQD	33	PF 68 copolymer	Luminescence at 1270 nm	Nenad K. Stanković et al. (2018a)
N-doped carbon dots	19	Coal	UV-Vis (DBPF)	Mingyu Li et al. (2017)

These techniques make use of probes that react with singlet oxygen, such as TMP, ABDA, and DBPF, and then measured the optical response. It's simple to detect singlet oxygen at 1270 nm because the bulk of CQDs possess visible-spectrum luminous. Due to the frequent absence of unpaired electrons in CQDs, measuring TEMPO via electron paramagnetic resonance (EPR) is also simple. Due to the overlap in the spectra between the CQDs and the probes, it may be challenging to evaluate photolabile probes using visible photoluminescence or UV-Vis.

7.6　CYTOTOXICITY OF CQDs

Bagheri et al. (2018) discovered that CQDs were toxic to yeast cells in a dose-dependent way. At concentrations of 1–4 g mL^{-1}, carbon dots (CDs) produced from *Trapa bispinosa* peel extract demonstrated greater than 80% MDCK cell survival (Mewada et al., 2013). According to Lou et al., 1000 mg mL^{-1} of CDs made from aqueous extracts of Radix Puerariae Carbonisata showed 80% viability on blood-derived RAW 264.7 murine macrophage cells (J. Luo et al., 2019). Human hepatitis B cell lines (HpG2), human lung cancer cell lines (A549), human breast cancer cell lines (MDA-MB-231), and human cervical cancer cell lines (HeLa) all demonstrated better than 60% vitality on CDs made from ginger juice (C.-L. Li et al., 2014). One of the major drawbacks of CDs as photosensitizers was ROS generation, which could impair DNA molecule stability and cell signaling, leading to toxicity. Production of ROS and surface area are positively correlated. Furthermore, chemical properties such as size, solubility, pH, light wavelength, and surface functional groups have a significant influence on ROS levels (Fu, Xia, Hwang, Ray, & Yu, 2014).

Due to their low toxicity and photostability, GQDs show tremendous potential for use in photodynamic therapy (Ge et al., 2014; Rakovich & Rakovich, 2018). To reduce the levels of toxicity, the doping and co-doping techniques use nitrogen (N), boron (B), phosphorus (P), sulfur (S), or a combination of these elements (Y. Han et al., 2015; H. Li et al., 2015; Sadhanala & Nanda, 2016; J. Zhou et al., 2014). When thin films of CQDs were deposited in mouse embryonic fibroblast cell lines via Langmuir-Blodgett method, low-level cytotoxicity was observed (Stanković, Bodik, Šiffalovič, Kotlar, & Mičušik, 2018b). After 6 hours of exposure to blue light, these films' cytotoxicity slightly changed. NIH/3T3 cells were safe for CQDs/polyurethane nanocomposites, regardless of the extract content, according to cell viability studies on the NIH/3T3 and A549 cell lines (Kováčová et al., 2020). When the extract concentrations were 75 and 100%, the same nanocomposites only demonstrated minimal or moderate cytotoxicity toward A549 cells. Hela cells were not cytotoxic to the gamma-irradiated CQDs/polyurethane nanocomposite (Budimir et al., 2021). Only nanocomposites that had been exposed to 200 kGy of radiation and had extract concentrations of 75 or 100%, respectively, showed mild or moderate toxicity to U-87 MG cells. U-87 MG cells were generally more sensitive than HeLa cells.

7.7 ADVANTAGES OF CQDs IN COSMETIC INDUSTRY

CQDs valued by the cosmetics industry for a variety of reasons in the twenty-first century, taking into account the advancements in nanotechnology (Al Yahyai, Al-Lawati, & Hassanzadeh, 2022; Khan & Asmatulu, 2013; M. Son, S. W. Park, & Y. K. Jung, 2021a), including their use as active substances, transporters, or excipients. The main objectives of using CQDs in the formulation of cosmetic goods are to boost product effectiveness, improve penetration into deeper skin layers (because to their minute size and precise optical characteristics), reduce toxicity, and enhance the stability of active components (Hu et al., 2019; J. Liu, Li, & Yang, 2020b).

7.8 DERMATOLOGY AND COSMETICS USE CQDs MEDICATION DELIVERY SYSTEMS

The lipid bilayer that surrounds the core aqueous area in liposomes is often composed of phospholipids that are phosphatidylcholine-enriched (X. Wang, Yang, Chen, & Shin, 2008). Liposomes were globular, closed-colloidal vesicles. Phosphatidylcholine, a crucial component of liposomes, has long been used in skin and hair care products due to its moisturizing and conditioning qualities. In cosmeceuticals such as anti-aging and sunscreen products, hair treatments, and skin moisturizers that comprise synthetic and plant-based active ingredients, nanoliposomes are used (Kaur & Agrawal, 2007; Raza et al., 2014; Takahashi, Kitamoto, Asikin, Takara, & Wada, 2009). Solid lipid nanoparticles transform into solid, oily droplets of lipids stabilized by surfactants when heated to body temperature. Both lipophilic and hydrophilic drugs delivered using them often. Solid lipids and oils were combined to create nano-structured lipid carrier particles, which can hold more active chemicals per unit volume (Pardeike, Hommoss, & Müller, 2009). For skin and hair care, a compound with carbo-siloxane dendrimer was developed which has good water resistance, more shine, a perceptible feeling, and exceptional adhesive properties (Tournilhac & Simon, 2001). A lamellar phase of a non-ionic surfactant was layered around an aqueous cavity in niosomes, which were extremely small, unilamellar nanostructures with a size range of 10–100 nm. Niosomes have the potential to transport antioxidants through the skin, including ascorbic acid, resveratrol, and ellagic acid (Coviello et al., 2015; Pardakhty et al., 2012). In the size range of 471–565 nm, a slightly bigger niosome containing phytoderived antioxidants such resveratrol, alpha-tocopherol, and curcumin demonstrated better antioxidant benefit to the skin and increased skin penetration activity for cosmeceutical applications (Tavano, Muzzalupo, Picci, & de Cindio, 2014). Recently, scientists developed carbon nanomaterials containing vitamin E and ascorbic acid that displayed improved skin protection against premature aging due to their antioxidant characteristics, much to niosomes (Ito, Itoga, Yamato, Akamatsu, & Okano, 2010a; Y. Ito et al., 2010b). A non-toxic polymeric membrane encloses an inner liquid core at the nanoscale, forming a shell vesicular structure known as a nanocapsule. To increase the impact of its cosmetics, the French company L'Oreal developed nanocapsule-based cosmetic products for potential dermatological use in 1995 (Poletto, Beck, Guterres, Pohlmann, & Care, 2011). Strong antibacterial and antifungal activities in carbon nanomaterials have recently been demonstrated (T). They were widely used in cosmeceuticals products to make deodorants, face packs, and anti-aging creams. Moreover, CQDs are presently utilized in products including toothpaste, soap, face cream, food packaging, textiles, household appliances, disinfectants, and bandages for wounds (Moniruzzaman et al., 2022; M. H. Son et al., 2021b). Recent developments in the cosmeceuticals industry, namely in the skin care area, involved carbon nanotechnology.

7.9 APPLICATION OF CQDs IN COSMETICS

1. Anti-aging and sunscreen

   It's interesting to note that over the previous two years, research on graphene and CQDs (Feng et al., 2017; Hess et al., 2017; Xie et al., 2016) reveals that both materials have good compatibility with polymers and excellent anti-UV application results. It has been used in packaging made of polyethylene terephthalate (PET), specifically for CQDs, to prevent nutrition loss. Also, in comparison to GQDs, CQDs have been shown to be the most effective QDs as a replacement for industrial UV absorbers (Figure 7.5). This is due to their affordable prices and straightforward synthesis procedures. Even though it was claimed that CQDs could transmit visible light, their use in high transparency products such as packing bags and agricultural film was limited by their narrow-band absorption and poor UV absorption efficiency. The regulation of the absorption spectra, stabilities under varied pH values, temperatures, and UV radiation replicating practical conditions, dispersity

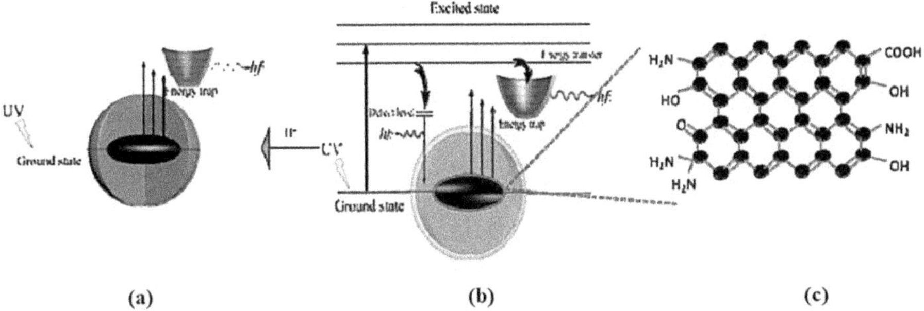

FIGURE 7.5 (a) UV absorbing mechanism of CQDs; (b) the UV absorption pathway of CQDs was activated by pH control when fluorescence was quenched. When CQDs with conjugated structures gather UV light, it converges into the energy trap and is then released as heat energy via pathways I and II. UV energy is transferred to the excited state in Route I, where it emits fluorescence and heat radiation; (c) the conjugated structure of CQDs (Hu et al., 2019).

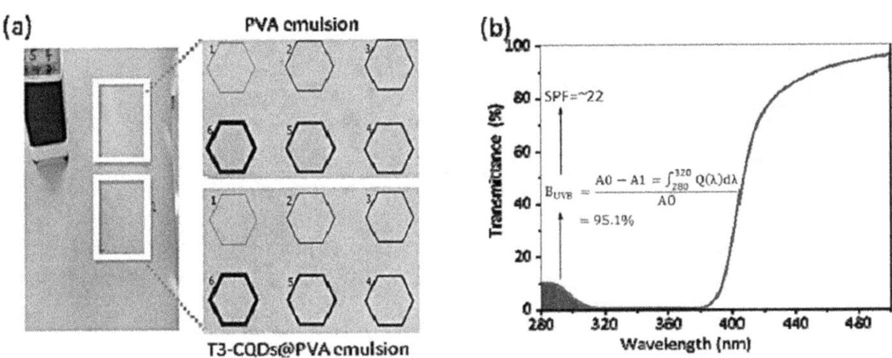

FIGURE 7.6 CQDs being used as an UV absorber in sunscreen formulation. (a) In order to determine whether and when skin redness emerged under UV light between 280 and 320 nm, PVA and T3-CQDs@PVA7 emulsion were coated on the body back with a coating weight of 2 mg/cm. Locations 1, 2, 3, 4, and 5 received radiation doses of 197, 246.25, 307.81, 480.96, and 601.20 w/cm^2, respectively; (b) in order to determine whether and when skin redness emerged under UV light between 280 and 320 nm, PVA and T3-CQDs@PVA7 emulsion were coated on the body back with a coating weight of 2 mg/cm. Locations 1, 2, 3, 4, and 5 received radiation doses of 197, 246.25, 307.81, 480.96, and 601.20 w/cm^2, respectively (Hu et al., 2019).

in different solvents, and alternative applications of CQDs as UV absorbers have sadly not been investigated. Moreover, it is yet unknown how QDs absorb UV light. CQDs and polyvinyl alcohol (PVA) composite films and emulsions with high UV fluorescence are employed as UV absorbers in anti-aging polymers and sunscreens. CQDs with N,N'bis(2-aminoethyl)-1,3-propanediamine @ PVA composite were added to sunscreens as a broad spectrum UV absorber to prevent human skin diseases caused by UV radiation (Figure 7.6) (Hu et al., 2019).

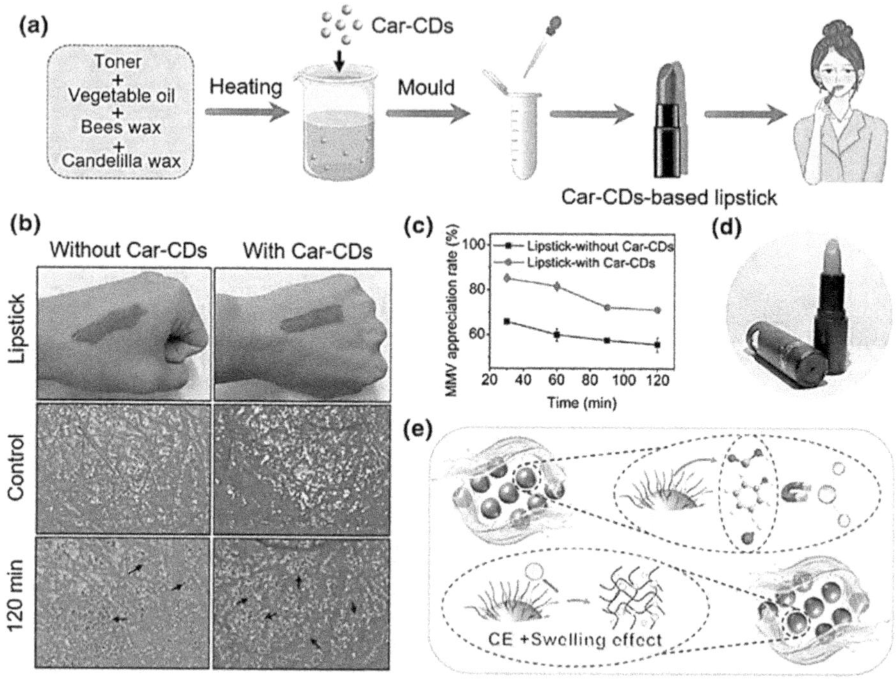

FIGURE 7.7 (a) Schematic representation of the moisturizing lipstick production process using car-CDs; (b) changes in the moisture content of the hands after using moisturizing lipstick; (c) After applied moisturizing lipstick, the curve of hand skin moisture changed; (d) images of prepared moisturizing lipstick; (e) ability of Car-CDs to retain moisture through a specific method (Dong et al., 2021).

2. **Moisturizing lipstick**

CQDs are highly hygroscopic in nature. Its capability is strongly related to its surface groups, which are primarily made up of hydroxyl and carboxyl groups. They can be employed as a possible humectant due to strong water solubility and abundance of surface functional groups.

A novel one-pot solvothermal approach used to create Car-CQDs which produced from carmine cochineal. Solvothermal synthesis, one of the most used synthesis techniques, has a number of benefits, including being affordable, simple to use, and especially good in producing CQDs from a variety of carbon-based precursors. Further testing of Car-CDs' ability to preserve moisture in human skin was done using the moisture measurement value method. An even more exciting development is the use of Car-CDs as a nanoadditive in moisturizing lipstick, suggesting a potential benefit for use in skin care and cosmetics (Figures 7.7 and 7.8) (Dong et al., 2021).

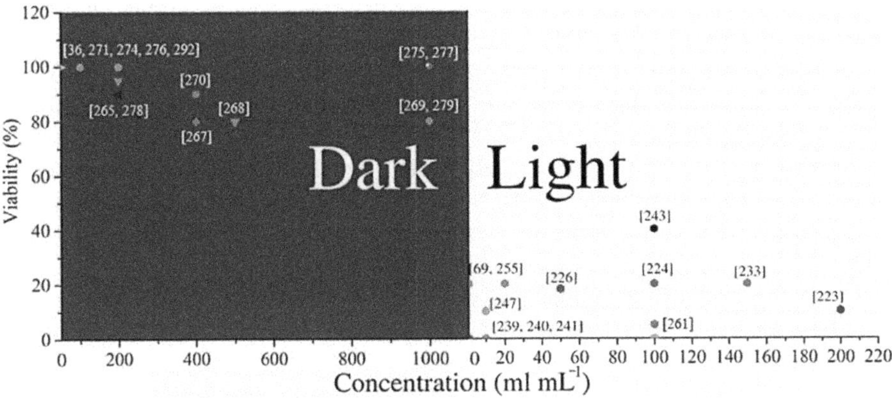

FIGURE 7.8 In the dark (violet) and exposed to light (yellow), cytotoxicity of carbon-based nanoparticles. The cytotoxicity values in relation to CQD doses, represented by dots in the graph (Jovanović et al., 2023).

7.10 FUTURE PROSPECTS AND CHALLENGES

In photodynamic therapy, CQDs have a very promising and broad future. Together with creation and advancement of this as innovative, effective PDT agents, new fields are also emerging. Hence, the creation of novel composites with self-sterilizing capabilities is a rapidly expanding field with potential uses in daily items, cosmetics, and medical equipment. There are various problems that need to be overcome before these carbonaceous nanoparticles are allowed in stores, medical facilities, and homes.

The first challenge was related to the differences in qualities of dots made using various synthetic methods. Here, how diverse optical properties demonstrate themselves in GQDs with the same size and structure have been explained (Tang et al., 2022; G. Yang et al., 2018; Y. Yang et al., 2021). More research on the structure required as the source of the photoluminescence of carbon-based nanoparticles is needed. The absence of unsolved mysteries involved perplexing scientists, resulting in a situation where each approach produces different dots, despite the fact that they appear structurally and morphologically similar. The structure underlying such particles had to be clarified using new experimental techniques.

The second concern relates to the cost, yields of production, and work-intensive purification. Low synthetic yields were typical for the production of carbon nanoparticles, and the dots were frequently separated by time-consuming dialysis. Production must be far more effective in order to be transmitted to industries.

The validity of techniques for ROS generation was another crucial issue. Dependability related to the optical characteristics of nanoparticles (J. Chen et al., 2020a). Although there were techniques for detecting various radicals created by illumination, these techniques were initially developed for the examination of molecules of photosensitizers. Nanoparticles had a wide range of characteristics; for example, they cannot dissolve but instead disperse. Absorbance and luminescence may alter as a result of this. Nanoparticles showed to increase cytokine and ROS generation within cells (Dutta et al., 2015; Qin et al., 2015), although PEG passivation improved the biocompatibility of GQDs and reduced the generation of ROS (Chandra, Deshpande, Shinde, Pillai, & Singh, 2014). Most investigations revealed that GQDs did not enter cell nuclei, which is associated with potential genotoxicity. Similar to this, in vitro research showed that CQDs depending on the dosage used were either innocuous or showed low toxicity toward various cell lines.

Figure 7.8 provided a summary of the toxicity of CQDs. The bulk of investigations have clearly shown that they are harmless in the absence of light but turn harmful when different light wavelengths are used.

The fact that it generated ROS when lighted is one of their most fascinating characteristics. When secure, non-lethal substances are exposed to light, they turn into deadly poisons. Both bacterial and cancerous cells have been shown to be affected by the toxic effects. These novel materials with exceptional qualities, along with others like chemical stability and adjustable solubility, open the door for new approaches:

- The formation of antimicrobial and anticancer drugs;
- Implementing innovative methods to treat certain conditions.
- Building the framework for novel goods for residential and medical use, such as antimicrobial plastics.

Compared to photofrin and hematoporphyrin, which exhibit dark cytotoxicity, cutaneous phototoxicity, and limited solubility, carbon-based dots have advantages (Iyer, Wolf, Zhukova, Padanilam, & Nguyen, 2018). Although though second-generation PSs (5-aminolevulinic acid, benzoporphyrin, chlorin, and phthalocyanine) are more soluble and less poisonous in the dark, poor stability proved a problem (Allison et al., 2004; Duchi et al., 2013). Third-generation PSs that combine carbon-based nanomaterials, liposomes, micelles, quantum dots, and dendrimers are currently being developed (Mfouo-Tynga, Dias, Inada, & Kurachi, 2021). The creation of new multifunctional nanosystems that serve as both therapeutic and bioimaging tools is facilitated by the development of carbon-based nanoparticles (Sharker, 2021).

7.11 CONCLUSION

Since the last few years, carbon nanomaterials like CQDs have gained tremendous attention and interest due to their incomparable and specific properties. Here, we explain their optical and anti-aging properties. We also explained here, the advantages of CQDs in cosmetic industry and dermatology. Earlier, researchers described the reactive oxygen species (ROS) generation via carbon nanomaterials (Dutta et al., 2015). The generation of ROS depends upon the size and shape of nanomaterials. Due to dot in size and shape CQDs also generated a low amount of ROS which makes them less toxic. Doping with other materials, has an effect on their toxicity, making them non-toxic. This property of CQDs enhanced their application in cosmetic industry specially in skin care, sunscreens, moisturizing lipsticks, etc. Lastly the future prospects and challenges of using CQDs in cosmetics and photosensitizers have been explained.

REFERENCES

Al Yahyai, I., Al-Lawati, H. A. J., & Hassanzadeh, J. (2022). Carbon dots-modified paper-based chemiluminescence device for rapid determination of mercury (II) in cosmetics. *Luminescence, 37*(7), 1087–1097. https://doi.org/10.1002/bio.4261

Alaghmandfard, A., Sedighi, O., Rezaei, N. T., Abedini, A. A., Khachatourian, A. M., Toprak, M. S., & Seifalian, A. (2021). Recent advances in the modification of carbon-based quantum dots for biomedical applications. *Materials Science Engineering: C 120*, 111756.

Aljohani, H., Ahmed, Y., El-Shafey, O., El-Shafey, S., Fouad, R., & Shoueir, K. (2018). Decolorization of turbid sugar juice from sugar factory using waste powdered carbon. *Applied Water Science 8*, 1–10.

Allison, R. R., Downie, G. H., Cuenca, R., Hu, X.-H., Childs, C. J., Sibata, C. H. J. P., & Therapy, P. (2004). Photosensitizers in clinical PDT. *Photodiagnosis Photodynamic Therapy 1*(1), 27–42.

Atabaev, T. S. (2018). Doped carbon dots for sensing and bioimaging applications: A minireview. *Nanomaterials 8*(5), 342.

Atta, A. M., El-Mahdy, G. A., Al-Lohedan, H. A., & Shoueir, K. R. (2015). Electrochemical behavior of smart N-isopropyl acrylamide copolymer nanogel on steel for corrosion protection in acidic solution. *International Journal of Electrochemical Science 10*(1), 870–882.

Azizi-Lalabadi, M., Hashemi, H., Feng, J., & Jafari, S. M. (2020). Carbon nanomaterials against pathogens; the antimicrobial activity of carbon nanotubes, graphene/graphene oxide, fullerenes, and their nanocomposites. *Advances in Colloid Interface Science 284*, 102250.

Bagheri, Z., Ehtesabi, H., Hallaji, Z., Latifi, H., & Behroodi, E. (2018). Investigation the cytotoxicity and photo-induced toxicity of carbon dot on yeast cell. *Ecotoxicology and Environmenta Safety, 161*, 245–250. https://doi.org/10.1016/j.ecoenv.2018.05.071

Bourlinos, A. B., Rathi, A. K., Gawande, M. B., Hola, K., Goswami, A., Kalytchuk, S., … Zboril, R. (2017). Fe(III)-functionalized carbon dots—Highly efficient photoluminescence redox catalyst for hydrogenations of olefins and decomposition of hydrogen peroxide. *Applied Materials Today, 7*, 179–184. https://doi.org/10.1016/j.apmt.2017.03.002

Budimir, M., Marković, Z., Vajdak, J., Jovanović, S., Kubat, P., Humpoliček, P., … Milivojević, D. (2021). Enhanced visible light-triggered antibacterial activity of carbon quantum dots/polyurethane nanocomposites by gamma rays induced pre-treatment. *Radiation Physics Chemistry, 185*, 109499.

Buglak, A. A., Filatov, M. A., Hussain, M. A., & Sugimoto, M. (2020). Singlet oxygen generation by porphyrins and metalloporphyrins revisited: A quantitative structure-property relationship (QSPR) study. *Journal of Photochemistry and Photobiology A: Chemistry, 403*, 112833. https://doi.org/10.1016/j.jphotochem.2020.112833

Chandra, A., Deshpande, S., Shinde, D. B., Pillai, V. K., & Singh, N. (2014). Mitigating the cytotoxicity of graphene quantum dots and enhancing their applications in bioimaging and drug delivery. *ACS Macro Letters 3*(10), 1064–1068.

Chauhan, P., Saini, J., & Chaudhary, S. (2020). Agarose waste derived toxicologically screened carbon dots as dual sensor: A mechanistic insight into luminescence and solvatochromic behaviour. *Nano-Structures Nano-Objects 24*, 100585.

Chen, B. B., Liu, Z. X., Zou, H. Y., & Huang, C. Z. (2016). Highly selective detection of 2, 4, 6-trinitrophenol by using newly developed terbium-doped blue carbon dots. *Analyst 141*(9), 2676–2681.

Chen, J., Wu, W., Zhang, F., Zhang, J., Liu, H., Zheng, J., … Zhang, J. (2020a). Graphene quantum dots in photodynamic therapy. *Nanoscale Advances* 2(10), 4961–4967.

Chen, Y., Cao, Y., Ma, C., & Zhu, J.-J. (2020b). Carbon-based dots for electrochemiluminescence sensing. *Materials Chemistry Frontiers* 4(2), 369–385.

Cheng, J., Wang, C.-F., Zhang, Y., Yang, S., & Chen, S. (2016). Zinc ion-doped carbon dots with stron yellow photoluminescence. *RSC Advances*, 6(43), 37189–37194. https://doi.org/0.1039/C5RA27808B

Coviello, T., Trotta, A., Marianecci, C., Carafa, M., Di Marzio, L., Rinaldi, F., … Matricardi, P. (2015). Gel-embedded niosomes: preparation, characterization and release studies of a new system for topical drug delivery. *Colloids Surfaces B: Biointerfaces 125*, 291–299.

Dong, C., Xu, M., Wang, S., Ma, M., Akakuru, O. U., Ding, H., … Bi, H. (2021). Fluorescent carbon dots with excellent moisture retention capability for moisturizing lipstick. *Journal of Nanobiotechnology*, 19(1), 299. https://doi.org/10.1186/s12951-021-01029-6

Duchi, S., Sotgiu, G., Lucarelli, E., Ballestri, M., Dozza, B., Santi, S., … Donati, D. (2013). Mesenchymal stem cells as delivery vehicle of porphyrin loaded nanoparticles: Effective photoinduced in vitro killing of osteosarcoma. *Journal of Controlled Release 168*(2), 225–237.

Dutta, T., Sarkar, R., Pakhira, B., Ghosh, S., Sarkar, R., Barui, A., & Sarkar, S. (2015). ROS generation by reduced graphene oxide (rGO) induced by visible light showing antibacterial activity: Comparison with graphene oxide (GO). *RSC Advances 5*(98), 80192–80195.

Ezati, P., Roy, S., & Rhim, J.-W. (2022). Pectin/gelatin-based bioactive composite films reinforced with sulfur functionalized carbon dots. *Colloids and Surfaces A: Physicochemical and Engineering Aspects*, 636, 128123. https://doi.org/10.1016/j.colsurfa.2021.128123

Feng, X., Zhao, Y., Jiang, Y., Miao, M., Cao, S., & Fang, J. (2017). Use of carbon dots to enhance UV-blocking of transparent nanocellulose films. *Carbohydrate Polymers 161*, 253–260.

Fisher, G. J., Kang, S., Varani, J., Bata-Csorgo, Z., Wan, Y., Datta, S., & Voorhees, J. J. (2002). Mechanisms of photoaging and chronological skin aging. *Archives of Dermatology 138*(11), 1462–1470.

Flores-Pacheco, A., Álvarez-Ramos, M. E., & Ayón, A. (2020). Down-shifting by quantum dots for silicon solar cell applications. In *Solar Cells and Light Management* (pp. 443–477): Elsevier.

Fu, P. P., Xia, Q., Hwang, H.-M., Ray, P. C., & Yu, H. (2014). Mechanisms of nanotoxicity: Generation of reactive oxygen species. *Journal of Food and Drug Analysis*, 22(1), 64–75. https://doi.org/10.1016/j.jfda.2014.01.005

Fulop, T., Khalil, A., & Larbi, A. (2012). The role of elastin peptides in modulating the immune response in aging and age-related diseases. *Pathologie Biologie 60*(1), 28–33.

Gai, W., Zhao, D. L., & Chung, T.-S. (2019). Thin film nanocomposite hollow fiber membranes comprising Na+-functionalized carbon quantum dots for brackish water desalination. *Water Research 154*, 54–61.

Gan, N., Shi, H., An, Z., & Huang, W. (2018). Recent advances in polymer-based metal-free room-temperature phosphorescent materials. *Advanced Functional Materials 28*(51), 1802657.

Ge, J., Jia, Q., Liu, W., Lan, M., Zhou, B., Guo, L., … Wang, P. (2016). Carbon dots with intrinsic theranostic properties for bioimaging. *Red-Light-Triggered Photodynamic/Photothermal Simultaneous Therapy In Vitro and In Vivo. 5*(6), 665–675. https://doi.org/10.1002/adhm.201500720

Ge, J., Lan, M., Zhou, B., Liu, W., Guo, L., Wang, H., … Zhou, H. (2014). A graphene quantum dot photodynamic therapy agent with high singlet oxygen generation. *Nature Communications 5*(1), 4596.

Gong, N., Wang, H., Li, S., Deng, Y., Chen, X.A., Ye, L., & Gu, W. (2014). Microwave-Assisted polyol synthesis of gadolinium-doped green luminescent carbon dots as a bimodal nanoprobe. *Langmuir*, 30(36), 10933–10939. https://doi.org/10.1021/la502705g

Guo, L., Li, L., Liu, M., Wan, Q., Tian, J., Huang, Q., ... Wei, Y. (2018). Bottom-up preparation of nitrogen doped carbon quantum dots with green emission under microwave-assisted hydrothermal treatment and their biological imaging. *Materials Science and Engineering: C, 84*, 60–66. https://doi.org/10.1016/j.msec.2017.11.034

Hamblin, M. R. (2018). Fullerenes as photosensitizers in photodynamic therapy: Pros and cons. *Photochemical & Photobiological Sciences, 17*(11), 1515–1533. https://doi.org/10.1039/C8PP00195B

Han, C., Xu, H., Wang, R., Wang, K., Dai, Y., Liu, Q., ... Xu, K. (2016). Synthesis of a multifunctional manganese(ii)–carbon dots hybrid and its application as an efficient magnetic-fluorescent imaging probe for ovarian cancer cell imaging. *Journal of Materials Chemistry B, 4*(35), 5798–5802. https://doi.org/10.1039/C6TB01250G

Han, Y., Tang, D., Yang, Y., Li, C., Kong, W., Huang, H., ... Kang, Z. (2015). Non-metal single/dual doped carbon quantum dots: a general flame synthetic method and electrocatalytic properties. *Nanoscale, 7*(14), 5955–5962.

Hess, S. C., Permatasari, F. A., Fukazawa, H., Schneider, E. M., Balgis, R., Ogi, T., ... Stark, W. J. (2017). Direct synthesis of carbon quantum dots in aqueous polymer solution: one-pot reaction and preparation of transparent UV-blocking films. *Journal of Materials Chemistry A 5*(10), 5187–5194.

Hsu, M.-F., & Chiang, B.-H. (2009). Stimulating effects of Bacillus subtilis natto-fermented Radix astragali on hyaluronic acid production in human skin cells. *Journal of Ethnopharmacology 125*(3), 474–481.

Hu, G., Lei, B., Jiao, X., Wu, S., Zhang, X., Zhuang, J., ... Liu, Y. (2019). Synthesis of modified carbon dots with performance of ultraviolet absorption used in sunscreen. *Optics Express, 27*(5), 7629–7641. https://doi.org/10.1364/OE.27.007629

Huang, G., Lin, Y., Zhang, L., Yan, Z., Wang, Y., & Liu, Y. (2019). Synthesis of sulfur-selenium doped carbon quantum dots for biological imaging and scavenging reactive oxygen species. *Scientific Reports, 9*(1), 19651. https://doi.org/10.1038/s41598-019-55996-w

Hui, W., Yang, Y., Xu, Q., Gu, H., Feng, S., Su, Z., ... Fang, J. (2020). Red-carbon-quantum-dot-doped SnO2 composite with enhanced electron mobility for efficient and stable perovskite solar cells. *Advanced Materials 32*(4), 1906374.

Iravani, S., & Varma, R. S. (2020). Green synthesis, biomedical and biotechnological applications of carbon and graphene quantum dots: A review. *Environmental Chemistry Letters 18*, 703–727.

Irshad, M., & Chaudhuri, P. (2002). Oxidant-antioxidant system: Role and significance in human body. *The Indian Journal of Experimental Biology.*

Ito, S., Itoga, K., Yamato, M., Akamatsu, H., & Okano, T. (2010a). The co-application effects of fullerene and ascorbic acid on UV-B irradiated mouse skin. *Toxicology 267*(1–3), 27–38.

Ito, Y., Warner, J. H., Brown, R., Zaka, M., Pfeiffer, R., Aono, T., ... Ardavan, A. (2010b). Controlling intermolecular spin interactions of La@ C 82 in empty fullerene matrices. *Physical Chemistry Chemical Physics 12*(7), 1618–1623.

Iyer, R., Wolf, J., Zhukova, D., Padanilam, D., & Nguyen, K. T. (2018). Nanomaterial based photo-triggered drug delivery strategies for cancer theranostics. In *Handbook of Nanomaterials for Cancer Theranostics* (pp. 351–391): Elsevier.

Jiang, F., Chen, D., Li, R., Wang, Y., Zhang, G., Li, S., ... Wang, C. J. N. (2013). Eco-friendly synthesis of size-controllable amine-functionalized graphene quantum dots with anti-mycoplasma properties. *5*(3), 1137–1142.

Jie, G., Zhou, Q., & Jie, G. (2019). Graphene quantum dots-based electrochemiluminescence detection of DNA using multiple cycling amplification strategy. *Talanta 194*, 658–663.

Jovanović, S., Marković, Z., Budimir, M., Prekodravac, J., Zmejkoski, D., Kepić, D., ... Marković, B. T. (2023). Lights and dots toward therapy: Carbon-based quantum dots as new agents for photodynamic therapy. *Pharmaceutics 15*(4), 1170.

Kandasamy, G. (2019). Recent advancements in doped/co-doped carbon quantum dots for multi-potential applications. *C, 5*(2), 24.

Kaur, I. P., & Agrawal, R. (2007). Nanotechnology: A new paradigm in cosmeceuticals. *Recent Patents on Drug Delivery Formulation 1*(2), 171–182.

Khan, W. S., & Asmatulu, R. (2013). Nanotechnology emerging trends, markets, and concerns. In *Nanotechnology Safety* (pp. 1–16): Elsevier.

Kim, K. W., Choi, T.-Y., Kwon, Y. M., & Kim, J. Y. H. (2020). Simple synthesis of photoluminescent carbon dots from a marine polysaccharide found in shark cartilage. *Electronic Journal of Biotechnology 47*, 36–42.

Kou, X., Jiang, S., Park, S.-J., & Meng, L.-Y. (2020). A review: Recent advances in preparations and applications of heteroatom-doped carbon quantum dots. *Dalton Transactions*, *49*(21), 6915–6938. https://doi.org/10.1039/D0DT01004A

Kováčová, M., Kleinová, A., Vajďák, J., Humpolíček, P., Kubát, P., Bodík, M., … Špitálský, Z. (2020). Photodynamic-active smart biocompatible material for an antibacterial surface coating. *Journal of Photochemistry Photobiology B: Biology 211*, 112012.

Kurtz, A., & Oh, S.-J. (2012). Age related changes of the extracellular matrix and stem cell maintenance. *Preventive Medicine*, *54*, S50–S56.

Labat-Robert, J., Fourtanier, A., Boyer-Lafargue, B., Robert, L. J. J. O. P., & Biology, P. B. (2000). Age dependent increase of elastase type protease activity in mouse skin: Effect of UV-irradiation. *Journal of Photochemistry Photobiology B: Biology 57*(2–3), 113–118.

Lan, M., Zhao, S., Zhang, Z., Yan, L., Guo, L., Niu, G., … Wang, P. (2017). Two-photon-excited near-infrared emissive carbon dots as multifunctional agents for fluorescence imaging and photothermal therapy. *Nano Research 10*, 3113–3123.

Lanzilotto, A., Kyropoulou, M., Constable, E. C., Housecroft, C. E., Meier, W. P., & Palivan, C. G. (2018). Porphyrin-polymer nanocompartments: Singlet oxygen generation and antimicrobial activity. *JBIC Journal of Biological Inorganic Chemistry*, *23*(1), 109–122. https://doi.org/10.1007/s00775-017-1514-8

Lee, K.-C., Lo, P.-Y., Lee, G.-Y., Zheng, J.-H., & Cho, E.-C. (2019). Carboxylated carbon nanomaterials in cell cycle and apoptotic cell death regulation. *Journal of Biotechnology 296*, 14–21.

Li, C.-L., Ou, C.-M., Huang, C.-C., Wu, W.-C., Chen, Y.-P., Lin, T.-E., … Chang, H.-T. (2014). Carbon dots prepared from ginger exhibiting efficient inhibition of human hepatocellular carcinoma cells. *Journal of Materials Chemistry B*, *2*(28), 4564–4571. https://doi. org/10.1039/C4TB00216D

Li, H., Kong, W., Liu, J., Liu, N., Huang, H., Liu, Y., & Kang, Z. (2015). Fluorescent N-doped carbon dots for both cellular imaging and highly-sensitive catechol detection. *Carbon 91*, 66–75.

Li, M., Chen, T., Gooding, J. J., & Liu, J. (2019). Review of carbon and graphene quantum dots for sensing. *ACS Sensors*, *4*(7), 1732–1748. https://doi.org/10.1021/acssensors. 9b00514

Li, M., Yu, C., Hu, C., Yang, W., Zhao, C., Wang, S., … Qiu, J. (2017). Solvothermal conversion of coal into nitrogen-doped carbon dots with singlet oxygen generation and high quantum yield. *Chemical Engineering Journal*, *320*, 570–575. https://doi.org/10.1016/ j.cej.2017.03.090

Lin, L., Luo, Y., Tsai, P., Wang, J., & Chen, X. (2018). Metal ions doped carbon quantum dots: Synthesis, physicochemical properties, and their applications. *TrAC Trends in Analytical Chemistry 103*, 87–101.

Lin, L., Song, X., Chen, Y., Rong, M., Wang, Y., Zhao, L., … Chen, X. (2015). Europium-decorated graphene quantum dots as a fluorescent probe for label-free, rapid and sensitive detection of Cu2+ and L-cysteine. *Analytica Chimica Acta 891*, 261–268.

Liu, J., Geng, Y., Li, D., Yao, H., Huo, Z., Li, Y., … Xu, W. (2020a). Deep red emissive carbonized polymer dots with unprecedented narrow full width at half maximum. *Advanced Materials 32*(17), 1906641.

Liu, J., Li, R., & Yang, B. (2020b). Carbon dots: A new type of carbon-based nanomaterial with wide applications. *ACS Central Science, 6*(12), 2179–2195. https://doi.org/10.1021/acscentsci.0c01306

Liu, M. L., Chen, B. B., Yang, T., Wang, J., Liu, X. D., & Huang, C. Z. (2017). One-pot carbonization synthesis of europium-doped carbon quantum dots for highly selective detection of tetracycline. *Methods Applications in Fluorescence 5*(1), 015003.

Liu, T., Li, N., Dong, J. X., Luo, H. Q., & Li, N. B. (2016a). Fluorescence detection of mercury ions and cysteine based on magnesium and nitrogen co-doped carbon quantum dots and IMPLICATION logic gate operation. *Sensors Actuators B: Chemical 231*, 147–153.

Liu, T., Li, N., Dong, J. X., Luo, H. Q., & Li, N. B. (2016b). Fluorescence detection of mercury ions and cysteine based on magnesium and nitrogen co-doped carbon quantum dots and IMPLICATION logic gate operation. *Sensors and Actuators B: Chemical, 231*, 147–153. https://doi.org/10.1016/j.snb.2016.02.141

Losso, J. N., Munene, C. N., Bansode, R. R., & Bawadi, H. A. (2004). Inhibition of matrix metalloproteinase-1 activity by the soybean Bowman–Birk inhibitor. *Biotechnology Letters 26*, 901–905.

Luo, J., Kong, H., Zhang, M., Cheng, J., Sun, Z., Xiong, W., ... Qu, H. (2019). Novel carbon dots-derived from radix puerariae carbonisata significantly improve the solubility and bioavailability of baicalin. *Journal of Biomedical Nanotechnology, 15*(1), 151–161. https://doi.org/10.1166/jbn.2019.2675

Luo, Q., Ding, H., Hu, X., Xu, J., Sadat, A., Xu, M., ... Bi, H. (2020). Sn4+ complexation with sulfonated-carbon dots in pursuit of enhanced fluorescence and singlet oxygen quantum yield. *Dalton Transactions, 49*(21), 6950–6956. https://doi.org/10.1039/D0DT01187H

Ma, Y., Chen, A. Y., Huang, Y. Y., He, X., Xie, X. F., He, B., ... Wang, X. Y. (2020). Off-on fluorescent switching of boron-doped carbon quantum dots for ultrasensitive sensing of catechol and glutathione. *Carbon, 162*, 234–244. https://doi.org/10.1016/j.carbon.2020.02.048

Maity, N., Nema, N. K., Abedy, M. K., Sarkar, B. K., & Mukherjee, P. K. (2011). Exploring Tagetes erecta Linn flower for the elastase, hyaluronidase and MMP-1 inhibitory activity. *Journal of Ethnopharmacology 137*(3), 1300–1305.

Manuskiatti, W., & Maibach, H. I. (1996). Hyaluronic acid and skin: wound healing and aging. *International Journal of Dermatology 35*(8), 539–544.

Markovic, Z., & Trajkovic, V. (2008). Biomedical potential of the reactive oxygen species generation and quenching by fullerenes (C60). *Biomaterials, 29*(26), 3561–3573. https://doi.org/10.1016/j.biomaterials.2008.05.005

Marković, Z. M., Labudová, M., Danko, M., Matijašević, D., Mičušík, M., Nádaždy, V., ... Todorović Marković, B. M. (2020). Highly efficient antioxidant f- and cl-doped carbon quantum dots for bioimaging. *ACS Sustainable Chemistry & Engineering, 8*(43), 16327–16338. https://doi.org/10.1021/acssuschemeng.0c06260

Mewada, A., Pandey, S., Shinde, S., Mishra, N., Oza, G., Thakur, M., ... Sharon, M. (2013). Green synthesis of biocompatible carbon dots using aqueous extract of Trapa bispinosa peel. *Materials Science and Engineering: C, 33*(5), 2914–2917. https://doi.org/10.1016/j.msec.2013.03.018

Mfouo-Tynga, I. S., Dias, L. D., Inada, N. M., & Kurachi, C. (2021). Features of third generation photosensitizers used in anticancer photodynamic therapy. *Photodiagnosis Photodynamic Therapy 34*, 102091.

Mohanty, A., Baaziz, W., Lafjah, M., Da Costa, V., & Janowska, I. (2018). Few layer graphene as a template for Fe-based 2D nanoparticles. *FlatChem 9*, 15–20.

Mohanty, A., & Janowska, I. (2019). Tuning the structure of in-situ synthesized few layer graphene/carbon composites into nanoporous vertically aligned graphene electrodes with high volumetric capacitance. *Electrochimica Acta 308*, 206–216.

Molaei, M. J. (2019). A review on nanostructured carbon quantum dots and their applications in biotechnology, sensors, and chemiluminescence. *Talanta 196*, 456–478.

Moniruzzaman, M., Dutta, S. D., Hexiu, J., Ganguly, K., Lim, K.-T., & Kim, J. (2022). Polyphenol derived bioactive carbon quantum dot-incorporated multifunctional hydrogels as an oxidative stress attenuator for antiaging and in vivo wound-healing applications. *Biomaterials Science 10*(13), 3527–3539.

Mukherjee, P. K., Maity, N., Nema, N. K., & Sarkar, B. K. (2011). Bioactive compounds from natural resources against skin aging. *Phytomedicine 19*(1), 64–73.

Pardakhty, A., Shakibaie, M., Daneshvar, H., Khamesipour, A., Mohammadi-Khorsand, T., & Forootanfar, H. (2012). Preparation and evaluation of niosomes containing autoclaved Leishmania major: a preliminary study. *Journal of Microencapsulation 29*(3), 219–224.

Pardeike, J., Hommoss, A., & Müller, R. H. (2009). Lipid nanoparticles (SLN, NLC) in cosmetic and pharmaceutical dermal products. *International Journal of Pharmaceutics 366*(1–2), 170–184.

Pirzado, A. A., Le Normand, F., Romero, T., Paszkiewicz, S., Papaefthimiou, V., Ihiawakrim, D., & Janowska, I. (2019). Few-layer graphene from mechanical exfoliation of graphite-based materials: Structure-dependent characteristics. *ChemEngineering 3*(2), 37.

Poletto, F. S., Beck, R. C., Guterres, S. S., Pohlmann, A. R. J. N., & Care, N. N. A. F. S. (2011). Polymeric nanocapsules: Concepts and applications. *Nanocosmetics Nanomedicines: New Approaches for Skin Care 49*–68.

Qin, Y., Zhou, Z.-W., Pan, S.-T., He, Z.-X., Zhang, X., Qiu, J.-X., … Zhou, S.-F. (2015). Graphene quantum dots induce apoptosis, autophagy, and inflammatory response via p38 mitogen-activated protein kinase and nuclear factor-κB mediated signaling pathways in activated THP-1 macrophages. *Toxicology 327*, 62–76.

Qu, S., Zhou, D., Li, D., Ji, W., Jing, P., Han, D., … Shen, D. (2016). Toward efficient orange emissive carbon nanodots through conjugated sp2-domain controlling and surface charges engineering. *Advanced Materials 28*(18), 3516–3521.

Rajamanikandan, S., Biruntha, M., & Ramalingam, G. (2022). Blue Emissive Carbon Quantum Dots (CQDs) from bio-waste peels and its antioxidant activity. *Journal of Cluster Science, 33*(3), 1045–1053. https://doi.org/10.1007/s10876-021-02029-0

Rakovich, A., & Rakovich, T. (2018). Semiconductor versus graphene quantum dots as fluorescent probes for cancer diagnosis and therapy applications. *Journal of Materials Chemistry B 6*(18), 2690–2712.

Raza, K., Shareef, M. A., Singal, P., Sharma, G., Negi, P., & Katare, O. P. (2014). Lipid-based capsaicin-loaded nano-colloidal biocompatible topical carriers with enhanced analgesic potential and decreased dermal irritation. *Journal of Liposome Research 24*(4), 290–296.

Ren, X., Liu, L., Li, Y., Dai, Q., Zhang, M., & Jing, X. (2014). Facile preparation of gadolinium(iii) chelates functionalized carbon quantum dot-based contrast agent for magnetic resonance/fluorescence multimodal imaging. *Journal of Materials Chemistry B, 2*(34), 5541–5549. https://doi.org/10.1039/C4TB00709C

Ristic, B. Z., Milenkovic, M. M., Dakic, I. R., Todorovic-Markovic, B. M., Milosavljevic, M. S., Budimir, M. D., … Trajkovic, V. S. (2014). Photodynamic antibacterial effect of graphene quantum dots. *Biomaterials, 35*(15), 4428–4435. https://doi.org/10.1016/j.biomaterials.2014.02.014

Rittié, L., & Fisher, G. J. (2002). UV-light-induced signal cascades and skin aging. *Ageing Research Reviews 1*(4), 705–720.

Rodríguez-Varillas, S., Fontanil, T., Obaya, Á. J., Fernández-González, A., Murru, C., & Badía-Laíño, R. (2022). Biocompatibility and antioxidant capabilities of carbon dots obtained from tomato (Solanum lycopersicum). *12*(2), 773.

Sadhanala, H. K., & Nanda, K. K. (2016). Boron-doped carbon nanoparticles: Size-independent color tunability from red to blue and bioimaging applications. *Carbon 96*, 166–173.

Šafranko, S., Stanković, A., Hajra, S., Kim, H.-J., Strelec, I., Dutour-Sikirić, M., … Jokić, S. (2021). Preparation of multifunctional N-Doped carbon quantum dots from citrus clementina peel: Investigating targeted pharmacological activities and the potential application for Fe3+ sensing. *14*(9), 857.

Sajid, P. A., Chetty, S. S., Praneetha, S., Murugan, A. V., Kumar, Y., & Periyasamy, L. (2016). One-pot microwave-assisted in situ reduction of Ag+ and Au3+ ions by Citrus limon extract and their carbon-dots based nanohybrids: a potential nano-bioprobe for cancer cellular imaging. *RSC Advances*, *6*(105), 103482–103490. https://doi.org/10.1039/C6RA24033J

Sharker, S. M. (2021). Nanoparticle for -photoresponsive minimal-invasive cancer therapy. *Cancer Nanotheranostics*, *2*, 201–216.

Shen, C. L., Lou, Q., Zang, J. H., Liu, K. K., Qu, S. N., Dong, L., & Shan, C. X. (2020). Near-infrared chemiluminescent carbon nanodots and their application in reactive oxygen species bioimaging. *Advanced Science 7*(8), 1903525.

Shen, J., Shang, S., Chen, X., Wang, D., & Cai, Y. (2017). Highly fluorescent N, S-co-doped carbon dots and their potential applications as antioxidants and sensitive probes for Cr (VI) detection. *Sensors and Actuators B: Chemical*, *248*, 92–100. https://doi.org/10.1016/j.snb.2017.03.123

Shi, Y., Liu, X., Wang, M., Huang, J., Jiang, X., Pang, J., … Zhang, X. (2019). Synthesis of N-doped carbon quantum dots from bio-waste lignin for selective irons detection and cellular imaging. *International Journal of Biological Macromolecules 128*, 537–545.

Shinoda, K., Suganami, A., Moriya, Y., Yamashita, M., Tanaka, T., Suzuki, A. S., … Tamura, Y. (2022). Indocyanine green conjugated phototheranostic nanoparticle for photodiagnosis and photodynamic therapy. *Photodiagnosis and Photodynamic Therapy*, *39*, 103041. https://doi.org/10.1016/j.pdpdt.2022.103041

Son, M., Park, S. W., & Jung, Y. K. (2021a). Antioxidant and anti-aging carbon quantum dots using tannic acid. *Nanotechnology*, *32*. https://doi.org/10.1088/1361-6528/ac027b

Son, M. H., Park, S. W., & Jung, Y. K. (2021b). Antioxidant and anti-aging carbon quantum dots using tannic acid. *Nanotechnology*, *32*(41), 415102. https://doi.org/10.1088/1361-6528/ac027b

Stanković, N. K., Bodik, M., Šiffalovič, P., Kotlar, M., & Mičušik, M. (2018a). Antibacterial and antibiofouling properties of light triggered fluorescent hydrophobic carbon quantum dots Langmuir–Blodgett thin films. *ACS Sustainable Chemistry Engineering 6*(3).

Stanković, N. K., Bodik, M., Šiffalovič, P., Kotlar, M., Mičušik, M., Špitalsky, Z., … Marković, Z. M. (2018b). Antibacterial and antibiofouling properties of light triggered fluorescent hydrophobic carbon quantum dots langmuir–blodgett thin films. *ACS Sustainable Chemistry & Engineering*, *6*(3), 4154–4163. https://doi.org/10.1021/acssuschemeng.7b04566

Su, W., Wu, H., Xu, H., Zhang, Y., Li, Y., Li, X., & Fan, L. (2020). Carbon dots: A booming material for biomedical applications. *Materials Chemistry Frontiers 4*(3), 821–836.

Takahashi, M., Kitamoto, D., Asikin, Y., Takara, K., & Wada, K. (2009). Liposomes encapsulating Aloe vera leaf gel extract significantly enhance proliferation and collagen synthesis in human skin cell lines. *Journal of Oleo Science 58*(12), 643–650.

Tan, Q., Kong, X., Guan, X., Wang, C., & Xu, B. (2020). Crystallization of zinc oxide quantum dots on graphene sheets as an anode material for lithium ion batteries. *CrystEngComm*, *22*(2), 320–329. https://doi.org/10.1039/C9CE01285K

Tang, S., Chen, D., Yang, Y., Wang, C., Li, X., Wang, Y., … Science, I. (2022). Mechanisms behind multicolor tunable Near-Infrared triple emission in graphene quantum dots and ratio fluorescent probe for water detection. *Journal of Colloid Interface Science 617*, 182–192.

Tavano, L., Muzzalupo, R., Picci, N., & de Cindio, B. (2014). Co-encapsulation of antioxidants into niosomal carriers: Gastrointestinal release studies for nutraceutical applications. *Colloids Surfaces B: Biointerfaces 114*, 82–88.

Tejwan, N., Saini, A. K., Sharma, A., Singh, T. A., Kumar, N., & Das, J. (2021). Metal-doped and hybrid carbon dots: A comprehensive review on their synthesis and biomedical applications. *Journal of Controlled Release 330*, 132–150.

Thulasi, S., Kathiravan, A., & Asha Jhonsi, M. (2020). Fluorescent carbon dots derived from vehicle exhaust soot and sensing of tartrazine in soft drinks. *ACS Omega 5*(12), 7025–7031.

Tournilhac, F., & Simon, P. (2001). Cosmetic or dermatological topical compositions comprising dendritic polyesters. In: Google Patents.

Trache, D., Thakur, V. K., & Boukherroub, R. (2020). Cellulose nanocrystals/graphene hybrids—a promising new class of materials for advanced applications. *Nanomaterials 10*(8), 1523.

Varsha Raveendran, P. T., & Renuka, N. K. (2022). Hydrothermal synthesis of biomass-derived carbon nanodots: Characterization and applications. *Materials Chemistry and Physics, 288*, 126236. https://doi.org/10.1016/j.matchemphys.2022.126236

Wang, J., Wei, J., Su, S., & Qiu, J. (2015). Novel fluorescence resonance energy transfer optical sensors for vitamin B 12 detection using thermally reduced carbon dots. *New Journal of Chemistry 39*(1), 501–507.

Wang, J., Xu, M., Wang, D., Li, Z., Primo, F. L., Tedesco, A. C., & Bi, H. (2019a). Copper-doped carbon dots for optical bioimaging and photodynamic therapy. *Inorganic Chemistry, 58*(19), 13394–13402. https://doi.org/10.1021/acs.inorgchem.9b02283

Wang, K.-H., Lin, R.-D., Hsu, F.-L., Huang, Y.-H., Chang, H.-C., Huang, C.-Y., & Lee, M.-H. (2006). Cosmetic applications of selected traditional Chinese herbal medicines. *Journal of Ethnopharmacology 106*(3), 353–359.

Wang, S., Ma, M., Liang, Q., Wu, X., Abbas, K., Zhu, J., … Bi, H. (2022). Single-atom manganese anchored on carbon dots for promoting mitochondrial targeting and photodynamic effect in cancer treatment. *ACS Applied Nano Materials, 5*(5), 6679–6690. https://doi.org/10.1021/acsanm.2c00716

Wang, X., Yang, L., Chen, Z., & Shin, D. M. (2008). Application of nanotechnology in cancer therapy and imaging. *CA: A Cancer journal for Clinicians 58*(2), 97–110.

Wang, X., Yang, P., Feng, Q., Meng, T., Wei, J., Xu, C., & Han, J. (2019b). Green preparation of fluorescent carbon quantum dots from cyanobacteria for biological imaging. *Polymers 11*(4), 616.

Wang, Y., & Hu, A. (2014). Carbon quantum dots: Synthesis, properties and applications. *Journal of Materials Chemistry C 2*(34), 6921–6939.

Wang, Y., Meng, H., Jia, M., Zhang, Y., Li, H., & Feng, L. (2016). Intraparticle FRET of Mn(ii)-doped carbon dots and its application in discrimination of volatile organic compounds. *Nanoscale, 8*(39), 17190–17195. https://doi.org/10.1039/C6NR05927A

Wary, K. K., Thakker, G. D., Humtsoe, J. O., & Yang, J. (2003). Analysis of VEGF-responsive genes involved in the activation of endothelial cells. *Molecular Cancer 2*(1), 1–12.

Wen, Y., Jia, Q., Nan, F., Zheng, X., Liu, W., Wu, J., … Wang, P. (2019). Pheophytin derived near-infrared-light responsive carbon dot assembly as a new phototheranotic agent for bioimaging and photodynamic *Therapy. 14*(12), 2162–2168. https://doi.org/10.1002/asia.201900416

Wu, W., Zhan, L., Fan, W., Song, J., Li, X., Li, Z., … Wu, M. (2015). Cu–N dopants boost electron transfer and photooxidation reactions of carbon dots. *Angewandte Chemie International Edition 54*(22), 6540–6544.

Xie, Z., Du, Q., Wu, Y., Hao, X., & Liu, C. (2016). Full-band UV shielding and highly daylight luminescent silane-functionalized graphene quantum dot nanofluids and their arbitrary polymerized hybrid gel glasses. *Journal of Materials Chemistry C 4*(41), 9879–9886.

Xu, Y., Jia, X.-H., Yin, X.-B., He, X.-W., & Zhang, Y.-K. (2014). Carbon quantum dot stabilized gadolinium nanoprobe prepared via a one-pot hydrothermal approach for magnetic resonance and fluorescence dual-modality bioimaging. *Analytical Chemistry, 86*(24), 12122–12129. https://doi.org/10.1021/ac503002c

Yang, G., Wu, C., Luo, X., Liu, X., Gao, Y., Wu, P., … Saavedra, S. S. (2018). Exploring the emissive states of heteroatom-doped graphene quantum dots. *The Journal of Physical Chemistry C 122*(11), 6483–6492.

Yang, Y., Tang, S., Chen, D., Wang, C., Gu, B., Li, X., … Aspects, E. (2021). Multifunctional red-emission graphene quantum dots with tunable light emissions for trace water sensing, WLEDs and information encryption. *Colloids Surfaces A: Physicochemical Engineering Aspects 622*, 126593.

Yokoi, T., Goto, T., Hara, M., Sekino, T., Seki, T., Kamitakahara, M., … Kawashita, M. (2021). Incorporation of tetracarboxylate ions into octacalcium phosphate for the development of next-generation biofriendly materials. *Communications Chemistry, 4*(1), 4. https://doi.org/10.1038/s42004-020-00443-5

Yu, C., Xuan, T., Chen, Y., Zhao, Z., Liu, X., Lian, G., & Li, H. (2016). Gadolinium-doped carbon dots with high quantum yield as an effective fluorescence and magnetic resonance bimodal imaging probe. *Journal of Alloys and Compounds, 688*, 611–619. https://doi.org/10.1016/j.jallcom.2016.07.226

Yuan, F., Li, S., Fan, Z., Meng, X., Fan, L., & Yang, S. (2016). Shining carbon dots: Synthesis and biomedical and optoelectronic applications. *Nano Today 11*(5), 565–586.

Yuan, F., Wang, Z., Li, X., Li, Y., Tan, Z.A., Fan, L., & Yang, S. (2017). Light-emitting diodes: bright multicolor bandgap fluorescent carbon quantum dots for electroluminescent light-emitting diodes (Adv. Mater. 3/2017). *Advanced Materials 29*(3).

Yuan, X., Liu, Z., Guo, Z., Ji, Y., Jin, M., & Wang, X. (2014). Cellular distribution and cytotoxicity of graphene quantum dots with different functional groups. *Nanoscale Research Letters 9*, 1–9.

Yuan, Y. H., Li, R. S., Wang, Q., Wu, Z. L., Wang, J., Liu, H., & Huang, C. Z. (2015). Germanium-doped carbon dots as a new type of fluorescent probe for visualizing the dynamic invasions of mercury(ii) ions into cancer cells. *Nanoscale, 7*(40), 16841–16847. https://doi.org/10.1039/C5NR05326A

Yue, J., Li, L., Jiang, C., Mei, Q., Dong, W.-F., & Yan, R. (2021). Riboflavin-based carbon dots with high singlet oxygen generation for photodynamic therapy. *Journal of Materials Chemistry B, 9*(38), 7972–7978. https://doi.org/10.1039/D1TB01291F

Zhang, D.-Y., Zheng, Y., Zhang, H., He, L., Tan, C.-P., Sun, J.-H., … Ji, L.-N. (2017). Ruthenium complex-modified carbon nanodots for lysosome-targeted one-and two-photon imaging and photodynamic therapy. *Nanoscale 9*(47), 18966–18976.

Zhang, M., Zhao, L., Du, F., Wu, Y., Cai, R., Xu, L., … Du, F. J. N. (2019). Facile synthesis of cerium-doped carbon quantum dots as a highly efficient antioxidant for free radical scavenging. *30*(32), 325101.

Zhang, Q., Xu, W., Han, C., Wang, X., Wang, Y., Li, Z., … Wu, M. (2018). Graphene structure boosts electron transfer of dual-metal doped carbon dots in photooxidation. *Carbon 126*, 128–134.

Zhao, S., Wu, S., Jia, Q., Huang, L., Lan, M., Wang, P., & Zhang, W. (2020). Lysosome-targetable carbon dots for highly efficient photothermal/photodynamic synergistic cancer therapy and photoacoustic/two-photon excited fluorescence imaging. *Chemical Engineering Journal, 388*, 124212. https://doi.org/10.1016/j.cej.2020.124212

Zhao, S., Yang, K., Jiang, L., Xiao, J., Wang, B., Zeng, L., … Lan, M. (2021). Polythiophene-based carbon dots for imaging-guided photodynamic therapy. *ACS Applied Nano Materials, 4*(10), 10528–10533. https://doi.org/10.1021/acsanm.1c02042

Zheng, M., Li, Y., Liu, S., Wang, W., Xie, Z., & Jing, X. (2016). One-pot to synthesize multifunctional carbon dots for near infrared fluorescence imaging and photothermal cancer therapy. *ACS Applied Materials Interfaces 8*(36), 23533–23541.

Zhou, J., Shan, X., Ma, J., Gu, Y., Qian, Z., Chen, J., & Feng, H. (2014). Facile synthesis of P-doped carbon quantum dots with highly efficient photoluminescence. *Rsc Advances 4*(11), 5465–5468.

Zhou, Y., Sharma, S. K., Peng, Z., & Leblanc, R. M. (2017a). Polymers in carbon dots: A review. *Polymers, 9*(2), 67.

Zhou, Y., Sun, H., Wang, F., Ren, J., & Qu, X. (2017b). How functional groups influence the ROS generation and cytotoxicity of graphene quantum dots. *Chemical Communications* *53*(76), 10588–10591.

Zhu, C., Yang, S., Sun, J., He, P., Yuan, N., Ding, J., … Xie, X. (2015a). Deep ultraviolet emission photoluminescence and high luminescece efficiency of ferric passivated graphene quantum dots: Strong negative inductive effect of Fe. *Synthetic Metals 209*, 468–472.

Zhu, S., Meng, Q., Wang, L., Zhang, J., Song, Y., Jin, H., … Yang, B. (2013). Highly photoluminescent carbon dots for multicolor patterning, sensors, and bioimaging. *Angewandte Chemie International Edition 52*(14), 3953–3957.

Zhu, S., Song, Y., Zhao, X., Shao, J., Zhang, J., & Yang, B. (2015b). The photoluminescence mechanism in carbon dots (graphene quantum dots, carbon nanodots, and polymer dots): Current state and future perspective. *Nano Research 8*, 355–381.

8 Synergizing Carbon Quantum Dots for Biomedical Imaging, Targeted Drug Delivery, and Photodynamic Therapy

Syed Ansar Ali, T. Saichand, Tanvi Shingote, Benny Harshitha, Srivalliputtur Sarath Babu, Ravichandiran Velyutham and Govinda Kapusetti

8.1 INTRODUCTION

In the rapidly advancing landscape of nanotechnology, the convergence of multidisciplinary sciences has paved the way for groundbreaking innovations with profound implications for biomedical applications. Among the myriad nanostructures that have emerged, carbon quantum dots (CQDs) have garnered significant attention due to their unique physicochemical properties and versatile applications. As the demand for non-invasive, high-resolution imaging techniques and targeted drug delivery systems continues to escalate, integrating CQDs into biomedical research holds tremendous promise. These nanoscale carbonaceous materials exhibit remarkable optical properties, biocompatibility, and facile surface functionalization, rendering them ideal candidates for advanced biomedical applications (1). Nanotechnology, as defined by size, is naturally broad, including fields of science as diverse as surface science, organic chemistry, molecular biology, semiconductor physics, energy storage, engineering, microfabrication, and molecular engineering. The associated research and applications are equally diverse, ranging from extensions of conventional device physics to completely new approaches based upon molecular self-assembly, from developing new materials with dimensions on the nanoscale to direct control of matter on the atomic scale. Chemistry, physics, materials science, biology, and medicine are all included in the interdisciplinary and multidisciplinary field of nanotechnology research (2).

DOI: 10.1201/9781003437857-10

Within the vast world of nanotechnology, quantum dots stand as diminutive marvels, wielding profound implications for diverse scientific disciplines and technological frontiers. At the nexus of quantum mechanics and materials science, these nanoscale semiconductors exhibit extraordinary properties, pushing the boundaries of what is conceivable in manipulating and utilizing light and matter. Quantum dots are nanosized crystalline structures, typically composed of semiconductor materials, where quantum confinement effects confine the motion of charge carriers in all three spatial dimensions (3). This confinement imparts quantum dots with exceptional and tunable optical properties, including size-dependent absorption and emission spectra and superior photochemical stability (4). The quantum dots' ability to emit light with high efficiency and in a range of colors, from ultraviolet to near-infrared, has positioned them as veritable luminous beacons in fields such as optoelectronics (5), imaging, and sensing. The synthesis of quantum dots spans a rich tapestry of methods, each tailored to control these nanocrystals' size, shape, and composition. From traditional colloidal synthesis to advanced approaches like epitaxial growth and microfabrication techniques (6), researchers have harnessed a diverse toolkit to sculpt quantum dots with precision.

As the narrative unfolds, the exploration extends to multifaceted applications that quantum dots have catalyzed across scientific disciplines. Quantum dots have become integral players in the realms of electronics, photonics (7), and, prominently, biomedicine. Their implementation in biological imaging, from fluorescence microscopy to in vivo imaging, has revolutionized the visualization of cellular and molecular processes. Furthermore, quantum dots have emerged as promising candidates for drug delivery, photothermal therapy, and diagnostics, capitalizing on their tailored optical properties and facile surface functionalization. With its comprehensive survey of quantum dots, this chapter aspires to provide readers with a nuanced understanding of the fundamental principles governing these nanoscale entities. From the quantum mechanical phenomena that underpin their unique behavior to the intricate dance of atoms in their synthesis and, finally, to the myriad applications spanning scientific disciplines, this exploration aims to be a beacon guiding scholars, researchers, and enthusiasts through the captivating world of quantum dots. In doing so, we unveil these diminutive yet potent entities' transformative potential, which continues redefining the boundaries of what is achievable at the intersection of quantum science and nanotechnology. Within the following pages, we embark on a journey through the fundamental characteristics of QDs, synthesis methodologies, and the underlying principles governing the interactions between CQDs and biological systems. The chapter will unravel the intricacies of leveraging CQDs as contrast agents for biomedical imaging modalities, shedding light on their potential to enhance diagnostic precision and enable early disease detection. Simultaneously, the exploration extends into the realm of nanodrug delivery and photodynamic treatment (PDT), where the unique attributes of CQDs offer an unprecedented opportunity to design and implement precision-targeted therapeutic interventions. From cellular uptake mechanisms to in vivo behavior, this chapter aims to provide a comprehensive understanding of the synergistic amalgamation of CQDs with biomedical applications.

8.2 QUANTUM DOTS AND THEIR FUNDAMENTAL CHARACTERISTICS

Quantum dots (QDs) are semiconductors with core-shell structures and a diameter typically ranging from 2 to 10nm (8). The quantum confinement effect (QCE) explains the structural characteristics and prominent properties of QDs. The word confinement means to confine the motion of a randomly moving electron to restrict its motion to specific energy levels, and quantum reflects the atomic realm of particles. QCE mainly deals with the energy of confined electrons. The energy levels of electrons will not remain continuous, as in the case of bulk materials compared to nanocrystals (9). Semiconducting nanomaterials exhibit fascinating properties when reducing their dimensionality from 2D to 1D to 0D. QCE occurs when reducing the size and shape of nanomaterials to less than 100–10 nm or even less. The QCE occurs only in semiconductor quantum dots because their optical, electrical, and bandgap properties are tunable concerning changes in particle size that lead to various applications (10). Electrons confined in one direction are called quantum wells, where electrons move in 2D and are quantized in 1D. Electrons are confined in two directions called quantum wires, where electrons move in 1D and 2D (11). Electrons are confined in three directions, called quantum dots, where electrons move in 0D and quantized 3D. It is essential to know about excitons because it is the first step to understanding quantum dots and the quantum confinement effect in semiconductors. Electrons shift from the valence band to the conduction band when light falls on semiconductors. As the electrons move from the lower-level valence band to the higher-level conduction band, the excited electrons in QDs leave a hole in the valence band. The absorption of light by the semiconductor material to create a bound electron-hole pair is called an exciton, or an electron-hole pair is a quasiparticle called an exciton. In an unconfined (bulk) semiconductor, an electron-hole pair is typically bound within a characteristic length called the Bohr exciton radius. The Bohr radius (a^O) varies from 2 to 50 nm depending on the material dielectric coefficient. The particle size, about the Bohr radius for nanostructured semiconductors, impacts the electron-wave function (12). The electron density states, energy gap, and discrete energy levels cause concerning changes in size in the bandgap. When bulk materials are smaller, the electron energy levels overlap rather than being distinct or continuous, but when nanoscale materials are more significant, the individual electron energy levels appear. confinement can be in 1D, 2D, and 3D. Quantum dots and quantum wells exhibit distinct physicochemical characteristics compared to 3D bulk solids because of the reduction in solid size, i.e., from 3D to 2D or 0D. Smaller semiconductor materials are good at providing the desired electrical, magnetic, optical, and chemical properties (13). The low-dimensional materials have distinct chemical and physical characteristics that are not present in their bulk materials. For example, structural changes, such as quantum-size effects, result from the confinement of electrons and holes to LDS. The quantum confinement effect (QCE) in zero-dimensional QDs is characterized by sizes smaller than or equal to the exciton radius predicted by Bohr's quantum mechanics theory. The result of direct recombination between the valence and conduction bands, made possible by the conjugated domain's small size, is band gap fluorescence. As a photosensitizer for photodynamic therapy (PDT) and as a nanocarrier for targeted drug delivery (chemotherapy) (14)

8.3 QUANTUM DOTS AND NANOTECHNOLOGY

Nanoparticles and quantum dots, both in the fascinating realm of nanotechnology, represent distinct classes of nanomaterials with unique properties and applications. While the terms are sometimes used interchangeably, it is essential to recognize the nuanced differences between nanoparticles and quantum dots, as each class offers its own set of advantages and limitations. Nanoparticles are a broad category encompassing particles with dimensions on the nanometer scale, typically ranging from 1 to 100 nanometers. They can be composed of various materials, including metals, metal oxides, polymers, and ceramics. The defining characteristic of nanoparticles is their size, allowing them to exhibit properties different from their bulk counterparts. This versatility in composition allows nanoparticles to serve myriad purposes, ranging from drug delivery and catalysis to imaging and sensors, due to their ability to interact with biological systems and materials at the nanoscale (15). Additionally, nanoparticle synthesis methods are often scalable, facilitating the production of substantial quantities for industrial applications.

In contrast, quantum dots represent a subset of nanoparticles that exhibit distinctive quantum mechanical properties resulting from their confined size. Typically composed of semiconductor materials like cadmium selenide or indium phosphide, quantum dots possess quantized energy levels that impart size-dependent optical and electronic characteristics. Notable advantages of quantum dots include tunable emission spectra, allowing precise adjustment of the emitted light color for applications such as biological imaging. Their high quantum yield and photostability make quantum dots well-suited for displays, sensors, and biological labeling applications. Distinguishing factors between nanoparticles and quantum dots include the manifestation of quantum confinement effects in the latter, where the size of the particle dictates its electronic and optical properties. Nanoparticles, in contrast, may or may not display such effects, depending on their composition and size. While nanoparticles can be crafted from various materials, quantum dots are typically semiconductor nanocrystals with specific material compositions.

Furthermore, quantum dots exhibit unique, size-dependent optical properties, setting them apart from other nanoparticles. In conclusion, nanoparticles and quantum dots represent diverse classes of nanomaterials, each offering distinctive advantages. The choice between them depends on the specific requirements of the intended application, with quantum dots often favored for applications demanding precise optical properties and quantum mechanical effects.

Colloidal quantum dots (QDs) have gained significant attention in recent decades due to their standard optical features linked to quantum confinement phenomena, in which their band gap may be controlled by modifying particle size. As a result of QD features such as photostability, brilliant luminescence, size-dependent PL, narrow emission, and broad absorption bands, colloidal QDs have received much interest during the last few decades (16). Carbon quantum dots are nanoparticles composed of carbon atoms. They have unique optical and electronic properties due to their small size and quantum confinement effects. Due to their biocompatibility, low toxic-ity, and tunable fluorescence properties, these dots have gained significant attention in various fields, such as bioimaging, sensing, and energy storage. For example, in bioimaging, CQDs can be used as contrast agents to enhance the visibility of specific tissues or cells in medical imaging techniques such as fluorescence or magnetic reso-nance imaging. Their small size allows them to easily penetrate biological barriers and target specific areas, providing accurate and detailed images for diagnosis (17). Biomedical imaging has evolved significantly with nanotechnology, and CQDs are gaining attention due to their tiny size, biocompatibility, and low toxicity. This chap-ter dives into recent progress in using CQDs for biomedical imaging, focusing on synergistic applications. We will explore how CQDs are made, how they can be mod-ified, and the impact of these factors on their optical properties. Additionally, we will examine the current state of CQD-based imaging techniques, their benefits, and potential challenges while looking ahead to future possibilities.

Synthesis and Surface Functionalization of CQDs: CQDs can be synthesized by various methods, such as top-down approaches (e.g., chemical oxidation, electro-chemical exfoliation, laser ablation, etc.) or bottom-up approaches (e.g., hydrothermal, microwave, solvothermal, etc.). The synthesis route can affect CQDs' physicochemi-cal properties and optical characteristics, such as size, shape, surface functionaliza-tion, quantum yield, and emission wavelength. Therefore, optimizing the synthesis parameters and selecting the appropriate precursors and solvents is essential to obtaining high-quality CQDs for specific biomedical applications (18). However, precursor materials, reaction conditions, and post-synthesis treatments affect CQD properties. The precursor materials are the carbon sources that are used to synthesize CQDs. They can be natural, synthetic, organic, inorganic, solid, liquid, or gaseous. The type and composition of the precursor materials can determine the carbon con-tent, functional groups, and heteroatoms of the CQDs. Citric acid, glucose, and urea are commonly used as precursors for obtaining highly luminescent CQDs (19, 20). The use of different precursors can also result in different morphologies and sizes of CQDs. For example, polyethylene glycol (PEG) as a precursor can produce spherical CQDs, while phenylenediamine can produce rod-shaped CQDs.

Reaction conditions are the parameters that control the synthesis process of CQDs, such as temperature, time, pressure, pH, solvent, catalyst, and microwave irradiation. The reaction conditions can affect the nucleation, growth, and aggrega-tion of the CQDs and their surface passivation and functionalization. For instance, increasing the temperature or time can increase the size and crystallinity of the CQDs, while decreasing the pH or adding a solvent can increase the solubility and stability of the CQDs (21). Different catalysts or microwave irradiation can also enhance the yield and quality of the CQDs. Iron oxide nanoparticles as a catalyst can produce CQDs with a high quantum yield and a narrow size distribution. In contrast, microwave irradiation can quickly produce CQDs with uniform size and shape (22).

Post-synthesis treatments are the methods that are used to purify, separate, and modify the CQDs after the synthesis process. They can include filtration, centrifuga-tion, dialysis, precipitation, washing, drying, annealing, and surface modification. The post-synthesis treatments can affect the purity, dispersity, and functionality of the CQDs. Filtration and centrifugation can remove the large aggregates and impurities from the CQDs, while dialysis and precipitation can separate them based on their size and charge. Washing and drying can remove the residual solvent and moisture from the CQDs, while annealing can improve the crystallinity and conductivity of the CQDs. Surface modification can introduce different functional groups or ligands to the CQDs, affecting their solubility, stability, properties, biocompatibility, and reactivity (23).

One of the ways to coat CQDs with biomolecules or polymers is to use surface functionalization techniques. Surface functionalization is the process of modifying the surface of CQDs with different functional groups or biomolecules to enhance their stability, biocompatibility, and specificity. Surface functionalization can also tune CQDs' optical properties and fluorescence behavior, making them more suitable for imaging (24). Figure 8.1 depicts various surface modifications and coatings for

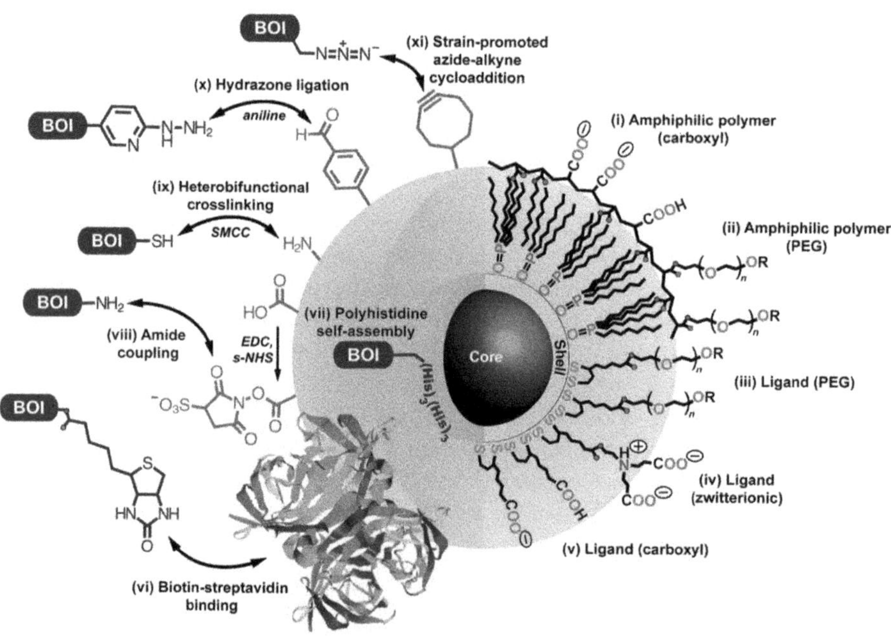

FIGURE 8.1 Illustrative overview of the chemistry of core-shell QDs. Coatings for aqueous solubility are as follows: (i) amphiphilic polymer coating with carboxyl(ate) groups; (ii) amphiphilic polymer coating with PEG oligomers; (iii) dithiol ligand with a distal PEG oligomer; (iv) dithiol ligand with a distal zwitterionic functionality; and (v) dithiol ligand with a distal carboxyl(ate) group. Common R groups include carboxyl, amine, and methoxy, although many others can be introduced (e.g., see vi, x, xi). Methods for conjugating biomolecules of interest (BOI) are as follows: (vi) biotin-streptavidin binding; (vii) polyhistidine self-assembly to the inorganic shell of the QD; (viii) amide coupling using EDC/s-NHS activation; (ix) heterobifunctional crosslinking using succinimidyl-4-(N-maleimidomethyl)cyclohexane-1-carboxylate (SMCC; structure not shown); (x) aniline-catalyzed hydrazone ligation; and (xi) strain-promoted azide–alkyne cycloaddition. The double arrows are intended to represent conjugation between the functional groups and, in principle, their interchangeability (not reaction mechanisms or reversibility) (30).

core shell QDs to improve aqueous solubility and to conjugate biomolecules of interest. Coating CQDs with polyethylene glycol (PEG) to improve their water solubility, biostability, and biocompatibility PEG can also reduce the aggregation and photoblinking of CQDs and increase their quantum yield and emission wavelength (25). Coating CQDs with chitosan, a natural polysaccharide, enhances their antibacterial and antifungal activity. Chitosan can also increase CQDs' fluorescence intensity and stability, enabling their pH-sensitive drug delivery (26). Coating CQDs with bovine serum albumin (BSA), a natural protein, to improve their biocompatibility, biodegradability, and bioavailability BSA can protect CQDs from oxidation and degradation and facilitate cellular uptake and targeting (27, 28). Coating CQDs with folic acid, a natural vitamin, increases their specificity and affinity for cancer cells. Folic acid can also improve the fluorescence and photostability of CQDs and enable their selective drug delivery and photodynamic therapy (29).

8.4 OPTICAL PROPERTIES AND IMAGING MODALITIES

CQDs optical properties, like size-dependent emission and photostability, are crucial for imaging. The optical properties of CQDs, especially their fluorescence, are affected by various factors, such as the synthesis method and parameters, such as the type, ratio, and concentration of precursors, the reaction time and temperature, the solvent, and the purification process. These factors can influence CQDs size, shape, surface functionalization, quantum yield, and emission wavelength (31). It also looks at combining CQDs with other agents for improved imaging contrast and sensitivity: the doping of CQDs with heteroatoms, such as nitrogen, sulfur, phosphorus, boron, etc. These atoms can introduce new energy levels and modify CQDs electronic structure and surface states, resulting in enhanced fluorescence intensity, stability, and tunable emission color (32). The external environment includes pH, temperature, solvent, metal ions, etc. These factors can affect CQDs' fluorescence behavior and properties, such as fluorescence quenching, enhancement, shifting, or switching.

CQDs have been widely used for various bioimaging applications, including fluorescence imaging of cells, tissues, organs, tumors, bacteria, viruses, etc. CQDs can serve as bright and stable fluorescent probes that can emit light in the range from the UV to the NIR region, covering different biological windows. CQDs can also be modified with different functional groups or biomolecules to improve their biocompatibility, biostability, and specificity for different biological targets. Multimodal imaging of different modalities, such as fluorescence, magnetic resonance, computed tomography, photoacoustic, etc. CQDs can be combined with other nanomaterials, such as metal nanoparticles, magnetic nanoparticles, graphene, etc., to achieve multifunctional and multimodal imaging (33–35). This can provide complementary and synergistic information for better diagnosis and therapy.

Sensing and biosensing of various analytes, such as metal ions, acids, proteins, biothiols, polypeptides, DNA and miRNA, water pollutants, hematin, drugs, vitamins, and other chemicals. CQDs can act as sensitive and selective sensors and biosensors based on different mechanisms, such as fluorescence quenching, static quenching, dynamic quenching, energy transfer, the inner filter effect, photo-induced electron transfer, and fluorescence resonance energy transfer (36, 37).

8.4.1 *In Vitro Imaging*

CQDs play a crucial role in cytological imaging within laboratory settings. Due to their small size and tunable fluorescence, they serve as ideal probes for tracking cellular structures (Figure 8.2), monitoring cellular processes, and investigating intracellular dynamics. Researchers commonly use CQDs to label specific cell organelles or biomolecules, enabling precise visualization and analysis under fluorescence microscopy. Another notable application of CQDs in vitro involves selectively targeting and labeling specific cells or cellular components. Functionalized CQDs, featuring surface modifications such as aptamers or antibodies, allow targeted binding to particular cell types. This capability is particularly advantageous for studying cellular interactions, identifying diseased cells, or tracking the delivery of therapeutic agents within cell cultures. CQDs serve as versatile imaging agents in various biological assays. Their integration into assays facilitates the detection of biomolecules, the assessment of cellular viability, and the monitoring of enzymatic activities. The unique optical properties of CQDs contribute to the sensitivity and precision of these assays, making them valuable tools in bioanalytical research (38–40).

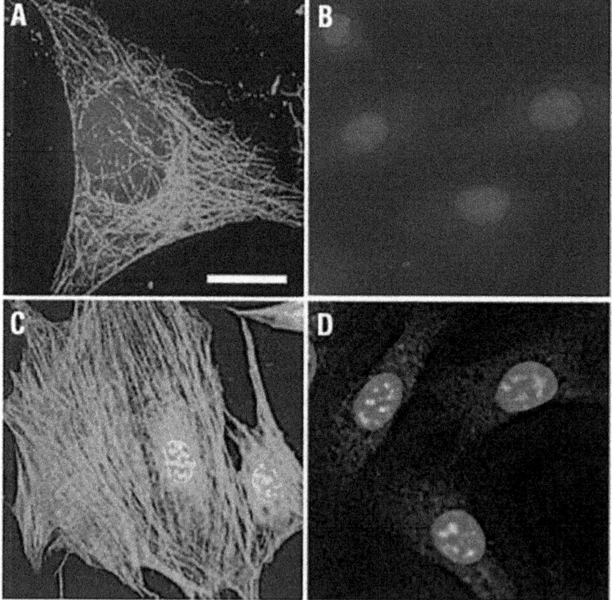

FIGURE 8.2 Staining of cytoskeleton fibers in 3T3 mouse fibroblast cells with QD-streptavidin. (A) Microtubules were labeled with monoclonal anti-α tubulin antibody, biotinylated anti-mouse IgG and QD 630–streptavidin (red). (B) Control for (A) without primary antibody. (C) Actin filaments were stained with biotinylated phalloidin and QD 535–streptavidin (green). (D) Control for (C) without biotin-phalloidin. The nuclei were counterstained with Hoechst 33342 blue dye. Filter sets ex 480 ± 20 nm/em 535 ± 10 nm and ex 560 ± 27.5 nm/em 635 ± 10 nm were used to observe signals of QD 535 and QD 630, respectively. Scale bar, 10 μm for (A), 24 μm for (B) through (D) (41).

***In Vivo* Imaging:** In the realm of in vivo imaging, CQDs have found significant applications, particularly in tumor imaging. Functionalized CQDs can be designed to selectively accumulate in tumor tissues, providing high-contrast imaging for early cancer detection (42). Their biocompatibility and low toxicity make them attractive candidates for long-term in vivo imaging studies. CQDs are explored for whole-body imaging studies to understand their biodistribution and pharmacokinetics, as shown in Figures 8.3 and 8.4.

Administered systemically in animal models, CQDs' fluorescence or other imaging signals can be tracked in real time. This information is crucial for assessing the

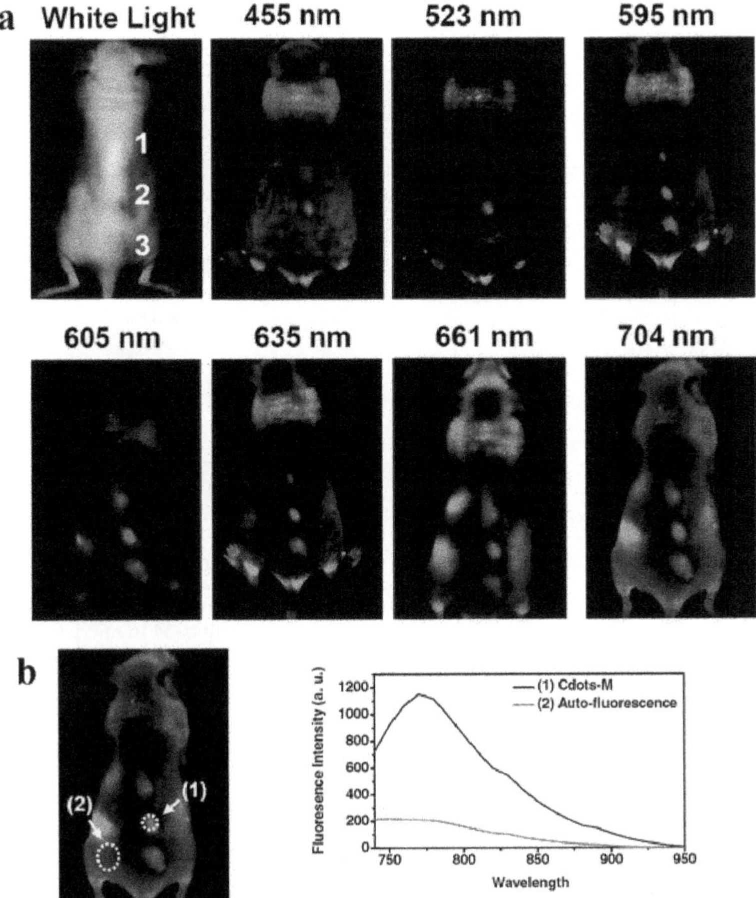

FIGURE 8.3 In vivo fluorescence imaging. Cdots-M represents Cdots from Multiwall Nanotubes (MWNTs) a) In vivo fluorescence images of a Cdots-M-injected mouse. The images were taken under various excitation wavelengths at 455, 523, 595, 605, 635, 661, and 704 nm. Red and green represent fluorescent signals of Cdots-M and the tissue autofluorescence, respectively. b) Signal-to-background separation of the spectral image taken under the NIR (704 nm) excitation. The Cdots fluorescence was well separated from the tissue autofluorescence background (43).

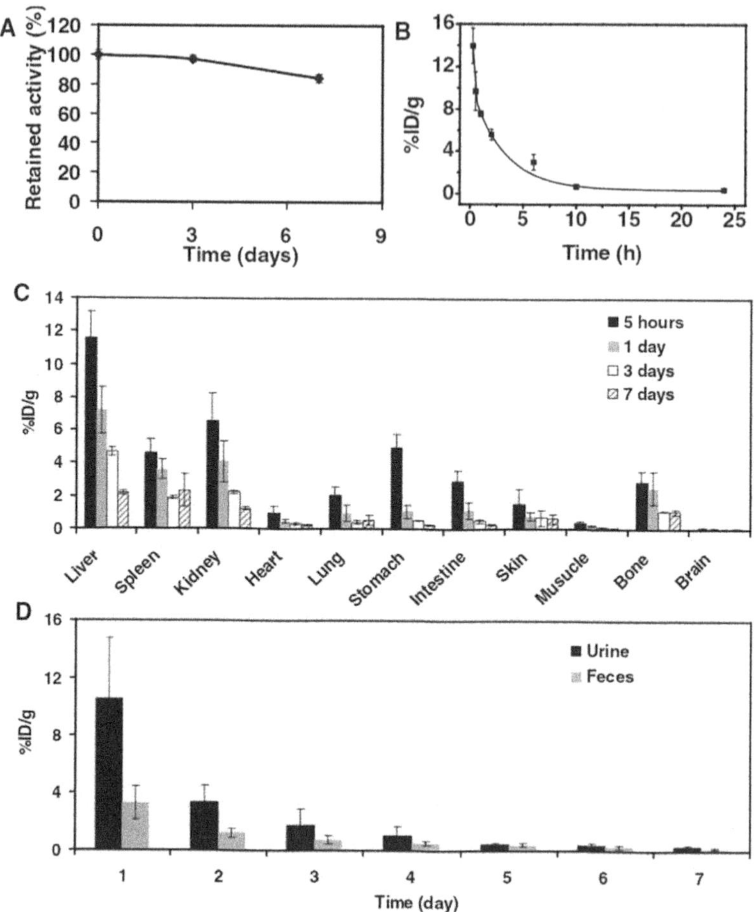

FIGURE 8.4 Pharmacokinetics and biodistribution of 125I-Cdots-M in mice. (A) The radio-labeling stability curve of 125I-Cdots-M in mouse plasma at 37°C. (B) The blood circulation curve of 125I-Cdots-M. (C) Time-dependent biodistribution of 125I-Cdots-M in female Balb/c mice. (D) Distribution of 125I-Cdots-M in urine and feces of Balb/c mice collected by metabolism cages (43).

safety and feasibility of CQDs for future clinical applications. CQDs are valuable for real-time monitoring of dynamic biological processes within living organisms. Examples include tracking the migration of immune cells, studying the circulatory system, or visualizing changes in cellular metabolism. The ability of CQDs to provide real-time imaging data contributes to a deeper understanding of complex biological phenomena. CQDs hold promise in theranostic applications, seamlessly combining diagnostic imaging with therapeutic functionalities. Functionalized CQDs can carry therapeutic payloads while simultaneously serving as imaging agents. This dual role allows for real-time monitoring of therapeutic interventions, making them valuable tools in personalized medicine (38–40).

8.5 TOXICITY, PHARMACOKINETICS, AND BIODISTRIBUTION OF QDs IN-VIVO

CQDs are a promising and versatile material for biomedical applications, especially bioimaging. However, before they can be used for clinical purposes, it is crucial to understand how they behave in the body, their distribution, pharmacokinetics, and any associated toxicity. Understanding the behavior of CQDs in vivo is essential for assessing their potential applications in medicine. Several key factors, including distribution, pharmacokinetics, and toxicity, are crucial in determining CQDs' biocompatibility and safety profile. Biodistribution refers to the spatial and temporal distribution of CQDs within the body after administration. The size, surface properties, and functionalization of CQDs influence their biodistribution. Studies have shown that smaller CQDs tend to have a more widespread distribution, and surface modifications can be tailored to enhance targeting to specific tissues or organs (44, 45). Various cells can internalize CQDs through endocytosis, and they can be localized in different cellular compartments, such as the cytoplasm, the nucleus, the mitochondria, or the lysosomes, depending on their size, surface charge, and functionalization. Biodistribution studies provide insights into where CQDs accumulate and how long they persist in various biological compartments (46). Depending on their size and surface properties, CQDs can be excreted from the body through different routes, such as urine, feces, bile, or sweat. Smaller CQDs (<5 nm) tend to be eliminated faster than larger ones (>10 nm), and hydrophilic CQDs tend to be cleared more efficiently than hydrophobic ones. Pharmacokinetics examines how the body processes a substance over time. For CQDs, this includes absorption, distribution, metabolism, and excretion (ADME). The small size of CQDs allows efficient absorption, and surface modifications can influence their circulation time. Understanding the pharmacokinetics of CQDs is crucial for determining the appropriate dosage, administration route, and frequency to achieve the desired therapeutic or imaging effects (47). Evaluating the toxicity of CQDs is a critical aspect of their biomedical applications. Biocompatibility is a notable advantage of CQDs, but potential adverse effects must be systematically assessed. Toxicity studies investigate whether CQDs induce any harmful effects on cells, tissues, or organs. CQDs have shown low toxicity and good biocompatibility in various in vitro and in vivo studies compared to conventional semiconductor quantum dots that contain heavy metals (48). CQDs have been reported to have no or minimal effects on cell viability, proliferation, differentiation, apoptosis, inflammation, oxidative stress, DNA damage, and immune response. Factors such as concentration, exposure duration, and surface functionalization play significant roles in determining the safety profile of CQDs. Comprehensive toxicity assessments are essential for ensuring the feasibility of CQDs in clinical settings.

The behavior of CQDs in the body has direct implications for their clinical applications. In the realm of biomedical imaging, understanding the biodistribution and pharmacokinetics of CQDs helps optimize imaging protocols for accurate and reliable results. Additionally, the low toxicity of CQDs positions them as promising candidates for therapeutic applications. Continued research is necessary to elucidate the behavior of CQDs in vivo further. Long-term studies can provide insights into the chronic effects of CQDs and their potential for cumulative toxicity.

Additionally, exploring innovative surface modifications and engineering strategies can enhance the biocompatibility of CQDs, opening new avenues for safe and effective clinical applications. In conclusion, a comprehensive understanding of how CQDs behave in the body, encompassing biodistribution, pharmacokinetics, and toxicity, is crucial for advancing their biomedical applications. This knowledge forms the foundation for developing CQDs as versatile medical tools, ranging from advanced imaging technologies to targeted therapeutic interventions.

Despite their promise, CQDs face challenges like long-term toxicity concerns, the need for standardized synthesis methods, and regulatory considerations. One of the challenges and opportunities for CQDs in bioimaging is understanding their fluorescence's origin and mechanism. Different theories have been proposed to explain the fluorescence of CQDs, such as the quantum confinement effect, surface state effect, carbon core effect, molecular state effect, etc. However, no consensus exists on the dominant factor determining CQDs' fluorescence. Moreover, the fluorescence of CQDs can be influenced by various external factors, such as pH, temperature, solvent, metal ions, etc. Therefore, it is necessary to investigate CQDs' fluorescence behavior and properties under different conditions and environments and elucidate the relationship between their structure and function. Another challenge and opportunity for CQDs in bioimaging is to improve their performance and functionality. Although CQDs have many advantages over other fluorescent probes, they still face limitations, such as low quantum yield, broad emission spectrum, aggregation-induced quenching, photoblinking, etc. These limitations can affect the sensitivity, resolution, contrast, and stability of bioimaging. Therefore, developing novel strategies and techniques to overcome these drawbacks and enhance CQDs' bioimaging quality and efficiency is desirable. Some possible approaches include doping, surface engineering, hybridization, functionalization, etc. The chapter critically assesses these issues and suggests future research directions. It highlights the potential of CQDs in biomedical and multimodal imaging, pointing toward a roadmap for overcoming current limitations.

8.6   CARBON QUANTUM DOTS AS TARGETED NANOCARRIERS

Over the past few years, death from cancer has grown to such an extent that in late 2022, it has been considered the worst, with almost 10 million recorded deaths. Success in cancer treatment depends highly on the stage at which it is detected, so an early diagnosis is imperative for effective treatment. Aiming at early diagnosis, scientists are actively looking for something compelling in this fight against cancer, creating a great demand for new approaches for cancer detection and monitoring in live cells. In hospitals, tissue biopsies, although laborious and invasive, are used as a diagnostic procedure (49). There are a variety of advantages to using nanoparticles (NPs) over other materials. The NPs might remain at the tumor site due to the increased permeability and retention (EPR) effect. Another reason why NPs should be preferred is because the surface of an NP may be specifically engineered to reduce non-specific absorption by the reticuloendothelial systems (50). Another feature is the high surface-area-to-volume ratio, which allows therapeutic compounds to be trapped efficiently and not destroyed by the microenvironment. Photothermal treatment (PTT), chemotherapy, gene therapy (GT), photodynamic therapy (PDT), and other monotherapies are commonly utilized to treat cancer. In navigating this exploration, we aim to not only elucidate the current state of the art but also to inspire future research endeavors that hold the key to unlocking the full potential of CQDs in advancing the frontiers of biomedical imaging and targeted drug delivery. As we embark on this intellectual voyage, we invite readers to delve into the intricate world of CQDs and witness the transformative impact they may wield in shaping the future of personalized medicine and therapeutic efficacy.

The landscape of cancer treatment and diagnostics is undergoing a revolutionary shift with the advent of nanomedicine, employing both large and small nanoparticles characterized by unique biological features. Quantum dots–drug conjugates used as a carrier for targeted drug delivery and gene therapy are shown in Figure 8.5. These nanocarriers exhibit remarkable capabilities in effectively binding, absorbing, and transporting imaging agents and anticancer drugs. Organic nanocarriers exemplify this transformative approach, including liposomes, lipids, dendrimers, carbon nano-tubes, emulsions, and synthetic polymers. Nanocarriers offer numerous advantages over traditional drug delivery systems, including enhanced adsorption capacity, increased surface area, improved reactivity, and a smaller overall size (51, 52).

The CQDs-CBP (carboplatin injectable solution) complex exhibits promising applications in chemotherapeutic cancer treatment due to its pH-dependent release behavior, enhanced permeability and retention (EPR) impact, negative surface charge, and a size of 77.44 nm. Biocompatibility testing on three T3-L1 cell lines (HT-29 and MCF-7) demonstrated minimal side effects during chemotherapy administration. The green nanoarchitecture-tonic system holds potential as a medication delivery device (54). Li and colleagues created a quantum dot (CQD)-based doxorubicin nanocarrier technology to boost captopril's therapeutic efficacy and enable 96-hour tracking of QD-drug biodistribution. In vitro tests on breast MCF-7 cancer cells revealed that the system, which featured a carbon dot-Glu-CD moiety attached to 5-aminolevulinic acid (5-ALA), significantly impaired the morphology and cytotoxicity of malignant cells. (55). Combining curcumin with chitosan, CQDs, and Fe_2O_3 has resulted in the development of a novel medication, addressing the challenges of poor solubility and rapid breakdown in circulation. This innovative formulation enhances loading efficiency, bioavailability, and encapsulation efficiency. The synthesized nanocomposite,

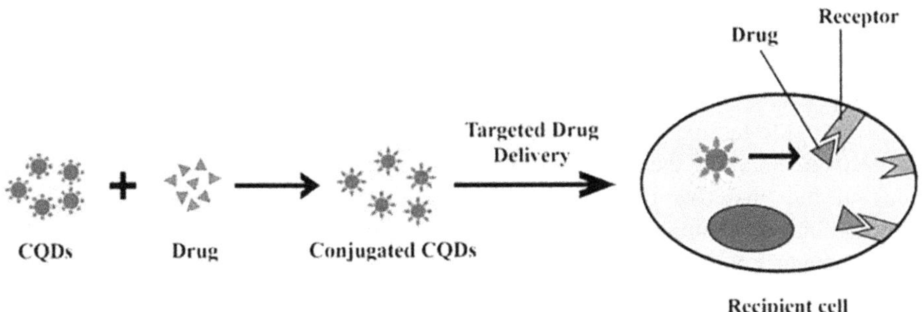

FIGURE 8.5 Schematic representation of the CQD-guided drug delivery system (53).

$CS/CQDs/Fe_2O_3$, emerges as a promising candidate for targeted cancer treatment, showcasing pH-dependent targeting and significantly decreasing cell survival. This approach to curcumin treatment represents a promising avenue in cancer therapy (56).

Studies on the therapeutic impact of CQD-RAW on Alzheimer's disease (AD) have used NIR irradiation. The compound's better photothermal characteristics explain Aβ1-42 deposition, while its surface N-containing functional groups inhibit Aβ aggregation. Experiments on in vitro cells validated CQD-RAW's great biosafety and capacity to impede Aβ1-42 neurotoxicity. Studies using immunohistochemistry and animals showed that AD mice's memory impairment was improved (58). The synthetic S-N-CQDs, formed through reduced glutathione and citric acid monohydrate, have proven efficient for detecting tetracycline antibiotics based on the IFE mechanism. These fluorescence sensors exhibit affordability, simplicity in fabrication, rapid response, precision, sensitivity, and remarkable selectivity. Given their favorable outcomes in actual samples and challenging conditions, these sensors are well-suited for food and drug analysis applications. The proposed technique holds promise for detecting tetracycline antibiotics (59). These carriers can target particular organs by modifying antibodies, aptamers, and other biological molecules. They facilitate the release and control of medications distinctively, elevating efficacy at lower doses, reducing adverse effects, and improving absorption and bioavailability. These carriers can modify membrane transport processes, enhance water solubility, and impede the rapid breakdown of medications by digestive enzymes. These modifications collectively contribute to increased medication effectiveness and reduced adverse effects.

Moreover, they can enhance drug delivery systems such as liposomes, micelles, and nanoparticles (60). An 81% drug loading in the Fe3O4@SiO2@alginate/CQDs nanohybrid is attributed to physical interactions such as hydrophobic, electrostatic, and stacking. Due to its magnetic and fluorescent qualities, it also exhibits a greater drug release rate at pH 5.5 than at pH 7.4, suggesting that it has the potential to be an excellent multifunctional nanocarrier for drug delivery systems and bioimaging in cancer treatment (61). Trichrome-tryptophan-sorbitol CQDs represent a potential anticancer nanotheranostic approach for the treatment of HCC. Using fluorescence imaging, green-emitting TC-WS-CQDs target HCC cells to provide early tumor surveillance. They also improve HCC prevention without medication administration by inducing autophagy via the p53-AMPK pathway. This strategy highlights a potential anticancer nanotherapeutic strategy by integrating diagnostics, targeting, and treatment (62). The m-phenylenediamine-CQD is an outstanding multifunctional delivery system characterized by its compact size, efficient cellular uptake, favorable biocompatibility, and integrated imaging capability. Notably, these m-CQDs exhibit the potential to facilitate the transportation of bioactive factors into the deeper zones of cartilage, enabling them to penetrate the dense surface layer and enhance the efficacy of the bioactive factors (63). Electrospun nanofibrous mats composed of chitosan-carbon quantum dot-titanium dioxide-graphene oxide (CS-CQD-TiO2-GO) are for wound healing applications. These nanofibers were uniformly and effectively integrated, exhibiting a tensile strength ranging from 3.8 to 9.0 MPa and a zeta potential of 68.7 nm. The mats displayed suitable cytocompatibility and effectively inhibited bacterial growth. In in vivo trials on mice, the composite mats demonstrated enhanced wound healing and reepithelization compared to the control group (64). Researchers have designed drug-loaded nanoparticles to target specific cancer cells and minimize harm to healthy ones during chemotherapy. These nanoparticles can effectively reach tumor locations, providing a targeted approach. The controlled release of medications from these nanoparticles ensures a prolonged therapeutic effect, reducing the necessity for frequent dosing. Additionally, using nanoparticles improves the solubility of medications with low water solubility, enhancing their bioavailability and overall efficacy in treating diseases. The application of cotransfected quantum dots and siRNA, along with the evaluation of transfection effectiveness and the construction of drug transporters with diverse physical properties, has led to the growing prominence of quantum dot-based medication delivery systems.

A similar concept is illustrated in Figure 8.6; HepG2 is a cell line derived from liver cancer cells. It works by interfering with the replication of cancer cells, ultimately leading to their death. An example is the doxorubicin nanocarrier system based on CQDs synthesized by Li et al., which exhibits significant cytotoxicity and morphological defects against cancer cells (65). When comparing the Arginine-CQD carboplex to the conventional "gold standard" PEI polyplex polycationic transfectant, the former exhibits lower toxicity and superior gene transfer capacity. Additionally,

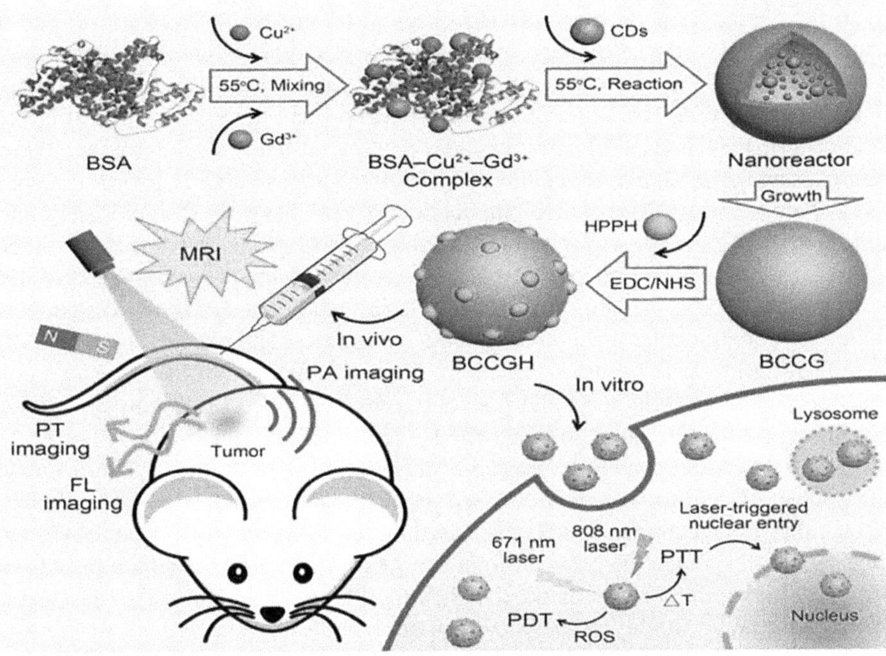

FIGURE 8.6 shows the CD-DOX conjugation in action. The amine group of DOX attaches to the carboxylic group of CD, and the CD-DOX conjugates are delivered to HL-7702 normal cells and HepG2 cancer cells. Because HepG2 cancer cells have a lower pH than HL-7702 normal liver cells, the CD–DOX conjugates will release DOX from these cells, but not from the former (57).

this cargo displays exceptional long-term stability in physiological media. The remarkable results, coupled with the photostable fluorescence capabilities of CQDs, expand the potential applications of this approach for controlled distribution and real-time monitoring (66). Zhou et al. developed a configuration involving mesoporous silica nanoparticles (MSNs) loaded with doxorubicin (DOX) and carbon dots. Upon imaging HeLa cells in vitro, the system exhibited robust green fluorescence (67).

The LAAM TC-CQDs model, elucidated in Figure 8.7, showcases quantum dots functioning as both nanocarriers and dyes for biomedical imaging of HeLa cells. Gene therapy addresses the root causes of diseases by introducing and expressing foreign DNA. Gene therapy's effectiveness relies on suitable gene vectors (67, 68). Nanoparticles and quantum dots (QDs), including CQDs, facilitate gene delivery through their biocompatibility, low toxicity, fluorescence emission, and stable photoluminescence. CQDs exhibit the capability to construct siRNA carriers and efficiently compact plasmid DNA for exceptional transfection efficiency. Through chondrogenesis from fibroblasts, they have generated nanoparticles with high solubility, low cytotoxicity, and fluorescence emission (69).

8.7   PHOTODYNAMIC TREATMENT (PDT) OF QDs

Von Tappeiner discovered "PDT" in 1903. He described PDT as a theranostic treatment for cancer. A photosensitizer (PS), light, and molecular oxygen are used to cause cellular and tissue damage, in which singlet oxygen is generated through a series of photo-induced processes and is believed to be the primary cytotoxic agent (71). Tappeiner used eosin as a photoactive PS to present the first results of PDT on skin cancer. PDT is used in cardiovascular therapy, restenosis, angioplasty, atherosclerosis, and other skin diseases such as condyloma, lupus vulgaris, psoriasis, syphilis, and skin cancers. The clinical application of PDT has grown significantly over time. The PDT concept was introduced in the early 1960s and advanced to clinical trials. Currently, PDT protocols are available for treating many types of cancer. PDT is now used to treat ovarian, prostate, dysplasia, papilloma, basal cell carcinomas, bone carcinomas, ocular melanoma, rheumatoid arthritis, and pancreatic cancer (72). It is also used to treat bacterial infections. He called this activity a "photodynamic reaction." Thomas Dougherty and his colleagues developed PDT with hematoporphyrin derivative (HPD) in the late 1970s (73). HPD administration followed by red light irradiation resulted in oxygen-dependent tissue reactions; it is now known that topical PDT is currently widely used to treat actinic keratosis. PSs are administered either intravenously or topically based on tumor location. PS is activated two days later by exposing the tissue to light energy of a specific wavelength, usually in the dye's maximum absorption band. When the PS absorbs light in the presence of molecular oxygen, highly reactive oxygen species destroy cancerous tissue, blood vessels, and pathogenic microorganisms. The PS can return to its ground state by emitting a photon (fluorescence) or an intersystem crossing (73), wherein the energy is lost as heat. PDT's primary purpose is to eliminate tumors without causing any harm to normal tissue. PDT has many advantages over conventional therapies but also has limitations such as low solubility; the excitation wavelength for PS is near-infrared (NIR); the inability to treat malignant tumors due to its localized nature;

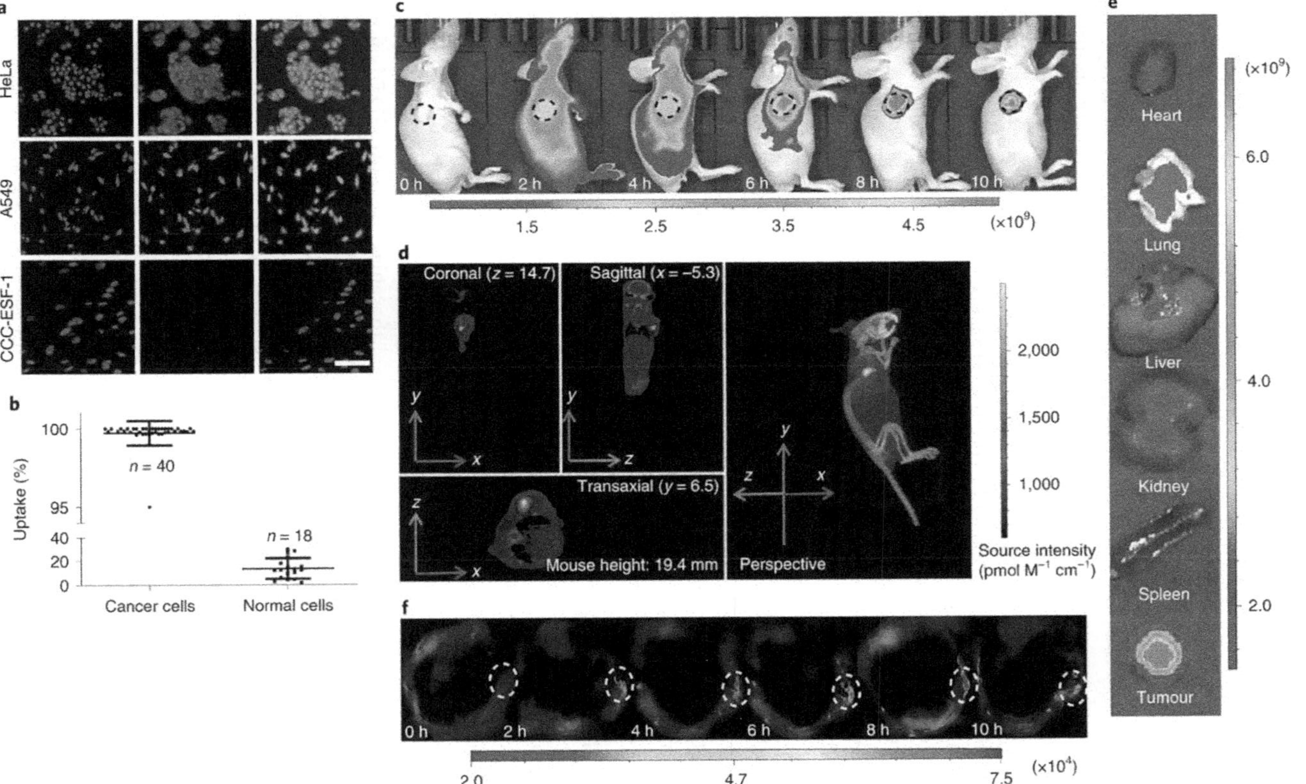

FIGURE 8.7   The investigation illustrates the impact of LAAM TC-CQDs on both cancerous and non-cancerous cells, employing LCSM images and flow cytometry. Furthermore, it elucidates the distribution of LAAM TC-CQDs in a mouse with a HeLa tumor, including a 3D reconstruction of the distribution. Ex vivo NIR fluorescence imaging and cross-sectional PA imaging were additionally employed to assess the influence of LAAM TC-CQDs on tumors and organs. The concentrations of LAAM TC-CQDs were standardized to ensure consistent in vivo PA signal (70).

and the burning sensation in surrounding healthy tissues. PS may be obtained in natural and synthetic forms, such as 5-ALA, MAOP (methyl amino levulinate), zinc phthalocyanine, tin etiopurpurin, and foscan, which have recently been produced. Phthalocyanine, chlorophyll, and porphyrin derivatives are the three main PS classes used in medical applications. Li and coworkers first produced the phthalocyanine nucleobase by combining excess 9-(2-bromoethyl) adenine with the precursor tetra-hydroxy phthalocyanine. Initially used as pigments in semiconductors, photoconductors, and other high-tech industries, the derivatives have also found use in material research. Phthalocyanines, as PS in PDT, are possible when hydrophilic groups are added to them. Because of the macrocycle structure's hydrophobicity and ability to aggregate (especially in ethanol), its solubility decreases. PSs are selected based on the porphyrin's structure (74). Porphyrin-based PSs are licensed for therapeutic use in the following indications: 5-ACA for penile cancer, gliomas, acne vulgaris, scan (head and neck cancer), photochlor, photofrin (lung cancer, cervical cancer, stomach cancer), visudyne (subfoveal choroidal, neovascularization), purlytin, and photolon (skin tumors, myopic maculopathy). Because of the high production of O_2 species and well-known chemistry, porphyrin-based PS is often used. PS fluorescence can immediately differentiate between healthy and cancerous tissues. Chlorine is more aromatic than porphyrins but does not fully round the structure. Chlorophyll is a magnesium-containing chlorine molecule that Snyder (USA) (1942) first used as a powerful potential treatment. Pheophorbide-a was the first chlorin derivative used for PDT; Allen identified the central element, chlorin e6, from the chlorin combinations that had minimal toxicity when supplied orally and intravenously (75).

8.8 PHOTOSENSITIZATION

When PS (photosensitizer) and visible light combine to form damaging reactive oxygen species, also called ROS, in the presence of oxygen (O2), this mechanism is known as photosensitization. When light enters a photosensitizer and creates highly active molecules, which are used for cancer treatment, the process is referred to as PDT, and it is minimally invasive and destroys target cells in the presence of oxygen. PDT has several advantages over conventional therapies. Because PDT is non-invasive, personalized, and can treat patients with repeated doses without causing resistance or going over total dose limitations (like with radiation), it has multiple benefits over traditional therapies. Furthermore, PDT recovers quickly and leaves little to no scars, allowing for outpatient treatment. Finally, PDT has not been associated with adverse effects (76).

8.9 TYPE I AND II MECHANISMS OF PDI

The mechanism of photosensitizer in cancer therapy involves a photosensitizer that absorbs a photon and gets moved into an excited singlet state when exposed to the light of a specific wavelength while it is in its ground state. The excited singlet state can be dissipated either by thermal decay or fluorescence emission. As an alternative, intersystem crossing allows the excited singlet state to transition to an excited triplet state at a lower energy. The photosensitizer can produce reactive species through

Type I and Type II reactions when in the excited triplet state. The photosensitizer transmits an electron to different receptor molecules in Type I PDT processes, producing free radicals such as the superoxide anion, hydroxyl radical, and hydrogen peroxide. When the excited triplet state photosensitizer reacts directly with molecular oxygen, reactive singlet oxygen is generated during Type II operations. The most pertinent Type II PDT procedures produce singlet oxygen, which causes the targeted tissue to be destroyed. Cancer cells are killed by both necrosis and apoptosis mechanisms, depending on the internal localization of the photosensitizer in the cell (76, 78, 79).

8.10 QUANTUM DOTS AS A PHOTOSENSITIZER

The diverse characteristics of CQDs contribute to their potential applications across various fields, particularly in bioimaging, drug delivery, chemical probing, and photon therapy. Their notable advantages include low cytotoxicity and strong biocompatibility (80). Many functional groups, such as thiol, carboxyl, hydroxyl, etc., are attached to the exterior of CQDs, which improves their performance in photodynamic treatment, photosensitization, biological imaging, targeted administration of drugs, as fluorescent markers for diagnosis and cell tracking, and biosensors. By explaining the origins and intent of CQDs (81). Carbon nanotubes, graphite, coal, natural biomass, and other materials may all be utilized to synthesize CQDs. Various functional groups or doping agents can also alter them to function more effectively. To enhance their functionality, certain functional groups or additives may modify CQDs. Depending on their size and structure, CQDs can emit fluorescence in various colors and absorb light in visible and ultraviolet (UV) ranges (82). In addition, an analysis of CQDs' in vivo properties is conducted to support their effectiveness as powerful drug delivery vehicles (83). They can function as photosensitizers that absorb light and transform that energy into other molecules, such as oxygen, to form reactive oxygen species (ROS) that can potentially destroy bacteria or cancerous cells. When exposed to visible light, CQDs can cause cancer cells or bacteria to pass away by producing reactive oxygen species (ROS) (84). According to some recent research, when exposed to visible light, *Caenorhabditis elegans* (*C. elegans*) models might undergo germline apoptosis when exposed to CQDs produced using the natural biomass of broccoli (85). Through polyamine interfacial modification, another study increased the effectiveness of CQDs as a photosensitizer for visible light (82). Reactive oxygen species (ROS), which can destroy pathogens and tumor cells, are produced by light-activated medications known as photosensitizers in PDT. Light-activated molecules are used in photodynamic therapy, a non-invasive treatment technique, to destroy unwell cells specifically. Because of their remarkable optical characteristics, CQDs have drawn interest as possible alternatives for improving PDT effectiveness. Idea delineated in Figure 8.8, The ability to absorb and emit light at wavelengths between the ultraviolet tand near-infrared allows efficient light absorption and energy transmission. Upon excitation, CQDs may produce reactive oxygen species (ROS), especially singlet oxygen, a critical mechanism for causing cell death in specific cancer cells. The ability to absorb and emit light at wavelengths between the ultraviolet and near-infrared allows efficient light absorption and energy transmission. Upon excitation, CQDs may produce reactive oxygen species (ROS),

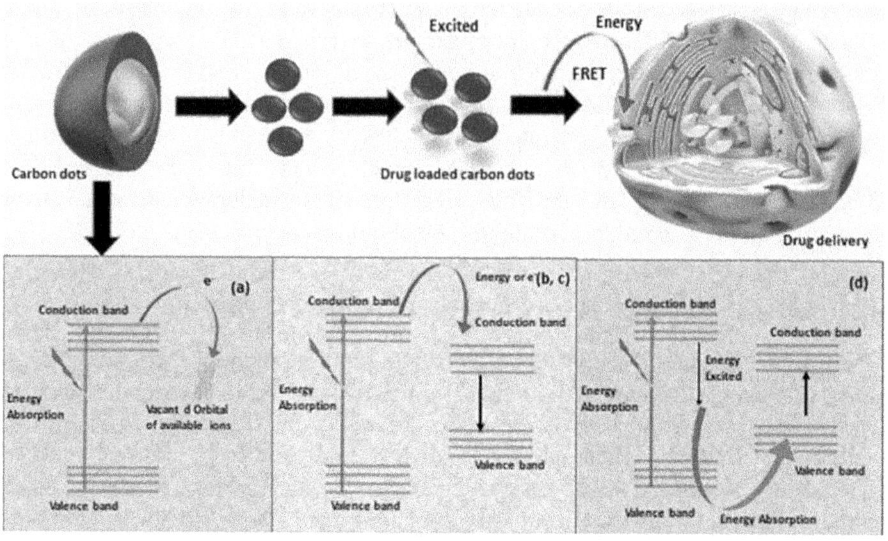

FIGURE 8.8 fluorescence quenching mechanism facilitating Drug delivery: a. PET (Photoinduced electron transfer) b. FRET (Forster resonance energy transfer) Quenching, c. SET (Surface energy transfer) Quenching, d. IFE (Inner filter effect) Quenching (77).

especially singlet oxygen, a critical mechanism for causing cell death in specific cancer cells (86). Soumya et al. used laser ablation and electrophoresis to synthesize single-walled carbon nanotubes (SWNTs). These substances are more reliable and ecologically friendly for medical applications since they are less hazardous, soluble in water, and free of heavy metals. Pillar-Little et al. discovered a high correlation between top-down synthesis's strong light-activated toxicity and CQDs' photodetection (PDT) efficiency. CQDs were studied by humans with prostate cancer by Petras and coworkers, who used them as in vitro photosensitizers for the production of reactive oxygen species (87). Su et al. synthesized magnetic CQDs and amine-functionalized CQDs conjugated with ampicillin, whereas Jiechao et al. produced C-dots having theranostic properties.

The evaluation of toxicity involved MTT and hemolytic assays, confirming the material's biocompatibility and non-toxic nature. To proceed with in vivo experiments, a mouse model of breast cancer was established by subcutaneously injecting 4T1 cells into the mouse's backside. Upon treatment, it was noted that exposure to light significantly reduced solid tumors in mice when treated with T-CDs. Additionally, analysis of the mice's tissue samples revealed no adverse effects on major organs post-TCD treatment. This study illustrates the potential of synthesized T-CDs to serve as a promising photosensitizer for cancer therapy as shown in Figure 8.9. According to Chowdhury et al., surface-functionalized and customized riboflavin CQDs may selectively destroy cancer cells by damaging their DNA via reactive oxygen species (ROS) (88). Tea polyphenol-derived CQDs (T-CDs) demonstrated dual red and blue fluorescence emission bands. They produced hydroxyl radicals when exposed to mildly visible LED light, suggesting that CQDs have potential as a photodetection agent in cancer treatment (89). With a coupled efficiency of about 50%, Chemen et al.

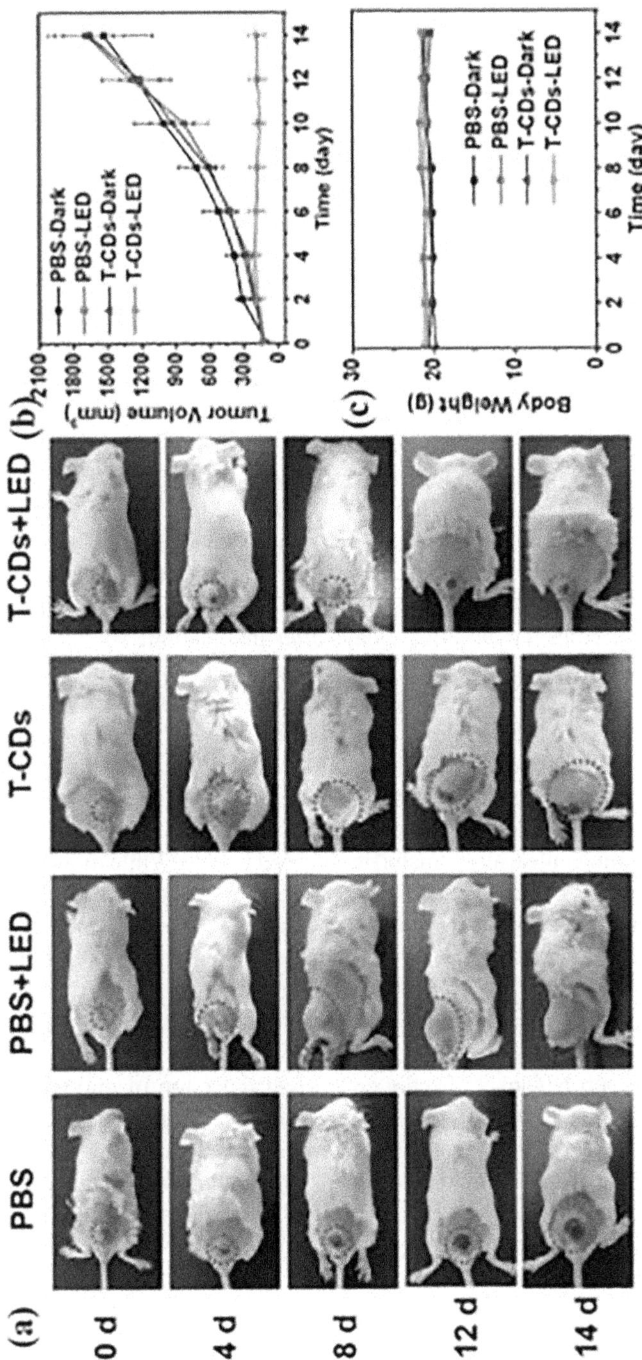

FIGURE 8.9 In vivo photodynamic therapy (a) Body weight changes in the indicated groups throughout the treatment; (b) quantitative evaluation of tumor volume at different time points; and (c) photographs of 4T1-tumor-bearing mice at various times and treatments (100).

developed a FRET system by covalently modifying Ce6 on the surface of green fluorescent CDs. Under 671 nm laser irradiation, the CDs-Ce6 system demonstrated increased phototoxicity, a more efficient rate of ROS generation, reduced dark toxicity, and more vibrant red fluorescence (90). Due to their high 1O2 generation, quantum yield (QY), and controlled synthesis, organic PSs such as phthalocyanine, hypocretin, and porphyrin have been combined with CDs for PDT of malignancies. The organic PSs' weak tumor-targeting abilities, limited water solubility, and ease of agglomeration are the disadvantages (91). Deep tumor treatment (PDT) may be more therapeutically effective for deeper tumors if functional materials with chemiluminescence or bioluminescence are used. Without an external light source, these materials may be used with molecular PSs and built-in chemiluminescence resonance energy transfer (CRET) or bioluminescence resonance energy transfer (BRET) systems to provide a high therapeutic effect for solid tumors. A system known as the CDs-Ce6 system combines Mg- and N-doped CDs with Ce6 to shift nearly all of the light energy to Ce6. FRET effectiveness is greatly increased by the proximity of CDs to Ce6 (92). Viral imaging CQDs are a good choice for bioimaging because of their aqueous solubility, biocompatibility, non-blinking, and physicochemical stability. Via single or multiple photon excitations, CQDs are easily absorbed by cells and allow for cell imaging. The level of doped nitrogen influences the intensity of CQD photoluminescence. Most CQDs have demonstrated the ability to enter the cell nucleus and illuminate the entire cell. Ehrlich ascites carcinoma cells (EAC) were isolated from the peritoneal cavity of adult female mice 7 days after inoculation. This cell suspension was then combined with a solution of CQDs and incubated for 30 minutes to explore the labeling of cells by CQDs. Surface passivation of CQDs results in high photoluminescence in both solid and liquid states, which is attributed to trapped surface energy. For instance, surface-passivated CQDs are a wavelength-tunable optical nanoprobe to target HeLa cell line cancer cells. Passivation involved various agents such as polyethylene glycol (PEG) chains, a copolymer of polyethyleneimine and polyethylene glycol, 4-armed PEG molecules, and transferrin-coupled CQDs. While most documented CQD-based cell imaging studies indicate CQDs are taken up by cells through endocytosis, there is limited evidence of substantial infiltration into the cell nucleus (93–95). Utilizing oxidized carbon nanotubes as the quencher facilitated the development of a FRET-based DNA detection technique. The detection limit for DNA was reduced to 75 pM, showcasing superior sensitivity compared to the previous method. Two CQDs emitting blue and green fluorescence were employed to craft two distinct DNA-functionalized nanoprobes, enabling the concurrent detection of multiple DNA targets. Through p-p interaction, these nanoprobes adhered to the surface of oxidized carbon nanotubes, effectively suppressing their fluorescence via the FRET process. The incorporation of graphene oxide as a quencher further enabled the simultaneous detection of diverse biomarkers, encompassing DNA and proteins, on this detection platform (96–98). TET, or triplet energy transfer, directly interacts with oxygen molecules to generate 1O2 through an energy transfer mechanism. This produced singlet oxygen (1O2) is employed in therapies and treatments, eliminating the need for an intermediary photosensitizer. For the TET process, quantum dots (QDs) must engage with ground-state triplet oxygen molecules (3O2), producing 1O2. Single-walled carbon nanotubes (SWNTs) are purified through laser ablation and electrophoresis.

The cost-effectiveness and straightforward synthesis procedures contribute to the gradual rise of CQDs as a novel addition to the nanocarbon material family (98, 99).

8.11 CHALLENGES AND FUTURE DIRECTIONS

Addressing the potential toxicity of CQDs remains a critical challenge. While these nanomaterials are generally considered biocompatible, comprehensive studies are needed to assess their long-term effects, potential accumulation, and biodegradability in vivo. Overcoming concerns related to toxicity is crucial for advancing CQDs from the laboratory to clinical applications. Achieving scalable production of CQDs with consistent quality poses a significant challenge. Standardizing synthesis methods and optimizing production processes are essential to ensuring reproducibility and reliability, especially when considering large-scale biomedical imaging and drug delivery applications. Understanding the in vivo behavior of CQDs, including their stability, circulation time, and biodistribution, is essential for their successful translation into clinical settings. Factors such as interactions with biological components and potential clearance pathways must be thoroughly investigated to optimize CQD performance and minimize unintended side effects. While integrating CQDs with PDT holds promise, challenges exist in optimizing the efficacy of light-activated therapeutic processes. Ensuring sufficient light penetration into target tissues and addressing potential limitations in the depth of PDT treatment are crucial considerations for enhancing therapeutic outcomes. Achieving high specificity in targeted drug delivery using CQDs remains a challenge. Fine-tuning the surface functionalization of CQDs to enhance their affinity for specific cells or tissues while minimizing off-target effects requires a nuanced approach. Strategies to overcome biological barriers and improve targeted drug release kinetics need further exploration.

Future research should focus on developing multifunctional CQDs as imaging agents and therapeutic carriers. Integration of various imaging modalities, such as combining fluorescence and magnetic resonance imaging, can enhance diagnostic accuracy and provide complementary information. Designing intelligent drug delivery systems that respond to specific stimuli, such as pH, temperature, or enzymatic activity, can further improve the precision of drug release at the target site. Investigating stimuli-responsive materials for coating CQDs holds promise for achieving controlled and triggered drug delivery. Conducting in-depth mechanistic studies to unravel CQDs' cellular and molecular interactions is essential. Understanding the intracellular fate of CQDs, including mechanisms of cellular uptake and subcellular localization, will contribute to optimizing their design for enhanced biomedical applications. Advancing CQDs from preclinical studies to clinical trials is a crucial future direction. Comprehensive validation of CQD-based technologies in relevant disease models and addressing regulatory challenges will be necessary to pave the way for their widespread clinical adoption. Encouraging collaborative efforts between researchers from diverse disciplines, including chemistry, biology, medicine, and engineering, will foster a holistic approach to addressing challenges and advancing the field. Cross-disciplinary collaboration can lead to innovative solutions and accelerate the translation of CQD technologies into practical clinical applications. In navigating these challenges and pursuing future directions, researchers can unlock the full potential of CQDs in revolutionizing biomedical imaging, precision-targeted drug delivery, and their integration with emerging therapeutic modalities such as Photodynamic Therapy. The journey toward overcoming these challenges and exploring new frontiers promises to reshape the landscape of nanomedicine and personalized healthcare.

8.12   CONCLUSION

Drawing together the threads of this exploration into the synergistic integration of CQDs for biomedical imaging and precision-targeted nanodrug delivery with a particular emphasis on their role in PDT, a panorama of transformative possibilities unfolds. The challenges and future directions elucidated herein underscore the multifaceted nature of this research frontier and emphasize the collaborative efforts required to unlock its full potential. The challenges posed by toxicity, scalability, and specificity in targeted drug delivery underscore the need for meticulous, interdisciplinary research. Addressing these challenges is imperative to translate CQD-based technologies into clinical applications safely. It serves as a catalyst for innovation and refinement in the ever-evolving field of nanomedicine. The identified future directions chart a course toward realizing more sophisticated and versatile applications. The prospect of developing CQDs with multifunctional capabilities, acting as both imaging agents and therapeutic carriers, heralds a new era in personalized medicine. Innovative drug delivery systems responsive to specific stimuli offer the promise of unprecedented control over drug release dynamics, ensuring maximal therapeutic efficacy while minimizing side effects.

The call for in-depth mechanistic studies and the imperative to advance CQDs from preclinical studies to clinical trials signal a commitment to robust scientific inquiry and the translation of beachside discoveries into bedside applications. The collaborative interdisciplinary research envisioned for the future reflects the recognition that the fusion of expertise from diverse fields is essential to comprehensively tackling CQD-based technologies' intricacies. As this chapter concludes, the journey through the synergistic realm of CQDs in biomedicine reveals the inherent promise and responsibility of harnessing nanotechnology for transformative healthcare solutions. The challenges posed are not impediments but rather invitations to innovation, prompting researchers to navigate uncharted territories and pioneer novel solutions. At the intersection of CQDs, biomedical imaging, precision-targeted drug delivery, and photodynamic therapy, the chapters of discovery are far from closed—they beckon us to turn the page and continue the narrative of groundbreaking advancements that hold the potential to reshape the landscape of healthcare in ways yet unimagined.

REFERENCES

1. Abdellatif, Ahmed AH, et al. "Biomedical applications of quantum dots: Overview, challenges, and clinical potential." *International Journal of Nanomedicine* (2022): 1951–1970.
2. Porter, Alan L., and Jan Youtie. "How interdisciplinary is nanotechnology?." *Journal of Nanoparticle Research* 11 (2009): 1023–1041.

3. Zhu, Shoujun, et al. "Photoluminescence mechanism in graphene quantum dots: Quantum confinement effect and surface/edge state." *Nano Today* 13 (2017): 10–14.

4. Stier, Oliver. "Electronic and optical properties of quantum dots and wires." (2005).

5. Zhang, Jian, et al. "Colloidal quantum dots: synthesis, composition, structure, and emerging optoelectronic applications." *Laser & Photonics Reviews* 17.3 (2023): 2200551.

6. Smith, Marcus J., et al. "Composite structures with emissive quantum dots for light enhancement." *Advanced Optical Materials* 7.4 (2019): 1801072.

7. Wang, Yaxin, et al. "Recent advances in synthesis and application of perovskite quantum dot based composites for photonics, electronics and sensors." *Science and Technology of Advanced Materials* 21.1 (2020): 278–302.

8. Soumya K, More N, Choppadandi M, Aishwarya DA, Singh G, Kapusetti G. A comprehensive review on carbon quantum dots as an effective photosensitizer and drug delivery system for cancer treatment. *Biomedical Technology.* 2023 December; 4:11–20.

9. Ramalingam, Gopal, et al. "Quantum confinement effect of 2D nanomaterials." *Quantum Dots-Fundamental and Applications.* IntechOpen, 2020.

10. Magnusson MH, Ohlsson BJ, Björk MT, Dick KA, Borgström MT, Deppert K, et al. Semiconductor nanostructures enabled by aerosol technology. *Front Phys (Beijing).* 2014 June 22;9(3):398–418.

11. Li, Jingbo, and Wang. "Comparison between quantum confinement effects of quantum wires and dots." *Chemistry of Materials* 16.21 (2004): 4012–4015.

12. Zipper, Elżbieta, Marcin Kurpas, and Maciej M. Maśka. "Wave function engineering in quantum dot–ring nanostructures." *New Journal of Physics* 14.9 (2012): 093029.

13. Li, Jinghong, and Jin Z. Zhang. "Optical properties and applications of hybrid semiconductor nanomaterials." *Coordination Chemistry Reviews* 253.23–24 (2009): 3015–3041.

14. Lo, Pui-Chi, Baozhong Zhao, Wubiao Duan, Wing-Ping Fong, Wing-Hung Ko, and Dennis KP Ng. Synthesis and in vitro photodynamic activity of mono-substituted amphiphilic zinc(II) phthalocyanines. *Bioorganic & Medicinal Chemistry Letters* 2007 February;17(4):1073–7.

15. Abdellatif, Ahmed AH, et al. "Biomedical applications of quantum dots: Overview, challenges, and clinical potential." *International Journal of Nanomedicine* (2022): 1951–1970.

16. Magesh V, Sundramoorthy AK, Ganapathy D. Recent advances on synthesis and potential applications of carbon quantum dots. *Frontiers in Materials* 2022 July 1;9.

17. Lim, Shi Ying, Wei Shen, and Zhiqiang Gao. Carbon quantum dots and their applications. *Chemical Society Reviews* 2015;44(1):362–81.

18. Wang, Ru, et al. "Recent progress in carbon quantum dots: Synthesis, properties and applications in photocatalysis." *Journal of Materials Chemistry A* 5.8 (2017): 3717–3734.

19. Yadav, Pradeep Kumar, et al. "Carbon quantum dots: Synthesis, structure, properties, and catalytic applications for organic synthesis." *Catalysts* 13.2 (2023): 422.

20. Magesh, Vasanth, Ashok K. Sundramoorthy, and Dhanraj Ganapathy. "Recent advances on synthesis and potential applications of carbon quantum dots." *Frontiers in Materials* 9 (2022): 906838.

21. Lim, Shi Ying, Wei Shen, and Zhiqiang Gao. "Carbon quantum dots and their applications." *Chemical Society Reviews* 44.1 (2015): 362–381.

22. Wang, Xiao, et al. "A mini review on carbon quantum dots: Preparation, properties, and electrocatalytic application." *Frontiers in Chemistry* 7 (2019): 671.

23. Moniruzzaman, Md, and Jongsung Kim. "Synthesis and post-synthesis strategies for polychromatic carbon dots toward unique and tunable multicolor photoluminescence and associated emission mechanism." *Nanoscale* 15.34 (2023): 13858–13885.

24. Karakoti, Ajay Singh, et al. "Surface functionalization of quantum dots for biological applications." *Advances in Colloid and Interface Science* 215 (2015): 28–45.

25. Juang, Ruey-Shin, et al. "Highly luminescent aggregate-induced emission from polyethylene glycol-coated carbon quantum dot clusters under blue light illumination." *Journal of Materials Chemistry C* 8.46 (2020): 16569–16576.

26. Janus, Łukasz, et al. "Chitosan-based carbon quantum dots for biomedical applications: Synthesis and characterization." *Nanomaterials* 9.2 (2019): 274.

27. Nakane, Yuko, et al. "Bovine serum albumin-coated quantum dots as a cytoplasmic viscosity probe in a single living cell." *Analytical Methods* 4.7 (2012): 1903–1905.

28. Lazim, Azwan Mat, Regina Sisika A. Sonthanasamy, and Tan Ling Ling. "Binding study of carbon dots to bovine serum albumin." *AIP Conference Proceedings*. Vol. 2111. No. 1. AIP Publishing, 2019.

29. Meng, He, et al. "Conjugates of folic acids with BSA-coated quantum dots for cancer cell targeting and imaging by single-photon and two-photon excitation." *JBIC Journal of Biological Inorganic Chemistry* 16 (2011): 117–123.

30. Petryayeva, Eleonora, W. Russ Algar, and Igor L. Medintz. "Quantum dots in bioanalysis: A review of applications across various platforms for fluorescence spectroscopy and imaging." *Applied Spectroscopy* 67.3 (2013): 215–252.

31. Yang, Hai-Li, et al. "Carbon quantum dots: Preparation, optical properties, and biomedical applications." *Materials Today Advances* 18 (2023): 100376.

32. Miao, Shihai, et al. "Hetero-atom-doped carbon dots: Doping strategies, properties and applications." *Nano Today* 33 (2020): 100879.

33. Zrazhevskiy, Pavel, Mark Sena, and Xiaohu Gao. "Designing multifunctional quantum dots for bioimaging, detection, and drug delivery." *Chemical Society Reviews* 39.11 (2010): 4326–4354.

34. Liao, Jinfeng, et al. "Multifunctional nanostructured materials for multimodal cancer imaging and therapy." *Journal of Nanoscience and Nanotechnology* 14.1 (2014): 175–189.

35. Rajamanickam, Karunanithi. "Multimodal molecular imaging strategies using functionalized nano probes." *Jouranl of Nanotechnology Research* 1 (2019): 119–135.

36. Li, Meixiu, et al. "Review of carbon and graphene quantum dots for sensing." *ACS Sensors* 4.7 (2019): 1732–1748.

37. Molaei, Mohammad Jafar. "Principles, mechanisms, and application of carbon quantum dots in sensors: A review." *Analytical Methods* 12.10 (2020): 1266–1287.

38. Chinnathambi, Shanmugavel, and Naoto Shirahata. "Recent advances on fluorescent biomarkers of near-infrared quantum dots for in vitro and in vivo imaging." *Science and Technology of Advanced Materials* 20.1 (2019): 337–355.

39. Tian, Xiumei, et al. "Carbon quantum dots: In vitro and in vivo studies on biocompatibility and biointeractions for optical imaging." *International Journal of Nanomedicine* (2020): 6519–6529.

40. Xu, Quan, et al. "Quantum dots in cell imaging and their safety issues." *Journal of Materials Chemistry B* 9.29 (2021): 5765–5779.

41. Wu, Xingyong, et al. "Immunofluorescent labeling of cancer marker Her2 and other cellular targets with semiconductor quantum dots." *Nature Biotechnology* 21.1 (2003): 41–46.

42. Pons, Thomas, et al. "In vivo imaging of single tumor cells in fast-flowing bloodstream using near-infrared quantum dots and time-gated imaging." *ACS Nano* 13.3 (2019): 3125–3131.

43. Tao, Huiquan, et al. "In vivo NIR fluorescence imaging, biodistribution, and toxicology of photoluminescent carbon dots produced from carbon nanotubes and graphite." *Small* 8.2 (2012): 281–290.

44. Su, Yuanyuan, et al. "In vivo distribution, pharmacokinetics, and toxicity of aqueous synthesized cadmium-containing quantum dots." *Biomaterials* 32.25 (2011): 5855–5862.

45. Tang, Yuan, et al. "The role of surface chemistry in determining in vivo biodistribution and toxicity of CdSe/ZnS core–shell quantum dots." *Biomaterials* 34.34 (2013): 8741–8755.

46. Tsoi, Kim M., et al. "Are quantum dots toxic? Exploring the discrepancy between cell culture and animal studies." *Accounts of Chemical Research* 46.3 (2013): 662–671.

47. Riviere, Jim E. "Pharmacokinetics of nanomaterials: An overview of carbon nanotubes, fullerenes and quantum dots." *Wiley Interdisciplinary Reviews: Nanomedicine and Nanobiotechnology* 1.1 (2009): 26–34.

48. Navarro-Ruiz, Maria Carmen, et al. "A systematic comparative study of the toxicity of semiconductor and graphitic carbon-based quantum dots using in vitro cell models." *Applied Sciences* 10.24 (2020): 8845.

49. Martins CSM, LaGrow AP, Prior JA V. Quantum dots for cancer-related miRNA monitoring. *ACS Sens*ory 2022 May 27;7(5):1269–99.

50. Bajpai, Sushant, Tiwary, Saurabh Kr, Sonker, Muskan, Joshi, Ayush, Gupta, Vishwas, Kumar, Yogendra, Shreyash, Nehil, and Biswas, Susham. Recent advances in nanoparticle-based cancer treatment: A review. *ACS Applied Nano Materials Journal* 2021 July 23;4(7):6441–70

51. Senapati S, Mahanta , AK, Kumar S, Maiti P. Controlled drug delivery vehicles for cancer treatment and their performance. *Signal Transduct Target Ther.* 2018 March 16;3(1):7.

52. Zhao MX, Zhu BJ. The research and applications of quantum dots as nano-carriers for targeted drug delivery and cancer therapy. *Nanoscale Research Letter* 2016 December 18;11(1):207.

53. Magesh, Vasanth, Ashok K. Sundramoorthy, and Dhanraj Ganapathy. "Recent advances on synthesis and potential applications of carbon quantum dots." *Frontiers in Materials* 9 (2022): 906838.

54. González-Reyna MA, Molina GA, Juarez-Moreno K, Rodríguez-Torres A, Esparza R, Estevez M. "Green nanoarchitectonics of carbon quantum dots from Cinchona Pubescens Vahl as targeted and controlled drug cancer nanocarrier." *Biomaterials Advances* 2023 October;153:213561.

55. Khan MS, Sheikh A, Abourehab MAS, Gupta N, Kesharwani P. Understanding the theranostic potential of quantum dots in cancer management. *Mater Today Communication* 2023 August;36:106424.

56. Zoghi M, Pourmadadi M, Yazdian F, Nigjeh MN, Rashedi H, Sahraeian R. Synthesis and characterization of chitosan/carbon quantum dots/Fe2O3 nanocomposite comprising curcumin for targeted drug delivery in breast cancer therapy. *International Journal of Biological Macromolecules* 2023 September;249:125788.

57. Zeng Q, Shao D, He X, Ren Z, Ji W, Shan C, et al. Carbon dots as a trackable drug delivery carrier for localized cancer therapy in vivo. *Journal of Materials Chemistry B.* 2016;4(30):5119–26.

58. Ye P, Li L, Qi X, Chi M, Liu J, Xie M. Macrophage membrane-encapsulated nitrogen-doped carbon quantum dot nanosystem for targeted treatment of Alzheimer's disease: Regulating metal ion homeostasis and photothermal removal of β-amyloid. *Journal of Colloid and Interface Science* 2023 November;650:1749–61.

59. Fan Y, Qiao W, Long W, Chen H, Fu H, Zhou C, et al. Detection of tetracycline antibiotics using fluorescent "Turn-off" sensor based on S, N-doped carbon quantum dots. *Spectrochimica Acta, Part A: Molecular and Biomolecular Spectroscopy* 2022 June;274:121033.

60. Molaei MJ, Salimi E. Magneto-fluorescent superparamagnetic $Fe^3O^4@SiO_2@$alginate/carbon quantum dots nanohybrid for drug delivery. *Materials Chemistry and Physics* 2022 September;288:126361.

61. Cai C, Huang JJ, Sano K, Zhu Y, Zhang Y, Wu Q, et al. A water-soluble corannulene with highly efficient ROS production. *Materials Chemistry and Physics* 2022 April;281:125885.

62. Wang Y, Chen J, Tian J, Wang G, Luo W, Huang Z, et al. Tryptophan-sorbitol based carbon quantum dots for theranostics against hepatocellular carcinoma. *Journal of Nanobiotechnology*. 2022 December 14;20(1):78.

63. Guo L, Duan Q, Wu G, Zhang B, Huang L, Xue J, et al. Novel multifunctional delivery system for chondrocytes and articular cartilage based on carbon quantum dots. *Sensors and Actuators B: Chemical* 2022 April;356:131348.

64. Norouzi F, Pourmadadi M, Yazdian F, Khoshmaram K, Mohammadnejad J, Sanati MH, et al. PVA-Based nanofibers containing chitosan modified with graphene oxide and carbon quantum dot-doped TiO_2 enhance wound healing in a rat model. *Journal of Functional Biomaterials* 2022 December 15;13(4):300.

65. Rezaei A, Hashemi E. A pseudohomogeneous nanocarrier based on carbon quantum dots decorated with arginine as an efficient gene delivery vehicle. *Scientific Reports* 2021 July 2;11(1):13790.

66. Seo J, Lee J, Lee C Bin, Bae SK, Na K. Nonpolymeric pH-Sensitive carbon dots for treatment of tumor. *Bioconjugate Chemistry* 2019 March 20;30(3):621–32.

67. Zhou J, Deng W, Wang Y, Cao X, Chen J, Wang Q, et al. Cationic carbon quantum dots derived from alginate for gene delivery: One-step synthesis and cellular uptake. *Acta Biomaterialia* 2016 September;42:209–19.

68. Wu YF, Wu HC, Kuan CH, Lin CJ, Wang LW, Chang CW, et al. Multi-functionalized carbon dots as theranostic nanoagent for gene delivery in lung cancer therapy. *Scientific Reports* 2016 February 16;6(1):21170.

69. Cao X, Wang J, Deng W, Chen J, Wang Y, Zhou J, et al. Photoluminescent cationic carbon dots as efficient non-viral delivery of plasmid SOX9 and chondrogenesis of fibroblasts. *Scientific Reports* 2018 May 4;8(1):7057.

70. Li S, Su W, Wu H, Yuan T, Yuan C, Liu J, et al. Targeted tumour theranostics in mice via carbon quantum dots structurally mimicking large amino acids. *Nature Biomedical Engineering* 2020 March 30;4(7):704–16.

71. Anas A, Sobhanan J, Sulfiya KM, Jasmin C, Sreelakshmi PK, Biju V. Advances in photodynamic antimicrobial chemotherapy. *Journal of Photochemistry and Photobiology C: Photochemistry Reviews*. 2021 December;49:100452.

72. Kim M, Jung H, Park H. Topical PDT in the treatment of benign skin diseases: Principles and new applications. *International Journal of Molecular Sciences* 2015 September 25;16(10):23259–78.

73. Yaghini E, Seifalian AM, MacRobert AJ. Quantum dots and their potential biomedical applications in photosensitization for photodynamic therapy. *Nanomedicine*. 2009 April;4(3):353–63.

74. Tedesco A, Rotta J, Lunardi C. Synthesis, photophysical and photochemical aspects of phthalocyanines for photodynamic therapy. *Current Organic Chemistry* 2003 January 1;7(2):187–96.

75. Liu Y, Zhang J, Zuo C, Zhang Z, Ni D, Zhang C, et al. Upconversion nano-photosensitizer targeting into mitochondria for cancer apoptosis induction and cyt c fluorescence monitoring. *Nano Research* 2016 November 1;9(11):3257–66.

76. Lovell JF, Liu TWB, Chen J, Zheng G. Activatable photosensitizers for imaging and therapy. *Chem Review* 2010 May 12;110(5):2839–57.

77. Nair A, Haponiuk JT, Thomas S, Gopi S. Natural carbon-based quantum dots and their applications in drug delivery: A review. *Biomedicine & Pharmacotherapy*. 2020 December;132:110834.

78. Ge J, Lan M, Zhou B, Liu W, Guo L, Wang H, et al. A graphene quantum dot photodynamic therapy agent with high singlet oxygen generation. *Nature Communications* 2014 August 8;5(1):4596.

79. Wu X, Abbas K, Yang Y, Li Z, Tedesco AC, Bi H. Photodynamic Anti-bacteria by carbon dots and their nano-composites. *Pharmaceuticals.* 2022 April 18;15(4):487.

80. Hasanzadeh A, Mofazzal Jahromi MA, Abdoli A, Mohammad-Beigi H, Fatahi Y, Nourizadeh H, et al. Photoluminescent carbon quantum dot/poly-l-Lysine core-shell nanoparticles: A novel candidate for gene delivery. *The Journal of Drug Delivery Science and Technology* 2021 Febuary;61:102118.

81. Shabbir H, Csapó E, Wojnicki M. Carbon quantum dots: The role of surface functional groups and proposed mechanisms for metal ion sensing. *Inorganics (Basel).* 2023 June 20;11(6):262.

82. Elsherbiny SM, Shao C, Acheampong A, Khalifa MA, Liu C, Huang Q. Green synthesis of broccoli-derived carbon quantum dots as effective photosensitizers for the PDT effect testified in the model of mutant *Caenorhabditis elegans. Biomater Science* 2022;10(11):2857–64.

83. Yadav PK, Chandra S, Kumar V, Kumar D, Hasan SH. Carbon quantum dots: Synthesis, structure, properties, and catalytic applications for organic synthesis. *Catalysts.* 2023 February 16;13(2):422.

84. Jung H, Sapner VS, Adhikari A, Sathe BR, Patel R. Recent progress on carbon quantum dots based photocatalysis. *Frontiers in Chemistry* 2022 April 25;10.

85. Ye KH, Wang Z, Gu J, Xiao S, Yuan Y, Zhu Y, et al. Carbon quantum dots as a visible light sensitizer to significantly increase the solar water splitting performance of bismuth vanadate photoanodes. *Energy & Environmental Science* 2017;10(3):772–9.

86. Karagianni A, Tsierkezos NG, Prato M, Terrones M, Kordatos K V. Application of carbon-based quantum dots in photodynamic therapy. *Carbon N Y.* 2023 January;203:273–310.

87. Alaghmandfard A, Sedighi O, Tabatabaei Rezaei N, Abedini AA, Malek Khachatourian A, Toprak MS, et al. Recent advances in the modification of carbon-based quantum dots for biomedical applications. *Materials Science and Engineering: C.* 2021 January;120: 111756.

88. Su X, Xu Y, Che Y, Liao X, Jiang Y. A type of novel fluorescent magnetic carbon quantum dots for cells imaging and detection. *Journal of Biomedical Materials Research Part A* 2015 December 26;103(12):3956–64.

89. Yang Y, Ding H, Li Z, Tedesco AC, Bi H. Carbon dots derived from tea polyphenols as photosensitizers for photodynamic therapy. *Molecules.* 2022 December 6;27(23):8627.

90. Song J, Gao X, Yang M, Hao W, Ji DK. Recent advances of photoactive near-infrared carbon dots in cancer photodynamic therapy. *Pharmaceutics.* 2023 Febraury 24;15(3):760.

91. Deshmukh S, Deore A, Mondal S. Ultrafast dynamics in carbon dots as photosensitizers: A review. *ACS Applied Nano Materials Journal* 2021 August 27;4(8):7587–606.

92. Sun Z, Zhang L, Wu F, Zhao Y. Photosensitizers for two-photon excited photodynamic therapy. *Advanced Functional Materials* 2017 December 3;27(48).

93. Lim SY, Shen W, Gao Z. Carbon quantum dots and their applications. *Chemical Society Reviews* 2015;44(1):362–81.

94. Zhang M, Wang W, Cui Y, Chu X, Sun B, Zhou N, et al. Magnetofluorescent Fe_3O_4/carbon quantum dots coated single-walled carbon nanotubes as dual-modal targeted imaging and chemo/photodynamic/photothermal triple-modal therapeutic agents. *Chemical Engineering Journal* 2018 April;338:526–38.

95. Pan Y, Yang J, Fang Y, Zheng J, Song R, Yi C. One-pot synthesis of gadolinium-doped carbon quantum dots for high-performance multimodal bioimaging. *Journal of Materials Chemistry B* 2017;5(1):92–101.

96. Qian ZS, Shan XY, Chai LJ, Ma JJ, Chen JR, Feng H. DNA nanosensor based on bio-compatible graphene quantum dots and carbon nanotubes. *Biosensors and Bioelectronics* 2014 October;60:64–70.

97. Feng H, Qian Z. Functional carbon quantum dots: A versatile platform for chemosensing and biosensing. *The Chemical Record.* 2018 May 24;18(5):491–505.

98. Juzeniene A, Moan J. The history of PDT in Norway. *Photodiagnosis and Photodynamic Therapy* 2007 March;4(1):3–11.

99. Baker SN, Baker GA. Luminescent carbon nanodots: Emergent nanolights. *Angewandte Chemie International Edition.* 2010 September 10;49(38):6726–44.

100. Yang Y, Ding H, Li Z, Tedesco AC, Bi H. Carbon dots derived from tea polyphenols as photosensitizers for photodynamic therapy. *Molecules.* 2022 December 6;27(23):8627.

9 Carbon Quantum Dots for Wound Healing and Wound Dressing

Shiji Mathew Abraham

9.1 INTRODUCTION

Skin is the largest organ of our body and is the chief barrier which protects us from injuries and microbial invasion. Skin is also responsible for maintaining the adequate levels of body fluids, electrolytes, and nutrients (Yu et al. 2016). Serious defects in skin can have a huge impact on people's health and life. The skin has developed a set of innate complex processes to protect and repair itself (Rodrigues et al. 2019). Wound healing is a complicated biological process which involves inflammation, hemostasis, restoration of the extracellular matrix (ECM), and cell proliferation (Y. Hao et al. 2020). Wound healing is an adaptive process which usually occurs naturally on its own, but an extensive full-thickness (chronic) wound may not always be quite easy to manage as it may lead to numerous complications such as infection, bleeding, inflammation, scarring, impaired healing, delayed angiogenesis, and in some cases may be even associated with amputation and death (Frykberg and Banks 2015; H. Wang et al. 2021). Wound healing process depends on external factors such as the level of oxygen, temperature and pH changes, and variation in enzymes (Bhattacharyya et al. 2022). Hence, for effective management of chronic wounds, timely and comprehensive wound diagnosis is essential.

Many strategies are being employed to manage wounds which include the use of wound dressings, instruments, cell therapy, and transplantation. The most common, simple, and cost-effective method for treating wounds is the application of suitable wound dressings. An ideal wound dressing must be efficient in preventing infection, maintaining moisture around the wound surface, promoting the rate of wound closure, and reducing scar formation (N. Dehghani et al. 2023). Nanomaterials have interesting features such as antibacterial property, good biocompatibility, and biodegradability that render them useful in various biomedical applications including their use as wound dressing materials. Nanomaterials when included in wound dressing can modify each stage of the wound healing process owing to their antibacterial, anti-inflammatory, pro-angiogenic, and proliferative characteristics (Naskar and Kim 2020). Hence, nanomaterials can be advantageous in overcoming all issues related to efficient wound healing.

Of the many nanomaterials explored, carbon quantum dots (CQDs) are potential candidates in designing antibacterial and smart wound dressing materials. One of the interesting features of CQDs apart from those mentioned in common among nano-materials is that they can be easily developed from natural precursors, are renewable, and cost-effective. This chapter focuses on the recent developments and applications of CQDs as wound dressing materials. A note on various wound healing processes and a discussion on the commonly adopted synthesis methods of CQDs are also included. Various forms of CQD-based wound dressing materials are also discussed in this chapter.

9.2 THE PROCESS OF WOUND HEALING

Wound healing is a complicated biological response of our body with respect to skin damages and it occurs through four main overlapping phases such as hemostasis, inflammation, proliferation and maturation (Figure 9.1) (Guo and DiPietro 2010).

9.2.1 HEMOSTASIS

Hemostasis is the first step of wound healing, which stops hemorrhage by the formation of blood clot. This stage may last for 2 days. During this stage, the clotting factors get released. Platelets come in contact with collagen, leading to activation and aggregation. An enzyme, thrombin causes the conversion of fibrinogen to a fibrin mesh, which strengthens the platelet and forms a firm clog, preventing further blood loss. This also forms structural foundation for the formation of future granulation tissue (Lux 2022; Ehtesabi and Nasri 2021).

9.2.2 INFLAMMATION

In this second phase of the healing process, the wound bed prepares for growing fresh tissues by eliminating bacteria and debris from the wound site. This is done with the help of a distinct group of white blood cells named neutrophils and some enzymes. As the neutrophils leave, the macrophages arrive and release growth factors, proteins, and

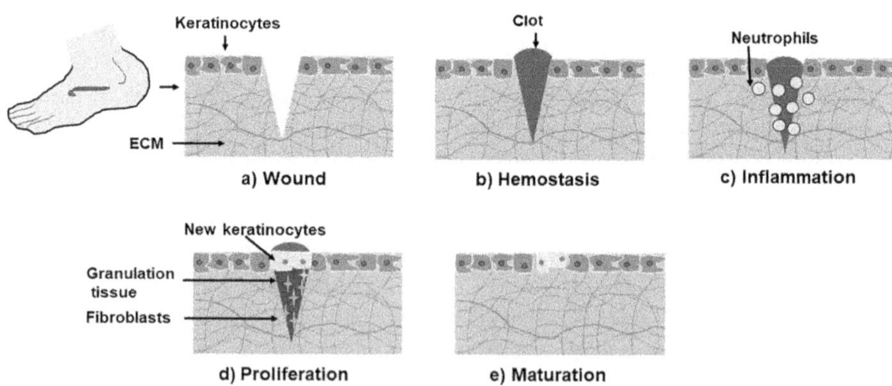

FIGURE 9.1   Schematic representation of the wound healing process.

Adapted and modified from Ehtesabi and Nasri 2021.

ROS. This stage lasts for around 7 days in acute and longer in chronic wounds and is often accompanied by inflammatory signs such as pain, redness, swelling, and heat.

9.2.3 PROLIFERATION

The third phase is marked by the filling and covering of the wound which occurs in three steps. The first step is named filling, where the wound bed is filled with granulation tissue formed by new blood vessels. The second step is contraction; where the contracted wound edges get stretched towards the center of the wound. During the third step, new keratinocytes arise from the wound bed and migrates towards the edge until the epithelium is covered. This phase usually lasts for 4–24 days.

9.2.4 MATURATION

The last phase is the maturation phase or the remodeling phase. During this phase, reorganization of collagen fibers as well as remodeling and maturation of the new tissue occurs, leading to a strong and flexible tissue. The duration of this phase varies according to the wound and may take 24 days to 2 years. As already mentioned, the healing process is complex and depends on varied local and systemic factors (Ehtesabi and Nasri 2021).

9.3 ROLE OF WOUND DRESSING IN HEALING PROCESS

A wound dressing is a covering that can be applied on the wound and help it heal by binding it with the surrounding tissue. Immediate covering up of a wound with a suitable dressing is vital as it prevents excessive blood loss and speeds up the restoration of the skin's integrity. An optimal wound dressing can also play an important role in accelerating the wound healing process by various ways. The wound dressing can act as a physical barrier between the external environment and the wound, control bleeding, retain moisture around the wound, absorb excess fluid from the wound surfaces, create a good gas exchange level, and protect the wound against infection and contamination. Biomaterial-based wound dressings have gained more popularity as they are less toxic, highly biocompatible, and non-allergic. They are available in various forms such as membranes, fibers, films, foams, gauzes, wafers, hydrogels, sponges, and tissue-engineered scaffolds (Shakiba-Marani and Ehtesabi 2023).

9.4 CARBON QUANTUM DOTS (CQDs) AS WOUND DRESSING MATERIAL

Carbon quantum dots are attractive carbon nanomaterials of sizes < 10 nm, which have excellent properties that enable them to be used for biomedical applications. Because of these attractive properties, CQDs are widely used as fluorescent probes (Huang et al. 2019; Shi et al. 2016) for bioimaging (Ding et al. 2018; Liu et al. 2018), in optoelectronic devices, in photocatalysis (Lu et al. 2017; Zhang et al. 2018), in anticounterfeiting printing (Gu et al. 2022), and in wound dressings. These properties include good biocompatibility (Ghirardello, Ramos-Soriano, and Galan 2021), low

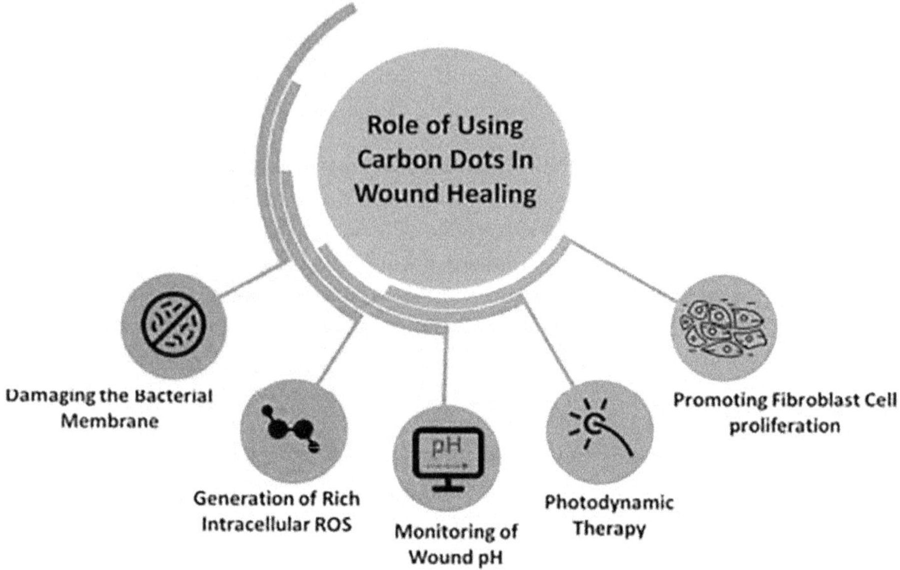

FIGURE 9.2   Schematic showing how CQDs aid in wound healing process.

Reprinted and reused with permission from Ehtesabi and Nasri 2021.

toxicity (Pormohammad et al. 2021), optical properties (Chan, Liu, and Hsiao 2019), good fluorescence, fluorescence stability, tunable emission (Anwar et al. 2019), good water solubility, photostability, chemical inertness, easy handling, eco-friendliness (Anwar et al. 2019), and moreover the presence of hydroxyl, carboxyl, and epoxy groups enables them to be modified into desirable multifunctional nanomaterials (Mahat et al. 2020; Y. Sun et al. 2022; Yoon et al. 2020). Furthermore, the derivatives of CQDs can induce damage to bacterial cells, induce oxidative stress, can monitor pH changes, and can promote fibroblast cell proliferation (H. Sun et al. 2014). Due to the antimicrobial property, CQDs are an important component included in wound dressing to compact bacterial infections. Also, the ability of CQDs to release reactive oxygen species (ROS) upon visible light irradiation further promotes antibacterial activity and speeds up sterilization, thereby enhancing wound healing. Moreover, the ROS generated can act as cell signaling mediators which can also promote the skin regeneration process (X. Hao et al. 2021). The role of CQDs as a component in wound healing material is depicted in Figure 9.2.

9.5   SYNTHESIS METHODS OF CQDs

CQDs can be synthesized by top down and bottom-up methods. Top-up technique involves the breakdown of carbon containing materials via physical, chemical, or electrochemical methods. Bottom-up methods involve gradual chemical unification of smaller organic molecules. The bottom-up approaches include pyrolytic methods, reverse micelle method, chemical oxidation, solvothermal and hydrolytic carbonization, template method, microwave-assisted method, etc. (Tajik et al. 2020). For the fabrication of CQDs for wound dressing applications, the mostly adopted synthesis methods include hydrothermal, pyrolytic, and microwave-assisted method.

Hydrothermal and solvothermal carbonization is an environmentally friendly, cost-effective, and non-toxic approach to produce carbon-based materials from a variety of precursors. In this method, a hydrous solution of the precursor is used as the reaction system in an enclosed container to generate carbon-based materials at desired high temperature and pressure conditions. A material which is insoluble or less soluble in normal condition is dissolved and recrystallized in this method (Y. Wang and Hu 2014). Another inexpensive approach where electromagnetic radiations with a wavelength of 1 mm to 1 m is employed for rapid synthesis of CQDs is called microwave-assisted method. The uniform heating of the microwave enables faster reaction and also reduces possible side reactions and byproducts (De Medeiros et al. 2019). Pyrolytic methods are another preferred method of CQD synthesis. Here the organic substances are subjected to physical and chemical alterations and decomposed in an inert atmosphere. This method is also simple to perform, affordable, and requires only less reaction time (Anirudh Sharma and Das 2019). Table 9.1 lists different CQD-based wound dressings and the method of synthesis adopted in each case.

9.6 FORMS OF CQD-BASED WOUND DRESSINGS

CQD-based wound dressing materials can be developed and applied in different forms; it could be either in the form of CQD-based bandages, hydrogels, sponges, patches, nanofiber scaffolds, and CQD-based injections. Even pH sensing or other stimuli-sensitive smart wound dressing materials can be developed using CQDs. We will investigate the details of each type of application and the mechanism of working.

9.6.1 CQD-BASED HYDROGEL PATCHES

Among the various functional wound dressings available, hydrogels have attracted intensive attention because of their advantages in facilitating diabetic wounds (H. Wang et al. 2021). In a recent study, a colorimetric sensor array was developed on polydimethylsiloxane microfluidic patch which could simultaneously detect five wound biomarkers such as glucose, urea, uric acid, pH, and total protein, thereby providing absolute assessment of infection and inflammation. Biogenic carbon dots were prepared using amino acids and polymers as the precursors by hydrothermal method. Enzyme-based and non-enzyme-based sensors used in this study enabled qualitative detection of multiple wound markers simultaneously within 15 mins and showed long-term wound monitoring. Furthermore, the CQD-based hydrogel patches exhibited good blood compatibility with a hemolysis rate lower than 8.99%, high detection accuracy with recovery rates of 91.5%–113.1% (Zheng et al. 2023) (Figure 9.3).

In another work, the wound healing activities of curcumin and curcumin-derived carbon dots (CurCDs) were compared. This study revealed that CurCDs which showed excellent properties such as improved solubility, stability, proliferative, pro-angiogenic, and antibacterial activity compared to that of curcumin, could be more beneficial in wound healing. For achievement of a sustained release of CurCD at the wound site, a protease responsive hydrogel (GHCD) was prepared using CurCD as a cross-linker (Anjana Sharma et al. 2022). The development of CurCDs and the

TABLE 9.1

Examples of CQD-based Wound Dressing Materials

Composite Label	Precursor for CQD Synthesis	Size of CQDs	Synthesis Method	Type of Material	In Vitro/ in Vivo	Healing Time	Functions Performed	References
-	*p*-phenylenediamine and polyethyleneimine	2.7± 0.5 nm	Solvothermal method		Both	12 days	Antibacterial activity against *S. aureus* and antioxidant activity for promoting wound healing	Qu et al. (2023)
CS/CQDs (5, 10, 15%)	Folic acid	-	Hydrothermal method		In vitro	-	Antibacterial activity against *S. aureus* and *E. coli*	Kazeminava et al. (2022)
SA-CD double-layer hydrogel	*Urtica dioica*	3.5 nm	Hydrothermal method		In vitro	3 days	Biocompatible, hemostatic and flexible, good mechanical and water barrier properties	Ebrahimi and Ehtesabi (2022)
LCDs	Levofloxacin		Hydrothermal method				Antibacterial activity against multidrug resistant bacteria	Zhang et al. (2018)
La@N-P-CQD/ PVA	5' adenosine disodium and Lanthanum chloride		Hydrothermal method				Antibacterial activity and better wound healing	M. Wang et al. (2022)
CS/PVA/QDs	Okra	-	Hydrothermal method		Both	72 hrs	Flexible and hemostatic	Shakiba-Marani and Ehtesabi (2023)
CS/SF/N-CQDs-α-TCP	Nitrogen-doped CQDs	-	Hydrothermal method		Both	12 days	Antibacterial, wound healing ability	S. Dehghani, Hosseini, and Regenstein (2018)
TCDs/CaO$_2$@ ZE	Tea				Both	10 days	Wound healing promoting property in diabetic rats	Dong et al. (2023)

Q-CQDs	Natural curcumin and 2, 3 epoxypropyl trimethylammonium chloride		Double thermal method			Infected wound healing ability	Zhang et al. (2018)
CurCD	Curcumin	4 nm		Both	14 days	Promoted wound healing and improved angiogenesis	Anjana Sharma et al. 2022)
ONCD	Onion peel powder	2–4 nm	Short microwave treatment	Both	2 weeks	Accelerated migration rate of fibroblasts, promoted faster healing of full thickness wound in rat model	Bankoti et al. (2017)
qCQDs	Dimethyl diallyl ammonium chloride and glucose	3 nm	One pot method	Both	14 days	Antibacterial activity and enhanced wound healing	C. Zhao et al. (2022)
LNZ-BCDs	Bovine serum albumin	4.5 ± 0.3 nm	Hydrothermal method	Both	48 h	Antibacterial activity against MRSA, enhanced cell proliferation and migration	Ghataty et al. (2023)
O-CDs/MCC		0.6–4.2 nm	Microwave-assisted hydrothermal method	In vitro	-	Wound pH monitoring	P. Yang et al. (2019)
Q-CQDs	Natural curcumin and 2, 3 epoxypropyl trimethylammonium chloride (GTA)	3.05 ± 0.95 nm	Microwave-assisted hydrothermal method	Both	14 days	Antibacterial property	Wu et al. (2022)
Nylon-11/ F-CDs	Forsythia	1.05–2.25 nm	Magnetic hyperthermia method	In vitro	3 days	Good cytocompatibility	Chen et al. (2022)

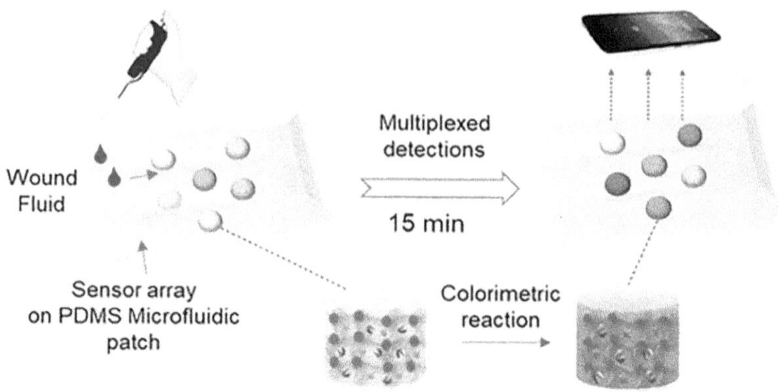

FIGURE 9.3   Working of carbon dot-doped hydrogel sensor patch.

Reprinted and reused with permission from Zheng et al. 2023. Copyright © 2023 American Chemical Society.

subsequent fabrication of protease responsive hydrogels are depicted in Figure 9.4. A comparative analysis using a skin excision model showed that GHCD sustained a faster wound closure with better angiogenesis and full restoration of the epithelium.

9.6.2   INJECTABLE HYDROGEL CQDs

Hydrogels can act as efficient wound dressings as they can maintain moisture around wounds, increase oxygen permeation, helps in cooling wounds, and alleviate injury pain. Injectable hydrogel wound dressings are promising materials with unique properties, such as capable of filling wounds or irregular spaces, sticking to wounds, and in situ coated drugs (X. Zhao et al. 2018). One of the disadvantages of hydrogels which limits its applications in wound dressings is the lack of elasticity which can be managed by developing self-healing hydrogels (Taylor and In Het Panhuis 2016). Mou et al. developed anionic CD31 and conjugated it with ε-polylysine to construct an injectable and self-healing hydrogel (CD-Plys) which possessed excellent biocompatibility, antibacterial activity against Gram-positive and Gram-negative bacteria, and accelerated wound healing with epithelization and enhanced angiogenesis. Glutaraldehyde was used as the precursor for development of the CQDs (Mou et al. 2022).

In another recent study, self-healing, injectable carbon-dot-based hydrogels were developed using ε-poly (L-lysine) as the precursor for carbon dots (PL-CD) together with oxidized dextran (ODA). This hydrogel material showed flexible injectability along with strong self-healing properties and excellent antibacterial properties against *S. aureus*. According to the study, the PL-CD@ODA hydrogel was found to be 100% bactericidal to *S. aureus* (X. Yang et al. 2021) (Figure 9.5).

In another approach to develop injectable CQD-based wound dressing materials, Li et al. used gentamycin sulfate and diammonium citrate as precursors for the synthesis of carbon dots. Then carboxymethyl chitosan was mixed with the developed

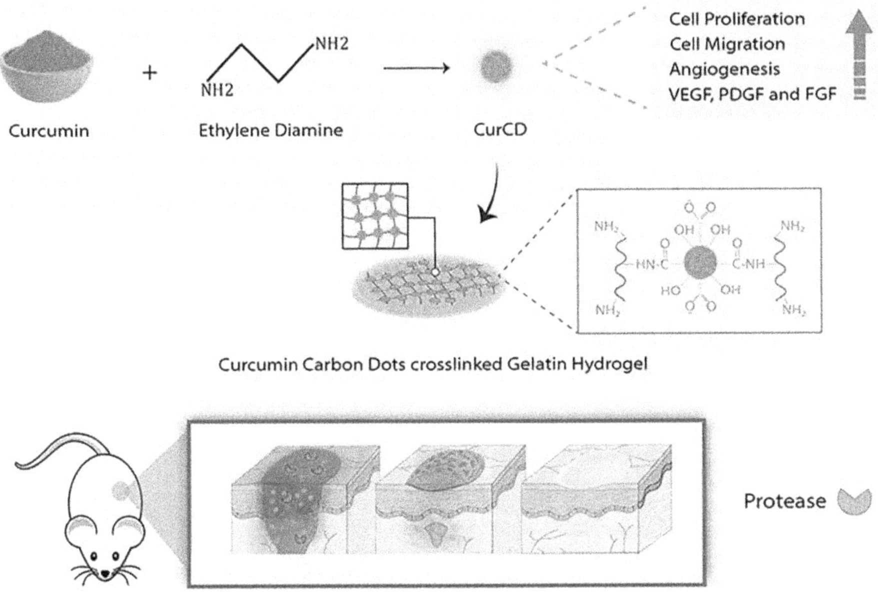

FIGURE 9.4   Wound healing property of curcumin carbon dot-crosslinked gelatin hydrogel. **Reprinted and reused with permission from (Anjana Sharma et al. 2022)**

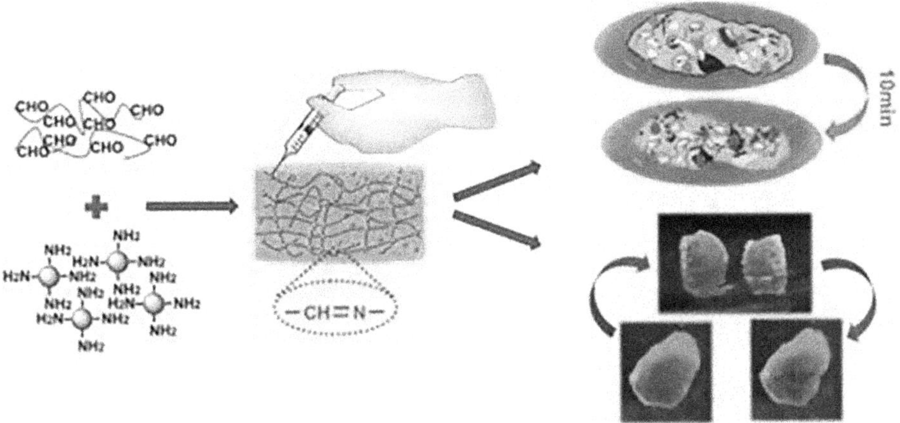

FIGURE 9.5   Self-healing and injectable CQD based hydrogel for wound healing application. **Reprinted and reused with permission from Yang et al. 2021.**

CQDs and then later reacted with oxidized dextran through a Schiff base linkage to form a hydrogel network. Besides being highly biocompatible, non-cytotoxic, and non-hemolytic, the injectable hydrogel exhibited multiple functionalities such as low drug resistance, inherent self-healing ability, stretchability, compressive property, anti-biofilm property, and pH-dependent release of CQDs (Figure 9.6) (Li et al. 2021).

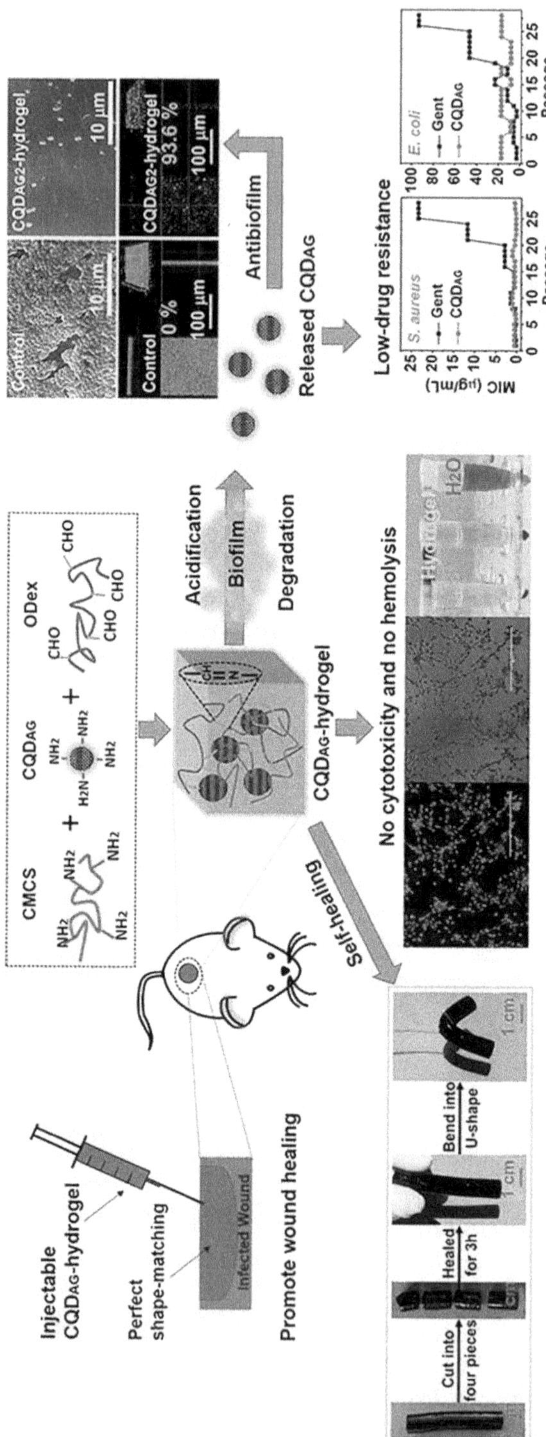

FIGURE 9.6 Illustration depicting the development of injectable CQD$_{AG}$ hydrogel and its multiple functions as wound dressing. Reprinted and reused with permission from Li et al. (2021). Copyright © 2023 Elsevier B.V.

9.6.3   pH-responsive CQD-based Dressings

Wound healing process can be delayed by infection. When a wound is infected with bacteria, there will be pH fluctuation at the wound site. Hence, an ideal wound dressing material must be able to prevent bacterial colonization as well as monitor pH to enable fast healing process. Monitoring of the pH of wounds is crucial for interpreting the wound status, as early identification of infection in wounds and non-healing wounds can enable timely administration of useful therapy (P. Yang et al. 2019). Numerous studies have focused on the development and application of pH-responsive CQD-based wound dressings. Most of the CQD-based pH detection systems are based on pH-induced single photoluminescence intensity change or fluorescence measurement (Ding et al. 2018).

A pH-responsive CQD-based smart drug delivery system composed of cotton patch nanocomposites incorporated with jute carbon dots was developed by Deb et al. Neem (*Azadirachta indica*) extract was used to exemplify the drug release study. The hybrid cotton-jute carbon dot patch showed two distinct release profiles at pH 5 and 7, with increased release at pH 5. This study proved that it could be applied as a potential wound healing material which is expected to enhance the release of the desired drug when the pH gets lowered as in the case of a bacterial infection in the wound, thereby accelerating the healing process (Deb, Konwar, and Chowdhury 2020) (Figure 9.7).

A recent study reported the development of a smart electrospun biosensing nanomaterial network based on polycaprolactone and CQDs for direct detection of *Staphylococcus aureus* in wounds (Pebdeni, Hosseini, and Barkhordari 2022). This

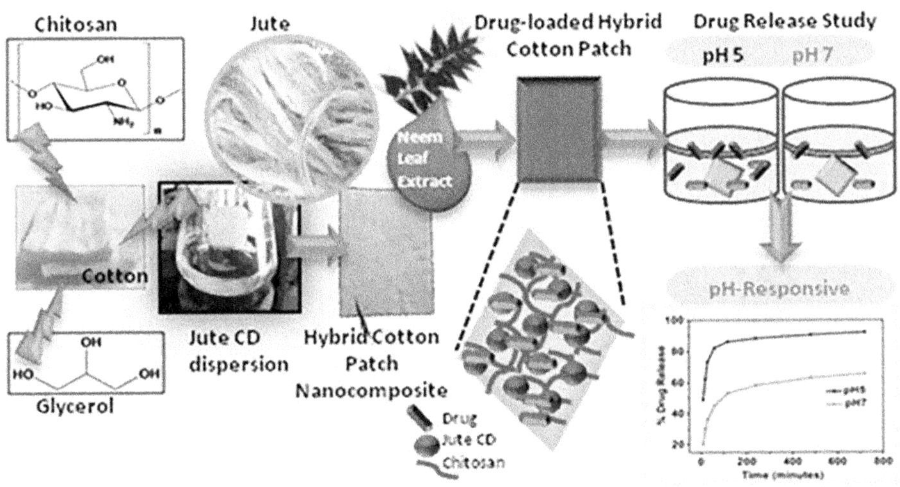

FIGURE 9.7   Graphical abstract showing the development and applications of jute carbon dot-cotton patch.

Reprinted and reused with permission from Deb, Konwar, and Chowdhury 2020.

biosensing platform worked based on the aptamers and the fluorescence property of CQDs. *S. aureus* was captured by the aptamers conjugated to the nanofiber network and then the sensitivity was measured in varying concentrations of bacteria which lead to enhancement of fluorescence emission under a UV lamp, which was observed with the naked eye.

9.6.4 CQD-BASED BANDAGES

Bandages are commonly used wound dressing materials. Many studies have reported on the development and effective applications of CQD-based bandages. Mou et al. prepared carbon dots from citric acid and ε-polylysine, and these carbon dots were incorporated into the PVA matrix to form a biocompatible, bandage-type dressing for wound healing. The developed bandages had excellent antibacterial activity against *E. coli* and *S. aureus*. When these bandages were pasted on wounds and removed after two days, complete wound closure was detected within 14 days (Mou et al. 2023) (Figure 9.8).

9.6.5 CQD-BASED SPRAY

In another recent work, positively charged CQDs were synthesized from *p*-phenylenediamine and polyethyleneimine by a one-pot solvothermal method. The CQDs exhibited excellent antibacterial properties against *S. aureus* and was also found to scavenge free radicals, protect wounds from oxidative stress, and heal wounds faster. The CQDs also expressed good biocompatibility in vitro and in vivo. Simple dropping or spraying of the developed CQDs into wound of a mouse model demonstrated effective wound healing without any side effects (Qu et al. 2023) (Figure 9.9).

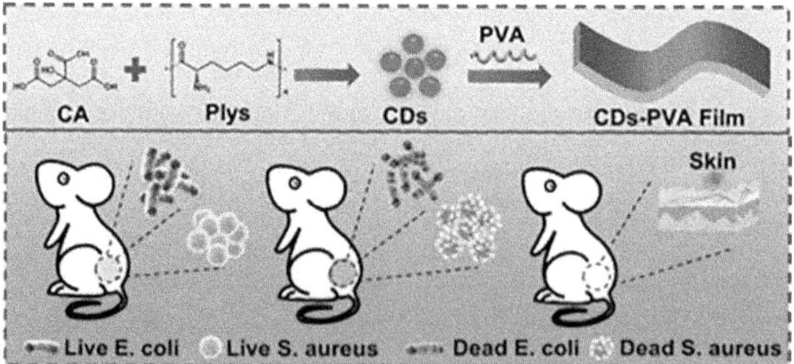

FIGURE 9.8 Schematic showing synthesis of CDs from citric acid and ε-polylysine and the development and applications of CDs-PVA film-based wound dressing material.

Reprinted and reused with permission from Mou et al. (2023). Copyright © 2023 American Chemical Society.

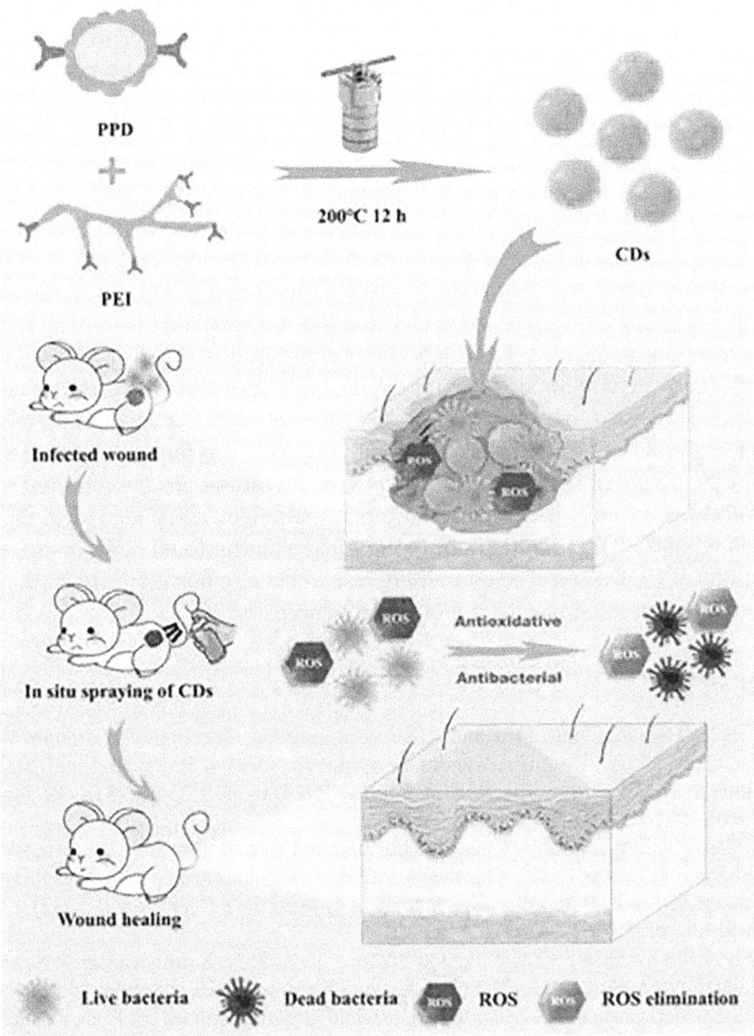

FIGURE 9.9 Synthesis and spraying of CQDs on mouse model for wound healing experiment.

Reprinted and reused with permission from (Qu et al. 2023). Copyright © 2023 American Chemical Society.

9.7 CONCLUSIONS AND FUTURE OUTLOOK

Wound healing research area has witnessed a very successful perspective owing to the intervention of CQDs. CQDs and its formulations have achieved a very prominent application in wound dressing area. CQDs are carbon-based tiny nanomaterials having a size range less than 10 nm. Multiple functionalities of CQDs in terms of high antibacterial activity, release of ROS, ability to monitor changes in wound pH as well as promotion of fibroblast cell proliferation increase their suitability as a faster wound healing material compared to others. CQDs also have the advantage of being synthesized from a variety of easily available precursors such as biomass waste, phytochemicals, and other natural resources. Moreover, CQDs can be formulated into hydrogels, adhesives, foams, sprays, or any other forms that can be suitable for application on wounds. This chapter includes the current literature and article reviews available on the novel applications of CQDs in wound healing process and compares the advantages of CQDs-based wound healing methods over conventional methods. Since the core and the surface functional groups contribute to most of the functionalities of CQDs, more clarification is needed on the structural analysis and the reaction mechanism of CQDs. Future research is highly recommended for exploring innovative methods for controlled development of CQDs. More emphasis is required to reveal other possibilities of CQDs as well as hybrid materials incorporating CQDs aiding in the wound healing process. Even though CQDs are proven to be safe by cytotoxicity assays, further *in vivo* investigations are required to probe the possibilities of any risk factors and other challenges associated with the use of CQDs on wounds. This chapter hopes to provide a strong foundation on the existing applications of CQDs and urge up-coming researchers to look on the unexplored possibilities of this promising zero-dimensional nanomaterial.

REFERENCES

Anwar, Sadat, Haizhen Ding, Mingsheng Xu, Xiaolong Hu, Zhenzhen Li, Jingmin Wang, Li Liu, et al. 2019. "Recent Advances in Synthesis, Optical Properties, and Biomedical Applications of Carbon Dots." *ACS Applied Bio Materials* 2 (6): 2317–38. https://doi.org/10.1021/acsabm.9b00112.

Bankoti, Kamakshi, Arun Prabhu Rameshbabu, Sayanti Datta, Bodhisatwa Das, Analava Mitra, and Santanu Dhara. 2017. "Onion Derived Carbon Nanodots for Live Cell Imaging and Accelerated Skin Wound Healing." *Journal of Materials Chemistry B* 5 (32): 6579–92. https://doi.org/10.1039/C7TB00869D.

Bhattacharyya, Swarup Krishna, Suvendu Nandi, Tamal Dey, Samit Kumar Ray, Mahitosh Mandal, Narayan Chandra Das, and Susanta Banerjee. 2022. "Fabrication of a Vitamin B12-Loaded Carbon Dot/Mixed-Ligand Metal Organic Framework Encapsulated within the Gelatin Microsphere for PH Sensing and In Vitro Wound Healing Assessment." *ACS Applied Bio Materials* 5 (12): 5693–5705. https://doi.org/10.1021/acsabm.2c00725.

Chan, Ming-Hsien, Ru-Shi Liu, and Michael Hsiao. 2019. "Graphitic Carbon Nitride-Based Nanocomposites and Their Biological Applications: A Review." *Nanoscale* 11 (32): 14993–3. https://doi.org/10.1039/C9NR04568F.

Chen, Xu, Ying Qin, Xinru Song, He Li, Yue Yang, Jiazhuang Guo, Tingting Cui, Jiafei Yu, Cai-Feng Wang, and Su Chen. 2022. "Green Synthesis of Carbon Dots and Their Integration into Nylon-11 Nanofibers for Enhanced Mechanical Strength and Biocompatibility." *Nanomaterials* 12 (19): 3347. https://doi.org/10.3390/nano12193347.

De Medeiros, Tayline V., John Manioudakis, Farah Noun, Jun-Ray Macairan, Florence Victoria, and Rafik Naccache. 2019. "Microwave-Assisted Synthesis of Carbon Dots and Their Applications." *Journal of Materials Chemistry C* 7 (24): 7175–95. https://doi.org/10.1039/C9TC01640F.

Deb, Ankita, Achyut Konwar, and Devasish Chowdhury. 2020. "PH-Responsive Hybrid Jute Carbon Dot-Cotton Patch." *ACS Sustainable Chemistry & Engineering* 8 (19): 7394–7402. https://doi.org/10.1021/acssuschemeng.0c01221.

Dehghani, Niloofar, Fatemeh Haghiralsadat, Fatemeh Yazdian, Fatemeh Sadeghian-Nodoushan, Nasrin Ghasemi, Fahime Mazaheri, Mehrab Pourmadadi, and Seyed Morteza Naghib. 2023. "Chitosan/Silk Fibroin/Nitrogen-Doped Carbon Quantum Dot/α-Tricalcium Phosphate Nanocomposite Electrospinned as a Scaffold for Wound Healing Application: In Vitro and in Vivo Studies." *International Journal of Biological Macromolecules* 238 (May): 124078. https://doi.org/10.1016/j.ijbiomac.2023.124078.

Dehghani, Samira, Seyed Vali Hosseini, and Joe M. Regenstein. 2018. "Edible Films and Coatings in Seafood Preservation: A Review." *Food Chemistry* 240 (February): 505–13. https://doi.org/10.1016/j.foodchem.2017.07.034.

Ding, Hui, Ji-Shi Wei, Peng Zhang, Zi-Yuan Zhou, Qing-Yu Gao, and Huan-Ming Xiong. 2018. "Solvent-Controlled Synthesis of Highly Luminescent Carbon Dots with a Wide Color Gamut and Narrowed Emission Peak Widths." *Small* 14 (22): 1800612. https://doi.org/10.1002/smll.201800612.

Dong, Zhenyou, Junhui Yin, Xueqing Zhou, Suyun Li, Zhenyu Fu, Pei Liu, Longxiang Shen, and Wenyan Shi. 2023. "Natural and Biocompatible Dressing Unit Based on Tea Carbon Dots Modified Core-Shell Electrospun Fiber for Diabetic Wound Disinfection and Healing." *Colloids and Surfaces B: Biointerfaces* 226 (June): 113325. https://doi.org/10.1016/j.colsurfb.2023.113325.

Ebrahimi, Somaye, and Hamide Ehtesabi. 2022. "Fabrication of Double-Layer Alginate/Carbon Dot Nanocomposite Hydrogel for Potential Wound Dressing Application." *Materials Letters* 325 (October): 132806. https://doi.org/10.1016/j.matlet.2022.132806.

Ehtesabi, Hamide, and Reyhaneh Nasri. 2021. "Carbon Dot-Based Materials for Wound Healing Applications." *Advances in Natural Sciences: Nanoscience and Nanotechnology* 12 (2): 025006. https://doi.org/10.1088/2043-6262/abffc9.

Frykberg, Robert G., and Jaminelli Banks. 2015. "Challenges in the Treatment of Chronic Wounds." *Advances in Wound Care* 4 (9): 560–82. https://doi.org/10.1089/wound.2015.0635.

Ghataty, Dina Saeed, Reham Ibrahim Amer, Mai A. Amer, Mohamed F. Abdel Rahman, and Rehab Nabil Shamma. 2023. "Green Synthesis of Highly Fluorescent Carbon Dots from Bovine Serum Albumin for Linezolid Drug Delivery as Potential Wound Healing Biomaterial: Bio-Synergistic Approach, Antibacterial Activity, and In Vitro and Ex Vivo Evaluation." *Pharmaceutics* 15 (1): 234. https://doi.org/10.3390/pharmaceutics15010234.

Ghirardello, Mattia, Javier Ramos-Soriano, and M. Carmen Galan. 2021. "Carbon Dots as an Emergent Class of Antimicrobial Agents." *Nanomaterials* 11 (8): 1877. https://doi.org/10.3390/nano11081877.

Gu, Xuexin, Lingli Zhu, Dekui Shen, and Chong Li. 2022. "Facile Synthesis of Multi-Emission Nitrogen/Boron Co-Doped Carbon Dots from Lignin for Anti-Counterfeiting Printing." *Polymers* 14 (14): 2779. https://doi.org/10.3390/polym14142779.

Guo, S., and L.A. DiPietro. 2010. "Factors Affecting Wound Healing." *Journal of Dental Research* 89 (3): 219–29. https://doi.org/10.1177/0022034509359125.

Hao, Xiaoli, Lingling Huang, Chengfei Zhao, Sining Chen, Wanjing Lin, Yinning Lin, Lirong Zhang, et al. 2021. "Antibacterial Activity of Positively Charged Carbon Quantum Dots without Detectable Resistance for Wound Healing with Mixed Bacteria Infection." *Materials Science and Engineering: C* 123 (April): 111971. https://doi.org/10.1016/j.msec.2021.111971.

Hao, Yuanping, Wenwen Zhao, Liyu Zhang, Xi Zeng, Zhanyi Sun, Demeng Zhang, Peili Shen, et al. 2020. "Bio-Multifunctional Alginate/Chitosan/Fucoidan Sponges with Enhanced Angiogenesis and Hair Follicle Regeneration for Promoting Full-Thickness Wound Healing." *Materials & Design* 193 (August): 108863. https://doi.org/10.1016/j.matdes.2020.108863.

Huang, Shan, Erli Yang, Jiandong Yao, Xu Chu, Yi Liu, Yue Zhang, and Qi Xiao. 2019. "Nitrogen, Cobalt Co-Doped Fluorescent Magnetic Carbon Dots as Ratiometric Fluorescent Probes for Cholesterol and Uric Acid in Human Blood Serum." *ACS Omega* 4 (5): 9333–42. https://doi.org/10.1021/acsomega.9b00874.

Kazeminava, Fahimeh, Siamak Javanbakht, Mohammad Nouri, Pourya Gholizadeh, Parinaz Nezhad-Mokhtari, Khudaverdi Ganbarov, Asghar Tanomand, and Hossein Samadi Kafil. 2022. "Gentamicin-Loaded Chitosan/Folic Acid-Based Carbon Quantum Dots Nanocomposite Hydrogel Films as Potential Antimicrobial Wound Dressing." *Journal of Biological Engineering* 16 (1): 36. https://doi.org/10.1186/s13036-022-00318-4.

Li, Peili, Shuai Liu, Xu Yang, Shoukang Du, Wentao Tang, Weiwei Cao, Jinwei Zhou, Xuedong Gong, and Xiaodong Xing. 2021. "Low-Drug Resistance Carbon Quantum Dots Decorated Injectable Self-Healing Hydrogel with Potent Antibiofilm Property and Cutaneous Wound Healing." *Chemical Engineering Journal* 403 (January): 126387. https://doi.org/10.1016/j.cej.2020.126387.

Liu, JunJun, Daowei Li, Kai Zhang, Mingxi Yang, Hongchen Sun, and Bai Yang. 2018. "One-Step Hydrothermal Synthesis of Nitrogen-Doped Conjugated Carbonized Polymer Dots with 31% Efficient Red Emission for In Vivo Imaging." *Small* 14 (15): 1703919. https://doi.org/10.1002/smll.201703919.

Lu, Siyu, Laizhi Sui, Junjun Liu, Shoujun Zhu, Anmin Chen, Mingxing Jin, and Bai Yang. 2017. "Near-Infrared Photoluminescent Polymer-Carbon Nanodots with Two-Photon Fluorescence." *Advanced Materials* 29 (15): 1603443. https://doi.org/10.1002/adma.201603443.

Lux, Cassie N. 2022. "Wound Healing in Animals: A Review of Physiology and Clinical Evaluation." *Veterinary Dermatology* 33 (1): 91. https://doi.org/10.1111/vde.13032.

Mahat, Nur Akma, Siti Aisyah Shamsudin, Nora Jullok, and Akmal Hadi Ma'Radzi. 2020. "Carbon Quantum Dots Embedded Polysulfone Membranes for Antibacterial Performance in the Process of Forward Osmosis." *Desalination* 493 (November): 114618. https://doi.org/10.1016/j.desal.2020.114618.

Mou, Chengjian, Xinyuan Wang, Yanchao Liu, Zhigang Xie, and Min Zheng. 2023. "A Robust Carbon Dot-Based Antibacterial CDs-PVA Film as a Wound Dressing for Antibiosis and Wound Healing." *Journal of Materials Chemistry B* 11 (9): 1940–47. https://doi.org/10.1039/D2TB02582E.

Mou, Chengjian, Xinyuan Wang, Jiahui Teng, Zhigang Xie, and Min Zheng. 2022. "Injectable Self-Healing Hydrogel Fabricated from Antibacterial Carbon Dots and ε-Polylysine for Promoting Bacteria-Infected Wound Healing." *Journal of Nanobiotechnology* 20 (1): 368. https://doi.org/10.1186/s12951-022-01572-w.

Naskar, Atanu, and Kwang-sun Kim. 2020. "Recent Advances in Nanomaterial-Based Wound-Healing Therapeutics." *Pharmaceutics* 12 (6): 499. https://doi.org/10.3390/pharmaceutics12060499.

Pebdeni, Azam Bagheri, Morteza Hosseini, and Aref Barkhordari. 2022. "Smart Fluorescence Aptasensor Using Nanofiber Functionalized with Carbon Quantum Dot for Specific Detection of Pathogenic Bacteria in the Wound." *Talanta* 246 (August): 123454. https://doi.org/10.1016/j.talanta.2022.123454.

Pormohammad, Ali, Nadia K. Monych, Sougata Ghosh, Diana L. Turner, and Raymond J. Turner. 2021. "Nanomaterials in Wound Healing and Infection Control." *Antibiotics* 10 (5): 473. https://doi.org/10.3390/antibiotics10050473.

Qu, Xiaoqing, Chenxi Gao, Lei Fu, Yuefeng Chu, Jian-Hua Wang, Hongdeng Qiu, and Jia Chen. 2023. "Positively Charged Carbon Dots with Antibacterial and Antioxidant Dual Activities for Promoting Infected Wound Healing." *ACS Applied Materials & Interfaces* 15 (15): 18608–19. https://doi.org/10.1021/acsami.2c21839.

Rodrigues, Melanie, Nina Kosaric, Clark A. Bonham, and Geoffrey C. Gurtner. 2019. "Wound Healing: A Cellular Perspective." *Physiological Reviews* 99 (1): 665–706. https://doi.org/10.1152/physrev.00067.2017.

Shakiba-Marani, Robabeh, and Hamide Ehtesabi. 2023. "A Flexible and Hemostatic Chitosan, Polyvinyl Alcohol, Carbon Dot Nanocomposite Sponge for Wound Dressing Application." *International Journal of Biological Macromolecules* 224 (January): 831–39. https://doi.org/10.1016/j.ijbiomac.2022.10.169.

Sharma, Anirudh, and Joydeep Das. 2019. "Small Molecules Derived Carbon Dots: Synthesis and Applications in Sensing, Catalysis, Imaging, and Biomedicine." *Journal of Nanobiotechnology* 17 (1): 92. https://doi.org/10.1186/s12951-019-0525-8.

Sharma, Anjana, Vineeta Panwar, Navita Salaria, and Deepa Ghosh. 2022. "Protease-Responsive Hydrogel, Cross-Linked with Bioactive Curcumin-Derived Carbon Dots, Encourage Faster Wound Closure." *Biomaterials Advances* 139 (August): 212978. https://doi.org/10.1016/j.bioadv.2022.212978.

Shi, Bingfang, Yubin Su, Liangliang Zhang, Mengjiao Huang, Rongjun Liu, and Shulin Zhao. 2016. "Nitrogen and Phosphorus Co-Doped Carbon Nanodots as a Novel Fluorescent Probe for Highly Sensitive Detection of Fe^{3+} in Human Serum and Living Cells." *ACS Applied Materials & Interfaces* 8 (17): 10717–25. https://doi.org/10.1021/acsami.6b01325.

Sun, Hanjun, Nan Gao, Kai Dong, Jinsong Ren, and Xiaogang Qu. 2014. "Graphene Quantum Dots-Band-Aids Used for Wound Disinfection." *ACS Nano* 8 (6): 6202–10. https://doi.org/10.1021/nn501640q.

Sun, Yanan, Min Zhang, Bhesh Bhandari, and Chaohui Yang. 2022. "Recent Development of Carbon Quantum Dots: Biological Toxicity, Antibacterial Properties and Application in Foods." *Food Reviews International* 38 (7): 1513–32. https://doi.org/10.1080/87559129.2020.1818255.

Tajik, Somayeh, Zahra Dourandish, Kaiqiang Zhang, Hadi Beitollahi, Quyet Van Le, Ho Won Jang, and Mohammadreza Shokouhimehr. 2020. "Carbon and Graphene Quantum Dots: A Review on Syntheses, Characterization, Biological and Sensing Applications for Neurotransmitter Determination." *RSC Advances* 10 (26): 15406–29. https://doi.org/10.1039/D0RA00799D.

Taylor, Danielle Lynne, and Marc In Het Panhuis. 2016. "Self-Healing Hydrogels." *Advanced Materials* 28 (41): 9060–93. https://doi.org/10.1002/adma.201601613.

Wang, Heni, Zejun Xu, Meng Zhao, Guiting Liu, and Jun Wu. 2021. "Advances of Hydrogel Dressings in Diabetic Wounds." *Biomaterials Science* 9 (5): 1530–46. https://doi.org/10.1039/D0BM01747G.

Wang, Mingqian, Yutian Su, Yihan Liu, Ying Liang, Shishan Wu, Ninglin Zhou, and Jian Shen. 2022. "Antibacterial Fluorescent Nano-Sized Lanthanum-Doped Carbon Quantum Dot Embedded Polyvinyl Alcohol for Accelerated Wound Healing." *Journal of Colloid and Interface Science* 608 (February): 973–83. https://doi.org/10.1016/j.jcis.2021.10.018.

Wang, Youfu, and Aiguo Hu. 2014. "Carbon Quantum Dots: Synthesis, Properties and Applications." *Journal of Materials Chemistry C* 2 (34): 6921. https://doi.org/10.1039/C4TC00988F.

Wu, Lina, Yaoran Gao, Chengfei Zhao, Dandan Huang, Wenxin Chen, Xinhua Lin, Ailin Liu, and Liqing Lin. 2022. "Synthesis of Curcumin-Quaternized Carbon Quantum Dots with Enhanced Broad-Spectrum Antibacterial Activity for Promoting Infected Wound Healing." *Biomaterials Advances* 133 (February): 112608. https://doi.org/10.1016/j.msec.2021.112608.

Yang, Pei, Ziqi Zhu, Tao Zhang, Wei Zhang, Weimin Chen, Yizhong Cao, Minzhi Chen, and Xiaoyan Zhou. 2019. "Orange-Emissive Carbon Quantum Dots: Toward Application in Wound PH Monitoring Based on Colorimetric and Fluorescent Changing." *Small* 15 (44): 1902823. https://doi.org/10.1002/smll.201902823.

Yang, Xu, Peili Li, Wentao Tang, Shoukang Du, Meizhe Yu, Haojie Lu, Huaping Tan, and Xiaodong Xing. 2021. "A Facile Injectable Carbon Dot/Oxidative Polysaccharide Hydrogel with Potent Self-Healing and High Antibacterial Activity." *Carbohydrate Polymers* 251 (January): 117040. https://doi.org/10.1016/j.carbpol.2020.117040.

Yoon, Cheolsang, Kab Pil Yang, Jungwook Kim, Kyusoon Shin, and Kangtaek Lee. 2020. "Fabrication of Highly Transparent and Luminescent Quantum Dot/Polymer Nanocomposite for Light Emitting Diode Using Amphiphilic Polymer-Modified Quantum Dots." *Chemical Engineering Journal* 382 (February): 122792. https://doi.org/10.1016/j.cej.2019.122792.

Yu, Betty, Soo-Young Kang, Ariya Akthakul, Nithin Ramadurai, Morgan Pilkenton, Alpesh Patel, Amir Nashat, et al. 2016. "An Elastic Second Skin." *Nature Materials* 15 (8): 911–18. https://doi.org/10.1038/nmat4635.

Zhang, Jin, Xingzhong Yuan, Longbo Jiang, Zhibin Wu, Xiaohong Chen, Hou Wang, Hui Wang, and Guangming Zeng. 2018. "Highly Efficient Photocatalysis toward Tetracycline of Nitrogen Doped Carbon Quantum Dots Sensitized Bismuth Tungstate Based on Interfacial Charge Transfer." *Journal of Colloid and Interface Science* 511 (February): 296–306. https://doi.org/10.1016/j.jcis.2017.09.083.

Zhao, Chengfei, Xuewen Wang, Luying Yu, Lina Wu, Xiaoli Hao, Qicai Liu, Liqing Lin, et al. 2022. "Quaternized Carbon Quantum Dots with Broad-Spectrum Antibacterial Activity for the Treatment of Wounds Infected with Mixed Bacteria." *Acta Biomaterialia* 138 (January): 528–44. https://doi.org/10.1016/j.actbio.2021.11.010.

Zhao, Xin, Baolin Guo, Hao Wu, Yongping Liang, and Peter X. Ma. 2018. "Injectable Antibacterial Conductive Nanocomposite Cryogels with Rapid Shape Recovery for Noncompressible Hemorrhage and Wound Healing." *Nature Communications* 9 (1): 2784. https://doi.org/10.1038/s41467-018-04998-9.

Zheng, Xin Ting, Yingying Zhong, Huan Enn Chu, Yong Yu, Yu Zhang, Jiah Shin Chin, David Lawrence Becker, Xiaodi Su, and Xian Jun Loh. 2023. "Carbon Dot-Doped Hydrogel Sensor Array for Multiplexed Colorimetric Detection of Wound Healing." *ACS Applied Materials & Interfaces* 15 (14): 17675–87. https://doi.org/10.1021/acsami.3c01185.

10 Carbon Quantum Dots for Treating Viral Infections

*Neeta Gupta, Reena Rawat, Bhawana Jain,
Sanju Singh, Shraddha Vaishnav
and Shilpi Shrivastava*

10.1 INTRODUCTION

Throughout history, people have struggled with many diseases, such as plague, smallpox, swine flu, Ebola virus, human immunodeficiency virus (HIV), severe respiratory diseases (SARS), Middle East respiratory syndrome (MERS), corona and zika viruses, which paid a great price. It has a significant and negative influence on lives and wellbeing of billions of people. At the completion of 2019, a different and novel/new type of coronavirus, Severe Acute Respiratory Syndrome Coronavirus 2 (SARS-CoV-2) was first identified which then transmitted to the entire world. Today, the 2019 coronavirus (COVID-19), initiated by SARS-CoV-2, is a serious and continuing danger to human health. Virus causing COVID-19 is predicted to be among the deadliest viruses in history of humanity. In this exceptional worldwide crisis, the need and urgency to develop and produce effective vaccines and diagnostics has never been greater. Table 10.1 describes some of the most important diseases in life and their main treatment and diagnosis.

Singh, P. et al. (2021) described that nanotechnology possesses the prospective to create novel products and merchandises that can change every aspect of living and life. It remains to be accepted as one of the major six important technologies' that will change our lives in all aspects. Ge, Y. et al. (2014) explained that nanomedicine today casts an important part in patients' health and eminence of life, leading to many medical and medical applications such as screening, diagnosis, pain management, delivery of drugs, and development.

Lara, H. H. et al. (2010) explained the unique physical and chemical properties of various nanomaterials have emerged as new anti-inflammatory agents. They are also widely used in the identification of contagious diseases. Molaei, M. J. (2019) demonstrated over the past decade that CQDs have emerged as novel class of nanomaterials has attracted increased consideration due to their unique properties.

DOI: 10.1201/9781003437857-12

TABLE 10.1
Viruses and Their Diagnostic Techniques Reported

Virus	Infection	Method of Treatment	Diagnosis	References
SARS-CoV-2	COVID-19	Vaccines Antiviral agents/ drugs	RT-PCR using swab and sputum Blood test Antibody test	Krammer, F. (2020)
Ebola	Fever	Monoclonal antibodies	PCR ELISA IgM & IgG antibody detection specific to Ebola	Breman and Henderson (2002)
HIV	Acquired immune deficiency syndrome-AIDS	Anti-viral medicines HIV inhibitors HIV vaccines	PCR/viral-load assessment; ELISA; Finger/Swab test Western blot test	Pollard, A. J. Bijker (2021)
SARS	Severe acute respiratory syndrome	Anti-viral drugs Convalescent plasma and immunoglobulin	RT-PCR; Serology; ELISA	Craigie, J. & Wishart (1936)
MERS	Middle east respiratory syndrome	Anti-viral drugs	RT-PCR; Serology; ELISA; Immuno-fluorescence assay	Zulfiqar, H. F. et al. (2017)
Variola	Smallpox	Injections/vaccines Anti-viral drugs	Serum examination; Skin examination	Stockman, L. J. et al. (2006)

CQDs basically are extremely tiny and have a normal/average diameter of less than 10 nm, with high solubility in water, beautiful photoluminescence, photo-stability, exceptional biocompatibility, minimum/no toxicity, environmentally friendly and extraordinary sustainability, etc. Ting, D. (2018) studied that some CQD strains have strong immunity and ability against human coronaviruses, arteriviruses, noroviruses and herpes viruses. Barras, A. et al. (2016) reported that CQDs derived from a monomer (benzoxazine) are broad-spectrum drugs against flaviviruses and non-viral viruses.

Here in, we have presented a detailed as well as updated summary on the types, structures, synthesis, properties, and medical applications of CQDs, focusing on the basic and advanced mechanisms and parts in the diagnosis, avoidance/prevention, and management of different types of bacterial infection (Figure 10.1.).

Research into the utilization of CQDs to combat against COVID-19 has also been highlighted and discussed over time (Figure 10.2.).

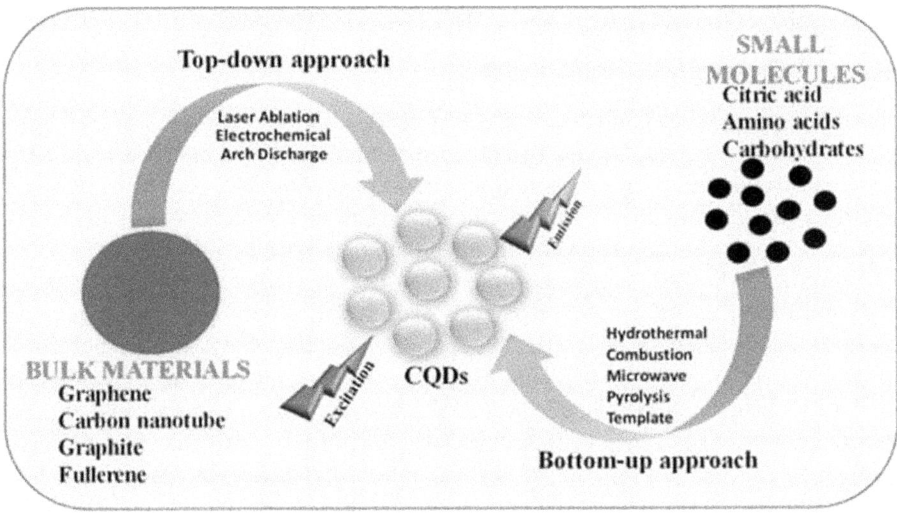

FIGURE 10.1 Typical methods used to synthesize carbon quantum dots [116].

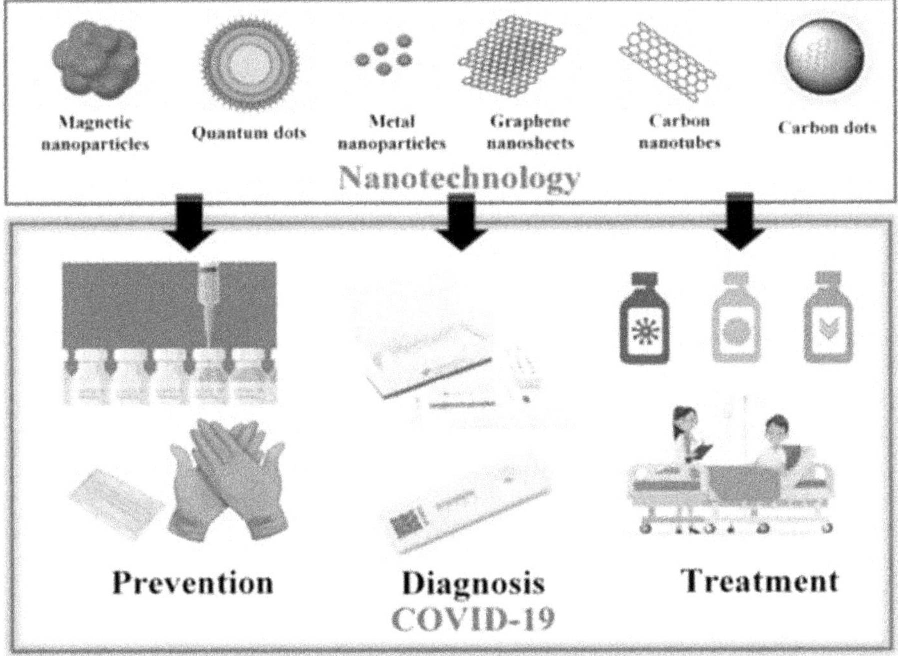

FIGURE 10.2 Nanotechnology applications for COVID-19 prevention, diagnosis, and therapy [117].

10.2 NANOMATERIALS AND DIFFERENT VIRUSES

10.2.1 Overall Viral Pathogenesis

Jones, J. E. et al. (2021) demonstrated that viruses on their own are advanced/progressed and have various strains. In a broad spectrum, the pathogenic processes comprise bacterial entrance, reproduction and transmission in vivo, tissue proliferation, and response to immunity. A deeper comprehension on the pathogenesis of the disease may support the development of anti-inflammatory drugs.

Dimitrov, D. S. (2004) explained different types of bacteria have different routes of entry, for example, through the respiratory tract, which is one of the most important routes through which bacteria enter the human body. Bacteria that enter the bodies through the respiratory tract can bind to precise receptors on epithelial cells. Cao, W. et al. (2020) studied SARS and SARS-CoV-2 and can bind to enzymes that are converted to angiotensin-2 (ACE-2). Conversely, few viruses can come into the body through the skin (such as the papilloma virus) or through the urogenital tract (such as G. herpes simplex virus 2 and HIV) or stomach viruses such as rotavirus and norovirus. After entering, the proliferating pathogenic virus can continue to remain local and/or turn to systemic by lymphatic and hematogenous ways. Rockx, B. et al. (2020) explained viruses like MERS, SARS, and SARS-CoV-2, which enter the human body via the respiratory tract, can spread very rapidly through the fluid/mucous stratum covering the epithelial surface, so the disease caused by these bacteria will heal and accelerate [28].

Acharya, S. (2020) demonstrated that different viruses have different infection patterns, mainly due to differences in the main sites of their replication and destruction (tissues/body). For example, SARS-CoV-2 can proliferate in the upper part of the respiratory tract and viscera as it uses ACE2 as its chief receptor, and ACE2 is mainly conveyed in the bloodstream, alveolar monocytes, macrophages, and endothelium. An infected person may or may not show symptoms of the disease. Hui, K. P.-Y. et al. (2022) studied diseases occur only when the immune system of host/virus is damaged. For instance, cells infected with SARS-CoV-2 cause an overproduction of cytokines that damage the respiratory organs and affect functioning of the lungs. Lukassen, S. et al. (2020) published single-cell RNA sequencing data show that the transmembrane protease serine protease 2 (TMPRSS2) is highly expressed in nasal epithelial cells, lungs, and bronchial branches, and is co-expressed with ACE2, which explains the tissue specificity of SARS-CoV-2. Mehta, P. et al. (2020) studied that after binding to ACE2 in airway epithelial cells, SARS-CoV-2 began to proliferate and move towards airways and alveolar epithelial cells. Rapid replication of SARS-CoV-2 in the lungs induces a potent immune cytokine response, leading to infiltration of lung-damaging cells. Giamarellos-Bourboulis, E. J. et al's. (2020) studies provided the symptoms of COVID-19 caused by SARS-CoV-2 which range from mild pneumonia to life-threatening breathing difficulties. In the latter, oxygenation is affected by lung inflammation, which is also a reflection of immune-induced host damage.

10.2.2 Disease Detection using Nanoparticles

Benzigar, M. R. et al. (2021) reported that there is no effective treatment for many pathogenic bacteria, and hence prompt and accurate diagnosis of the disease is crucial to prevent infection. However, current methods, including serological anti-body testing or reverse PCR, are sufficiently sensitive and specific to detect the virus in clinical specimens. Benzigar, M. R. et al. (2021) explained nanomaterials exhibit a variety of optical, electrical, magnetic and mechanical properties and are widely used in sensing and diagnostics. Yadavalli, T. et al. (2018) showed that metal and metal oxide nanoparticles such as gold nanoparticles (AuNPs), silver nanoparticles (AgNPs), aluminum nanoparticles (AlNPs), and iron oxide nanoparticles have been successfully used for disease detection. Nanobiohybrid systems contain and combine one or more biomolecules (e.g., DNA, RNA, antibodies, antigens, and peptides derived from bacteria and metal nanoparticles are often collected and used). In this way, surface functionalization and tunable physicochemical properties can be obtained easily, quickly, with high precision, without labels and/or multiple detection methods. Negahdari, B.et al. (2019) reported the use of AuNPs as biosensors for HBV (hepatitis B) detection, the use of $MoS_2@Cu_2O$-Pt nanohybrids as enzyme-mimetic tags for HBsAg detection, and the use of gold-plated metal oxide nanoparticles. It is used for the diagnosis of HBV based on HBV DNA analysis.

Jia, Z. et al. (2019) reported on metal and magnetic nanoparticles, other nanomaterials such as carbon nanotubes (CNTs) and silicon dioxide nanoparticles (SiNPs) which have also been used for disease detection. Some researchers have designed and developed NiCo-based metal-organic frameworks (such as $NiCo_2O_4$-CoO@CNTs) to detect HIV-1 and found that the system has high electrochemical performance, biocompatibility, and strong biocompatibility for DNA analysis. Chunduri, L. A. A. et al. (2017) explained the system can capture human blood samples with good stability and reproducibility. It was reported that streptavidin-labeled and europium-doped fluorescent SiNPs can be used to detect HIV-1 p24 antigen with improved specificity, about 1000 times higher than color ELISA.

10.2.3 Nanoparticles as Antibiotics

Nasrollahzadeh, M. et al. (2020) demonstrated that available antibiotics still face deficiencies and problems such as opposition, adverse effects, narrow range, and economical burdens. Advanced nanomaterials that can enter cells and inhibit viral replication have been used successfully not only as antibody carriers but also as antibodies themselves. Xu, X. et al. (2004) researched that some nanoparticles are capable of reducing the risk of drug reactions and have an extensive variety of properties for use as anti-inflammatory agents. Mintz, K. J. et al. (2019) explained that nanoparticles can attack and kill bacteria with photothermally or photocatalytically persuaded reactive oxygen species (ROS). In general, various metals, metal oxides, and hybrid nanoparticles have been successfully synthesized and used in chemical reactions.

10.3 CARBON QUANTUM DOTS (CQDs)

Feng, H. and Qian (2018) studied carbon quantum dots (CQDs), also known as carbon dots (CDs), are a new fluorescent subclass in the class of carbon-based nanomaterials and have an average size of usually less than 10 nm. Ming, H. et al. (2012)

performed experiments, in which a mixture of new fluorescent nanoparticles was isolated during purification of single-walled carbon nanotubes. Since then, different CQDs have been prepared by various methods. Zheng, X. T. et al. (2015) showed that further progress has been made in various aspects such as derivation/modification and functionalization. Tao, S. et al. (2019) studied some advanced properties such as unique optical and electrical properties, chemical stability, good biocompatibility, low cost and flexibility, CQDs hold great promise in many applications, especially biomedical applications. CQDs can also be made from a variety of natural materials, giving them some unique features such as green planning and economical use.

10.3.1 STRUCTURES AND TYPES OF CARBON QUANTUM DOTS

Liu, J. et al. (2020c) explained there is some controversy about the concept of CQD; it is generally accepted that CQDs are zero-dimensional nanomaterials containing carbon and functional groups on the surface and the size of CQDs is generally in the range of 2–10 nm. While the inner structure contains sp2 and sp3 hybridized carbon atoms, while the outer structure contains sp3 hybrid carbon atoms. Considering their chemical structure, CQDs encompass many forms. Although there is no standard classification for CQDs in the literature based on their carbon core structure and morphology, carbon dots can be divided into CQDs, graphite-structured CQDs, carbonized polymer dots (CPDs), and C_3N_4 crystallization core CQDs.

Muthamma, K. et al. (2021) showed that spherical and monolithic carbon-based nanoparticle CQDs are the most reported. And the most important feature of CQDs is their size-dependent photoluminescence. Compared to graphite, the X-ray diffraction (XRD) pattern of CQDs shows two characteristic peaks at 22.59° and 18.20°; this indicates the presence of amorphous carbon and hexagonal carbon.

Liu, R. et al. (2009) studied that under certain conditions, nitrogen atoms can join the carbon core of CQDs to form specific nitride structures (g-C_3N_4 or β-C_3N_4). Tepliakov, N. V. et al (2019) explained when the nitrogen additive in the product reaches a certain threshold, the main structure of CQD changes, turning into carbon nitride nanocrystals. C_3N_4 core CQDs generally show good optical properties and photocatalytic activity. Graphene quantum dots (GQDs) are a class of carbon nanomaterials containing π-conjugated communities. They have a graphene lattice structure and contain one or more graphene layers less than 5 nm thick.

Ajith M. P. et al. (2022) compared with conventional CQDs, GQDs have more sp2 crystalline carbon atoms and fewer crystal defects. In Raman spectroscopy, GQDs show graphene-like D and G bands, but have higher ID/IG numbers due to more sp3 hybridized carbon at the edges. Due to the small size of GQDs, quantum confinement and edge effects become important. Therefore, GQDs have a non-zero gap, while large graphene nanosheets often show a zero-width gap. These features give GQDs the same electrical and optical properties as other CQDs.

Tajik, S. et al. (2020) reported that CPD is a new concept proposed to describe CQDs with a highly dehydrated cross-linked polymer framework. Zuo, P. et al. (2016) explained that during the synthesis reaction, intermediates go through complex processes such as polymerization, dehydration, and carbonization, eventually obtaining polymer/carbohybrid structures. For this reason, CPD is sometimes considered a special type of CQD. CPD can be converted to CQD by controlled carbonization. One of the main differences between CQDs and CPDs is the photoluminescence process. The optical properties of CPDs are usually determined by the emission constant. CPDs contain many subfluorophores such as double bonds and single coordinate heteroatoms. Tan, X. et al. (2015) demonstrated that these subfluorophores exhibit poor photoluminescence due to intramolecular rotation and vibration. Enhanced photoluminescent properties can be seen in CPD due to the limitation of intramolecular rotation and vibration due to chemical crosslinking or physical aggregation. There is controversy over whether CQDs have a general crystal structure.

Yu, H. et al. (2016) reported in previous studies that CQDs are mostly amorphous and exhibit different patterns based on XRD. However, Brisebois, P. P. and Siaj (2020) explained CQDs can be used as crystalline materials by selecting appropriate synthetic methods and starting materials. In recent years, it has been reported that most CQDs have a crystalline structure. The core of CQDs can be monocrystalline or polycrystalline. More importantly, the optical properties of CQDs are affected by their crystal structure.

Lu, Q. et al. (2017) explained CQDs have sp3 hybridized amorphous carbon cores. However, sp2 hybrid domains can be created under special conditions. In sp3 hybridized carbon atoms, the valence electrons are attached to stable σ bonds and are only sensitive to high-energy ultraviolet light, whereas in sp2 hybridized carbon atoms, valence electrons are delocalized in all regions and therefore have broad absorption in the visible spectral range. In addition, amorphous CQDs are more sensitive to photobleaching than crystalline CQDs, indicating that the photostability is close to that of CQDs.

10.3.2 Synthesis of Carbon Quantum Dots

da Silva Souza et al. (2018) reported several synthesis methods for synthesis of CQDs that possess dissimilar properties (physical and chemical). Addition of these can be done with utmost simplicity by manipulating reactants/antibodies. For cases involving carbon for synthesis, the process of CQDs could be broadly divided into "top-down" and "bottom-up" methodologies. Liu, Y. et al. (2020) reported "Top-down" methods are usually physical or chemical methods for producing small CQDs via exfoliation from bulky carbon sources like carbon-fibers, activated-carbon, carbon-nanotubes (CNTs), and rods of graphite. The "bottom-up" approach contains glucose, citric acid, folic acid, etc. It starts with small molecular carbon sources, and few recent reports regarding the synthesis of CQDs are relevant to the use of different carbons with different synthetic yields and applications. "Top-Down" Method: In general, the formation of CQDs by the separation of multidimensional huge precursors of carbon is considered "top-down". Methods include chemical and laser ablation, electrochemical carbonization, and hydro-thermal or solvothermal or oxidative pyrolysis (Figure 10.3).

de Medeiros, T. V. et al. (2019) reported that the cheap carbonaceous raw constituents are often employed as precursors. Owing to the straightforward synthesis process, it is also possible to mass-produce CQDs. In distinction, CQDs are simple to clean by electrochemical carbonization. In the electrochemical process, CQDs can

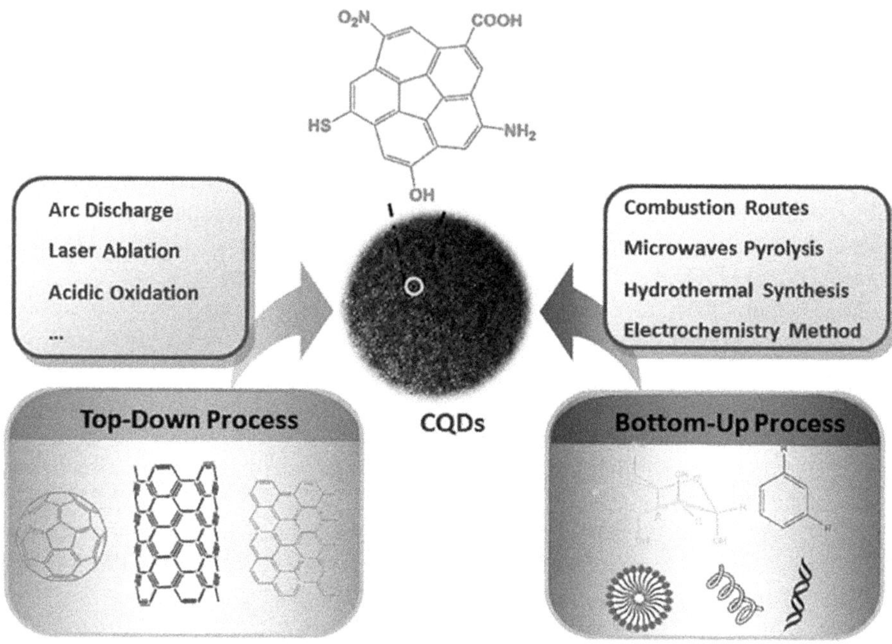

FIGURE 10.3 The standard procedures for creating CQDs [118].

be exfoliated straight from electrodes of graphite beneath the influence of electric field-induced redox reactions in electrochemical cells. This approach contributes to the inexpensive and easy synthesis of CQDs. By adjusting parameters such as electrolyte content as well as the current used, CQDs with diverse physicochemical properties could be achieved.

Priecel, P. and Lopez-Sanchez (2019) used for synthesizing CQDs. The first technique was to employ laser to cut carbon material (like glass) into water, and the next method was to cut carbon-powder (like carbon powder, graphite-powder) which is suspended in aqueous solution. By using the method of laser-ablation, the bone tissue is destroyed by photothermal evaporation and Coulomb scattering in the field of laser energy. Therefore, more carbon decomposes into smaller CQDs. Laser ablation is considered as a simple and green technique with high-purity products. However, during the manufacturing process, the solution is prone to clouding, resulting in loss of laser power that affects the performance of the CD. Also, because the volume of the liquid is more in comparison to the amount of the electricity, the reaction usually fails; the negative material will be removed later. Papaioannou, N. et al. (2019) studied chemical oxidation, sometimes referred to as the Hummers method, uses strong oxidizing agents (e.g., hydrogen peroxide, nitric and sulfuric acids) for treatment of carbon precursors at low temperatures to synthesize CQDs. In general, carbon monoxide can be a polymer material (e.g., G. graphene) or small molecules (such as sucrose). This method has the advantages of simple use, higher efficiency, and shorter time.

In another research, a group of GQDs was initially prepared by the hydrothermal process. Next, these GQDs are placed in distilled H_2O and microwaved in a microwave oven for around 5 min. As a result, GQDs showed higher efficacy and the QY of GQDs increased from 21.0% to 34%, which increased by 6% after treatment. This improvement can be explained by the elongation of the π-conjugated system and the inhibition of non-radiative processes. The hydrothermal method is another method based on the "bottom-up" approach. The reaction of different COs in high-temperature hydrothermal reactors is generally considered environmentally friendly, controllable, and cost-effective. Qu, D. et al. (2014) studied in the case of microwave-assisted irradiation technique, formation of CQDs in this methodology occurs in four steps/phases: decomposition, aromatization/polymerization, nucleation, and growth. Firstly, the carbonaceous precursors like amino acids, fructose, glucose, etc. experience dehydration as well as polymerization for the formation of solids and sugars. Nucleation of CQD occurs when the cluster reaches its critical supersaturation point. At the same time, aromatics diffuse to the particle surface and cause the development of functionalized entities on the surfaces of CQD. Lastly, with the progress in reactions, the reaction intermediates are converted to full CQDs which have a narrow distribution of particle size. The efficiency of CQDs which are fabricated using hydrothermal methodology depends on the time of reaction, temperature, and reactants used.

On extending the reaction time from 2 to 24 hours at a wavelength of 11 nm, it was seen that there was an increase in the amount of nitrogen atoms doped in the core of carbon when the time was increased. An increase in the QY was also seen to increase from 58% to 81%. It was also observed that the QY of the synthesized CQDs was sensitive to temperatures. The shift in the temperature to either higher or lower than the optimum, there was a decrease in the QY in the opposite way respectively. The selection of reactants can affect the optical characteristics of CQDs. CQDs that are synthesized from citric acid and primary amines exhibited the uppermost degree of nitrogen doping and photoluminescence intensity compared to those synthesized from secondary and tertiary amines.

10.3.3 Properties of Carbon Quantum Dots

As a favorable functional nanomaterial, the utmost attractive property of CQDs is the optical characteristics. Lim, S. Y. et al. (2015) explained that due to the chain structure in the chemical assembly of CQDs, the absorption spectra of CQDs largely shows visible light in the ultraviolet section and its tail extends into the visible light range. A synthetic container has been reported for the production of complete emitting color CQDs. Subsequently upon purification by silica gel chromatography, CQDs showed luminescence which was excitation-independent and ranged from blue to red. Gan, Z. et al. (2016) studied that upon UV excitation, CQDs could emit fluorescent emission. In general, synthesized intact CQDs initially does not show fluorescent characteristics. Nevertheless, CQDs can show excellent fluorescence properties after crosslinking with polar moieties. A previous study suggested excitation wavelength dependence for emission intensity and wavelength. Isnaeni, Herbani, Y. et al. (2018) demonstrated that with an increase in the excitation wavelength, there is a shift in the wavelength of emission from the long wavelength region, and hence the emission is able to cover all the visible region. Yet, few latest studies showed that some sort of CQDs can cause an emission in light at certain wavelengths upon excitation.

Wu, Y.-F. et al. (2016) explained the fluorescent characteristics of CQDs can be affected by certain parameters. In general, as the content of CQDs increases, the main energy can change from the transition of π-π* energy to transition of n-π* energy and from the surface-surface interactions between CQDs [95]. Buchs, G. et al. (2018) studied the surface energy of the CQDs will be reduced, resulting in a shorter lifetime of fluorescence. Additionally, the dimensions of CQDs affect the fluorescent characteristics of CQDs. In general, photoluminescent wavelengths show a redshift with increasing size. Liu, Y. et al. (2020) defined the mechanism of luminescence of CQDs is still uncertain. The phenomenon of luminescence could be attributed to many factors, like effects due to dimensions of quantum, structure of crystal, surface condition, functional regions, and functional groups.

Generally, all CQDs which are synthesized require either passivation or oxidation of surface for modification of fluorophore. Zhao, P. Zhu (2018) studied the CQDs surface often contains functional entities having oxygen and are usually hydrophilic. The hydrophilic characteristics of CQDs will depend on the reactants and the synthesis methodology. CQDs that are derived from precursors that are soluble tend to be very hydrophilic because the functional entities of the precursors are deposited on the surface of the CQDs while fabrication is done. In contrast, CQDs that are derived using insoluble materials can be water soluble after some cross-linking and modifications.

Yao, H. et al. (2018) showed that compared to conventional quantum dots containing heavy metals, CQDs showed improved solubility in water as well as biocompatibility, as observed in various studies on cytotoxicity. For instance, Nair et al. showed that GQDs were generated by a sonochemical microwave heating system and then verified for cytotoxicity by the MTT method using the HeLa cell track. No cytotoxicity was observed in the high-dose GQDs treatment assembly. Wang, Haitao et al. (2019) studied both sorts of CQDs displayed decent biocompatibility for normal breast cell-lines as well as breast cancer-cells with cell viabilities of > 85% and > 90% respectively, at a concentration of 200 mg mL^{-1}. The raw materials that can be used to create CQDs come from a variety of sources, from synthetic materials to natural materials. Few CQDs exist naturally in environment and interact with the human body.

Qu, K. et al. (2013) studied the processes of formation as well as the cytotoxicity of CQDs that were produced in sheep. Through the roasting procedure, the proteins, lipids, and simple carbohydrates of mutton undergo a high-temperature decomposition and carbonization process to become CQDs. The study found that CQDs from sheep roasted at high temperatures exhibited greater cytotoxicity than sheep roasted at low temperatures. Overall, however, CQDs showed low cytotoxicity (over 90% survival at 2 mg mL^{-1} concentration) and exhibited better biocompatibility in experiments. Most importantly, CQDs have the ability to scavenge free radicals to protect HepG2 cells from H_2O_2-induced oxidative damage.

10.3.4 Biomedical Solicitation of CQDs

He, Y.-S. et al. (2012) studied biomolecular revealing plays an imperative character in ailment diagnosis, management, and medical investigation. Recently, CQDs have been described for application in researches related to biomolecular studies. A new method using CQDs to detect dopamine concentrations in the blood was reported. They form CQDs with specific catechol entities that can interact with Fe^{3+} to form quinone groups on the surface, thereby quenching CQDs. Yang, L. et al. (2018) reported when dopamine is added to the body, it reacts with Fe^{3+} and restores fluorescence, preventing the reaction between Fe^{3+} and CQDs. In this way, dopamine concentration can be determined by plotting a standard curve between dopamine content and fluorescence change. In this study, the limit of detection of dopamine was reached at 68 nM. An improved CQD-based fluorescence method for dopamine detection was subsequently reported. They created a fluorescent probe by combination of CQDs and gold nanoclusters, where CQDs act as energizers and gold nanoclusters act as energy acceptors. Due to the presence of dopamine, fluorescence resonance energy exchange is inhibited and results in fluorescence reduction of gold nanoclusters and return of fluorescence of CQDs. Thus, dopamine concentration could be calculated by quantifying the strength of dual different emission wavelengths. The test has a lower limit of 2.9 nM and a wider variety of 5–180 nM.

Besides microscopic recognition, CQDs could be used for the revealing of biological macromolecules and bacteria also. Singh, S. et al. (2017) explained the technique is very profound and can identify S. aureus at concentrations between 1 and 200 CFU mL^{-1}. Owing to the excellent biocompatibility, solubility in water as well as the fluorescent behavior, CQDs could explore new bioimaging probes with some productive results. Peng et al. reported the functional CQDs were generated using a hydrothermal method which could bind petrified bone with high affinity as well as specificity. They tested the animals with zebra-fish and found CQDs were efficaciously absorbed in the gastric cavity. At the same time, CQDs show additional potential for targeted drug release. In another study, Liu et al. described an advanced bioimaging approach using red-emissions of CQDs to attain single-photon and two-photon images. The CQDs are formed by conjugated aromatic molecules of amine in the vicinity of oxidative radical chemicals. In comparison to shorter wavelength at the infrared (750–950 nm), long wavelength infrared photons penetrate deep into tissue, providing deep, high sensitivity in vivo bioimaging. The resulting CQDs exhibit red light with a high QY of 84% at 615 nm and a narrow emission line width.

The outcomes indicated that CQDs could be precisely affected in the lysosomal region and an optimistic luminescent field was witnessed at the injection site. In two-photon bioimaging means, CQDs exhibit upconversion fluorescence that emits a characteristic signal under excitation of 1050 and 1150 nm infrared light. Therefore, the depth of image effortlessly exceeds 200 μm, and the maximum depth of penetration reaches 500 μm. CQDs were primed by a hydrothermal method by the use of m-phenylenediamine and L-cysteine. The resulting CQDs exhibit nucleolar targeting potential across multiple cell-lines. The ability of the target was attributed to selective binding to RNA molecules due to the unique chemistry of CQDs. A platform for delivery of drug was equipped by conjugating protoporphyrin IX to CQDs. In comparison with free protoporphyrin IX, the platform for drug delivery based on CQDs exhibited overall improvements in tumor targeting efficacy, circulation of blood, retention of tumor, toxicology, and antitumor efficacy. Singh et al. 2017 developed hydrogels of CQDs-DNA for continuous delivery of drugs and monitoring. The initial step is functionalization of CQDs with 5'-phosphorylated DNA molecules to form CQD-DNA complexes. In the second step, the structure of the DNA is changed by regulating the solution's pH, resulting in a left-to-gel transition. Lastly, encapsulation of CQDs-DNA by doxorubicin (DOX) by adsorption electrostatically.

10.4 SOLICITATION OF CQDs FOR INHIBITING AND TREATING VIRAL INFECTION

With many developments and innovations in recent years, nanotechnology has changed our lives and redefined many medical/medical fields like diagnosis, treatment, drug delivery, and construction. Because of the unique and cutting-edge properties, the possibilities of CQDs in drug delivery, gene delivery, phototherapy, and radiation therapy have been explored and applied. Various studies showed that some CQDs displayed lower toxicology and high immunogenicity against brain tumors.

10.4.1 Virus Penetration and Uncoating

The lifespan of viruses and animal crowds could be broadly classified into 3 steps: (1) infection and uncoating; (2) no contamination or coating; (3) no contamination and coating. (2) Virus replication and assembly; (3) Virus release [106]. The initial step is normally thought to start with the supplement of the entering virus to the host cell.

The virus may then inject its genetic substantially in the cell or the virus may enter the cell membrane by the endocytic route. Because infection can only occur when the virus has parasitized in the brain, preventing the virus from attaching and invading is considered a good strategy for preventing disease. Some CQDs have been shown to have anti-viral/anti-inflammatory properties. Their inhibitory activity against disease depends on the chemical makeup, composition, shape, and size of the CQDs. For instance, it is seen that it can obstruct the interaction among the cells and bacteria, thereby inhibiting invasion of virus.

Fahmi et al. (2016) described that CQDs modified with boronic acid can act as penetration inhibitors against HIV infection. Rendering to earlier studies, boronic acid can cause glycopeptides and glycoproteins to interact specifically with HIV. CQDs were first synthesized by pyrolysis of citric acid. Because of their most common groups, like hydroxyl and carboxylate entities, carboxyphenylboronic acids can act on surfaces.

The resultant CQDs were later tested against HIV in MOLT-4 cells. They can disrupt the interaction between HIV and MOLT-4 cell membranes by binding gp120, a glycoprotein expressed on the HIV envelope and responsible for binding to human target cells. At the peak of the CQDs, the boronic acid domain of the CQDs reacted with the 1,2-cis-diol domain of gp120 to form tetravalent boronic acid diester ring complexes. Therefore, boronic acid-modified CQDs have excellent antibacterial activity with an IC50 value of 26.7 mg mL^{-1}.

More importantly, CQDs derived from benzoxazine monomer have recently been reported to be broad-spectrum inhibitors against some life-threatening viruses (Japanese encephalitis, Zika, and dengue viruses) and non-viruses (swine parvovirus and adeno-associated virus). Their broad-spectrum antiviral ability is attributed to the binding of CQDs to the virus, which interferes with the interaction between the virus and the cell. In addition to targeting bacteria, CQDs can also bind to the surface of cell membranes and block bacterial virus type 1 (HSV-1) infections.

Compared with other antibacterial nanoparticle-based inhibitors such as tannic acid modified silver nanoparticles, dextran sulfate and poly-L-lysine, the synthesized CQDs exh More importantly, CQDs derived from benzoxazine monomers have recently been reported to target some life-threatening diseases (Japanese encephalitis, Zika virus, and dengue virus) and non-communicable diseases (swine parvovirus and adeno-associated virus). Broad spectrum inhibitors. Tannic acid modified silver nanoparticles, dextran sulfate and poly-L-lysine, the synthesized CQDs exhibited higher antibacterial activity.

To further reveal the anti-inflammatory effect, the researchers evaluated the zeta potential changes of cells and bacteria before and after CQD incubation. Cultivation of sterile CQDs did not reduce bacterial zeta potential, whereas incubation of CQDs with mammalian cells resulted in significant changes in zeta potential. Fascinatingly, the authors additionally investigated the part of the boronic acid group in the immune system. Fructose was used for the conversion of boronic acid moiety to a five-ring ester, this was followed by a virus inhibition test. CQDs treated with fructose have also been shown to prevent hepatitis. This suggests that interfering with bacterial entry can be achieved by binding CQDs to receptors of cell surface devoid of the requirement for boronic acid moieties.

CQD can also be used in combination with some existing anti-inflammatory drugs to enhance the therapeutic effect. Aung et al. 2020 CQDs with a boronic acid center and graphene-like structure were produced by the hydrothermal method. According to some previous studies, boronic acid-modified CQDs have again shown efficacy in preventing invasion of HIV. This potent inhibitory capability is accredited to the binding of the boronic acid domain to gp120 via hydrogen bonding as well as covalent bonding. CQDs are obtained continuously with durival, a multidrug inhibitor with nucleoside reverse transcriptase activity, to process the sample to achieve better therapeutic results.

The collective complexes displayed better antibacterial activity. As we all know, HIV is a retrovirus which uses T-cells as its host and can easily produce antibodies. Therefore, survival and life expectancy can be significantly improved with early treatment. A cock-tail of different drugs that perform on diverse targets is called Highly Active Antiretroviral Therapy (HAART) and is among of the most operative ways to prevent HIV.

10.4.2 Interference with Viral Biosynthesis

When the viral genome enters the cell, translation or transcription of the viral genome begins, which is followed by viral protein and genome biosynthesis. During the work, giant bacteria are created and aggregated. Besides the interference with viral attachment and entry, CQDs may also protect against contagion by inhibiting viral biogenesis. Inazzo et al. (2018) examined the possibility of employing GQDs loaded with drugs as non-nucleoside reverse transcriptase inhibitors (NNRTIs) for the management of HIV [111].

Using multiwalled carbon nanotubes (MWCNTs) as the carbon source, monodispersed GQDs with prolonged acidic oxidation and exfoliation were synthesized. Surface of GQDs has been improved with carboxyl entities and crack constancy has been increased. Next, two NNRTIs, CHI499 and CDF119, were attached to the surfaces of the GQDs by means of esterification, respectively. Conjugation of GQDs to NNRTIs has been shown to be an effective combination compared to free drug. The combination of CQD and CHI499 greatly enhanced the anti-inflammatory activity, the conjugate complex of CDF119 and GQD showed the opposite trend (IC50 of 4.05 ± 0.33 vs. 43, IC50.3 $\pm$ 17), with or without GQD). These results can be accredited to the chemical configuration of GQDs and NNRTIs. Compared with the imide bond found in the GQDs-CDF119 complex, the amide bond present in the GQD-CHI499 complex is more easily cleaved as a result of displacement of the sulfonamide leaving group, which enables simple drug delivery in disease. Furthermore, as an addition to acting as a drug loading platform, CQDs also exhibit some level of anti-inflammatory action. The polycarboxylate nature of GQD can constrain reverse transcriptase activity by preventing the virus from binding to cells.

Ju et al. 2020 developed a CQD platform for gene delivery which was useful for the treatment of Kaposi sarcoma-associated herpes virus (KSHV) infection [112]. The synthesized CQDs were modified using antisense-locked nucleic acid (LNA) oligonucleotides. After CQDs are taken up by cells, LNA oligonucleotides bind to particular bacterial RNAs which leads to RNase H-mediated deprivation of viral RNAs.

Some recently discovered anti-inflammatory agents have previously been discovered for the synthesis of anti-inflammatory CQDs. Tong et al. described a method to combine glycyrrhizinate-based CQDs (Gly-CQDs) with anti-inflammatory potential [20]. The authors used glycyrrhizic acid, a Chinese herb with immunomodulatory properties, as a lead to synthesize CQDs by a hydrothermal approach.

Gly-CQD exhibits high antibacterial activity, inhibiting the growth of bacteria having a magnitude which had 5 orders. According to the study, the antiviral effect of Gly-CQDs could be activated by the following mechanisms: (1) inhibiting virus invasion and replication; (2) inhibiting virus replication; (3) inhibiting virus-induced reactive oxygen species (ROS) production; (4) regulating the expression of antibodies; (5) Promoting interferon production. According to transmission electron microscopy (TEM) and Fourier transform infrared spectroscopy (FTIR) results, Gly-CQDs were found to contain glycyrrhizic acid and most of the larger functional groups that are beneficial for immunity. In addition, the poor water solubility and serious side effects usually associated with glycyrrhizic acid are reduced when Gly-CQDs are used.

Lin et al. (2019) described an antiviral CQD using curcumin against enteroviruses [113]. Curcumin is a natural compound that has been identified to possess anti-inflammatory characteristics [114]. CQDs were produced by use of a straightforward drying method that can be carried out in one step. In the work, curcumin heating was done in an oven (muffle) for 2 hours at 120°C–210°C and then sonicated to produce an orange or brown residue. Subsequently, refined curcumin-based CQDs (Cur-CQDs) were attained by centrifugation and filtration.

At elevated temperatures, curcumin can get dehydration as well as condensed which is followed by pyrolysis and carbonization to form sp2 hybridized carbon nuclei. The surface of Cur-CQDs retains a tiny fraction of curcumin or polymer-like curcuminoids. Cur-CQDs unveiled lower cytotoxicity and improved immunogenicity compared to curcumin.

In divergence, more than 95% of diseased mice treated with Cur-CQDs could survive for a minimum period of 1 month. Immunological assay showed that Cur-CQDs can prevent viral contamination by interference with viral attachment as well as replication. The superior anti-inflammatory properties of Cur-CQDs over curcumin can be explained by changes in chemical arrangement during the synthesis. Spectrometry analysis showed that many entities like guaiacol, anisol, and 1-hexatriene are present on the surfaces of Cur-CQDs. Better hydrophilicity and higher concentration of antiviral active constituents of Cur-CQDs will contribute to their antiviral properties.

10.4.3 Strengthens the Immune System

The immune coordination is important for the body's immune structure. Many studies recently have shown that CQDs are capable of stimulating the immune system and improving particular immunity. The quaternary ammonium cationic CQDs may perform as a material to facilitate presentation of antigen and stimulate the immune system. In the research, high-quality CQDs were fabricated by a hydrothermal protocol using bisquaternary ammonium salt (BQAS) as the starting substance.

Ovalbumin (OVA) was used as standard antigen, which could be absorbed into CQDs by means of physical adsorption. To activate the immune system, antibodies are usually produced by antigen bestowing cells (APCs), which are capable of activating T-cells and specifically produce antibodies. However, minor antigens can face the difficulties related to weak immunity and difficulty uptake by APCs. In contrast, a strong cellular uptake was observed for OVA-dependent CQDs. Additionally, the CQDs produced in this study revealed potent anti-inflammatory properties. Mice vaccinated with OVA-CQD complexes secreted up to 60 times more OVA-specific IgG than mice treated with OVA alone. Antibody secretion may take longer than 8 weeks.

In addition, CQD adjuvants can enhance immunity which is cell mediated. As per the consequences of cytometry analysis, it was seen that mice treated with OVA-CQD displayed more OVA-specific CD4+ and CD8+ T cell propagation, with a 1–2-fold increase in proliferation of splenocyte. Thus, CQD adjuvants can support both humoral and cellular immunity. Nevertheless, the mechanisms of the effects remain unclear.

A study focused on some modified CQDs which showed immunomodulatory potential. CQDs were obtained by hydrothermal technique using glucose and tetraethylenepentamine as raw materials. Subsequently, ricin-binding subunit B (RTB), subunits of the protein ricin, is transported to CQDs by the process of absorption. Nanoparticles of CQDs-RTB were supplemented to macrophages. Therefore, no production by macrophages increases at a given dose. In addition, the cells can conceal many cytokines, TNF-α, and IL-6.

In comparison to free RTB, CQDs-RTB nanoparticles displayed the best efficacy in controlling the immunity of body. It can be attributed to the size of the CQDs-RTB nanoparticles because the ratio of size to bacteria is more easily recognized and internalized by APCs. Pseudorabies virus (PRV) and porcine reproductive and respiratory syndrome virus (PRRSV) were chosen as DNA virus and RNA virus models, respectively. Synthetic CQDs exhibited antiviral action against PRV and PRRSV by triggering the type I interferon response. As a glycoprotein that has anti-inflammatory properties, type I interferons (IFN-a and IFN-b) initiate intracellular gesturing pathways that lead to the manifestation of IFN-stimulated genes. After CQD injection, increased expression of interferon-associated mRNA was observed, indicating a positive effect on virus replication by activation of the type I interferon responses.

10.5 CONCLUSIONS

CQDs were reported for the first time in the year 2004, since then they have gained immense attention owing to their exceptional characteristics such as electrical, thermal, mechanical, optical, and various others. These excellent materials can be prepared in a simple and quick way by top-down approach and bottom-up approach by employing various carbon sources. CQDs have been successful in many medical applications like as biosensing, bioimaging, drug-delivery and gene-delivery, photothermal therapy, and lately in disease diagnosis, disease attack, and management/treatment. Over the last decade, a lot of efforts have been focused on the improvement of CQDs, which include synthetic methods, cleaning methods, functionalization, and efficiency. Nevertheless, there are still few difficulties to be overcome. For instance, it is challenging to assemble few CQDs efficiently and effectively and predicting the reproducibility their physical characteristics. An enhanced comprehension on the association among photoluminescence and surface passivation is required.

CQDs are used successfully as functional nanoscale materials in disease diagnosis as well as electrochemical detection and may replace or improve the performance of traditional assays used in disease detection bioassays. In an unprecedented reaction to the COVID-19 epidemic, CQDs have revealed promising potential in facilitating a good and accurate understanding of various pathogenic organisms such as SARS-CoV-2 and linked to bacterial biosynthesis. They enhance the immune system, especially against some dangerous and communicable diseases. With further enhancements and a better understanding of CQDs, the planning process that is better and greener (e.g., microwave-based methods) can be produced using low-cost materials and carbon monoxide, allowing products to be produced and reducing batch-to-batch variability.

REFERENCES

Aung, Y. Y., Kristanti, A. N., Khairunisa, S. Q., Nasronudin, N., & Fahmi, M. Z. (2020). Inactivation of HIV-1 infection through integrative blocking with amino phenylboronic acid attributed carbon dots. *ACS Biomaterials Science & Engineering*, 6(8), 4490–4501. doi:10.1021/acsbiomaterials.0c00508

Acharya, S. (2020). The COVID-19 pandemic: Theories to therapies. *Advances in Infectious Diseases*, 10(03), 16–28. doi:10.4236/aid.2020.103003

Barras, A., Pagneux, Q., Sane, F., Wang, Q., Boukherroub, R., Hober, D., & Szunerits, S. (2016). High efficiency of functional carbon nanodots as entry inhibitors of herpes simplex virus type 1. *ACS Applied Materials & Interfaces*, 8(14), 9004–9013. doi:10.1021/acsami.6b01681

Benzigar, M. R., Bhattacharjee, R., Baharfar, M., & Liu, G. (2021). Current methods for diagnosis of human coronaviruses: Pros and cons. *Analytical and Bioanalytical Chemistry*, 413(9), 2311–2330. doi:10.1007/s00216-020-03046-0

Brisebois, P. P., & Siaj, M. (2020). Harvesting graphene oxide – years 1859 to 2019: A review of its structure, synthesis, properties and exfoliation. *Journal of Materials Chemistry. C, Materials for Optical and Electronic Devices*, 8(5), 1517–1547. doi:10.1039/c9tc03251g.

Breman, J. G., & Henderson, D. A. (2002). Diagnosis and management of smallpox. *The New England Journal of Medicine*, 346(17), 1300–1308. doi:10.1056/NEJMra020025.

Buchs, G., Bercioux, D., Mayrhofer, L., & Gröning, O. (2018). Confined electron and hole states in semiconducting carbon nanotube sub-10 nm artificial quantum dots. *Carbon*, 132, 304–311. doi:10.1016/j.carbon.2018.02.031

Cao, W., & Li, T. (2020). [Review of COVID-19: Towards understanding of pathogenesis]. *Cell Research*, 30(5), 367–369. doi:10.1038/s41422-020-0327-4.

Craigie, J., & Wishart, F. O. (1936). The complement-fixation reaction in variola. *Canadian Public Health Journal*, 27(8), 371–379. http://www.jstor.org/stable/41977469

Chunduri, L. A. A., Kurdekar, A., Haleyurgirisetty, M. K., Bulagonda, E. P., Kamisetti, V., & Hewlett, I. K. (2017). Femtogram level sensitivity achieved by surface engineered silica nanoparticles in the early detection of HIV infection. *Scientific Reports*, 7(1), 7149. doi:10.1038/s41598-017-07299-1

de Medeiros, T. V., Manioudakis, J., Noun, F., Macairan, J.-R., Victoria, F., & Naccache, R. (2019). Microwave-assisted synthesis of carbon dots and their applications. *Journal of Materials Chemistry. C, Materials for Optical and Electronic Devices*, 7(24), 7175–7195. doi:10.1039/c9tc01640f

da Silva Souza, D. R., Caminhas, L. D., de Mesquita, J. P., & Pereira, F. V. (2018). Luminescent carbon dots obtained from cellulose. *Materials Chemistry and Physics*, 203, 148–155. doi:10.1016/j.matchemphys.2017.10.001

Dimitrov, D. S. (2004). Virus entry: Molecular mechanisms and biomedical applications. *Nature Reviews. Microbiology*, 2(2), 109–122. doi:10.1038/nrmicro817

Fahmi, M. Z., Sukmayani, W., Khairunisa, S. Q., Witaningrum, A. M., Indriati, D. W., Matondang, M. Q. Y., … Kameoka, M. (2016). Design of boronic acid-attributed carbon dots on inhibits HIV-1 entry. *RSC Advances*, 6(95), 92996–93002. doi:10.1039/c6ra21062g

Fang, L., Wu, M., Huang, C., Liu, Z., Liang, J., & Zhang, H. (2020). Industrializable synthesis of narrow-dispersed carbon dots achieved by microwave-assisted selective carbonization of surfactants and their applications as fluorescent nano-additives. *Journal of Materials Chemistry. A, Materials for Energy and Sustainability*, 8(40), 21317–21326. doi:10.1039/d0ta07252d

Feng, H., & Qian, Z. (2018). Functional carbon quantum dots: A versatile platform for chemosensing and biosensing. *Chemical Record* (New York, N.Y.), 18(5), 491–505. doi:10.1002/tcr.201700055.

Gan, Z., Xu, H., & Hao, Y. (2016). Mechanism for excitation-dependent photoluminescence from graphene quantum dots and other graphene oxide derivates: Consensus, debates and challenges. *Nanoscale*, 8(15), 7794–7807. doi:10.1039/c6nr00605a

Granich, R., Crowley, S., Vitoria, M., Lo, Y.-R., Souteyrand, Y., Dye, C., … Williams, B. (2010). Highly active antiretroviral treatment for the prevention of HIV transmission. *Journal of the International AIDS Society*, 13(1), 1. doi:10.1186/1758-2652-13-1

Ge, Y., Li, S., Wang, S., & Moore, R. (Eds.). (2014). *Nanomedicine: Principles and Perspectives*. Springer.

Giamarellos-Bourboulis, E. J., Netea, M. G., Rovina, N., Akinosoglou, K., Antoniadou, A., Antonakos, N., … Koutsoukou, A. (2020). Complex immune dysregulation in COVID-19 patients with severe respiratory failure. *Cell Host & Microbe*, 27(6), 992–1000.e3. doi:10.1016/j.chom.2020.04.009

He, Y.-S., Pan, C.-G., Cao, H.-X., Yue, M.-Z., Wang, L., & Liang, G.-X. (2018). Highly sensitive and selective dual-emission ratiometric fluorescence detection of dopamine based on carbon dots-gold nanoclusters hybrid. *Sensors and Actuators B, Chemical*, 265, 371–377. doi:10.1016/j.snb.2018.03.080

Hui, K. P.-Y., Cheung, M.-C., Lai, K.-L., Ng, K.-C., Ho, J. C.-W., Peiris, M., … Chan, M. C.-W. (2022). Role of epithelial-endothelial cell interaction in the pathogenesis of severe acute respiratory syndrome Coronavirus 2 (SARS-CoV-2) infection. *Clinical Infectious Diseases: An Official Publication of the Infectious Diseases Society of America*, 74(2), 199–209. doi:10.1093/cid/ciab406.

Isnaeni, Herbani, Y., & Suliyanti, M. M. (2018). Concentration effect on optical properties of carbon dots at room temperature. *Journal of Luminescence*, 198, 215–219. doi:10.1016/j.jlumin.2018.02.012

Jia, Z., Ma, Y., Yang, L., Guo, C., Zhou, N., Wang, M., Zhang, Z. (2019). NiCo2O4 spinel embedded with carbon nanotubes derived from bimetallic NiCo metal-organic framework for the ultrasensitive detection of human immune deficiency virus-1 gene. *Biosensors & Bioelectronics*, 133, 55–63. doi:10.1016/j.bios.2019.03.030

Jones, J. E., Le Sage, V., & Lakdawala, S. S. (2021). Viral and host heterogeneity and their effects on the viral life cycle. *Nature Reviews: Microbiology*, 19(4), 272–282. doi:10.1038/s41579-020-00449-9

Krammer, F. (2020). SARS-CoV-2 vaccines in development. *Nature*, 586(7830), 516–527. doi:10.1038/s41586-020-2798-3.

Lara, H. H., Ayala-Nuñez, N. V., Ixtepan-Turrent, L., & Rodriguez-Padilla, C. (2010). Mode of antiviral action of silver nanoparticles against HIV-1. *Journal of Nanobiotechnology*, 8(1), 1. doi:10.1186/1477-3155-8-1.

Liu, J., Li, R., & Yang, B. (2020c). Carbon dots: A new type of carbon-based nanomaterial with wide applications. *ACS Central Science*, 6(12), 2179–2195. doi:10.1021/acscentsci.0c01306

Liu, R., Wu, D., Liu, S., Koynov, K., Knoll, W., & Li, Q. (2009). An aqueous route to multicolor photoluminescent carbon dots using silica spheres as carriers. *Angewandte Chemie (International Ed. in English)*, 48(25), 4598–4601. doi:10.1002/anie.200900652

Liu, Y., Huang, H., Cao, W., Mao, B., Liu, Y., & Kang, Z. (2020b). Advances in carbon dots: from the perspective of traditional quantum dots. *Materials Chemistry Frontiers*, 4(6), 1586–1613. doi:10.1039/d0qm00090f

Lim, S. Y., Shen, W., & Gao, Z. (2015). Carbon quantum dots and their applications. *Chemical Society Reviews*, 44(1), 362–381. doi:10.1039/c4cs00269e

Liu, Y., Gou, H., Huang, X., Zhang, G., Xi, K., & Jia, X. (2020a). Rational synthesis of highly efficient ultra-narrow red-emitting carbon quantum dots for NIR-II two-photon bioimaging. *Nanoscale*, 12(3), 1589–1601. doi:10.1039/c9nr09524a

Lu, Q., Wu, C., Liu, D., Wang, H., Su, W., Li, H., … Yao, S. (2017). A facile and simple method for synthesis of graphene oxide quantum dots from black carbon. *Green Chemistry: An International Journal and Green Chemistry Resource: GC*, 19(4), 900–904. doi:10.1039/c6gc03092k

Lukassen, S., Chua, R. L., Trefzer, T., Kahn, N. C., Schneider, M. A., Muley, T., … Eils, R. (2020). SARS-CoV-2 receptor ACE2 and TMPRSS2 are primarily expressed in bronchial transient secretory cells. *The EMBO Journal*, 39(10), e105114. doi:10.15252/embj.20105114

M. P. Ajith, Pardhiya, S., & Rajamani, P. (2022). Carbon dots: An excellent fluorescent probe for contaminant sensing and remediation. *Small*, 18(15), e2105579. doi:10.1002/smll.202105579

Mehta, P., McAuley, D. F., Brown, M., Sanchez, E., Tattersall, R. S., Manson, J. J., & HLH Across Speciality Collaboration, UK. (2020). COVID-19: Consider cytokine storm syndromes and immunosuppression. *Lancet*, 395(10229), 1033–1034. doi:10.1016/S0140-6736(20)30628-0

Mintz, K. J., Zhou, Y., & Leblanc, R. M. (2019). Recent development of carbon quantum dots regarding their optical properties, photoluminescence mechanism, and core structure. *Nanoscale*, 11(11), 4634–4652. doi:10.1039/c8nr10059d

Ming, H., Ma, Z., Liu, Y., Pan, K., Yu, H., Wang, F., & Kang, Z. (2012). Large scale electrochemical synthesis of high quality carbon nanodots and their photocatalytic property. *Dalton Transactions (Cambridge, England: 2003)*, 41(31), 9526–9531. doi:10.1039/c2dt30985h

Muthamma, K., Sunil, D., & Shetty, P. (2021). Carbon dots as emerging luminophores in security inks for anti-counterfeit applications: An up-to-date review. *Applied Materials Today*, 23(101050), 101050. doi:10.1016/j.apmt.2021.101050

Molaei, M. J. (2019). Carbon quantum dots and their biomedical and therapeutic applications: A review. *RSC Advances*, 9(12), 6460–6481. doi:10.1039/c8ra08088g

Nasrollahzadeh, M., Sajjadi, M., Soufi, G. J., Iravani, S., & Varma, R. S. (2020). Nanomaterials and nanotechnology-associated innovations against viral infections with a focus on coronaviruses. *Nanomaterials (Basel, Switzerland)*, 10(6), 1072. doi:10.3390/nano10061072

Negahdari, B., Darvishi, M., & Saeedi, A. A. (2019). Gold nanoparticles and hepatitis B virus. *Artificial Cells, Nanomedicine, and Biotechnology*, 47(1), 469–474. doi:10.1080/2169 1401.2018.1546185.

Papaioannou, N., Titirici, M.-M., & Sapelkin, A. (2019). Investigating the effect of reaction time on carbon dot formation, structure, and optical properties. *ACS Omega*, 4(26), 21658–21665. doi:10.1021/acsomega.9b01798

Pollard, A. J., & Bijker, E. M. (2021). A guide to vaccinology: From basic principles to new developments. *Nature Reviews: Immunology*, 21(2), 83–100. doi:10.1038/s41577-020-00479-7

Payne, S. (2017). Viral pathogenesis. In *Viruses* (pp. 87–95). doi:10.1016/b978-0-12-803109-4.00009-x

Priecel, P., & Lopez-Sanchez, J. A. (2019). Advantages and limitations of microwave reactors: From chemical synthesis to the catalytic valorization of biobased chemicals. *ACS Sustainable Chemistry & Engineering*, 7(1), 3–21. doi:10.1021/acssuschemeng.8b03286

Qu, D., Zheng, M., Zhang, L., Zhao, H., Xie, Z., Jing, X., ... Sun, Z. (2014). Formation mechanism and optimization of highly luminescent N-doped graphene quantum dots. *Scientific Reports*, 4(1), 5294. doi:10.1038/srep05294

Qu, K., Wang, J., Ren, J., & Qu, X. (2013). Carbon dots prepared by hydrothermal treatment of dopamine as an effective fluorescent sensing platform for the label-free detection of iron(III) ions and dopamine. *Chemistry (Weinheim an Der Bergstrasse, Germany)*, 19(22), 7243–7249. doi:10.1002/chem.201300042

Rockx, B., Kuiken, T., Herfst, S., Bestebroer, T., Lamers, M. M., Oude Munnink, B. B., Haagmans, B. L. (2020). Comparative pathogenesis of COVID-19, MERS, and SARS in a nonhuman primate model. *Science* (New York, N.Y.), 368(6494), 1012–1015. doi:10.1126/science.abb7314

Singh, P., Singh, D., Sa, P., Mohapatra, P., Khuntia, A., & Sahoo, S. K. (2021). Insights from nanotechnology in COVID-19: Prevention, detection, therapy and immunomodulation. *Nanomedicine (London, England)*, 16(14), 1219–1235. doi:10.2217/nnm-2021-0004

Singh, S., Mishra, A., Kumari, R., Sinha, K. K., Singh, M. K., & Das, P. (2017). Carbon dots assisted formation of DNA hydrogel for sustained release of drug. *Carbon*, 114, 169–176. doi:10.1016/j.carbon.2016.12.020

Stockman, L. J., Bellamy, R., & Garner, P. (2006). SARS: Systematic review of treatment effects. *PLoS Medicine*, 3(9), e343. doi:10.1371/journal.pmed.0030343

Tao, S., Feng, T., Zheng, C., Zhu, S., & Yang, B. (2019). Carbonized polymer dots: A brand new Perspective to recognize luminescent carbon-based nanomaterials. *The Journal of Physical Chemistry Letters*, 10(17), 5182–5188. doi:10.1021/acs.jpclett.9b01384

Tan, X., Li, Y., Li, X., Zhou, S., Fan, L., & Yang, S. (2015). Electrochemical synthesis of small-sized red fluorescent graphene quantum dots as a bioimaging platform. *Chemical Communications (Cambridge, England)*, 51(13), 2544–2546. doi:10.1039/c4cc09332a

Tajik, S., Dourandish, Z., Zhang, K., Beitollahi, H., Van Le, Q., Jang, H. W., & Shokouhimehr, M. (2020). Carbon and graphene quantum dots: A review on syntheses, characterization, biological and sensing applications for neurotransmitter determination. *RSC Advances*, 10(26), 15406–15429. doi:10.1039/d0ra00799d

Tepliakov, N. V., Kundelev, E. V., Khavlyuk, P. D., Xiong, Y., Leonov, M. Y., Zhu, W., Rukhlenko, I. D. (2019). Sp2-sp3-hybridized atomic domains determine optical features of carbon dots. *ACS Nano*, 13(9), 10737–10744. doi:10.1021/acsnano.9b05444

Ting, D., Dong, N., Fang, L., Lu, J., Bi, J., Xiao, S., & Han, H. (2018). Multisite inhibitors for enteric coronavirus: Antiviral cationic carbon dots based on curcumin. *ACS Applied Nano Materials*, 1(10), 5451–5459. doi:10.1021/acsanm.8b00779.

Wang, Haitao, Xie, Y., Na, X., Bi, J., Liu, S., Zhang, L., & Tan, M. (2019). Fluorescent carbon dots in baked lamb: Formation, cytotoxicity and scavenging capability to free radicals. *Food Chemistry*, 286, 405–412. doi:10.1016/j.foodchem.2019.02.034

Wang, Hua, Sun, C., Chen, X., Zhang, Y., Colvin, V. L., Rice, Q., … Yu, W. W. (2017). Excitation wavelength independent visible color emission of carbon dots. *Nanoscale*, 9(5), 1909–1915. doi:10.1039/c6nr09200d

Weiss, C., Carriere, M., Fusco, L., Capua, I., Regla-Nava, J. A., Pasquali, M., … Delogu, L. G. (2020). Toward nanotechnology-enabled approaches against the COVID-19 pandemic. *ACS Nano*, 14(6), 6383–6406. doi:10.1021/acsnano.0c03697

Wu, Y.-F., Wu, H.-C., Kuan, C.-H., Lin, C.-J., Wang, L.-W., Chang, C.-W., & Wang, T.-W. (2016). Multi-functionalized carbon dots as theranostic nanoagent for gene delivery in lung cancer therapy. *Scientific Reports*, 6(1), 21170. doi:10.1038/srep21170

Xu, X., Ray, R., Gu, Y., Ploehn, H. J., Gearheart, L., Raker, K., & Scrivens, W. A. (2004). Electrophoretic analysis and purification of fluorescent single-walled carbon nanotube fragments. *Journal of the American Chemical Society*, 126(40), 12736–12737. doi:10.1021/ja040082h

Yadavalli, T., & Shukla, D. (2017). Role of metal and metal oxide nanoparticles as diagnostic and therapeutic tools for highly prevalent viral infections. *Nanomedicine: Nanotechnology, Biology, and Medicine*, 13(1), 219–230. doi:10.1016/j.nano.2016.08.016

Yang, L., Deng, W., Cheng, C., Tan, Y., Xie, Q., & Yao, S. (2018). Fluorescent immunoassay for the detection of pathogenic bacteria at the single-cell level using carbon dots-encapsulated breakable organosilica nanocapsule as labels. *ACS Applied Materials & Interfaces*, 10(4), 3441–3448. doi:10.1021/acsami.7b18714

Yao, H., Zhao, W., Zhang, S., Guo, X., Li, Y., & Du, B. (2018). Dual-functional carbon dot-labeled heavy-chain ferritin for self-targeting bio-imaging and chemo-photodynamic therapy. *Journal of Materials Chemistry. B, Materials for Biology and Medicine*, 6(19), 3107–3115. doi:10.1039/c8tb00118a

Yu, H., Li, X., Zeng, X., & Lu, Y. (2016). Preparation of carbon dots by non-focusing pulsed laser irradiation in toluene. *Chemical Communications (Cambridge, England)*, 52(4), 819–822. doi:10.1039/c5cc08384b

Zhao, P., & Zhu, L. (2018). Dispersibility of carbon dots in aqueous and/or organic solvents. *Chemical Communications (Cambridge, England)*, 54(43), 5401–5406. doi:10.1039/c8cc02279h

Zheng, X. T., Ananthanarayanan, A., Luo, K. Q., & Chen, P. (2015). Glowing graphene quantum dots and carbon dots: Properties, syntheses, and biological applications. *Small*, 11(14), 1620–1636. doi:10.1002/smll.201402648

Zulfiqar, H. F., Javed A. Sumbal, Afroze, B., Ali, Q., Akbar, K., …Husnain, T. (2017). HIV diagnosis and treatment through advanced technologies. *Frontiers in Public Health*, 5, 32. doi:10.3389/fpubh.2017.0003255.

Zuo, P., Lu, X., Sun, Z., Guo, Y., & He, H. (2016). A review on syntheses, properties, characterization and bioanalytical applications of fluorescent carbon dots. *Mikrochimica Acta*, 183(2), 519–542. doi:10.1007/s00604-015-1705-3

11 Carbon Quantum Dots and 3D Printing Technology

Alireza Kaviani and Zohreh Riahi

11.1 INTRODUCTION

In recent years, additive manufacturing (AM) has emerged as a cutting-edge technology that has reshaped the manufacturing industry. Unlike many traditional manufacturing processes that involve subtracting material to create a desired shape, AM takes a "bottom-up" approach, constructing objects layer by layer (Patel & Chen, 2022). This innovative approach has opened up new possibilities across various industrial applications. AM offers unparalleled versatility and flexibility, allowing for the creation of highly customized components and products. The technology has found applications in fields ranging from aerospace and automotive to healthcare and consumer goods. One of the key strengths of AM lies in its ability to work with a wide range of materials. Manufacturers can produce parts and objects using metallic, ceramic, polymeric, composite and hybrid materials. This adaptability in material selection enables the development of innovative products with enhanced both physical and mechanical properties. Beyond traditional materials, AM has paved the way for the creation of advanced materials (Butt, 2020; Wohlers & Caffrey, 2010). Moreover, the integration of nanomaterials into 3D printing has led to the development of innovative, versatile and multifunctional hybrid materials with various applications in biomedical, electronic, optical and energy storage devices (Hales et al., 2020; Jain et al., 2021; Paramasivam et al., 2021). That is why AM is a powerful tool in the hands of engineers and designers seeking to push the boundaries of what is possible in manufacturing.

One of the outstanding evolutions in the field of nanotechnology is the development of quantum dots (QDs). QDs are a type of fluorescent semiconductor nanoparticles typically ranging in diameter from 2 to 10 nanometers (Walling et al., 2009). These nanosized particles have captured significant attention from researchers over the past two decades due to their intriguing physical and chemical characteristics. The size of these quantum dots, along with shape, impurities, defects and surface coating, serves a crucial role in determining their optical properties, absorbance and photoluminescence (Gidwani et al., 2021; Timoshenko, 2023). The name "quantum dots" represents their quantum confinement effect, and subsequently, optical characteristics. Quantum confinement arises when electrons are restricted to a space on the

DOI: 10.1201/9781003437857-13

same scale as their de Broglie wavelength. Due to energy level splitting in QDs, an increase in the semiconductor band gap occurs as the size of the nanocrystal decreases. This causes a blue shift in the absorption and emission spectra (García de Arquer et al., 2021).

Semiconductor quantum dots have been the subject of extensive research for many years due to their strong and adjustable fluorescence emission characteristics, making them suitable for applications in biosensing (J. Li & Zhu, 2013) and bioimaging (Martynenko et al., 2017). However, they have certain disadvantages. For instance, their high toxicity stemming from the utilization of heavy metals during their production. Heavy metals are known to be highly toxic even at relatively low concentrations, which could hinder any potential in biomedical applications. This led to the development of carbon quantum dots (CQDs) as an alternative to semiconductor quantum dots. CQDs offer several advantages, including low toxicity, biocompatibility, affordability, chemical inertness, and similar fluorescence properties (S. Li et al., 2021b; B. Wang & Lu, 2022; Xia et al., 2019).

To date, scientists have successfully integrated various organic and inorganic nanomaterials, such as carbon nanotubes (Gnanasekaran et al., 2017), metallic nanoparticles (Clarissa et al., 2022; Zarei et al., 2023) and graphene (H. Guo et al., 2019), into the additive manufacturing process. For next-generation nanocomposites requiring additive manufacturing, QDs are ideal options due to their excellent solution processability, wide range of material- and size-dependent properties, and unique optical and emissive properties. QDs have been used in 3D printing to create optoelectrical materials (K. Liang et al., 2022b), advanced light-emitting devices (Kong et al., 2014) and even electrodes for lithium storage (C. Zhang et al., 2018). Toward the progress of fabricating QDs incorporated advanced materials using 3D-printing technologies, a wide spectrum of applications like handheld smartphone platforms for sensing applications to cell and ion imaging, photoinitiation, antibacterial and anticounterfeiting applications have been covered.

In this chapter, we begin by offering a brief introduction to AM processes, including the various types and technologies with which CQDs have been integrated. Following that, key characteristics of carbon dots (CDs), which are critical for 3D-printing, are covered. Then, the diverse applications of carbon within AM technologies, particularly in the field of sensing, imaging, polymerization and various other applications, are discussed.

11.2　AN OVERVIEW ON 3D PRINTING TECHNOLOGY

Having had an immense effect on both the industrial and commercial worlds, 3D printing technology has advanced substantially since it was initially developed over 50 years ago (Attaran, 2017; Choong, 2022).

Additive manufacturing, commonly referred to as 3D printing, is the "process of joining materials to make parts from 3D model data, usually layer upon layer, as opposed to subtractive manufacturing and formative manufacturing methodologies" according to the International Organization for Standardization (ISO)/American Society for Testing and Materials (ASTM) 52900:2015 standard. The standard categorizes additive manufacturing processes into seven distinct categories: (1) binder jetting (BJ); (2) directed energy deposition (DED); (3) material extrusion (MEX); (4) material jetting (MJ); (5) powder bed fusion (PBF); (6) sheet lamination (SL); and (7) vat photopolymerization (VPP), as depicted in Figure 11.1.

Based on the state of the precursor materials, two groups of AM methods can be classified: (1) fusion-based processes like DED, PBF which use energy to melt or fuse materials together to create a final product and (2) non-fusion-based processes like BJ, MJ and SL (Maleksaeedi et al., 2018). Each process is unique in terms of the materials that can be processed and the material properties that can be obtained. Different technologies, which are still being researched and refined, are utilized in each of the seven major process categories. Stereolithography (SLA) and digital light processing (DLP) for VPP, fused deposition modeling (FDM) for MEX, direct metal deposition (DMD) for DED, laminated object manufacturing (LOM) for SL, color jet 3D printing (CJP) for BJ, polyjet for MJ, and selective laser sintering (SLS) and

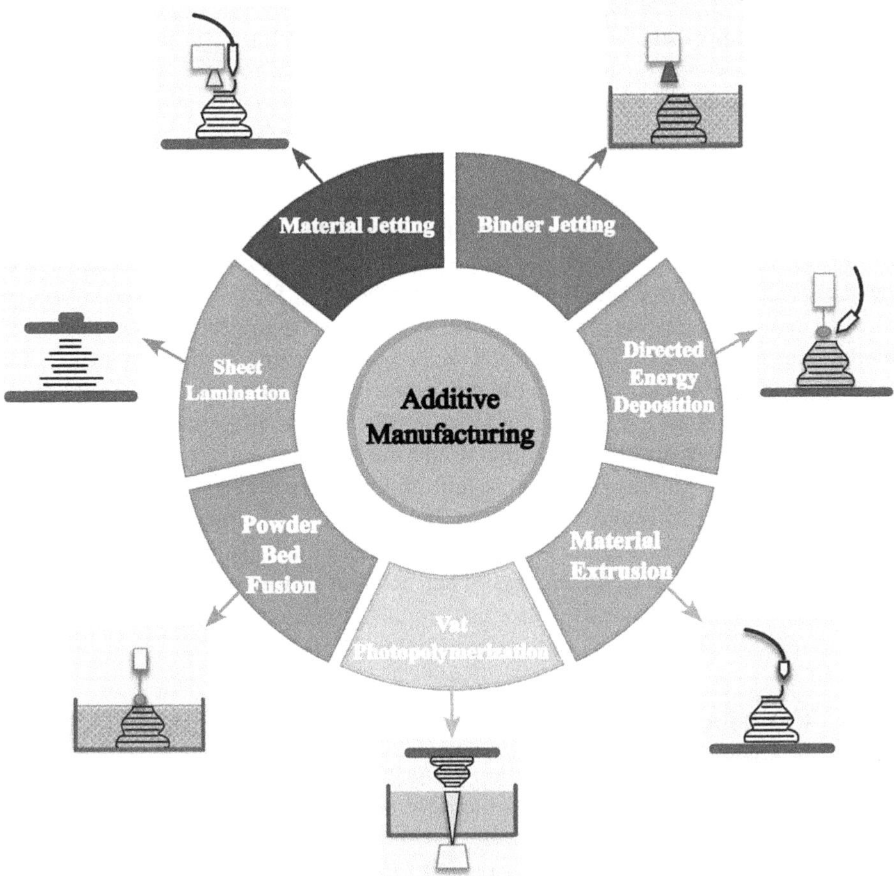

FIGURE 11.1 Seven additive manufacturing processes and corresponding schematics of how a 3D printed part is made.

Schematics are reproduced from Dilberoglu et al. (2017).

selective laser melting (SLM) for PBF are examples of representative 3D printing processes (Suh et al., 2020).

When compared to conventional manufacturing techniques, AM offers significant advantages. For example, AM uses wire, powder, sheet and other feedstocks that are selectively fused or joined together to manufacture a component from designed 3D models (Gibson et al., 2021). With a number AM technologies, it is possible to design and directly construct a complex product from a variety of materials, including metal, ceramic and polymer, with good dimensional precision. A 3D printer possesses the capability to produce a diverse array of shapes with each fabrication process, which stands in stark contrast to the limited shape spectrum achievable by traditional manufacturing machinery (Attaran, 2017). Utilizing a layered approach, a 3D printer can concurrently produce complex objects such as doors with integrated interlocking hinges, eliminating the need for subsequent assembly. This reduction in assembly requirements contributes to the streamlining of supply chains and labor and transportation saving cost, while simultaneously reducing environmental pollution associated with shorter supply chains. Since operational guidance for a 3D printer primarily derives from a design file, less operator expertise compared to, for example, injection molding machines when producing objects of equivalent complexity is needed (Gupta et al., 2019). The accessibility to unskilled manufacturing opens new ways for business models and offers innovative production solutions, particularly in challenging or remote environments. Additionally, when considering production space per unit volume, 3D printers outperform traditional manufacturing machinery. Moreover, when configured with a mobile printing apparatus, a 3D printer can manufacture objects larger in size than itself. AM processes, for instance, specialized in metallic materials generate minimal waste byproducts compared to traditional metal manufacturing methods. Therefore, all investigations came to the conclusion that AM could exert the least negative effects on the natural environment (Kumar et al., 2019; Mostafaei et al., 2021). Furthermore, as the field of multimaterial 3D printing evolves, it offers opportunities to blend and combine diverse raw materials. As a consequence, this yields an extensive and largely unexplored palette of materials with unique properties and functionalities. In this regard, a key aspect of the development of 3D-printed nanomaterials, especially quantum dots, is the creation of "functionalized" materials. Researchers have been actively investigating the incorporation of different additives and modifications to printable materials with an eye on enabling 3D printing of materials with required properties.

11.3   KEY FEATURES OF CARBON DOTS (CDs) FOR 3D-PRINTING

Carbon dots, a relatively recent addition to the carbon family, have gained significant attention for their outstanding and adjustable photoluminescence (PL), high quantum yield (QY), low toxicity, small size, good biocompatibility and abundant, cost-effective sources (Lei et al., 2022; J. Liu et al., 2020). These qualities have made CDs valuable in numerous applications, including biomedicine, environmental pollution control, sensing, catalysis, imaging, optoelectronic devices, and anti-counterfeiting (M. Han et al., 2018; Long et al., 2021; B. Wang & Lu, 2022; J. Xu et al., 2022). The evolution of CD-based materials can be divided into three distinct stages, Discovery stage (2004–2006), Initial development stage (2007 to 2011) (Sun et al., 2006) and Exponentially developing stage of CDs (from 2011 onward). In particular, there has been a growing trend of incorporating CDs into 3D printing precursor materials. Additionally, several cost-effective large-scale production methods for CQDs were reported during the last phase (L. Chen et al., 2023; Zhu et al., 2020).

It has been reported that CDs consist of quasi-spherical carbon nanoparticles with a crystalline core composed of a mixture of sp2 and sp3 carbons (S. Li et al., 2021b). The significant number of surface groups and polymer chains, such as carboxyl, hydroxyl, and amine functionalities, contribute to their exceptional water solubility and ease of blending with other materials without experiencing phase separation issues. Additionally, the abundant functional groups allow for straightforward modifications of CDs with various organic or polymeric molecules, making them promising candidates for diverse sensor and imaging applications (Jiang et al., 2015). The covalent carbon skeleton structure also enhances the stability of CDs, which, for instance, is crucial for biomedical applications (J. Xu et al., 2022). In comparison to organic dyes and some traditional quantum dots containing cadmium or lead, CDs not only demonstrate superior light stability like photoblinking, resistance to light-induced decomposition and photobleaching and a high photoluminescence quantum yield but also exhibit lower toxicity, reduced costs and outstanding biocompatibility (Lei et al., 2022; Macairan et al., 2022). The properties of CDs are determined by both their precursors and the synthesis method used, resulting in a wide variety of CDs. These synthesis approaches are generally categorized as top-down and bottom-up methods (Xia et al., 2019) (B. Wang et al., 2023a).

One of the groundbreaking features of CDs, which has found extensive use in 3D printing applications, is their optical properties. As previously mentioned, CDs exhibit a wide range of optical characteristics owing to their diverse structures. In the early years of CD research, the focus was primarily on their fluorescence emission properties, including emission wavelength, color, and brightness. However, some unique and more fascinating optical phenomena were often overlooked. In the field of 3D printing technology, these properties have proven to be highly influential in the fabrication of advanced devices such as portable smartphone-integrated 3D-printed sensors (D. Li & Wang, 2023; Solanki et al., 2022). These photoluminescence properties can be classified into various subcategories:

- Up-conversion Photoluminescence (PL): Unlike traditional PL properties, up-conversion PL involves the absorption of two or more photons with longer wavelengths and the emission of light with shorter wavelengths. This property has been extensively investigated for diverse applications, including photocatalysis and live-cell imaging (Deng et al., 2021; W. Zhang et al., 2019).
- Stimulus Response: Due to the diversity of CD structures and their physical and chemical properties, researchers have developed CDs that respond to various stimuli such as pressure, temperature, environmental factors and pH levels. These CD-based materials show broad potential applicability as light emitting diodes, as transparent fluorescent thin films, in biosensing and in cell imaging (Durrani et al., 2023; C. Li et al., 2020; Q. Wang et al., 2019).

- Aggregation-Induced Emission (AIE): AIE materials are a relatively recent development with significant research and application potential. AIE properties in CDs are evident when transitioning from liquid to solid states, from low concentration to high concentration, and from a dispersed state to a highly aggregated one. This phenomenon stands in stark contrast to aggregation-caused quenching. In the case of AIE, the luminescence becomes more intense as larger aggregates form. This property holds potential for various applications, including the detection of organic molecules and metal ions, latent fingerprint recognition, optoelectronic devices, and solar concentrators and biological purposes (Arshad et al., 2021; L. Li et al., 2021).

- Charge and energy transfer: When exposed to light, CDs have the capability to function as either electron donors or electron acceptors. They readily interact with the surrounding environment and surface-modified ligands. This facilitates charge and energy transfer processes. For instance, fluorescence resonance energy transfer (FRET) mechanism is one of the widely used mechanisms in biosensing field. This process can transmit photo excitation energy from a donor fluorophore to an acceptor fluorophore through intermolecular long-range dipole–dipole coupling (Dai et al., 2014; W. Gao et al., 2022).

11.4 APPLICATION OF CDs AND 3D-PRINTED MATERIALS

11.4.1 Sensing Applications

As part of traditional sensing methods, a number of practical techniques, including laser spectroscopy, gas chromatography, liquid chromatography, electrochemical method and mass spectrometry, have been utilized for detecting and quantifying volatile organic compounds, gases, and chemicals (Pröfrock & Prange, 2012; Wong & Khor, 2019). While these techniques demonstrate high sensitivity, they heavily rely on large instruments for detection, have high cost and complex procedures. In contrast to these methods, test strips offer simplicity, speed, real-time performance and visual detection (Kim et al., 2015). However, they are restricted to qualitative analysis and cannot perform quantitative detection. To address these issues, smartphones can play a part and convert visual information into numerical data for analysis. Generally, smartphones have been widely integrated with various sensors, including sensor chips, handheld detectors and test strips (Chandra Kishore et al., 2022). While a growing trend in designing smartphone test paper devices for detection purposes can be observed, these sensors are mainly employed for liquid analysis and struggle with gas collection and detection. CD-based sensing systems, on the other hand, have been designed for on-site and real-time analysis. They can be categorized into two main approaches, namely additive and subtractive manufacturing (Yat et al., 2022). 3D printing techniques offer versatility by producing products with diverse properties using various substrate materials. This presents an opportunity to design low-cost sensors and arrays, which could potentially address challenges related to material detection. Various configurations were employed to develop these portable devices.

As an example, one such portable device was designed to enable the attachment of a smartphone to a dark chamber for measuring fluorescence emission in controlled lighting conditions. This chamber was then linked to a cell holder in which the sample was positioned within a plastic cuvette, as depicted in Figure 11.2A. Additionally, the cell holder featured a light-emitting diode (LED) emitting light at a 90-degree angle relative to the smartphone camera, and this whole setup was used for collecting data. To connect the 3D printable capture device (as seen in Figure 11.2B), which is commonly printed using FDM technique, to the smartphone, a bracket was used, which was affixed to the plastic cover to standardize the distance between the cuvette and the camera lens. Once the cuvette was in place, the light source was activated, and the camera settings remained fixed until the analysis was completed. In another design, a compact handheld device, connected to a miniature smartphone through 3D-printing technology, has been introduced for on-site quantification. This device incorporates an imaging dark box integrated with optical components, as illustrated in Figure 11.2C. The attachment consists of four main components: an optical filter,

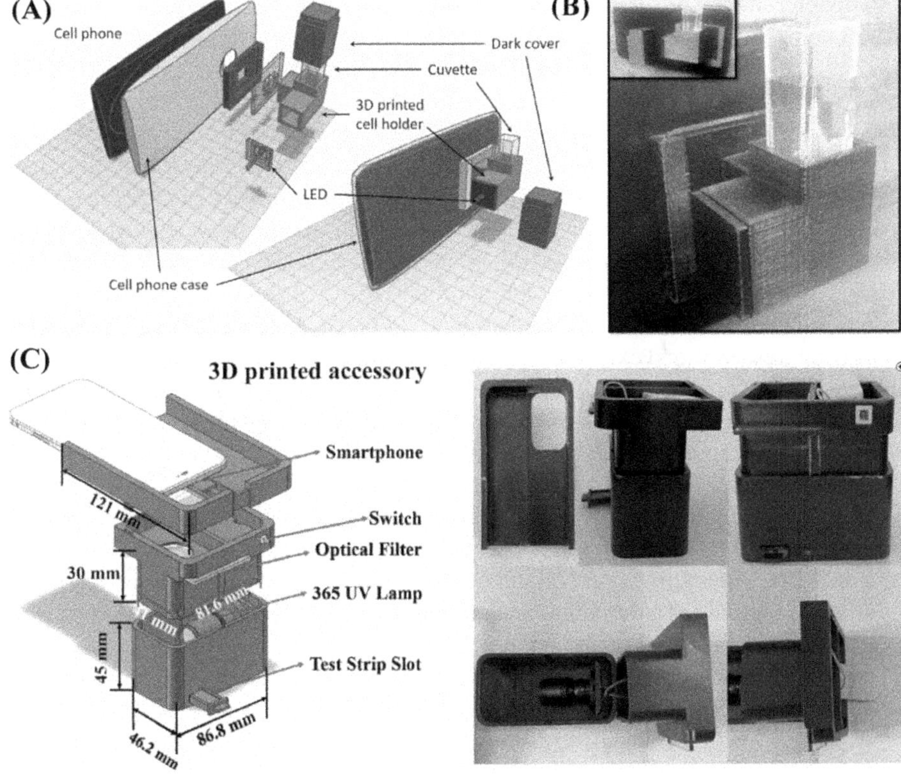

FIGURE 11.2 (a): the schematic representation detailing the distinct components integrated into the portable device (Uriarte et al., 2021), (b): a real photograph showcases the physical appearance of the devised apparatus (Vidal et al., 2020) and (c): schematic depiction of a designed handheld 3D printed device at different angles (Chang et al., 2023).

a slot for the sample, a UV light and a detachable dark enclosure to interface with the phone's camera. This handheld device offers several advantages like adjustment of the shooting distance and eliminating interference from surrounding light (Chang et al., 2023).

The recent focus on detecting trace amounts of food contamination, food nutrition and additives, water pollutants, and pesticide residues using advanced systems stems from the pressing issue of food safety, environment and human health protection (Solanki et al., 2022). For instance, according to the World Health Organization (WHO), there is a staggering global estimate of 600 million cases of foodborne diseases and 420,000 deaths annually as a result of consuming unsafe food worldwide, and this number is most likely underestimated (WHO, n.d.). Some efforts have been undertaken to practically achieve a highly sensitive, dependable and rapid sensing using 3D-printed smartphone-based devices. In case of pesticides, a nanosensor was fabricated in the first step by embedding N-doped CDs within a porphyrin metal–organic framework (N-CDs@PCN-222) through an in situ process. This nanosensor was designed to enable dual-mode detection of glyphosate (GLP) as an herbicide using ratiometric fluorescence (RF) and a colorimetric approach on a portable smartphone-integrated platform. The portable platform for smartphone-integrated colorimetric detection of GLP was assembled by integrating the sensor with both a smartphone and a 3D-printed mini-device. The construction of the smartphone-integrated platform utilized FDM technique (X. Luo et al., 2022). Another major concern within the environmental system and food stems from the extensive residues of antibiotics, which are commonly employed as medications and agents for stimulating growth (Arsène et al., 2022; J. Chen et al., 2019). Guo et al. (2023) employed a ratiometric approach to detect and differentiate four distinct tetracyclines: doxycycline (DOX), chlortetracycline (CTC), oxytetracycline (OTC) and tetracycline (TC). They synthesized dual-excitation carbon dots (DE-CDs) through microwave radiation of melamine and o-phenylenediamine (OPD). These DE-CDs exhibited robust yellow fluorescence and exceptional stability. Furthermore, concentration-dependent dual-excitation phenomenon, where varying the DE-CD concentration led to a split and shift in the excitation peaks toward 385 nm and 465 nm, is observed. By utilizing 3D printing technology, they developed a smartphone-integrated, on-site sensing device with a self-calibration feature. To detect another antibiotic, a fluorescent nanoprobe was produced for both qualitative and quantitative assessment of Amoxicillin (AMO). This innovative probe utilized environmentally friendly red carbon dots (RCDs) and blue carbon dots (BCDs). A chemical reaction that promoted hydrogen bonding led to an immediate increase in the intensity of the blue fluorescence emitted by the BCDs, along with a noticeable change in color from red to blue. This portable and user-friendly device demonstrated an exceptionally short detection time and an impressive level of sensitivity (Table 11.1.) (L. Li et al., 2023).

Liu et al. (2022) introduced a handheld multifunctional smartphone platform which integrated with FDM 3D printing technology and has been developed for real-time determination of azodicarbonamide (ADA) and glutathione (GSH). ADA present in flour can undergo simple decomposition into semi-carbazide and biuret compounds, which are genotoxic and carcinogenic. On the other hand, GSH, a cellular antioxidant, can combine with certain compounds containing ketones and

TABLE 11.1

Comparison of different CD-based 3D printed handheld smartphone-based sensing platforms in terms of the types of CDs, AM techniques, sensing substances, linear range and detection limit

Type of Carbon Dots	AM Technique	Sensing Substances	Linear Range	Detection Limit	References
R- and B- CDs	FDM	Amoxicillin (AMO)	0–6 µM	2.39 nM	L. Li et al. (2023b)
R- and B- CDs	FDM	Nitrite	2.5–600 µM	0.8 µM	H. Liang et al. (2022a)
Nitrogen doping carbon quantum dots (N-CDs)	FDM	Ag+	0.7–36 µM	83 nM	Tang et al. (2022)
Silicon doped Carbon quantum dots (SiCQDs)	FDM	Ascorbic acid (AA)	0–3 µM	18.12 nmol/L	C. Li et al. (2023a)
Dual-excitation carbon quantum dots	FDM	Doxycycline (DOX)	0.061–80 µM (DOX)	61 nM (DOX)	G. Guo et al. (2023)
		chlortetracycline (CTC)	0.072–105 (CTC)	72 nM (CTC)	
		oxytetracycline (OTC)	0.088–110 (OTC)	88 nM (OTC)	
		tetracycline (TC)	0.115–80 (TC)	115 nM (TC)	
N-CDs	DLP	Lysine	25–300 mM	16 mM	Ding et al. (2023)
CDs	FDM	F$^-$	150–1200 µM	7.998 µM	Yan et al. (2023)
N,P-CDs	FDM	glutathione (GSH)	0 – 28 µM (GSH)	`21.41 (GSH)	Shi et al. (2023)
		Mn(VII)	0–40 µM (Mn(VII))	24.49 nM (Mn(VII))	
CDs	FDM	Free chlorine	20–500 µg L^{-1}	6 µg L^{-1}	Uriarte et al. (2021)
N-CDs	Not mentioned	glyphosate (GLP)	0.01–6.67 mg/L	9.06 µg/L	X. Luo et al. (2022)
N-CDs	FDM	Hg^{2+}	0 µM–125 µM	0.024 µM	Chang et al. (2023)
R-CDs	FDM	Acetone	1.0–50.0 mM	2.62 µM	F. Yang et al. (2021)
B-CDs	SLA	GSH	0.1–200 µM (GSH)	0.07 µM (GSH)	T. Liu et al. (2022)
		Azodicarbonamide (ADA)	0.5–160 µM (ADA)	0.09 (ADA)	

unsaturated aldehydes, leading to the formation of toxic metabolites. The introduced system utilized RF nanoprobes comprising B-CDs and O-phenylenediamine (OPD) as indicators. In response to Ag^+ stimulation, nonfluorescent OPD was transformed into 2,3-diaminophenazine (OxOPD), emitting strong fluorescence at 562 nm. Simultaneously, the BCDs, acting as a responsive unit with low toxicity and high fluorescence, experienced quenching by OxOPD via FRET mechanism. This resulted in a distinctive RF response. Upon the addition of ADA, GSH was oxidized to GSSG (glutathione disulfide) so that Ag^+ ions were released. Consequently, BCD fluorescence was re-quenched by ADA while OxOPD fluorescence was reinstated. Figure 11.3A illustrates the determination mechanisms of GSH and ADA using deep learning strategies.

In another study, visual quantitative detection of GSH and Mn(VII) using a continuous change in fluorescence color was done by utilizing ratiometric fluorescent N,P co-doped carbon dots (N,P-CDs) embedded in a paper strip, along with a smartphone and a 3D-printed accessory to enhance the methodology. A color recognition app on the smartphone precisely determined the RGB values from the resulting fluorescence color variations (Shi et al., 2023).

In addition to addressing food contamination concerns, a similar approach was applied for on-site monitoring of food nutrition. A smart point-of-care sensor was created, comprising 3D printed accessories, a smartphone and a fluorescent paper chip. This sensor was developed by printing silicon-doped carbon dots (SiCDs)-Fe^{3+} as ink onto filter paper. In this setup, Si-CDs emitted a robust fluorescence signal that was quenched by Fe^{3+}, and then restored by ascorbic acid (AA) due to the release of -NH_2/-OH groups and the introduction of defects on SiCDs. With relative standard deviations ranging from 0.79% to 2.31%, it was confirmed that the sensor achieved satisfactory accuracy (C. Li et al., 2023a). Taking advantage of 3D printing technology, a fluorescence sensor was utilized for the visual detection of nitrite, a common food additive and preservative. This detection process involved the use of B- and R-CDs RF probes. In the presence of nitrite, a reaction occurred where nitrite interacted with the amino group on B-CDs to produce diazo compounds. This reaction led to the quenching of fluorescence in B-CDs. Meanwhile, R-CDs served as a reference signal in this detection system. The portable and integrated sensor was applied to detect nitrite in preserved meat and pickles, and the recovery rate fell within the range of 94.0% to 105% (H. Liang et al., 2022a).

In the aquatic environment, mercury ion (Hg^{2+}) is considered to be one of the most hazardous pollutants due to its toxic effects on human health and the environment. In terms of drinking water and wastewater discharge, the World Health Organization (WHO) recommends a maximum concentration of 1 g/L and 5 g/L for Hg^{2+} (Tene et al., 2022). One 3D-printed handheld detection platform integrated with a nitrogen-doped CD test strip exhibited a highly linear relationship between the R/B value and Hg^{2+} concentration and low detection limit (Table 11.1.). It was deduced that the fluorescence quenching of N-CDs induced by Hg^{2+} is attributed to dynamic quenching. This dynamic quenching phenomenon may arise due to the potential of oxygen and nitrogen functional groups present in the N-CDs, synthesized as per the preparation procedure, to form chelate complexes with Hg^{2+}. These interactions might involve an unoccupied orbital of Hg^{2+}. This leads to the formation of new complexes.

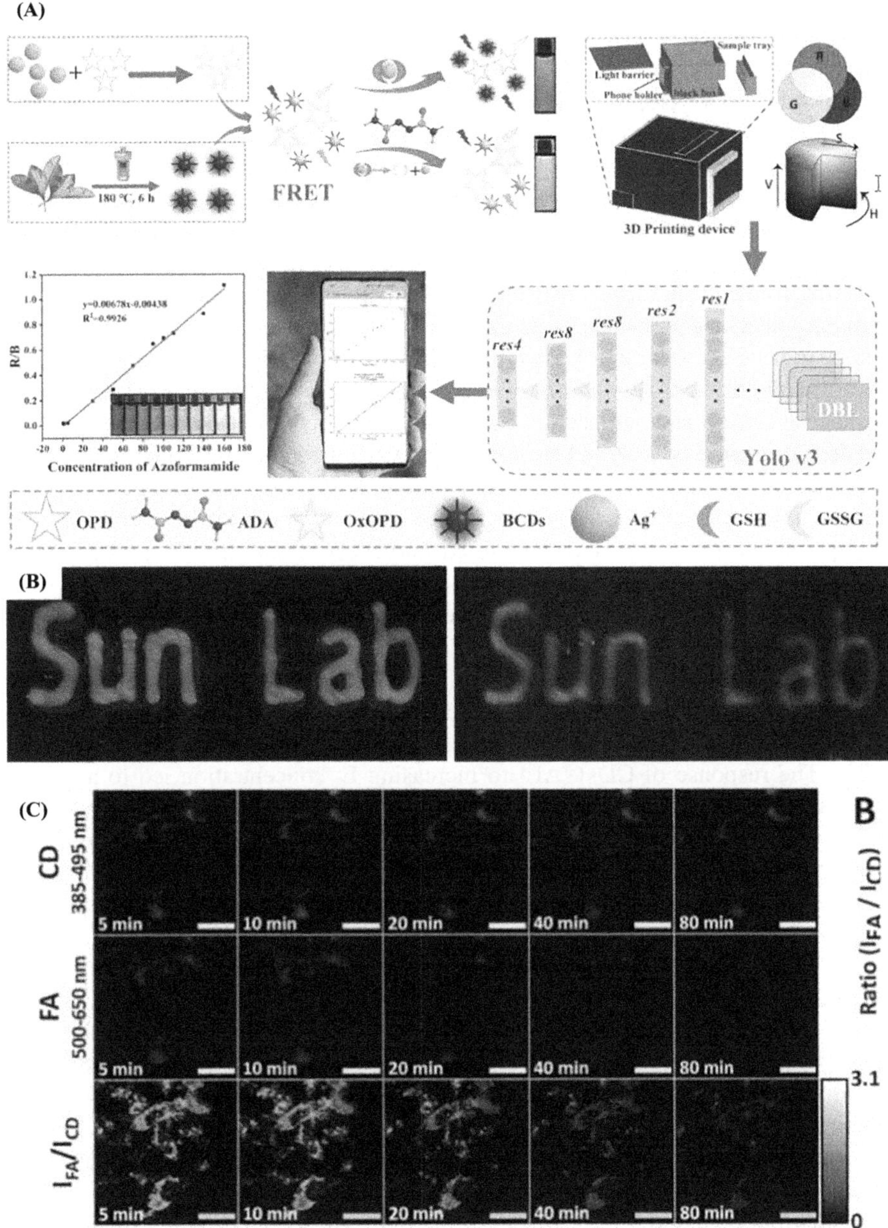

FIGURE 11.3 (a): Utilizing deep learning strategies, RF nanoprobes, and 3D printing technology for the determination of GSH and ADA (T. Liu et al., 2022), (b): the 3D-printed CQD@MIPs shown in two distinct scenarios: with the inclusion of pure water (left) and in the presence of a 20 μM DMHF aqueous solution (Right). These images were taken under the irradiation of a 450 nm LED lamp (reproduced from (X. Yang et al., 2020)) and (c): The potential for real-time monitoring of pH changes within live ASCs (Adipose-derived Stem Cells) located in Baghdadite scaffold, incubated with CD-based fluorescent nanoprobe and subjected to a high-concentration K+ buffer with a pH of 5, along with the addition of 10 μM nigericin.

Furthermore, beyond this finding, the developed platform was effectively employed for the accurate quantitative detection of Hg^{2+} within real water samples and biological systems (Chang et al., 2023). A smartphone-assisted sensing platform for detecting Ag^+ was also developed using fluorescent N-CDs produced through hydrothermal treatment with *Lycium ruthenicum* serving as carbon and nitrogen sources (Tang et al., 2022). For demonstrating its practicality and accuracy, the fluorescent probe's effectiveness was confirmed through testing in lake water, where the spiked recoveries of Ag^+ ranged from 98.99% to 104.19%. Another portable analytical device based on 3D printing and smartphone technology was also designed for the purpose of detecting free chlorine levels in water. Chlorination is commonly used to disinfect drinking water and improve its quality. Formation of disinfection byproducts and change in taste and odor are the two main disadvantages of the chlorination process. Regarding byproducts, two common types associated with chlorination are trihalomethanes (THMs) and haloacetic acids (HAAs). The compounds have reproductive and developmental effects, and are considered to be carcinogens (Gopal et al., 2007). In the developed setup, the fluorescence emission of CDs, synthesized from citric acid and urea, was influenced by the quenching effect induced by free chlorine. The smartphone's camera captured the altered fluorescence, and the 3D-printed device facilitated this connection. By processing the images through the RGB color system, a strong relationship was observed between the CDs signal and the concentration of free chlorine. This connection enabled accurate determination with low detection limits (Uriarte et al., 2021). Fluoride ions (F^-) were also successfully detected using an artificial intelligence-powered smartphone-based handheld detection platform which was comprised of 3D-printed accessory and $CDs@Al^{3+}$ test strip (Yan et al., 2023). The response of $CDs@Al^{3+}$ to increasing F^- concentration led to a gradual decrease in red emission and a corresponding increase in the ratio of a newly emerging green band. This was accompanied by a continuous shift in fluorescence color from red to green. This mechanism was harnessed to develop a RF paper sensor capable of visually recognizing F^-. The sensor demonstrated a low limit of detection and a broad linear range (Table 11.1.).

Another portable smartphone-based device was fabricated utilizing FDM printing technology for a RF sensing system, aimed at monitoring ketosis through the detection of acetone (F. Yang et al., 2021). This system featured a blue organic molecule (2-HCA) as the sensing component and R-CDs as the internal fluorescence standard. Moreover, it exhibited the potential to non-invasively monitor gaseous acetone levels in human breath which offers a painless way for diabetes diagnosis. Lysine, which is an essential amino acid, was successfully detected using a blue-emissive CD-entrapped microfluidic chip fabricated through DLP technology (Ding et al., 2023). This smartphone-based point-of-care testing platform required only a small sample volume of 3 mL and could provide test results within a quick 3-minute timeframe. It was effectively applied to swine serum samples, consistently delivering accurate results. The platform boasted several advantages, including ease of use, fast response, cost-effectiveness, minimal blood collection volume, and reduced stress for swine during the testing process.

Apart from smartphone-based systems, another approach has been employed to detect signaling molecules involved in the quorum sensing processes in foodborne pathogens. These auto-inducers play a significant role in influencing the virulence of foodborne pathogens and serve as indicators for monitoring the activity of spoilage bacteria (Rutherford & Bassler, 2012). Due to the ability of multicolored CDs to analyze many pathogens with high sensitivity in a single analytical run and the simplicity of conjugating the CDs structure with different bioreceptors, CD-based fluorescence techniques appear promising (L. Xu et al., 2017). Based on the mentioned merits, an environmentally friendly composite utilizing molecularly imprinted polymers (MIPs) was fabricated through a straightforward sol-gel technique, which includes long-wavelength emitting CDs. This composite was designed for fluorescent detection of AHLs as a signaling molecule. The CQD@MIP sensor exhibited a low detection limit of 0.067 µM which was effectively applied in AHL analysis within bacterial supernatants. Photo-crosslinked methacrylylated gelatin combined with CQD@MIPs as the printing ink was used in extrusion-based 3D bioprinters. As it can be seen from Figure 11.3B, the fluorescence intensity of DMHF, which has chemical structure similar to AHLs, exhibited a decline under the LED lamp illumination. This rapid AHL detection method, which has high sensitivity, low cost and simple operation, could replace frequently used chromatographic methods (Fekete et al., 2007).

Sensory systems encompass a broader scope than merely identifying substances. This holds especially true within biomedical applications, where intracellular pH (pHi) assumes a key role in the regulation of various cellular physiological processes (Casey et al., 2010; J. Han & Burgess, 2010). Beyond conventional methodologies for sensing intracellular pH (pHi), two-photon excitable probes possess the unique capability to simultaneously harness the energy of two near-infrared photons. This confers several advantages, including reduced susceptibility to interference from background species, diminished risk of photodamage to cellular structures and tissues, prolonged observation periods and increased penetration depth. Recent endeavors have shifted focus toward comprehending cellular behavior within more representative 3D in vitro cultures, as opposed to the conventional two-dimensional (2D) in vitro setups. The rationale behind this shift lies in the fact that 2D cultures overlook the complex interactions between cells and the 3D ECM environment present in vivo, thereby necessitating a more comprehensive approach to studying cell behavior. With this regard, Lesani et al. (2022) introduced two-photon RF nanoprobes based on CDs. The synthesized CDs were modified with fluoresceinamine, serving as a secondary responsive fluorophore, which facilitated the development of a ratiometric nanoprobe. This fluorescent ratiometric CD-based probe displayed outstanding sensitivity, specificity and reversibility to pH fluctuations. This investigation was conducted within a 3D bioactive Baghdadite ceramic scaffold that had been fabricated using SLA technique. The 3d-printed scaffold containing CDs effectively serve a dual purpose: firstly, as a two-photon fluorescence imaging agent for noninvasive monitoring of live cells (Figure 11.4D); secondly, as a two-photon ratiometric nanoprobe capable of providing real-time visualization and quantification of cytoplasmic pH levels in living cells in vitro and in vivo (Figure 11.3C).

11.4.2 Imaging Applications

Image-guided therapy refers to the use of medical imaging techniques to guide and monitor therapeutic procedures in real-time. It allows for precise targeting of damaged or diseased tissue and provides feedback on the effectiveness of the treatment.

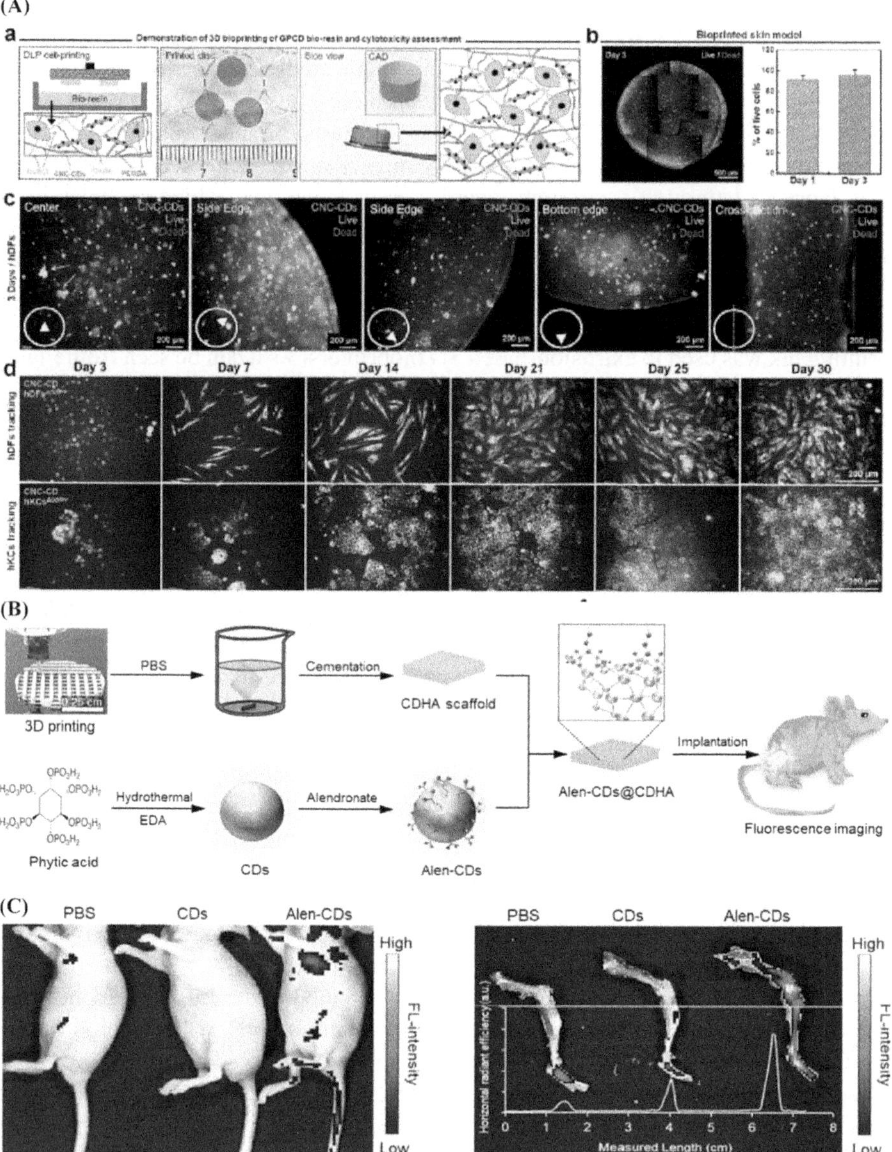

FIGURE 11.4 A: 3D Bioprinting and Dynamic Cell Tracking in Models with GPCD Bio-Resin. (a) Schematic depiction of the bioprinting process, involving precise printing of cells mixed with GPCD bio-resin, (b) Representative Live/Dead imaging of a full-thickness skin model using hDFs after 3 days of incubation, with quantification data, (c) Fluorescence microscopy (FL) images of hDFs at different positions within the hydrogel, showing hydrogel surface staining due to T-CNC@CDs. Insets indicate cell positions, (d) Dynamic tracking of hDFs and hKCs within the bioprinted hydrogel over a 30-day period (Dutta et al., 2023).

(Continued)

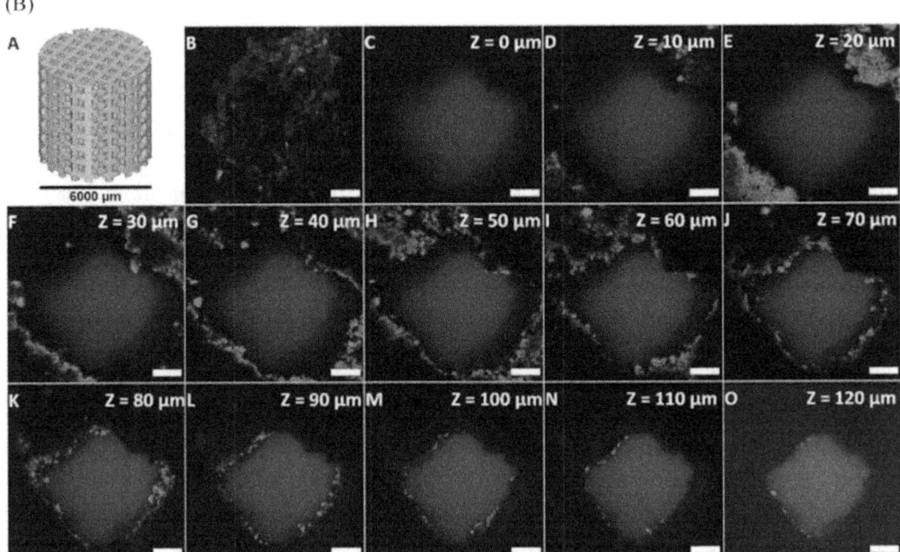

FIGURE 11.4 (CONTINUED) B: schematic depiction of fluorescence imaging using Alen-CDs@CDHA scaffolds in balb/c nude mice. C: The figure includes fluorescence images of balb/c nude mice that were administered PBS, CDs, and Alen-CDs, as well as fluorescence images of dissected legs from balb/c nude mice that received PBS, CDs, and Alen-CDs injections (K. K. Lee et al., 2023). D: a) Schematic of the microstructure of cylindrical Baghdadite scaffold (diameter: 6 mm) with a cubic internal architecture with 50% porosity and 300 μm pore size. b) Overlay of DIC and two-photon fluorescence images and (c-o) two-photon excited Z-stack images of the Baghdadite scaffold seeded with ASCs after incubation with FACD (800 μg/mL) for 24 h (from 0 to 120 μm; Δz = 10 μm, Scale: 100 μm).

The methods used for monitoring tumors, wounds, or surgical implants through minimally invasive procedures have predominantly relied on conventional imaging technologies like X-ray fluoroscopy, computed tomography (CT), ultrasound (US), or magnetic resonance imaging (MRI) (C. Wang et al., 2018). However, these methods necessitate advanced equipment and energy-intensive devices. In contrast, the fluorescent imaging technique has garnered significant interest in the area of medical diagnostics. Carbon dots possess relevant characteristics like small size, capability in emitting multiple colors, outstanding resistance to photodegradation, minimal damage to cells and strong compatibility with biological systems. That is why in early studies of CDs, they were used for fluorescence imaging of cells using both single-photon and multiphoton excitation (P. G. Luo et al., 2014; J. Zhang & Yu, 2016). Given the aforementioned points, the integration of CD-based self-tracking systems into biomedical implants becomes extremely desirable for research in image-guided tissue regeneration (Gibbs, 2012). In this regard, a hydrogel was developed using 2,2,6,6-(tetramethylpiperidin-1-yl)oxyl (TEMPO)-oxidized nanocellulose (T-CNCs) and CDs (Dutta et al., 2023). The resulting T-CNC@CDs were then incorporated into a liquid bio-resin containing gelatin methacryloyl (GelMA) and polyethylene glycol diacrylate (GPCD) for DLP bioprinting. This approach aimed to enable the dynamic tracking of cells during bioprinting. Human dermal fibroblasts (hDFs) were employed to bioprint full-thickness skin and blood vessel structures as a proof of concept. Utilizing the distinctive fluorescence property of T-CNC@CDs, human skin cells could be effectively monitored within the GPCD hydrogel for a duration of up to 30 days following the bioprinting process. This technique facilitated the creation of in vitro models that accurately recreated the natural microenvironment of both skin and blood vessels. Importantly, these bioprinted constructs exhibited prolonged tracking capabilities without any degradation or harm, underscoring the viability and durability of the method (Figure 11.4A).

In vivo bone imaging allows us to visualize, assess and measure bone structure, regeneration and health in living organisms. These techniques provide critical information for bone tissue engineering, osteoporosis assessment and other bone-related studies (Fragogeorgi et al., 2019). In pursuit of this objective, a novel composite material for bone replacement was fabricated which involved combining alendronate-conjugated CDs (referred to as Alen-CDs) with scaffolds made of calcium-deficient hydroxyapatite (CDHA). Thanks to its effective therapeutic effects in treating diverse bone-related diseases and its remarkable ability to strongly bind to bone tissues in living organisms, Alendronate was chosen for conjugation with CDs. The unique feature of this composite was its dual capability such as deactivating osteoclasts and enabling fluorescence imaging. CDHA scaffolds designed to resemble elements of bone structure were produced using a paste extruding 3D-deposition system (K. K. Lee et al., 2023). To monitor the effectiveness of different scaffolds, they were implanted under the epidermal tissues of balb/c nude mice. Following a 24-hour implantation period, a strong fluorescence signal was detected in the case of Alen-CDs@CDHA scaffold, while no fluorescence signal was observed in mice implanted without CDs (Figure 11.4 B&C).

Bioimaging of metallic ions in biological systems has emerged as a crucial technique in understanding their roles and impacts within living organisms. Metallic ions play diverse roles in biological processes, including enzymatic activities, signal transduction and oxidative stress. Detecting and monitoring these ions can provide insights into their distribution, concentration and interactions which can shed light on their physiological and pathological implications (Xue et al., 2022). Due to their distinctive electron transfer properties, N-CDs exhibit a strong selectivity for Fe^{3+} ions. Therefore, N-CDs were utilized for bioimaging of Fe^{3+} in Hela cells (Zhou et al., 2022). In another study, N-CDs were used for Hg^{2+} imaging applications (Chang et al., 2023). Upon the introduction of Hg^{2+}, a pronounced and clear blue FL signal became distinctly visible within HeLa cells. This was accompanied by persistent reduction in the red FL signal.

A streamlined approach was adopted for generating CDs with long wavelength emission (Saranti et al., 2022). These CDs were then combined with a polylactic acid (PLA)-based filament with bioactive glass (bioglass® 45S5). This nanocomposite material was then employed to 3D-printed scaffolds utilizing the FDM technique. Due to the potential influence of PLA on photoluminescence, it is anticipated that as PLA degrades and hydroxyapatite (HAp) forms a decrease in photoluminescence signals could be observed as the process advances. In another word, a portion of the luminescence diminishes or becomes obscured over time due to the development of a hydroxyapatite-like layer on the composite's surface following immersion in simulated body fluid (SBF). This observation suggests the feasibility of monitoring the healing process using bioimaging with CDs incorporated bioactive scaffold.

11.4.3 Polymerization Applications

Radical polymerization (RP) is a type of chain-growth polymerization that involves the formation of free radicals as reactive intermediates. It is one of the most widely used methods for producing synthetic polymers, such as polyethylene, polypropylene, polystyrene, and polyvinyl chloride and contributes to approximately 50% of the global annual synthetic polymer production, which amounts to around 334 million tons (Y. Gao et al., 2020). Radical polymerization can be initiated by various sources, such as heat, light or chemical initiators. The initiators produce radicals that can attack the double bonds of vinyl monomers and add them to the growing polymer chain. The chain propagation continues until two radicals combine and terminate the reaction. The resulting polymers have a wide range of molecular weights and dispersity, depending on the reaction conditions and the type of monomers used (Matyjaszewski & Davis, 2002).

Photoinitiated polymerization methods have become widespread in various industrial sectors, including coatings, adhesives, inks and microelectronics over the last few decades since they are efficient, energy saving, economical, environmentally friendly and enabling (Yagci et al., 2010). During photoinitiated polymerization, free radicals or other reactive species are generated by photoirradiation, thereby initiating the polymerization process. The photoinitiator assumes a significant role in the polymerization process. A photoinitiator, or a system of photoinitiators, is characterized as a molecule or a combination of molecules that, upon light absorption, starts the polymerization reaction (Shirai, 2015). In recent years, the utilization of innovative photoinitiators (PIs), particularly Quantum PIs, for free-radical polymerization has captured substantial interest from the scientific community. Thanks to their accurately adjustable properties based on structural and surface manipulation, quantum-confined nanoscale crystals with semiconductor characteristics, have attracted huge attention for their potential application in photopolymerization (Shukla et al., 2021; Waiskopf et al., 2021).

Utilizing 3D printing alongside localized photopolymerization enables the additive manufacturing of objects with micro/nanoscale precision. Nonetheless, the commonly employed radical polymerization techniques are typically suited for non-aqueous systems. Thus, the advancement of three-dimensional printing within aqueous environments becomes crucial. This is particularly significant due to the highly efficient polymerization process achievable in water, specifically through additive manufacturing methods. Emerging biomedical applications like tissue engineering scaffolding, intelligent drug delivery systems and shape-memory polymers greatly benefit from this approach (Jain et al., 2021). An additional limitation of existing commercial photoinitiators (PIs) is their exclusive compatibility with the UV light spectrum. This poses a challenge for certain specialized applications like 3D bioprinting and biomedicine, where ensuring the safety of both the light source and materials is paramount (M. Lee et al., 2020). To address this concern, it becomes imperative to create visible-light initiators that possess favorable biocompatibility and a degree of water solubility. CDs have the dual characteristics of being both water-soluble and amenable to manipulation for initiating photochemical reactions under visible light (Meng et al., 2019; Tomal et al., 2021). Technically speaking, for optimal performance, for example in typical DLP 3D printers, PIs should ideally absorb light within the range of 385 to 405 nm in order to efficiently generate free radicals (Pawar et al., 2017; H. Wang et al., 2021). However, CDs exhibit relatively weak absorbance at 405 nm. To enhance their light absorption capabilities, it may become necessary to modify the chemical structure of the carbon skeleton. One of the promising strategies to achieve this is through the introduction of heteroatoms such as nitrogen, phosphorus, boron, sulfur, etc. via doping. Huang et al. (2022) synthesized N-CDs using urea and sodium citrate. These initiators exhibited a robust absorption band at 406.5 nm in a diluted water solution, which aligns closely with the emission spectrum of the light source found in the majority of commercial 3D printers. To further enhance the photoinitiation process, coinitiators such as triethylamine (TEA) and neopentyl glycol (NPG) are introduced into the resin formulation. As depicted in Figure 11.5A, in the presence of these coinitiators, the photo-generated electrons or holes can participate in oxidation or reduction reactions with TEA and NPG, respectively, leading to the formation of active species. These active species play a crucial role in abstracting hydrogen atoms or undergoing decarboxylation reactions, ultimately resulting in the formation of highly efficient initiating radicals. This cooperative action between CDs and coinitiators significantly improves the overall photoinitiation performance of the resin system. By employing both DLP and extrusion-based 3D printing techniques and two monomers, namely PEGDA400 and GelMA, the possibility of using the CD-2/NPG photoinitiation system for innovative applications in 3D printing was also investigated. All the printed 3D structures exhibit exceptional resolution and well-defined edges (Figure 11.5B a and b). Remarkably, these structures exhibit yellow fluorescence when excited. The inherent fluorescence of the printed structures introduces the possibility of broader application avenues like fluorescence tracing and ion detection.

In another attempt (Tomal et al., 2021), CDs were fabricated from citric acid and doped with nitrogen and sulfur to act as universal photosensitizers for iodonium salts. These CDs can trigger the light-induced cationic polymerization of different types of monomers, such as vinyl, epoxy and acrylates. The initiating system containing CDs was used for cationic photopolymerization to make hydrogel materials by VPP printing process. A photocurable cationic resin based on a vinyl monomer, tri(ethylene glycol) divinyl ether (TEGDVE) was used for 3D printing experiments performed under a laser source of light (405 nm). The resin contained an IOD/N-doped-CA-CD initiating system. As shown in Figure 11.5C, a printout with a C-DOT inscription was obtained. The inscription had a remarkable thickness of ~0.5 mm and a high spatial resolution (limited only by the laser diode beam size: 50 μm spot). As mentioned earlier, a major challenge in 3D printing of hydrogel materials, especially for bio-medical application, is in choosing a suitable photosensitive composition and an initiating system type that can be easily dissolved in an aqueous media. For such a reason, the hydrogel materials with a specific structure were synthesized from the

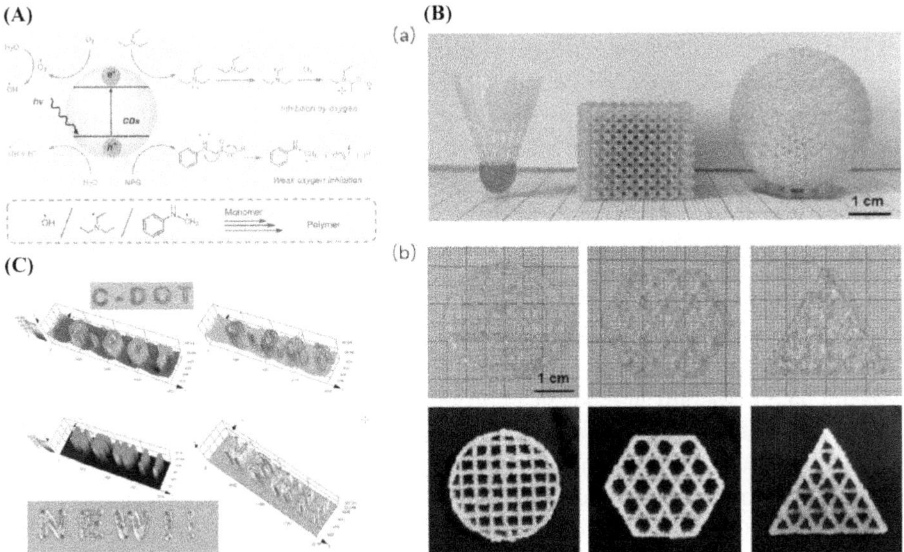

FIGURE 11.5 A: schematic of the proposed mechanism of CDs as visible light photoinitiators, including the excitation of CDs, generation of electron-hole pairs, oxidation of water to form hydroxyl radicals, reduction of residual oxygen to produce superoxide radicals and the role of coinitiators in enhancing the initiation process. B: Structures produced through DLP 3D printing (represented as (a)) and extrusion-based 3D printing (represented as (b)) (X. Huang et al., 2022). C: The 3D inscription depicted is formed through the cationic photopolymerization process. In this process, tetraethylene glycol divinyl ether (TEGDVE) is used as a monomer. This polymerization is initiated by a two-component photoinitiating system composed of N-doped-CDs at a concentration of 0.2 wt% and iodine at a concentration of 2 wt% (top) and 3D hydrogel inscription achieved through the process of free-radical photopolymerization. The involves using a mixture of HEA (hydroxyethyl acrylate) and water in a 1:1 weight ratio. To initiate the photopolymerization, a two-component photoinitiating system (CDs at a concentration of 0.2 wt% and IOD (iodine)) is employed (bottom) (Tomal et al., 2021).

acrylate monomer HEA and water in equal mass proportions, along with the initiator system IOD/CDs. This printed material represents exemplary optical resolution and a thickness of around 2.5 mm using low-intensity visible light emitted by LEDs (Figure 11.5C). These technologies also hold significant promise for biomedical applications, such as the *in situ* and 3D printed fabrication of hydrogels, all while utilizing secure visible light sources.

One of the challenges of radical polymerization is to control the molecular structure and architecture of the polymers. Since the radicals are highly reactive and indiscriminate, they can cause unwanted side reactions, such as chain transfer, branching, and cyclization. These reactions affect the properties and performance of the polymers. To overcome this problem, various techniques have been developed to regulate the radical reactivity and improve the polymerization control. Some examples are controlled radical polymerization (CRP) (Pan et al., 2016), reversible-deactivation radical polymerization (RDRP) (Destarac, 2018) and radical ring-opening polymerization (rROP) (Tardy et al., 2017).

CRP is a method that uses reversible activation/deactivation mechanisms to control the number and lifetime of active radicals. This allows for a better control over the molecular weight and dispersity of the polymers, as well as the possibility to synthesize complex architectures such as block copolymers, star polymers and graft polymers. Some examples of CRP techniques are atom transfer radical polymerization (ATRP), nitroxide-mediated polymerization (NMP) and reversible addition-fragmentation chain transfer (RAFT) polymerization (Pan et al., 2016). For more than 25 years, ATRP has been utilized to create polymers with preset molecular weights (MW), narrow MW distribution, architecture and functionality. During atom transfer radical addition reactions, the chain initiation and chain propagation steps are involved in living polymerization process in which chain breaking reactions are reversible (Krys & Matyjaszewski, 2017). Particularly in photo-ATRP, the atom transfer involves a radical halogen atom, and the reaction is catalyzed by a transition metal. However, the traditional approach imparts barrier for 3D-priting on account of two main reasons: the polymerization process in typical photo-ATRP systems is slow, which hinders the efficiency and speed of 3D printing. The other reason is that 3D printing is typically performed under open-air conditions, which exposes the printing process to oxygen. Oxygen inhibits the polymerization reaction, preventing the resin from fully curing and resulting in incomplete or weakly bonded layers (Quan et al., 2020). Semiconductor QDs possess the capability to generate electron-hole pairs upon exposure to light, thereby they can serve as proficient sources of either electron donation or electron acceptance in photomediated ATRP (Y. Huang et al., 2018; Wu et al., 2017). The enhancement of photoinduced electron transfer can be achieved by introducing additional sacrificial hole scavengers. This prolongs the active lifespan of photoexcited QDs, enabling more efficient electron transfer (Hutton et al., 2016). This not only depletes oxygen in the environment but also imparts improved oxygen tolerance to the reaction system. Apart from that, when compared to other types of QDs, nitrogen-doped QDs exhibited superior catalytic efficacy in the context of visible-light-induced atom transfer radical polymerization (ATRP). In a study (Qiao et al., 2022), this oxygen-tolerant, rapid polymerization system induced by visible light was developed. A DLP 3D printer introduced spatially controlled polymerization by digitally masking the violet LED light source (max = 405 nm). Upon optimization, the polymerization process could attain a monomer conversion exceeding 90% within 1 minute, while maintaining a polymer polydispersity index (PDI) below 1.25. To demonstrate the efficacy of the catalyzed aqueous photo-ATRP system using CQs for 3D printing, various complex geometric shapes were successfully printed, including four square prisms, four cylinders with progressively reduced dimensions and complex-shaped pyramids (Figure 11.6A). The printed objects illustrate desired resolution, evident in the well-defined edges and corners of the pyramid surfaces, which closely resemble the original model. Furthermore, the printed hydrogel pyramids displayed intense yellow fluorescence when exposed to ultraviolet light, which underscores the successful synthesis of functional hydrogel with fluorescence attributes via DLP 3D printing.

In addition to polymerization techniques for hydrogel formation, the interaction between nanoparticles (NPs) and polymers stands as a vital factor in creating nanocomposite (NC) hydrogels, which can impact characteristics like microstructure,

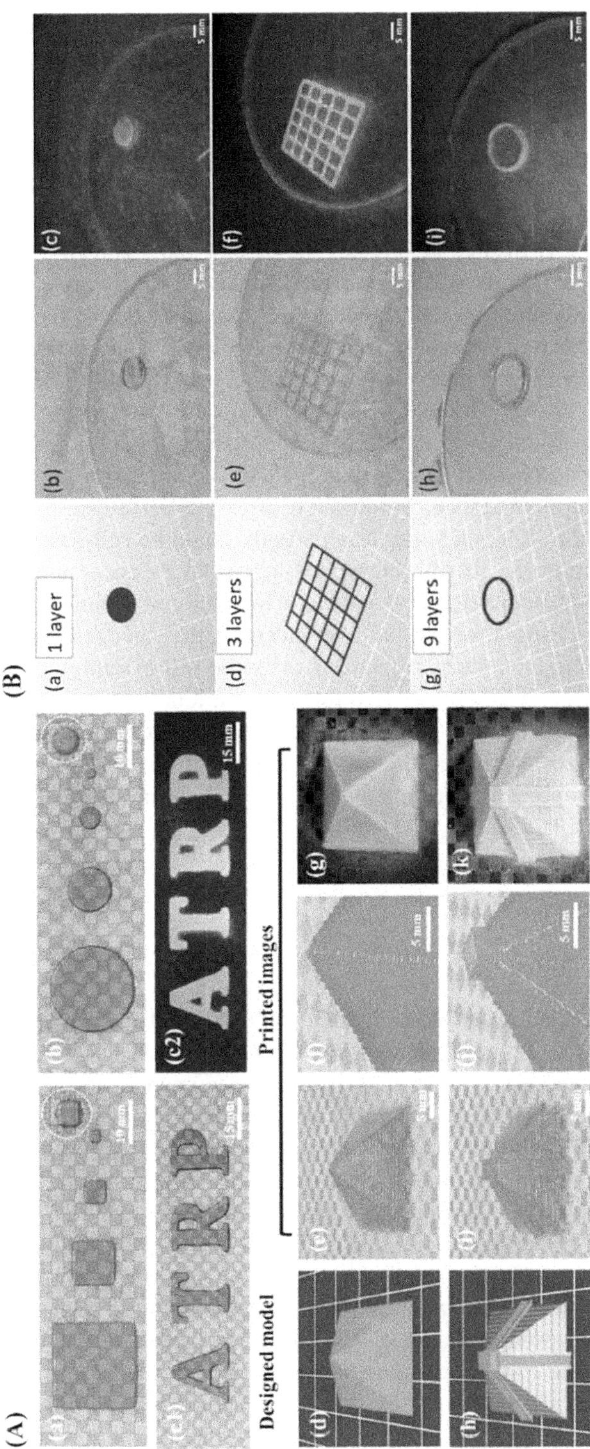

FIGURE 11.6   A: Various 3D printed objects and their details, (a) Displays square prisms with decreasing dimensions from 20 mm down to 2.5 mm, all with a thickness of 1 mm, (b) Shows printed cylinders with dimensions decreasing from 20 mm to 2.5 mm in diameter, also with a thickness of 1 mm, (c1) an optical image of the printed word "ATRP" under natural light, and (c2) the same word under ultraviolet light, (d, h) Features models of a simple pyramid and a Mayan pyramid, (e, i) presents panoramic photos of the 3D printed objects, (f, j) Provides close-up views, highlighting the clear and high-resolution details of the printed objects and (g, k) displays optical images of the two printed pyramids under ultraviolet light (Qiao et al., 2022). B: Images of 3D-printed patterns using PDA30@CD hydrogels, (a, d, g) initial 3D models used for printing, including a solid round shape, rectangular grid and a ring, (b, e, h) the resulting 3D-printed structures, (c, f, i) the appearance of the 3D-printed structures when exposed to UV light (C. H. Lu & Yeh, 2022).

mechanical strength and swelling behavior (T. Chen et al., 2018). In this context, Dynamic bonds, known for their unique attributes and adaptability, reap the benefits of dynamic bonds at the interface, which can enhance stress relaxation at the interface and consequently improve the mechanical properties of NC hydrogels (C.-H. Lu et al., 2021). These dynamic bonds in the form of Schiff base reactions were employed in a systematic study conducted on the interaction between amine-functionalized CDs and polydextran aldehyde (PDA) polymers (C. H. Lu & Yeh, 2022). This interaction was subsequently utilized in the creation of 3D-printed structures using an extrusion-based 3D printer. 3D-printed patterns of the rectangular grid, solid round shape and ring structure were produced (Figure 11.6B) so that under UV light, these structures showed strong fluorescence. Modulating the properties of the hydrogel was easily performed by adjusting either the size or the quantity of functional groups present on CDs. Simultaneously, the introduction of distinct quantities of functional aldehyde groups onto polydextran through oxidation offers an easily controllable method. This approach is particularly suitable for mass production and practical to finely tune the characteristics of the resulting hydrogel. By combining a photocurable monomer based on vanillin and CDs, bio-based resins were developed for DLP 3D printing. When exposed to UV light, the CDs partially could be self-assembled into micrometric fibers within the thermoset matrix during DLP processing. This phenomenon was elucidated by considering that the UV light induces a partial reduction of the CDs, which brings about the formation of electrostatic, van der Waals and π-π stacking interactions. These interactions, in turn, drive the self-assembly of CDs into robust fibers. The incorporation of CDs also formed additional secondary interactions within the thermoset composite. For the above reasons, along with the presence of Schiff-base linkages, CDs significantly contributed to preserving the composite's mechanical properties during mechanical reprocessing and chemical recycling (Liguori et al., 2023).

11.4.4 Other Applications

In the initial phases of utilizing CDs-containing 3D-printed materials, the primary focus lies in printing decorative and sample products. These serve as showcases to visualize the potential applications in future industrial products. These envisioned applications include probes designed for environmental and medical purposes, UV light converters and also sunglasses. One of the earliest documented instances of investigating the incorporation of CDs into a 3D printed photoluminescent material was conducted in 2018, in which orange CDs were incorporated into sodium polyacrylate (SPA) to create an ink suitable for SLA 3D printing technique (Zhou et al., 2018). The integration of O-CDs prevents excessive self-aggregation, which enables the preservation of photoluminescence (PL) in the solid state. Additionally, even when coated with photopolymer resin, the composite material maintains its long emission wavelength, thus minimizing interference from both the light source and the resin itself. The 3D printed Statue of Liberty specimen emitted a vibrant orange fluorescence, while the control scattered blue light (Figure 11.7.A).

The combination of CDs and printing methodologies extends beyond polymeric materials. Liquid metal (LM) and its alloys possess distinctive physicochemical

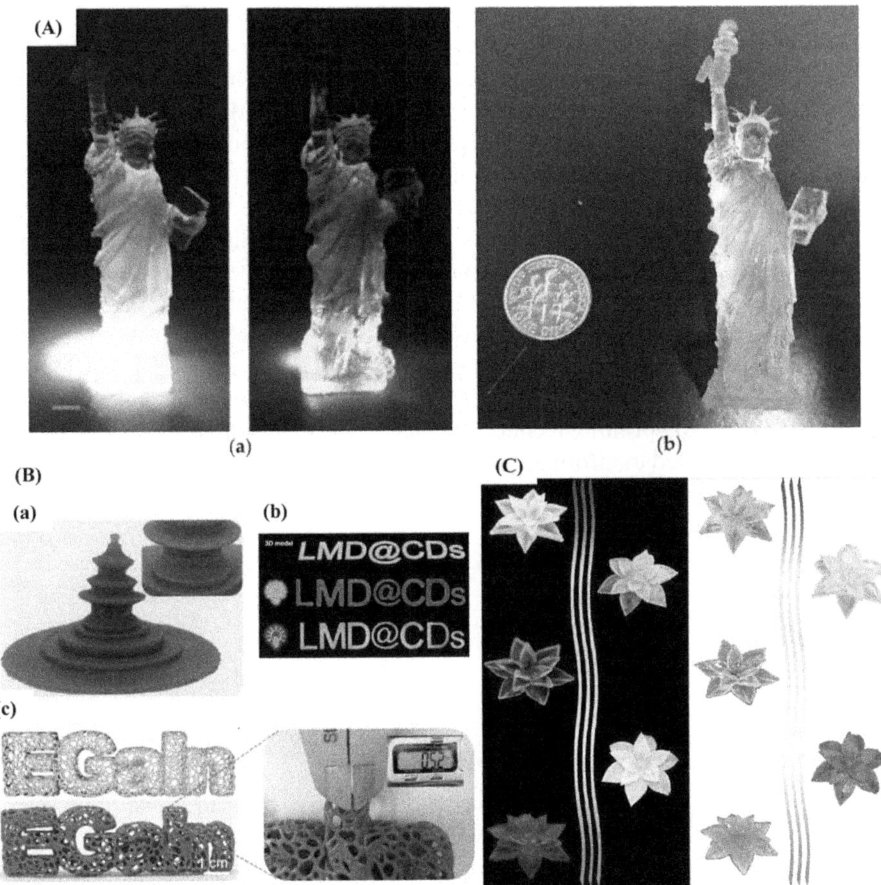

FIGURE 11.7 A: the 3D printed the Statue of Liberty using two different materials, (a) on the left side, O-CDs are employed, on the right side, a control material is used (scale bar = 5 cm), (b) size comparison of the printed specimen with a US dime (Zhou et al., 2018). B: (a) Panorama photos and a close-up of the Temple of Heaven produced through DLP 3D printing using LMD@CDs in the resin, (b) image of printed "LMD@CDs" word under natural light (middle) and ultraviolet light (bottom), (c) the 3D printed object of the complex hollow structure named "EGaIn". C: Images of 3D-printed flower lanterns created using a specialized patterning technique. The photographs on the right depict the flowers under daylight conditions, while those on the left show them when illuminated at 365 nm irradiation (Ai et al., 2023).

attributes that have gained prominence as emerging and functional materials over the past decade. The liquid metal alloy known as eutectic gallium/indium (EGaIn) embodies both metallic properties and liquid flowability, owing to its low viscosity at or slightly below room temperature. These features hold potential for innovative platforms across diverse applications due to its high thermal and electrical conductivity, as well as superior mechanical characteristics. In an endeavor to harness these qualities (L. Wang et al., 2023b), uniform LM droplets featuring nanolevel particle dimensions were synthesized using the Pickering miniemulsion technique facilitated by CDs.

After optimization, the LM droplets encapsulating CDs (LMD@CDs) found application as functional additives in the 3D/4D printing of hydrogels and cross-linked DLP resins. This system demonstrated its efficacy in fabricating intricate models like the Temple of Heaven and hollow structures, all exhibiting remarkable resolution (Figure 11.7.B (a,c)). Furthermore, the printed objects displayed consistent and robust blue fluorescence emission when subjected to 365 nm UV light (Figure 11.8B (b)). The light absorption characteristics of LMD@CDs played a dual role: enhancing printing precision and inducing variance in cross-linking density during the subsequent curing phase. Due to the photothermal properties of the LM and the observed variations in cross-linking density between the soft hydrogel, the 3D printed objects can demonstrate responsive behaviors when exposed to both water and NIR laser irradiation (Figure 11.8). This suggests a promising future for 4D printing of LMD@CD-based materials, where objects can dynamically respond to environmental stimuli.

Both CDs and 3D printing technologies have also demonstrated their capabilities in applications related to information encryption and anticounterfeiting. These applications are becoming increasingly critical in many high-value items like electronic

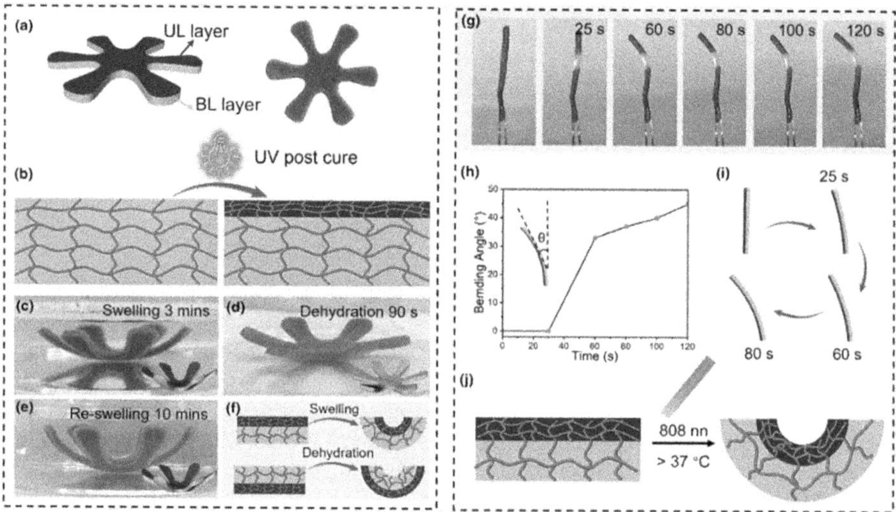

FIGURE 11.8 The swelling and desolvation processes along with near-infrared (NIR)-induced actuation of a material fabricated through DLP 3D printing with spatially resolved light doses (a) the designed geometrical features (on the left) and a top view of the printed petal object (on the right), (b) schematic of the dual-gradient effect achieved through post-curing under UV light, (c) depiction of the petal with the layer exposed to a higher light dose on top (UL, dark blue) after being submerged in water for 3 minutes, (d) after 90 seconds of dehydration, the same petal, now flipped and swollen, with the layer exposed to a lower light dose on top (BL, sky blue), (e) re-swelling of the petal in water after 10 minutes, with the UL layer on top, (f) a schematic of the transformation of the petal during the swelling and desolvation process, (g) capturing the state of LMD@CDs-striped composite hydrogel under 808 nm NIR laser stimulation, (h) the bending angles of the LMD@CDs composite hydrogel under NIR, (i) simulated bending angles and a scheme illustrating the actuation achieved through NIR and (j) deformation of petal when exposed to NIR irradiation (L. Wang et al., 2023b).

components, documents, agrochemicals, pharmaceuticals, jewelry and fashion items (Haider et al., 2022; Kalytchuk et al., 2018). A wide range of strategies have been developed to prevent counterfeiting, utilizing different materials and methods for authentication. Among these strategies, fluorescent anticounterfeiting techniques have gained prominence. These involve the use of various fluorescent materials such as organic fluorescent dyes, polymer dots, rare earth materials, inorganic quantum dots and CDs (Yu et al., 2021). CDs stand out due to their advantageous qualities including minimal toxicity, customizable optical properties based on size, shape and composition, and their ability to be produced through straightforward and cost-effective synthetic processes (Ren et al., 2022). Chitosan-based solid-state CDs (C-SS-CDs) were utilized as a color conversion layer with yellow fluorescence, yielding a 90% production rate of C-SS-CDs. These C-SS-CDs were then combined with epoxy resin and a curing agent to create composite materials, which were subsequently applied onto a 450 nm semiconductor chip to construct a White LED (WLED). The resulting WLED boasted color rendering index more than 90. Moreover, the C-SS-CDs/epoxy resin composites demonstrated applicability in 3D printing by generating distinct yellow solid-state luminescence when exposed to UV light across various 3D printing models (Ni et al., 2022). Another three-dimensional cellular structure was constructed through the direct writing process by combining siloxane with N-CDs and acrylate as photosensitive reagents. This process involved the introduction of UV light so that it can be a flexible optical device for anticounter-feiting measures using additive manufacturing (Zhou et al., 2022).

CDs offer a range of possibilities for colored displays, from wide-color-gamut displays to laser imaging and dynamic holographic display (Yoshinaga et al., 2021; Y. Zhang et al., 2023). Yet, due to the technical complexities associated with preparing solid-state fluorescence (SSF) CDs, the utilization of CDs in colored displays has been limited by aggregation-caused quenching (Ru et al., 2022). A breakthrough was achieved by functionalizing CDs with precisely structured salicylaldehyde (SA)-type ligands (Ai et al., 2023). This innovative approach led to the attainment of polychromatic SSF characteristics when subjected to UV excitation. By capitalizing on the beneficial effects of AIE and the abundant surface sites available for modification on CDs, it becomes feasible to mitigate or eliminate aggregation-caused quenching, thereby enabling the realization of multicolor SSF. In order to demonstrate the practical potential of SSF CD, illumination devices with three-dimensional (3D) lotus flower lanterns with seven vibrant colors were constructed using the optical properties of AIEgens-CDs (Figure 11.7.C). These findings exemplify the creation of a diverse array of luminescent objects and present the promising commercial prospects for their application in optical lamps.

Another study investigated the antibacterial effects of copper CDs (Cu-CDs) in 3D-printed PLA-based scaffolds (Azadmanesh et al., 2021). These scaffolds also contained hyaluronic acid, chitosan and rosmarinic acid. Unlike plain PLA scaffolds, the nanocomposite scaffolds displayed notable antibacterial properties against two bacterial types. In another word, all three compounds (CDs, copper CDs, and copper CDs with rosmarinic acid) exhibited antibacterial activity against Gram-positive bacterium *S. aureus* and Gram-negative bacterium *E. coli*. The minimum inhibitory concentration (MIC) values were 75 µg/ml for CDs, 20 µg/ml for copper CDs and

0.08 µg/ml for copper CDs combined with rosmarinic acid. The entire nanocomposite material showed excellent biocompatibility and contributed to an enhanced wound healing process.

An eye-opening approach involved the synergy of CDs and 3D printing to enhance combustion performance. This was achieved through the utilization of the FDM technique. By introducing gel-like CDs into the paraffin matrix at a mass ratio of 1%, remarkable improvements were observed compared to ABS/pure paraffin samples (Oztan et al., 2021). The CD addition led to an 11% increase in regression rate and an 8.5% increase in combustion efficiency values. These enhancements were achieved despite a compromise in mechanical properties. The improved combustion characteristics in the CD-loaded fuel grains were ascribed to factors including reduced viscosity, increased particle entrainment, heightened specific surface area and enhanced catalytic activity.

11.5 SUMMARY AND OUTLOOK

CDs and AM have emerged and attracted significant attention recently, both being potential alternatives to traditional semiconductor quantum dots and conventional manufacturing methods, respectively. Reaping the benefits from seven key processes that offer advantages such as flexible design with reduced expertise requirements, rapid prototyping, cost savings and the ability to create complex products, AM is addressed as one of the most significant scientific breakthroughs of the 20th century. Additionally, owing to its low toxicity, eco-friendliness, cost-effectiveness, and straightforward synthesis routes, coupled with unique optical properties and the capacity for surface modification, CDs have found numerous applications in areas like chemical and biosensing, bioimaging, photocatalysis and nanomedicine. As the integration of CQDs and AM continues to evolve, a wide variety of 3D-printed advanced functional materials has been produced. These systems are spreading from handheld smartphone platforms for sensing applications to cell and ion imaging, photoinitiation, antibacterial and anticounterfeiting applications. These groundbreaking advancements collectively demonstrate the potential for developing functional devices across fields ranging from food and the environment to biology and everyday consumer products.

The future of 3D printing technology based on CDs is poised to advance by focusing on optimization of the optical properties of CDs. Ongoing research efforts might be directed toward enhancing and broadening the optical capabilities of CDs. This endeavor includes the synthesis of CDs with high quantum yields, near-infrared (NIR) emission capabilities and prolonged phosphorescence. In the context of mass-producing 3D printing precursor materials, the production of high-quality CDs in substantial quantities remains a big challenge. Consequently, a focus will be placed on devising solutions to address these production challenges. Concerning AM, by developing or modifying advanced technologies, further improving could be carried out in order to enhance the resolution of complex structures, especially in ultrafast polymerization. The future outlook for these technologies appears promising, offering exciting possibilities for further innovation and practical applications.

REFERENCES

Ai, L., Song, Z., Nie, M., Yu, J., Liu, F., Song, H., Zhang, B., Waterhouse, G. I. N., & Lu, S. (2023). Solid-state fluorescence from carbon dots widely tunable from blue to deep red through surface ligand modulation. *Angewandte Chemie - International Edition*, *62*(12). https://doi.org/10.1002/anie.202217822

Arsène, M. M. J., Davares, A. K. L., Viktorovna, P. I., Andreevna, S. L., Sarra, S., Khelifi, I., & Sergueïevna, D. M. (2022). The public health issue of antibiotic residues in food and feed: Causes, consequences, and potential solutions. *Veterinary World*, *15*(3), 662.

Arshad, F., Pal, A., & Sk, M. P. (2021). Aggregation-induced emission in carbon dots for potential applications. *ECS Journal of Solid State Science and Technology*, *10*(2), 21001.

Attaran, M. (2017). The rise of 3-D printing: The advantages of additive manufacturing over traditional manufacturing. *Business Horizons*, *60*(5), 677–688. https://doi.org/10.1016/j.bushor.2017.05.011

Azadmanesh, F., Pourmadadi, M., Zavar Reza, J., Yazdian, F., Omidi, M., & Haghirosadat, B. F. (2021). Synthesis of a novel nanocomposite containing chitosan as a three-dimensional printed wound dressing technique: Emphasis on gene expression. *Biotechnology Progress*, *37*(4). https://doi.org/10.1002/btpr.3132

Butt, J. (2020). Exploring the Interrelationship between Additive Manufacturing and Industry 4.0. In *Designs* (Vol. 4, Issue 2). https://doi.org/10.3390/designs4020013

Casey, J. R., Grinstein, S., & Orlowski, J. (2010). Sensors and regulators of intracellular pH. *Nature Reviews Molecular Cell Biology*, *11*(1), 50–61.

Chandra Kishore, S., Samikannu, K., Atchudan, R., Perumal, S., Edison, T. N. J. I., Alagan, M., Sundramoorthy, A. K., & Lee, Y. R. (2022). Smartphone-operated wireless chemical sensors: A review. *Chemosensors*, *10*(2), 55.

Chang, D., Li, L., Dong, X., Shi, H., Wang, S., Zhao, Z., Lv, L., Yang, Y., & Shi, L. (2023). Dual photoluminescence emission carbon dots for ratiometric optical dual-mode and smartphone-integrated visual detection of mercury ion. *Journal of Environmental Chemical Engineering*, *11*(2), 109425. https://doi.org/10.1016/j.jece.2023.109425

Chen, J., Ying, G.-G., & Deng, W.-J. (2019). Antibiotic residues in food: Extraction, analysis, and human health concerns. *Journal of Agricultural and Food Chemistry*, *67*(27), 7569–7586.

Chen, L., Wang, C., Liu, C., & Chen, S. (2023). Facile access to fabricate carbon dots and perspective of large-scale applications. *Small*, *19*(31), 2206671.

Chen, T., Hou, K., Ren, Q., Chen, G., Wei, P., & Zhu, M. (2018). Nanoparticle–polymer synergies in nanocomposite hydrogels: From design to application. *Macromolecular Rapid Communications*, *39*(21), 1800337.

Choong, Y. Y. C. (2022). *Chapter 4 - Additive manufacturing for digital transformation* (C. D. Patel & C.-H. B. T.-D. M. Chen (eds.); pp. 145–182). Elsevier. https://doi.org/10.1016/B978-0-323-95062-6.00002-4

Clarissa, W. H.-Y., Chia, C. H., Zakaria, S., & Evyan, Y. C.-Y. (2022). Recent advancement in 3-D printing: Nanocomposites with added functionality. *Progress in Additive Manufacturing*, *7*(2), 325–350.

Dai, H., Shi, Y., Wang, Y., Sun, Y., Hu, J., Ni, P., & Li, Z. (2014). A carbon dot based biosensor for melamine detection by fluorescence resonance energy transfer. *Sensors and Actuators B: Chemical*, *202*, 201–208.

Deng, Y., Chen, M., Chen, G., Zou, W., Zhao, Y., Zhang, H., & Zhao, Q. (2021). Visible–ultraviolet upconversion carbon quantum dots for enhancement of the photocatalytic activity of titanium dioxide. *ACS Omega*, *6*(6), 4247–4254.

Destarac, M. (2018). Industrial development of reversible-deactivation radical polymerization: Is the induction period over? *Polymer Chemistry*, *9*(40), 4947–4967. https://doi.org/10.1039/c8py00970h

Dilberoglu, U. M., Gharehpapagh, B., Yaman, U., & Dolen, M. (2017). The role of additive manufacturing in the era of Industry 4.0. *Procedia Manufacturing*, *11*(June), 545–554. https://doi.org/10.1016/j.promfg.2017.07.148

Ding, C., Chen, X., Chen, X., Liu, Y., Xia, M., He, Z., Kang, Q., & Yan, X. (2023). Point-of-care testing for lysine concentration in swine serum via blue-emissive carbon dot-entrapped microfluidic chip. *Animal Nutrition*, *12*, 236–244. https://doi.org/10.1016/j.aninu.2022.08.017

Durrani, S., Yang, Z., Zhang, J., Wang, Z., Wang, H., Durrani, F., Wu, F.-G., & Lin, F. (2023). Nucleus-targeting pH-Responsive carbon dots for fast nucleus pH detection. *Talanta*, *252*, 123855. https://doi.org/10.1016/j.talanta.2022.123855

Dutta, S. D., Patil, T. V., Ganguly, K., Randhawa, A., Acharya, R., Moniruzzaman, M., & Lim, K. T. (2023). Trackable and highly fluorescent nanocellulose-based printable bio-resins for image-guided tissue regeneration. *Carbohydrate Polymers*, *320*(April), 121232. https://doi.org/10.1016/j.carbpol.2023.121232

Fekete, A., Frommberger, M., Rothballer, M., Li, X., Englmann, M., Fekete, J., Hartmann, A., Eberl, L., & Schmitt-Kopplin, P. (2007). Identification of bacterial N-acylhomoserine lactones (AHLs) with a combination of ultra-performance liquid chromatography (UPLC), ultra-high-resolution mass spectrometry, and in-situ biosensors. *Analytical and Bioanalytical Chemistry*, *387*(2), 455–467. https://doi.org/10.1007/s00216-006-0970-8

Fragogeorgi, E. A., Rouchota, M., Georgiou, M., Velez, M., Bouziotis, P., & Loudos, G. (2019). In vivo imaging techniques for bone tissue engineering. *Journal of Tissue Engineering*, *10*, 2041731419854586.

Gao, W., Xiang, S., Bai, M., Ruan, Y., Zheng, J., Cao, X., Xu, Y., Chen, Y., & Weng, W. (2022). Carbon dot crosslinking towards mechanochemically and photochemically induced fluorescence resonance energy transfer. *Polymer*, *257*, 125278.

Gao, Y., Zhou, D., Lyu, J., Sigen, A., Xu, Q., Newland, B., Matyjaszewski, K., Tai, H., & Wang, W. (2020). Complex polymer architectures through free-radical polymerization of multivinyl monomers. *Nature Reviews Chemistry*, *4*(4), 194–212. https://doi.org/10.1038/s41570-020-0170-7

García de Arquer, F. P., Talapin, D. V., Klimov, V. I., Arakawa, Y., Bayer, M., & Sargent, E. H. (2021). Semiconductor quantum dots: Technological progress and future challenges. *Science*, *373*(6555), eaaz8541.

Gibbs, S. L. (2012). Near infrared fluorescence for image-guided surgery. *Quantitative Imaging in Medicine and Surgery*, *2*(3), 177–187. https://doi.org/10.3978/j.issn.2223-4292.2012.09.04

Gibson, I., Rosen, D., Stucker, B., Khorasani, M., Gibson, I., Rosen, D., Stucker, B., & Khorasani, M. (2021). Materials for additive manufacturing. *Additive Manufacturing Technologies*, 379–428.

Gidwani, B., Sahu, V., Shukla, S. S., Pandey, R., Joshi, V., Jain, V. K., & Vyas, A. (2021). Quantum dots: Prospectives, toxicity, advances and applications. *Journal of Drug Delivery Science and Technology*, *61*, 102308. https://doi.org/10.1016/j.jddst.2020.102308

Gnanasekaran, K., Heijmans, T., Van Bennekom, S., Woldhuis, H., Wijnia, S., De With, G., & Friedrich, H. (2017). 3D printing of CNT-and graphene-based conductive polymer nanocomposites by fused deposition modeling. *Applied Materials Today*, *9*, 21–28.

Gopal, K., Tripathy, S. S., Bersillon, J. L., & Dubey, S. P. (2007). Chlorination byproducts, their toxicodynamics and removal from drinking water. *Journal of Hazardous Materials*, *140*(1), 1–6. https://doi.org/10.1016/j.jhazmat.2006.10.063

Guo, G., Li, T., Zheng, Q., Tang, S., Hu, H., Wang, X., & Chen, D. (2023). Dual-excitation carbon dots-based lateral flow visual sensing device for ratiometric determination and discrimination of tetracyclines in food. *Sensors and Actuators B: Chemical*, *395*(July), 134523 https://doi.org/10.1016/j.snb.2023.134523

Guo, H., Lv, R., & Bai, S. (2019). Recent advances on 3D printing graphene-based composites. *Nano Materials Science*, *1*(2), 101–115.

Gupta, V., Nesterenko, P., & Paull, B. (2019). An introduction to 3D printing. *3D Printing in Chemical Sciences: Applications across Chemistry*. London, UK: *The Royal Society of Chemistry*, 1–21.

Haider, A. A., Cun, Y., Bai, X., Xu, Z., Zi, Y., Qiu, J., Song, Z., Huang, A., & Yang, Z. (2022). Anti-counterfeiting applications by photochromism induced modulation of reversible upconversion luminescence in TiO 2: Yb 3+, Er 3+ ceramic. *Journal of Materials Chemistry C, 10*(16), 6243–6251.

Hales, S., Tokita, E., Neupane, R., Ghosh, U., Elder, B., Wirthlin, D., & Kong, Y. L. (2020). 3D printed nanomaterial-based electronic, biomedical, and bioelectronic devices. *Nanotechnology, 31*(17), 172001.

Han, J., & Burgess, K. (2010). Fluorescent indicators for intracellular pH. *Chemical Reviews, 110*(5), 2709–2728.

Han, M., Zhu, S., Lu, S., Song, Y., Feng, T., Tao, S., Liu, J., & Yang, B. (2018). Recent progress on the photocatalysis of carbon dots: Classification, mechanism and applications. *Nano Today, 19*, 201–218.

Huang, X., Shi, M., Zhai, H., Zhang, Y., Zhang, Y., & Zhao, Y. (2022). Nitrogen-doped carbon dots as visible light initiators for 3D (bio)printing. *Polymer Chemistry, 14*(3), 268–276. https://doi.org/10.1039/d2py01324j

Huang, Y., Zhu, Y., & Egap, E. (2018). Semiconductor quantum dots as photocatalysts for controlled light-mediated radical polymerization. *ACS Macro Letters, 7*(2), 184–189.

Hutton, G. A. M., Reuillard, B., Martindale, B. C. M., Caputo, C. A., Lockwood, C. W. J., Butt, J. N., & Reisner, E. (2016). Carbon dots as versatile photosensitizers for solar-driven catalysis with redox enzymes. *Journal of the American Chemical Society, 138*(51), 16722–16730.

Jain, K., Shukla, R., Yadav, A., Ujjwal, R. R., & Flora, S. J. S. (2021). 3D printing in development of nanomedicines. *Nanomaterials, 11*(2), 420.

Jiang, K., Sun, S., Zhang, L., Lu, Y., Wu, A., Cai, C., & Lin, H. (2015). Red, green, and blue luminescence by carbon dots: Full-color emission tuning and multicolor cellular imaging. *Angewandte Chemie, 127*(18), 5450–5453.

Kalytchuk, S., Wang, Y., Poláková, K., & Zboril, R. (2018). Carbon dot fluorescence-lifetime-encoded anti-counterfeiting. *ACS Applied Materials & Interfaces, 10*(35), 29902–29908.

Kim, G., Lim, J., & Mo, C. (2015). A review on lateral flow test strip for food safety. *Journal of Biosystems Engineering, 40*(3), 277–283.

Kong, Y. L., Tamargo, I. A., Kim, H., Johnson, B. N., Gupta, M. K., Koh, T.-W., Chin, H.-A., Steingart, D. A., Rand, B. P., & McAlpine, M. C. (2014). 3D printed quantum dot light-emitting diodes. *Nano Letters, 14*(12), 7017–7023.

Krys, P., & Matyjaszewski, K. (2017). Kinetics of atom transfer radical polymerization. *European Polymer Journal, 89*, 482–523.

Kumar, L. J., Pandey, P. M., & Wimpenny, D. I. (2019). *3D printing and additive manufacturing technologies* (Vol. 311). Springer.

Lee, K. K., Raja, N., Yun, H. Suk, Lee, S. C., & Lee, C. S. (2023). Multifunctional bone substitute using carbon dot and 3D printed calcium-deficient hydroxyapatite scaffolds for osteoclast inhibition and fluorescence imaging. *Acta Biomaterialia, 159*, 382–393. https://doi.org/10.1016/j.actbio.2023.01.028

Lee, M., Rizzo, R., Surman, F., & Zenobi-Wong, M. (2020). Guiding lights: Tissue bioprinting using photoactivated materials. *Chemical Reviews, 120*(19), 10950–11027. https://doi.org/10.1021/acs.chemrev.0c00077

Lei, M., Zheng, J., Yang, Y., Yan, L., Liu, X., & Xu, B. (2022). Carbon dots-based delayed fluorescent materials: Mechanism, structural regulation and application. *Iscience*.

Lesani, P., Singh, G., Lu, Z., Mirkhalaf, M., New, E. J., & Zreiqat, H. (2022). Two-photon ratiometric carbon dot-based probe for real-time intracellular pH monitoring in 3D environment. *Chemical Engineering Journal, 433*(P3), 133668. https://doi.org/10.1016/j.cej.2021.133668

Li, C., Qin, Z., Wang, M., Liu, W., Jiang, H., & Wang, X. (2020). Manganese oxide doped carbon dots for temperature-responsive biosensing and target bioimaging. *Analytica Chimica Acta, 1104*, 125–131.

Li, C., Xu, X., Wang, F., Zhao, Y., Shi, Y., Zhao, X., & Liu, J. (2023a). Portable smartphone platform integrated with paper strip-assisted fluorescence sensor for ultrasensitive and visual quantitation of ascorbic acid. *Food Chemistry, 402*(August 2022), 134222. https://doi.org/10.1016/j.foodchem.2022.134222

Li, D., & Wang, J. (2023). Semiconductor/carbon quantum dot-based hue recognition strategy for point of need testing: A review. *ChemistryOpen, 12*(4), e202200165.

Li, J., & Zhu, J.-J. (2013). Quantum dots for fluorescent biosensing and bio-imaging applications. *Analyst, 138*(9), 2506–2515.

Li, L., Shi, L., Jia, J., Eltayeb, O., Lu, W., Tang, Y., Dong, C., & Shuang, S. (2021a). Red fluorescent carbon dots for tetracycline antibiotics and pH discrimination from aggregation-induced emission mechanism. *Sensors and Actuators B: Chemical, 332*, 129513.

Li, L., Yang, L., Lin, D., Xu, S., Mei, C., Yu, S., & Jiang, C. (2023b). Hydrogen-bond induced enhanced emission ratiometric fluorescent handy needle for visualization assay of amoxicillin by smartphone sensing platform. *Journal of Hazardous Materials, 444*(PA), 130403. https://doi.org/10.1016/j.jhazmat.2022.130403

Li, S., Li, L., Tu, H., Zhang, H., Silvester, D. S., Banks, C. E., Zou, G., Hou, H., & Ji, X. (2021b). The development of carbon dots: From the perspective of materials chemistry. *Materials Today, 51*(December), 188–207. https://doi.org/10.1016/j.mattod.2021.07.028

Liang, H., Wang, Y., Zhang, L., Cao, Y., Guo, M., Yu, Y., & Lin, B. (2022a). Construction of integrated and portable fluorescence sensor and the application for visual detection in situ. *Sensors and Actuators B: Chemical, 373*(August), 132764. https://doi.org/10.1016/j.snb.2022.132764

Liang, K., Wang, R., Huo, B., Ren, H., Li, D., Wang, Y., Tang, Y., Chen, Y., Song, C., & Li, F. (2022b). Fully printed optoelectronic synaptic transistors based on quantum dot–metal oxide semiconductor heterojunctions. *ACS Nano, 16*(6), 8651–8661.

Liguori, A., Garfias González, K. I., & Hakkarainen, M. (2023). Unexpected self-assembly of carbon dots during digital light processing 3D printing of vanillin Schiff-base resin. *Polymer, 283*(June). https://doi.org/10.1016/j.polymer.2023.126252

Liu, J., Li, R., & Yang, B. (2020). Carbon dots: A new type of carbon-based nanomaterial with wide applications. *ACS Central Science, 6*(12), 2179–2195. https://doi.org/10.1021/acscentsci.0c01306

Liu, T., Chen, S., Ruan, K., Zhang, S., He, K., Li, J., Chen, M., Yin, J., Sun, M., Wang, X., Wang, Y., Lu, Z., & Rao, H. (2022). A handheld multifunctional smartphone platform integrated with 3D printing portable device: On-site evaluation for glutathione and azodicarbonamide with machine learning. *Journal of Hazardous Materials, 426* (September 2021), 128091. https://doi.org/10.1016/j.jhazmat.2021.128091

Long, C., Jiang, Z., Shangguan, J., Qing, T., Zhang, P., & Feng, B. (2021). Applications of carbon dots in environmental pollution control: A review. *Chemical Engineering Journal, 406*, 126848. https://doi.org/10.1016/j.cej.2020.126848

Lu, C.-H., Yu, C.-H., & Yeh, Y.-C. (2021). Engineering nanocomposite hydrogels using dynamic bonds. *Acta Biomaterialia, 130*, 66–79.

Lu, C. H., & Yeh, Y. C. (2022). Synthesis and processing of dynamic covalently crosslinked polydextran/Carbon dot nanocomposite hydrogels with tailorable microstructures and properties. *ACS Biomaterials Science and Engineering, 8*(10), 4289–4300. https://doi.org/10.1021/acsbiomaterials.2c00873

Luo, P. G., Yang, F., Yang, S.-T., Sonkar, S. K., Yang, L., Broglie, J. J., Liu, Y., & Sun, Y.-P. (2014). Carbon-based quantum dots for fluorescence imaging of cells and tissues. *Rsc Advances, 4*(21), 10791–10807.

Luo, X., Huang, G., Li, Y., Guo, J., Chen, X., Tan, Y., Tang, W., & Li, Z. (2022). Dual-modes of ratiometric fluorescent and smartphone-integrated colorimetric detection of glyphosate by carbon dots encapsulated porphyrin metal–organic frameworks. *Applied Surface Science*, *602*(July), 154368. https://doi.org/10.1016/j.apsusc.2022.154368

Macairan, J.-R., de Medeiros, T. V., Gazzetto, M., Yarur Villanueva, F., Cannizzo, A., & Naccache, R. (2022). Elucidating the mechanism of dual-fluorescence in carbon dots. *Journal of Colloid and Interface Science*, *606*, 67–76. https://doi.org/10.1016/j.jcis.2021.07.156

Maleksaeedi, S., Meenashisundaram, G. K., Lu, S., Salehi, M., & Jun, W. (2018). Hybrid binder to mitigate feed powder segregation in the inkjet 3D printing of titanium metal parts. *Metals*, *8*(5), 322.

Martynenko, I. V., Litvin, A. P., Purcell-Milton, F., Baranov, A. V., Fedorov, A. V., & Gun'Ko, Y. K. (2017). Application of semiconductor quantum dots in bioimaging and biosensing. *Journal of Materials Chemistry B*, *5*(33), 6701–6727.

Matyjaszewski, K., & Davis, T. P. (2002). *Handbook of Radical Polymerization*.

Meng, W., Bai, X., Wang, B., Liu, Z., Lu, S., & Yang, B. (2019). Biomass-derived carbon dots and their applications. *Energy & Environmental Materials*, *2*(3), 172–192.

Mostafaei, A., Elliott, A. M., Barnes, J. E., Li, F., Tan, W., Cramer, C. L., Nandwana, P., & Chmielus, M. (2021). Binder jet 3D printing—Process parameters, materials, properties, modeling, and challenges. *Progress in Materials Science*, *119*(May 2020), 100707. https://doi.org/10.1016/j.pmatsci.2020.100707

Ni, J., Huang, X., Bai, Y., Zhao, B., Han, Y., Han, S., Xu, T., Si, C., & Zhang, C. (2022). Resistance to aggregation-caused quenching: chitosan-based solid carbon dots for white light-emitting diode and 3D printing. *Advanced Composites and Hybrid Materials*, *5*(3), 1865–1875. https://doi.org/10.1007/s42114-022-00483-6

Oztan, C., Ginzburg, E., Akin, M., Zhou, Y., Leblanc, R. M., & Coverstone, V. (2021). 3D printed ABS/paraffin hybrid rocket fuels with carbon dots for superior combustion performance. *Combustion and Flame*, *225*, 428–434. https://doi.org/10.1016/j.combustflame.2020.11.024

Pan, X., Tasdelen, M. A., Laun, J., Junkers, T., Yagci, Y., & Matyjaszewski, K. (2016). Photomediated controlled radical polymerization. *Progress in Polymer Science*, *62*, 73–125. https://doi.org/10.1016/j.progpolymsci.2016.06.005

Paramasivam, G., Palem, V. V., Sundaram, T., Sundaram, V., Kishore, S. C., & Bellucci, S. (2021). Nanomaterials: Synthesis and applications in theranostics. *Nanomaterials*, *11*(12), 3228.

Patel, C. D., & Chen, C. H. (2022). Digital manufacturing: The Industrialization of "Art to Part" 3D Additive Printing. In *Digital Manufacturing: The Industrialization of "Art to Part" 3D Additive Printing*. https://doi.org/10.1016/C2020-0-02835-5

Pawar, A. A., Halivni, S., Waiskopf, N., Ben-Shahar, Y., Soreni-Harari, M., Bergbreiter, S., Banin, U., & Magdassi, S. (2017). Rapid three-dimensional printing in water using semiconductor-metal hybrid nanoparticles as photoinitiators. In *Nano Letters* (Vol. 17, Issue 7, pp. 4497–4501). https://doi.org/10.1021/acs.nanolett.7b01870

Pröfrock, D., & Prange, A. (2012). Inductively coupled plasma–mass spectrometry (ICP-MS) for quantitative analysis in environmental and life sciences: A review of challenges, solutions, and trends. *Applied Spectroscopy*, *66*(8), 843–868.

Qiao, L., Zhou, M., Shi, G., Cui, Z., Zhang, X., Fu, P., Liu, M., Qiao, X., He, Y., & Pang, X. (2022). Ultrafast visible-light-induced ATRP in aqueous media with carbon quantum dots as the catalyst and its application for 3D printing. *Journal of the American Chemical Society*, *144*(22), 9817–9826. https://doi.org/10.1021/jacs.2c02303

Quan, H., Zhang, T., Xu, H., Luo, S., Nie, J., & Zhu, X. (2020). Photo-curing 3D printing technique and its challenges. *Bioactive Materials*, *5*(1), 110–115. https://doi.org/10.1016/j.bioactmat.2019.12.003

Ren, S., Liu, B., Wang, M., Han, G., Zhao, H., & Zhang, Y. (2022). Highly bright carbon quantum dots for flexible anti-counterfeiting. *Journal of Materials Chemistry C, 10*(31), 11338–11346.

Ru, Y., Waterhouse, G. I. N., & Lu, S. (2022). Aggregation in carbon dots: Special Issue: Emerging Investigators. *Aggregate, 3*(6), e296.

Rutherford, S. T., & Bassler, B. L. (2012). Bacterial quorum sensing: Its role in virulence and possibilities for its control. *Cold Spring Harbor Perspectives in Medicine, 2*(11), a012427.

Saranti, A., Tiron-Stathopoulos, A., Papaioannou, L., Gioti, C., Ioannou, A., Karakassides, M. A., Avgoustakis, K., Koutselas, I., & Dimos, K. (2022). 3D-printed bioactive scaffolds for bone regeneration bearing carbon dots for bioimaging purposes. *Smart Materials in Medicine, 3*(August 2021), 12–19. https://doi.org/10.1016/j.smaim.2021.11.002

Shi, L., Feng, J., Li, X., Zhou, W., Zhang, G., Zhang, Y., Zhang, C., & Shuang, S. (2023). Handheld detection strategy: Real-time on-site assay of Mn(VII) and GSH integrating ratiometric fluorescent carbon dots paper strip, smartphone, and 3D-printed accessory. *Sensors and Actuators B: Chemical, 375*(July 2022), 132871 https://doi.org/10.1016/j.snb.2022.132871

Shirai, M. (2015). Photoinitiated polymerization. In *Encyclopedia of Polymeric Nanomaterials* (pp. 1579–1585). Springer Berlin Heidelberg: Berlin, Heidelberg.

Shukla, S., Pandey, P. C., & Narayan, R. J. (2021). Tunable quantum photoinitiators for radical photopolymerization. *Polymers, 13*(16), 1–20. https://doi.org/10.3390/polym13162694

Solanki, R., Patra, I., Kumar, T. C. H. A., Kumar, N. B., Kandeel, M., Sivaraman, R., Turki Jalil, A., Yasin, G., Sharma, S., & Abdulameer Marhoon, H. (2022). Smartphone-based techniques using carbon dot nanomaterials for food safety analysis. *Critical Reviews in Analytical Chemistry*, 1–19.

Suh, Y. J., Lim, T. H., Choi, H. S., Kim, M. S., Lee, S. J., Kim, S. H., & Park, C. H. (2020). 3D printing and nir fluorescence imaging techniques for the fabrication of implants. *Materials, 13*(21), 1–18. https://doi.org/10.3390/ma13214819

Sun, Y.-P., Zhou, B., Lin, Y., Wang, W., Fernando, K. A. S., Pathak, P., Meziani, M. J., Harruff, B. A., Wang, X., & Wang, H. (2006). Quantum-sized carbon dots for bright and colorful photoluminescence. *Journal of the American Chemical Society, 128*(24), 7756–7757.

Tang, S., Chen, D., Guo, G., Li, X., Wang, C., Li, T., & Wang, G. (2022). A smartphone-integrated optical sensing platform based on Lycium ruthenicum derived carbon dots for real-time detection of Ag+. *Science of the Total Environment, 825*, 153913. https://doi.org/10.1016/j.scitotenv.2022.153913

Tardy, A., Nicolas, J., Gigmes, D., Lefay, C., & Guillaneuf, Y. (2017). Radical ring-opening polymerization: Scope, Limitations, and Application to (Bio)Degradable Materials. *Chemical Reviews, 117*(3), 1319–1406. https://doi.org/10.1021/acs.chemrev.6b00319

Tene, T., Arias Arias, F., Guevara, M., Nuñez, A., Villamagua, L., Tapia, C., Pisarra, M., Torres, F. J., Caputi, L. S., & Vacacela Gomez, C. (2022). Removal of mercury(II) from aqueous solution by partially reduced graphene oxide. *Scientific Reports, 12*(1), 6326. https://doi.org/10.1038/s41598-022-10259-z

Timoshenko, V. Y. (2023). Quantum dots: Optical properties. In *Reference Module in Materials Science and Materials Engineering*. Elsevier. https://doi.org/10.1016/B978-0-323-90800-9.00177-3

Tomal, W., Świergosz, T., Pilch, M., Kasprzyk, W., & Ortyl, J. (2021). New horizons for carbon dots: Quantum nano-photoinitiating catalysts for cationic photopolymerization and three-dimensional (3D) printing under visible light. *Polymer Chemistry, 12*(25), 3661–3676. https://doi.org/10.1039/d1py00228g

Uriarte, D., Vidal, E., Canals, A., Domini, C. E., & Garrido, M. (2021). Simple-to-use and portable device for free chlorine determination based on microwave-assisted synthesized carbon dots and smartphone images. *Talanta, 229*(March). https://doi.org/10.1016/j.talanta.2021.122298

Vidal, E., Lorenzetti, A. S., Aguirre, M. Á., Canals, A., & Domini, C. E. (2020). New, inexpensive and simple 3D printable device for nephelometric and fluorimetric determination based on smartphone sensing. *RSC Advances, 10*(33), 19713–19719. https://doi.org/10.1039/d0ra02975k

Waiskopf, N., Magdassi, S., & Banin, U. (2021). Quantum photoinitiators: Toward emerging photocuring applications. *Journal of the American Chemical Society, 143*(2), 577–587. https://doi.org/10.1021/jacs.0c10554

Walling, M. A., Novak, J. A., & Shepard, J. R. E. (2009). Quantum dots for live cell and *in vivo* imaging. In *International Journal of Molecular Sciences*, 10(2), 441–491. https://doi.org/10.3390/ijms10020441

Wang, B., & Lu, S. (2022). The light of carbon dots: From mechanism to applications. *Matter, 5*(1), 110–149. https://doi.org/10.1016/j.matt.2021.10.016

Wang, B., Waterhouse, G. I. N., & Lu, S. (2023a). Carbon dots: mysterious past, vibrant present, and expansive future. *Trends in Chemistry*.

Wang, C., Wang, Z., Zhao, T., Li, Y., Huang, G., Sumer, B. D., & Gao, J. (2018). Optical molecular imaging for tumor detection and image-guided surgery. *Biomaterials, 157*, 62–75. https://doi.org/10.1016/j.biomaterials.2017.12.002

Wang, H., Zhang, B., Zhang, J., He, X., Liu, F., Cui, J., Lu, Z., Hu, G., Yang, J., Zhou, Z., Wang, R., Hou, X., Ma, L., Ren, P., Ge, Q., Li, P., & Huang, W. (2021). General one-pot method for preparing highly water-soluble and biocompatible photoinitiators for digital light processing-based 3D printing of hydrogels. *ACS Applied Materials & Interfaces, 13*(46), 55507–55516. https://doi.org/10.1021/acsami.1c15636

Wang, L., Zhang, J., Zhang, X., Shi, G., He, Y., Cui, Z., Zhang, X., Fu, P., Liu, M., Qiao, X., & Pang, X. (2023b). High colloidal stable carbon dots armored liquid metal nanodroplets for versatile 3D/4D Printing through Digital Light Processing (DLP). *Energy & Environmental Materials*, 1–7. https://doi.org/10.1002/eem2.12609

Wang, Q., Zhang, S., Wang, B., Yang, X., Zou, B., Yang, B., & Lu, S. (2019). Pressure-triggered aggregation-induced emission enhancement in red emissive amorphous carbon dots. *Nanoscale Horizons, 4*(5), 1227–1231.

WHO. (n.d.). *Estimating the burden of foodborne diseases*. https://www.who.int/activities/estimating-the-burden-of-foodborne-diseases

Wohlers, T., & Caffrey, T. (2010). Additive manufacturing state of the industry. *Wohlers Report*.

Wong, S.-F., & Khor, S. M. (2019). State-of-the-art of differential sensing techniques in analytical sciences. *TrAC Trends in Analytical Chemistry, 114*, 108–125.

Wu, X., Lv, X., Wang, J., Sun, L., & Yan, Y. (2017). Surface molecular imprinted polymers based on Mn-doped ZnS quantum dots by atom transfer radical polymerization for a room-temperature phosphorescence probe of bifenthrin. *Analytical Methods, 9*(31), 4609–4615.

Xia, C., Zhu, S., Feng, T., Yang, M., & Yang, B. (2019). Evolution and synthesis of carbon dots: From carbon dots to carbonized polymer dots. *Advanced Science, 6*(23). https://doi.org/10.1002/advs.201901316

Xu, J., Ning, J., Wang, Y., Xu, M., Yi, C., & Yan, F. (2022). Carbon dots as a promising therapeutic approach for combating cancer. *Bioorganic & Medicinal Chemistry, 72*, 116987. https://doi.org/10.1016/j.bmc.2022.116987

Xu, L., Lu, Z., Cao, L., Pang, H., Zhang, Q., Fu, Y., Xiong, Y., Li, Y., Wang, X., Wang, J., Ying, Y., & Li, Y. (2017). In-field detection of multiple pathogenic bacteria in food products using a portable fluorescent biosensing system. *Food Control, 75*, 21–28. https://doi.org/10.1016/j.foodcont.2016.12.018

Xue, S.-S., Pan, Y., Pan, W., Liu, S., Li, N., & Tang, B. (2022). Bioimaging agents based on redox-active transition metal complexes. *Chemical Science*.

Yagci, Y., Jockusch, S., & Turro, N. J. (2010). Photoinitiated polymerization: Advances, challenges, and opportunities. *Macromolecules, 43*(15), 6245–6260. https://doi.org/10.1021/ma1007545

Yan, L., Zhang, B., Zong, Z., Zhou, W., Shuang, S., & Shi, L. (2023). Artificial intelligence-integrated smartphone-based handheld detection of fluoride ion by Al^{3+}-triggered aggregation-induced red-emssion enhanced carbon dots. *Journal of Colloid and Interface Science, 651*(June), 59–67. https://doi.org/10.1016/j.jcis.2023.07.125

Yang, F., Yang, L., Xu, L., Guo, W., Pan, L., Zhang, C., Xu, S., Zhang, N., Yang, L., & Jiang, C. (2021). 3D-printed smartphone-based device for fluorimetric diagnosis of ketosis by acetone-responsive dye marker and red emissive carbon dots. *Microchimica Acta, 188*(9). https://doi.org/10.1007/s00604-021-04965-0

Yang, X., Sun, J., Cui, F., Ji, J., Wang, L., Zhang, Y., & Sun, X. (2020). An eco-friendly sensor based on CQD@MIPs for detection of N-acylated homoserine lactones and its 3D printing applications. *Talanta, 219*(March), 121343. https://doi.org/10.1016/j.talanta.2020.121343

Yat, Y. D., Foo, H. C. Y., Tan, I. S., Lam, M. K., & Lim, S. (2022). Carbon dots and miniaturizing fabrication of portable carbon dots-based devices for bioimaging, biosensing, heavy metals detection and drug delivery applications. *Journal of Materials Chemistry C.*

Yoshinaga, T., Shinoda, M., Iso, Y., Isobe, T., Ogura, A., & Takao, K. (2021). Glycothermally synthesized carbon dots with narrow-bandwidth and color-tunable solvatochromic fluorescence for wide-color-gamut displays. *ACS Omega, 6*(2), 1741–1750.

Yu, X., Zhang, H., & Yu, J. (2021). Luminescence anti-counterfeiting: From elementary to advanced. *Aggregate, 2*(1), 20–34.

Zarei, M., Shabani Dargah, M., Hasanzadeh Azar, M., Alizadeh, R., Mahdavi, F. S., Sayedain, S. S., Kaviani, A., Asadollahi, M., Azami, M., & Beheshtizadeh, N. (2023). Enhanced bone tissue regeneration using a 3D-printed poly (lactic acid)/Ti6Al4V composite scaffold with plasma treatment modification. *Scientific Reports, 13*(1), 3139.

Zhang, C., Shen, K., Li, B., Li, S., & Yang, S. (2018). Continuously 3D printed quantum dot-based electrodes for lithium storage with ultrahigh capacities. *Journal of Materials Chemistry A, 6*(41), 19960–19966.

Zhang, J., & Yu, S.-H. (2016). Carbon dots: Large-scale synthesis, sensing and bioimaging. *Materials Today, 19*(7), 382–393.

Zhang, W., Jia, L., Guo, X., Yang, R., Zhang, Y., & Zhao, Z. (2019). Green synthesis of up-and down-conversion photoluminescent carbon dots from coffee beans for Fe^{3+} detection and cell imaging. *Analyst, 144*(24), 7421–7431.

Zhang, Y., Wang, J., Wang, L., Fu, R., Sui, L., Song, H., Hu, Y., & Lu, S. (2023). Carbon dots with blue-to-near-infrared lasing for colorful speckle-free laser imaging and dynamical holographic display. *Advanced Materials*, 2302536.

Zhou, Y., Mintz, K. J., Oztan, C. Y., Hettiarachchi, S. D., Peng, Z., Seven, E. S., Liyanage, P. Y., De La Torre, S., Celik, E., & Leblanc, R. M. (2018). Embedding carbon dots in superabsorbent polymers for additive manufacturing. *Polymers, 10*(8), 1–12. https://doi.org/10.3390/polym10080921

Zhou, Y., Zhang, S., Li, S., Wei, L., & Zhang, L. (2022). Multifunctional N doped carbon dots for cellular sensing, light-emitting-diode, and additive manufacturing. *Materials Letters, 325*(July), 14–17. https://doi.org/10.1016/j.matlet.2022.132838

Zhu, Z., Cheng, R., Ling, L., Li, Q., & Chen, S. (2020). Rapid and large-scale production of multi-fluorescence carbon dots by a magnetic hyperthermia method. *Angewandte Chemie International Edition, 59*(8), 3099–3105.

12 Carbon Quantum Dots for Bioimaging

Anuja A Vibhute and Arpita Pandey-Tiwari

12.1 INTRODUCTION

Carbon quantum dots (CQDs) are an important class of fluorescent molecules. CQDs have physiochemical and biomedical properties, including biocompatibility, low toxicity, small size, chemical inertness, as well as exhibit promising optical properties. They have tunable emission spectra, broad excitation spectra, and high photostability (M. L. Liu et al., 2019a; Vibhute et al., 2023).

CQDs have gained importance in nanochemistry, which has led to the identification of applications, particularly in the field of biomedicine. Due to their advantages, CQDs have enormous potential in the fields of biology and medicine. Moreover, to expand usefulness in biological applications like bioimaging, biosensing, drug delivery, and nanomedicine, electrocatalysis CQDs has been used in research (Vibhute, Patil, et al., 2022). Due to excellent photoluminescence property of CQDs, they are used in bioimaging (Pandey & Bodas, 2020; Vibhute, Nille, et al., 2022). For efficient bioimaging, CQDs must have adequate brightness, imaging sensitivity, and photostability. They can also withstand the biodegradation brought on by different enzymes (Lin et al., 2019).

The surface functionalization and type of CQD is the key point to image human cells, fungi, and bacteria, and also visualize intracellular structures of cells such as nuclei, mitochondria, etc. CQD's low cytotoxicity is unrelated to the source of raw materials utilized to make them. Also, they do not alter the shape of the cell (Molkenova et al., 2020). However, various cell or tissue types have distinctive forms and compositions, as well as associated biomarkers on the membrane or in the cytoplasm, which cause a particular reaction to foreign nanoparticles (Speranza, 2021).

The chapter summarizes the bioimaging applications of CQDs including imaging of various ions, molecules, organelles, and cells. Each imaging part has been given a through description therein.

12.2 CARBON QUANTUM DOTS FOR BIOIMAGING

The advancements in bioimaging aim to communicate the possibilities as well as the challenges in bioimaging, bringing together several fields, outlining remaining constraints, and outlining solutions, hopefully creating new opportunities for

DOI: 10.1201/9781003437857-14

understanding cells and treating diseases. To comprehend different intracellular processes, imaging probes are essential. They must, however, easily enter cells, be tiny (ideally less than 10 nm), and interact with a particular compartment or biochemical.

Fluorescent CQDs are perfect in this regard because of their small size. CQDs have demonstrated excellent potential to be used as probes for analyzing biological systems due to their special properties, which include their ability to tune surface functions, superior photostability, high brightness, notable biocompatibility, and spontaneous penetration capabilities. This makes CQDs particularly appealing for imaging-guided biomedical applications (Geng et al., 2018; J. Zhang & Yu, 2016). They can also be functionalized to target specific intracellular elements, chemicals, or biomolecules, such as glutathione, amino acids, and DNA, as well as intracellular structures including lysosomes, mitochondria, and nuclei.

The key fluorescent CQD-based probes created for imaging different intracellular components/chemicals are listed in Table 12.1. Further details on these applications are provided in this section.

12.2.1 Imaging of Intracellular Ions

The metal ions and reactive oxygen species have specific intracellular role. So, assessing specific intracellular activity and imaging of ions are essential. For the selective capture of these ions, appropriately functionalized carbon dots are employed. CQDs have been combined with metals like gadolinium, which lessens their toxicity to organs and also stop their leakage (Q. Jiang et al., 2021). Cancer and other illnesses can arise when Fe^{3+} ion levels are abnormal. The majority of the fluorescence sensors for Fe^{3+} ion detection being developed now are based on CQDs.

Gao et al. have demonstrated N-[3-(trimethoxysilyl) propyl]ethylenediamine (DAMO) functionalized CQDs for sensitive detection of Fe^{3+} in living cells and zebrafish. A more significant finding revealed that the combination of CQDs and Fe^{3+} (CQDs/Fe^{3+}) could effectively distinguish between cancerous and normal cells based on the reductive environment of cancerous cells, particularly the variation in cellular glutathione (GSH) *in vitro* and *in vivo* (Figure 12.1), offering a quick method for cancer diagnosis (Gao et al., 2018). Similarly, for the fluorescence detection of Fe^{3+} ions in cervical cancer, carbon dots with nitrogen and sulfur co-doping made from cellulose-based biowaste were used (C. Cheng et al., 2019).

Potassium (K^+) fluorescent nanoprobes and the cationic liposome 1,2-dioleoyl-3-trimethylammonium-propanechloride (DOTAP) together stained hERG-HEK293 cells. The results of the screening of hERG channel inhibitors using K^+ fluorescent nanoprobes were consistent with those obtained using the conventional patch-clamp method and commercially available thallium ion (Tl^+) fluorescent probe test kits (Pan et al., 2021).

Intracellular pH sensing was done with pH-sensitive CQDs for better understanding of a cell's activity, which is done by estimating the internal pH of living cells. Nitrogen-doped Shiitake mushroom-derived CQDs were employed for intracellular pH sensing (W. J. Wang et al., 2016). Figure 12.2 shows that yellow emissive CQDs were used for monitoring full range of intracellular pH variations (S. Zhang et al., 2020).

TABLE 12.1

An Overview of Intracellular Imaging Probes Using Fluorescent Carbon Dots

S. No	Carbon Source	Conjugated Biomolecule, Nanoprobe Size	Imaging Probe	References
1.	Glycerol and a silane molecule	Nitrogen doping, ~6.1 nm	Fe^{3+}	Gao et al. (2018)
2.	(3-aminopropyl) triethoxysilane (APTES)	3.5 ± 0.5 nm	Mitochondria	Gao et al. (2017)
3.	p-phenylenediamine	4-formylbenzeneboronic acid, ~1.73 nm	Cell nucleus	Phukan et al. (2022)
4.	Citric acid	Poly ethylene glycol,	Cell nucleus	Yang et al. (2015)
5.	Citric acid	N,N-dimethylaniline, 2~0.4 nm	Lysosome	Guo et al. (2020)
6.	Konjac flour	magnetic mesoporous silica nanoparticles	Mitochondria	Y. Zhang et al. (2015)
7.	o-phenylenediamine	(3-Carboxyprop-1-yl) (triphenyl) phosphonium bromide, 3–8 nm	Peroxynitrite in mitochondria	X. Wu et al. (2017)
8.	2,4-dihydroxybenzaldehyde, 2,3-dimethylbenzothiazole iodide	–, 6.78 ± 0.3 nm	RNA	Yin et al. (2020)
9.	m-phenylenediamine, 1,2,3-propanetricarboxylic acid	–, 4.34 ± 1.13 nm	ClO^- in cell nucleus	H. Wu et al. (2021)
10.	L-tryptophan, L-phenylalanine	DNA, 4.8 nm	MFC-7, HepG 2 cells	Z. Wang et al. (2016)
11.	Lotus root	Glutathione, 1–3.8 nm	Human bladder cancer T24 cells	Yu et al. (2019)
12.	$CdSO_4$, C. sinensis plant leaves	–, 2–5 nm	A549 lung cancer cell	Shivaji et al. (2018)
13.	Sucrose, oil acid	–, ~1.84 nm	16HBE cells	B. Chen et al. (2013)
14.	Polyolefin waste	–, 1.5–3.5 nm	MDA-MB 468 cell	Kumari et al. (2018)
15.	Citric acid-urea/neutral red-triethyl amine	MnO_2 nanosheet/MnO_2 nanoflower, ~5 nm	Glutathione	He et al. (2015)
16.	2-azidoimidazole	–, 5.0 nm	Cysteine	Tang et al. (2017)
17.	Gram shells	–, 3–5 nm	Escherichia coli	Das et al. (2017)
18.	Aconitic acid	–, 1.6 nm	Targeted imaging of folate receptor overexpressed cancer cells	Qian et al. (2018)
19.	Tartaric acid, urea	–, 3 nm	Multicolor cell imaging	Konar et al. (2019)
20.	Folic acid	Stearic acid-g-polyethyleneimine, –	Triple Negative Breast Cancer	Sarkar et al. (2021)
21.	Citric acid, Folic acid	Bevacizumab,	Magnetic resonance imaging of hepatocellular carcinoma	Maghsoudinia et al. (2021)

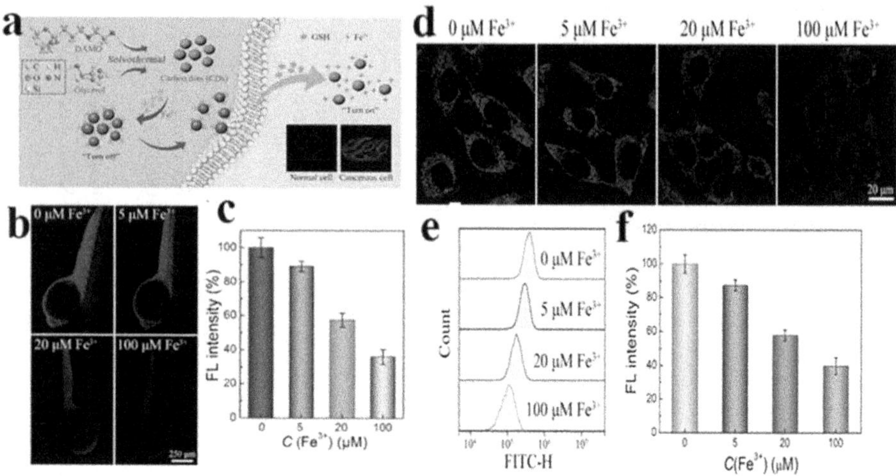

FIGURE 12.1 (a) Graphical representation of Fe^{3+} ion detection, (b) CLSM images of zebrafish treated with CDs (200 mg/mL) for 4 h, and then incubated with 0, 5, 20, or 100 mM Fe3þ for 2 h. (c) The corresponding average fluorescence statistics of the CLSM images in (b). (d) CLSM images of HeLa cells treated with CDs (50 mg/mL) for 10 min, and then incubated with 0, 5, 20, or 100 mM Fe^{3+} for 30 min. The confocal images were taken after washing the cells with PBS thrice. (e) Flow cytometry analysis of the cellular fluorescence after treatment with 0, 5, 20, and 100 mM Fe^{3+} for 30 min, respectively. (f) The corresponding statistics of the flow cytometric results in (e).

Reprinted with permission from reference (C. Cheng et al., 2019) Copyright 2018 Elsevier Publication.

12.2.2 Imaging of Intracellular Molecules

Molecular imaging enables observation, characterization, and quantification of biological processes occurring at the cellular and subcellular levels in healthy live humans, including patients. CQDs are utilized in the detection and management of conditions such as cancer, heart disease, Alzheimer's disease, and Parkinson's disease, as well as gastrointestinal, lung, bone, renal, and thyroid issues. For the imaging-based detection of DNA, RNA, amino acids, and glutathione, various functional carbon dots have been devised. For example, CQD-gold nanoparticles have been used for intracellular imaging of cancer-derived exosomes (X. Jiang et al., 2018).

Matai et.al synthesized self-assembled fluorescent hybrids for epirubicin delivery and intracellular imaging using hydroxyl-functionalized CQDs with anionic terminus and cationic acetylated G5 Poly (amido amine) (G5- Ac85) dendrimers (Matai et al., 2015). Dual emissive CQDs were used for imaging of lysine and pH (Figure 12.3) (Song et al., 2017). m-phenylenediamine-derived CQDs (m-CQDs) were used for real-time monitoring of cellular RNA dynamics during apoptosis, mitosis, and proliferation for several hours and up to 3 days, demonstrating their long-term imaging applicability.

The performance of m-CQDs for imaging nucleolar RNA in cells is superior to SYTO RNA Select, as shown by the distinct differences between the signals of the

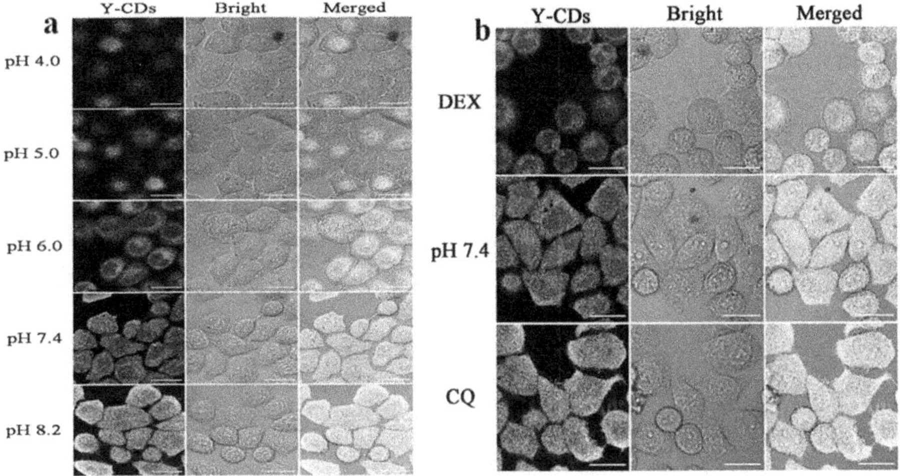

FIGURE 12.2 (a) Confocal fluorescence images of 40 mg/mL Y-CDs incubated with SMMC7721 cells in high-Kþ HEPES-buffered solution in the presence of nigericin at different pH levels. (b) Confocal microscopy analysis of SMMC-7721 cells treated with CQ and DEX. Excitation wavelength for Y-CDs: 458 nm; emission collection.

Reprinted with permission from reference (C. Cheng et al., 2019) Copyright 2020 Elsevier Publication.

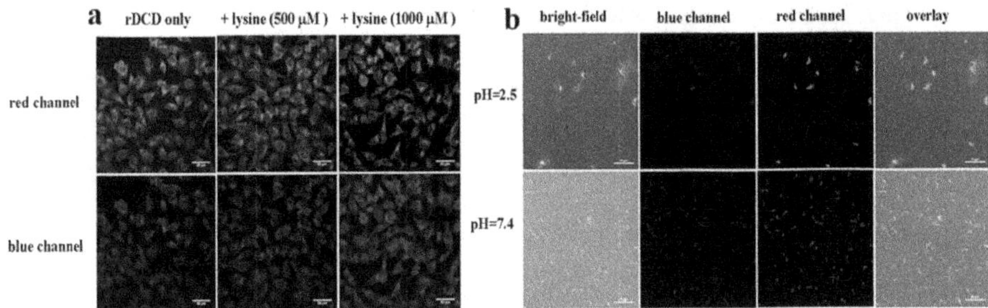

FIGURE 12.3 (a) Representative fluorescence images of HeLa cells treated with different concentrations of lysine in red and blue channels. HeLa cells were incubated with dCDs (100 µg/mL) for 3 h with concentrations of lysine (0, 500, and 1000 µM). Scale bar is 50 µm. (b) Visualization of pH changes in *E. coli* by confocal laser scanning microscopy at pH 2.5 and 7.4. The excitation wavelength was 405 nm.

Reprinted with permission from reference (C. Cheng et al., 2019) Copyright 2018 ACS Publication.

nucleus and the nucleoli (Figure 12.4) (Y. Cheng et al., 2018). As a result of interacting with intracellular RNA, the principle that distinguishes the CQDs from the molecular beacon involves increased fluorescence. Similar to this, imaging of RNA that bonds with intracellular RNA by "π-π" stacking is done using carbon dots made of m-phenylenediamine.

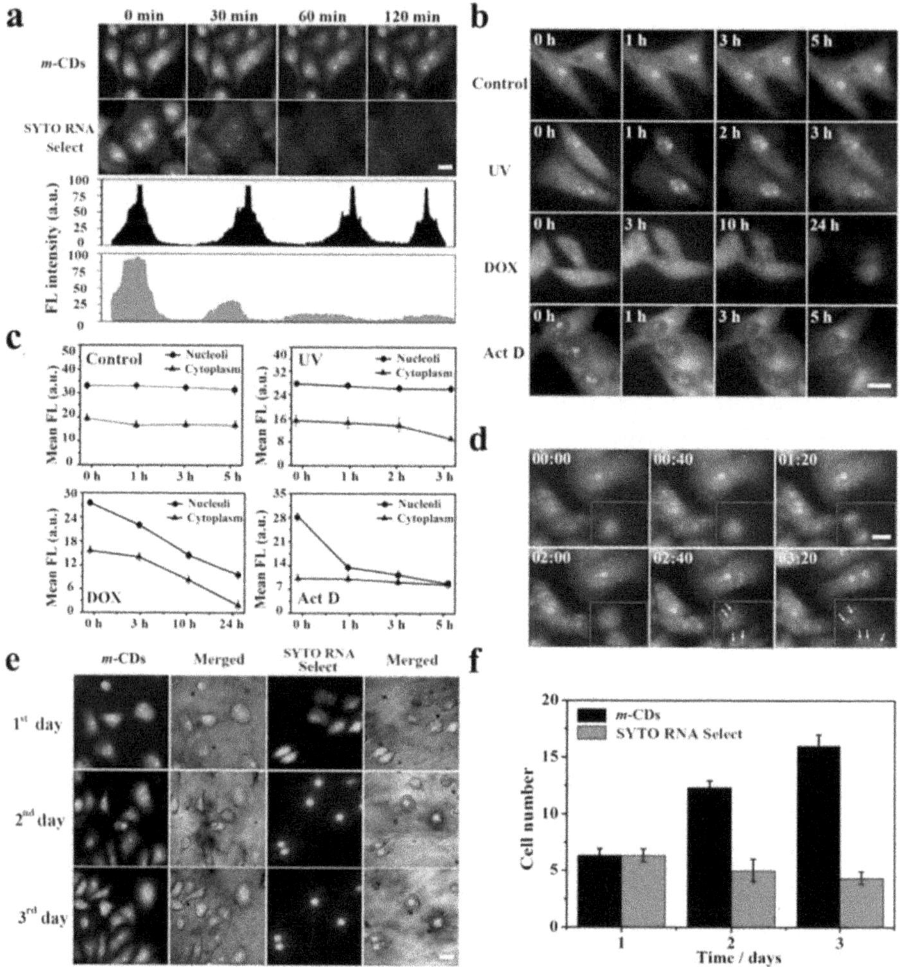

FIGURE 12.4 Long-term in situ imaging of cellular RNA with m-CDs. (a) Time-lapsed imaging of RNA by m-CDs and SYTO RNA Select (upper) and corresponding fluorescence intensity (lower). (b) Time-lapse imaging of RNA in HEp-2 cells after treatment with different apoptosis-inducing strategies. (c) Corresponding mean fluorescence intensity of m-CDs in nucleoli (dot) and cytoplasm (triangle) of b. (d) Time-lapse fluorescence imaging of RNA in HEp-2 cells during mitosis after incubation with m-CDs. Red boxes indicate the cells during mitosis. (e, f) Long time-lapse imaging of RNA in HEp-2 cells using m-CDs and SYTO RNA Select in the range of 0-3 days (e) and corresponding cell numbers. (f) All images are representative of replicate experiments (n=5).

Reprinted with permission from reference (Y. Cheng et al., 2018) Copyright 2018 ACS Publication.

12.2.3 Imaging of Intracellular Organelles

The endocytosis mechanism is primarily responsible for the internalization of fluorescent CQDs. For internalization target-specific functionalization or other methods are used to achieve specificity, either by inherent functional groups on the CQDs that were conserved from prior generations. Since different organelles have varied internal biochemistry and membrane properties, targeting the internalization or membrane of the organelle requires CQDs with specific properties. The specific properties include size, functional groups, biocompatibility, and an appropriate surface charge. The endocytosis mechanism is being followed by the labelling of various organelles with CQDs and monitoring using a variety of fluorescence techniques, such as multicolor imaging, ratiometric imaging, fluorescence quenching, and pH-dependent emission.

CQDs functionalized with weak positively charged or pH-dependent amino groups are found to target lysosomes. For example, by just combining p-benzoquinone and ethanediamine at ambient temperatures, the functional preservation strategy method yields new functional CQDs with emerald emission. These CQDs can dynamically target the lysosome and sensitively respond to the lysosomal pH *in vitro* (Q. Q. Zhang et al., 2018).

CQDs functionalized with naphthalimide derivatives have been used to image and track endogenous formaldehyde in lysosomes in living cells. Endocytosis of the naphthalimide derivative-functionalized CQDs appears to take place through clathrin and caveolae-mediated pathways, which are active transportation processes. The addition of weakly basic amino groups on the CQDs further improves the effectiveness of lysosome targeting (S. Chen et al., 2019).

Figure 12.5 (i) shows firstly reported lysosome-targeting CQDs that enable the concoction of a quick second-level incubation with a wash-free procedure which have potential for long-period tracking of lysosomes *in vivo*. The co-localization studies using CDs and synthetic colors MitoTracker Deep Red FM and LysoTracker Deep Red (commercial lysosomal dyes) (commercial mitochondrial dyes), NucRed Live 647 (nuclear dyes), using commercial colors were done (Qin et al., 2020).

It is possible that energy-dependent mechanisms including micropinocytosis, caveolae, and clathrin are involved in the uptake of CQDs by cells before they are transported to lysosomes. As a result, the majority of CQDs belonging to different functional groups can temporarily localize in lysosomes. Although the lysosome-labeling efficiency of CQDs with high surface amino group abundance is superior, they can also target the endoplasmic reticulum.

Highly positively charged or a mixture of positively and negatively charged CQDs target the nucleus and nucleolus (Zhu et al., 2019). While several CQDs can stain nucleoli in living cells, nucleolar staining dyes such as SYTO RNASelect are more suitable for fixed cells. Despite the fact that the nucleolus-labeling CQDs have been used for subcellular labelling, thermal sensing, and photothermal treatment applications, their use in diagnostic imaging of the nuclei, including the transformation processes, immune activation processes, and assessment of chemodrug treatment, has not been demonstrated (Han et al., 2019; Zhu et al., 2019).

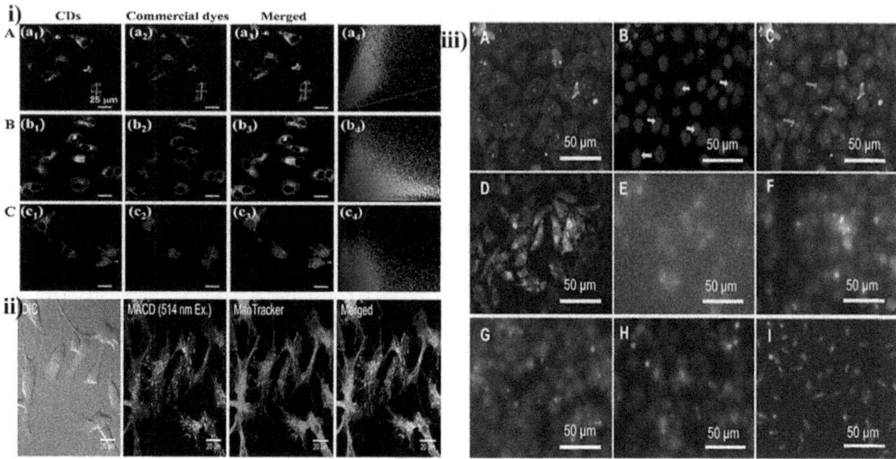

FIGURE 12.5 (i) Colocalization imaging of HeLa cells incubated with A) 30 µgml^{-1} CDs for 10 min and co-stained with 100 nM LysoTracker Deep Red, B) 100 nM MitoTracker Deep Red FM and, C) 2 drops mL^{-1} NucRed, (a$_1$), (b$_1$), and (c$_1$) are confocal images of CDs for 20 min. (a$_2$), (b$_2$), and (c$_2$) are images of commercial dyes. (a$_3$), (b$_3$), and (c$_3$) are images of CDs and commercial dyes. (a$_4$), (b$_4$), and (c$_4$) are the correlation plots of CDs and commercial dyes intensities. (ii) The green-to-yellow MACDs were found to be present mainly in mitochondria, as determined by their co-localization with MitoTracker. (iii) The fluorescence image of HeLa cells incubated with CDs: EDA 1: 2 and Hoechst 33342, (A) for blue bright excitation, (B) for UV bright excitation, (C) for overlap of (A) and (B). (D) Stained with SYTO RNA-select green fluorescent dye, (E) incubated with 400 µg/mL of CDs, (F) EDA, and (G) CA and PEI with CA: EDA 1: 0.5 and (H) 1: 2 for 24 h. (I) The fluorescence images of LN229 incubated with 400 µg/mL of CDs for 4 h.

(i) (Reprinted by permission from reference (Y. Cheng et al., 2018) Copyright 2018ACS Publication), (ii) (Reprinted by permission from reference Zhi et al., 2018) Copyright 2018 ACS NANOPublication), (iii) (Reprinted with permission from reference (Zhu et al., 2019) Copyright 2019PLOS ONE Publication).

Negatively charged CQDs made from m-phenylenediamine and L-cysteine were used by Hua et al. to demonstrate nucleolus targeting while serving as a vehicle for delivering drugs (Hua et al., 2018). Since CQDs and RNA have opposite charges, an electrostatic connection between them as the cause of nucleolus targeting can be excluded. The CQDs' interaction with DNA and RNA molecules gives them the ability to stain nucleoli, which causes them to be enriched there (Sun et al., 2016). Han et al. suggested a CQD-based imaging probe that is selective for dsDNA and ssRNA and has the extraordinary capacity to pass through a variety of biological barriers in living cells (Han et al., 2019).

In order to localize mitochondria, a variety of CQDs have been developed, most of which are based on the fluorescence quenching caused by free radicals and chemical species like peroxynitrite (Hua et al., 2017; Y. Wang et al., 2019; X. Wu et al., 2017, 2018). It has been proven that single-layered graphene CQDs with high yellow fluorescence, which are produced by the thermal condensation of perylene tetracarboxylic anhydride and polyethyleneimine, have good targeting ability for mitochondria (J. H. Liu et al., 2018). Malic acid derived CDs (MACDs) were used for the intracellular mitochondria imaging of Oncorhynchus mykiss (rainbow trout) epithelial gill cells (Figure 12.5 (ii)) (Zhi et al., 2018).

The endoplasmic reticulum (ER) can be imaged using minor changes in amine-functionalized CQDs with lipophilic molecules such as lauryl amine, because the endocytosis mechanism differs (E et al., 2021). The lauryl amine-functionalized CQDs have hydrophobic alkyl groups on surface, which accelerate endocytosis mediated by lipid rafts results in internalization and intracellular localization in the ER. A hydrothermal method was employed by Shuang et al. to create pH-responsive CQDs from citric acid and urea that were further functionalized with lauryl amine to demonstrate bioimaging of lysosomes and the ER. (Shuang et al., 2018).

Jiang et al. 2018 demonstrated bioimaging and monitoring of cancer-derived exosomes inside cells with tumor-specific antibodies attached to gold CQDs. CQDs were prepared with citric acid and L-cysteine targeting ability toward the Golgi apparatus. Even though several CQDs with thiol functional groups and an L-stereo structure have been employed to target the Golgi apparatus (Wei et al., 2023; M. Yuan et al., 2017; X. Zhang et al., 2022), a precise targeting mechanism is still not known.

12.2.4 IMAGING OF CELLS

Cancer cell, stem cell, and neuron imaging using CQDs was found helpful in exploring the development, diagnosis and treatment of cancers and neurological diseases, and also their potential use *in vivo* imaging applications. The functionalized CQDs can penetrate into various types of respective cancer cells and they are monitored by fluorescence imaging (M. L. Liu et al., 2019b; F. Yuan et al., 2015). The unique recognition method is mostly reliant on the interaction between functional CQDs and the surface groups of cancer cells. Glioma cells could be precisely tracked by polyethylene glycol CQDs synthesized from glucose and glutamic acid precursors. These polyethylene glycol CQDs identified the angiopep-2 surface group with higher sensitivity for imaging gliomas in comparison to healthy brain tissues (Ruan et al., 2014).

H. Liu et al. (2018) have developed nitrogen-doped CQDs that enabled imaging of cancer cells and folate receptor-mediated cellular uptake. In addition, hyaluronan-conjugated nitrogen-doped CQDs were prepared for bioimaging of tumor cells, which illustrates their potential use as carriers in targeted drug delivery (Figure 12.6 i, ii) (Karakoçak et al., 2021).

Stem cells contribute to bone repair, skin renewal, and neurorepair. Imaging of stem cells using CQDs is possible through endocytosis mechanism and a concentration-dependent manner. CQDs synthesized by bottom-up approach have been used for umbilical cord-derived mesenchymal stem cell imaging (Yan et al., 2018). Human bone marrow-derived mesenchymal stem cell imaging has been carried out by Kundrotas et al. using carboxylate QDs (Figure 12.6 iii) (Kundrotas et al., 2019). Gadolinium (III)-functionalized fluorescent carbon dots (Gd-CDs) synthesized by Chen and co-workers exhibited strong and stable fluorescence with excitation-independent emission behavior, promoting mesenchymal stem cell imaging (H. Chen et al., 2016).

To improve imaging of the nervous system, various methods were used. Nanoparticle-based imaging of the brain structure, neuron activity, and neurochemistry is in great demand. Natural porphyra polysaccharide CQDs were employed for neuronal induction from ectodermal mesenchymal stem cells via highly efficient non-viral gene delivery (J. Chen et al., 2017). These results demonstrated the potential of CQDs as a safe and efficient gene delivery system for adult neural stem cells. The potential for the development of useful techniques in the central nervous system for clinical diagnosis and therapy is very good with carbon dots having spontaneous penetration capabilities combined with special functional modification based on the distinctive neural membrane lipids and proteins. Li and coworkers developed a novel method of siRNA delivery into nerve cell (SK-N-SH) and also found electrostatic interaction-produced QD-PEG/siRNA nanoplexes, which suppressed the BACE1 gene linked to Alzheimer's disease (Figure 12.6 iv) (Li et al., 2012).

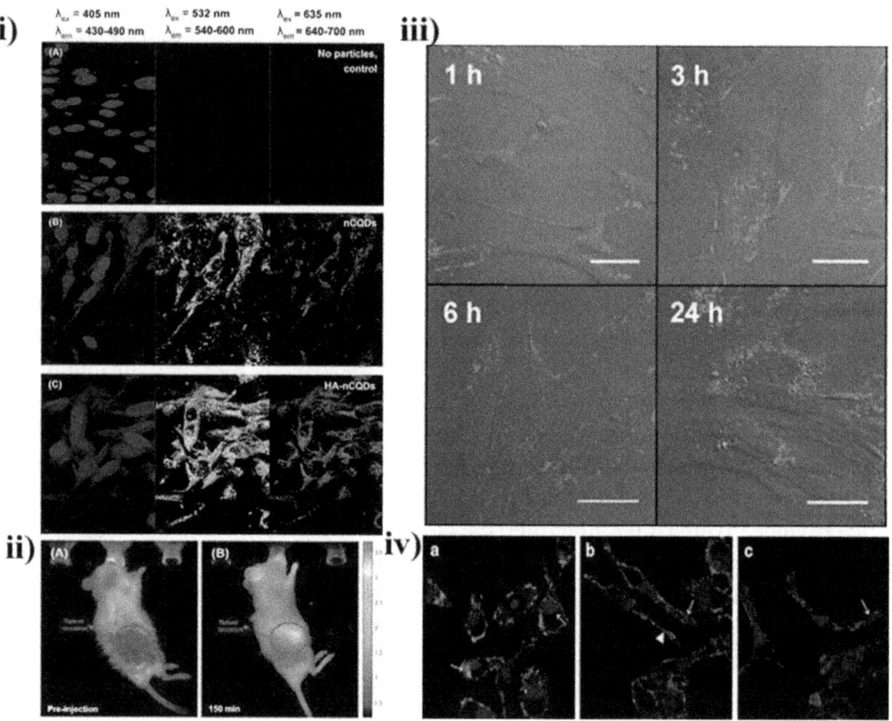

FIGURE 12.6 **(i)** Confocal microscopy images of ARPE-19 cells exposed to 0.6 mg/mL nCQDs, with and without HA conjugation. The cell nuclei were stained with DAPI. **(ii)** *In vivo* fluorescence images of mice bearing patient-derived WHIM4 tumor cells after intravenous injections of HA-nCQDs, **(iii)** MSC morphology and intracellular distribution of QDs after various times of incubation. Red color exhibits QD distribution in MSC culture. **iv)** LSM images of SK-N-SH cells cultured for 10 days. (a) siRNAs were released from QDs and retained their cytoplasmic distribution (arrow). (b, c) The cells sent out many neurites which contained a number of QDs under the axomembrane (arrow) and siRNAs within the axoplasm (arrow head) after QD-PEG/siRNAs transfection.

(ii) (Reprinted with permission from reference (Karakoçak et al., 2021) Copyright 2021 ACS Publication), (iii) (Reprinted with permission from reference (Kundrotas et al., 2019) Copyright 2019 BMC Publication), (iv) (Reprinted with permission from reference (Li et al., 2012) Copyright 2012 Molecular Therapy-Nucleic Acids Publication).

12.3 SUMMARY AND FUTURE PROSPECTS

The chapter summarizes the use of CQDs in bioimaging applications. Bioimaging with CQDs has various benefits, including photostability, biocompatibility, simplicity of synthesis and functionalization, low cost, multicolor emission, small size, and quick uptake. The reactive groups and surface functionalization give CQDs an advantage of biocompatibility, making them appropriate for bioimaging applications. The smaller size of CQDs gives high-resolution cell images compared to organic dyes. The preparation of small CQDs is thus significant with single and narrow fluorescence emission. Due to their superior photostability and simplicity of manufacturing, CQDs act as alternatives to organic dyes for certain imaging.

The specific synthesized CQDs with selective surface functionalization have high affinity toward cell types and organelles. CQDs for labelling or targeted delivery of medication can be produced without the need of any targeting agent or fluorophore. Producing CQDs with specific targeting features clear design principles are still lacking; labelling is typically accomplished through a system of trial and error. The very stable fluorescent CQDs for cell proliferation monitoring and tracking subsequent generations of cell division is still challenging.

By referring to the challenges of highly stable and extremely targeted CQDs for the bioimaging. Also, CQDs with high quantum yields in the near infrared and infrared areas are required. For this, the way can be cleared for advanced CQDs based bioimaging to have a long future.

ACKNOWLEDGMENTS

The research acknowledges the support from the intramural university project (project no DYPES/DU/R&D/2023/1164), D. Y. Patil Education Society, Kolhapur, India. The authors are also thankful to MJPRF given by Mahatma Jyotiba Phule Research and Training Institute.

REFERENCES

Chen, B., Li, F., Li, S., Weng, W., Guo, H., Guo, T., Zhang, X., Chen, Y., Huang, T., Hong, X., You, S., Lin, Y., Zeng, K., & Chen, S. (2013). Large scale synthesis of photoluminescent carbon nanodots and their application for bioimaging. *Nanoscale*, *5*(5). https://doi.org/10.1039/c2nr32675b

Chen, H., Wang, L., Fu, H., Wang, Z., Xie, Y., Zhang, Z., & Tang, Y. (2016). Gadolinium functionalized carbon dots for fluorescence/magnetic resonance dual-modality imaging of mesenchymal stem cells. *Journal of Materials Chemistry B*, *4*(46). https://doi.org/10.1039/c6tb01422d

Chen, J., Wang, Q., Zhou, J., Deng, W., Yu, Q., Cao, X., Wang, J., Shao, F., Li, Y., Ma, P., Spector, M., Yu, J., & Xu, X. (2017). Porphyra polysaccharide-derived carbon dots for non-viral co-delivery of different gene combinations and neuronal differentiation of ectodermal mesenchymal stem cells. *Nanoscale*, *9*(30). https://doi.org/10.1039/c7nr03327c

Chen, S., Jia, Y., Zou, G. Y., Yu, Y. L., & Wang, J. H. (2019). A ratiometric fluorescent nanoprobe based on naphthalimide derivative-functionalized carbon dots for imaging lysosomal formaldehyde in HeLa cells. *Nanoscale*, *11*(13). https://doi.org/10.1039/C9NR00039A

Cheng, C., Xing, M., & Wu, Q. (2019). A universal facile synthesis of nitrogen and sulfur co-doped carbon dots from cellulose-based biowaste for fluorescent detection of Fe^{3+} ions and intracellular bioimaging. *Materials Science and Engineering C, 99*. https://doi.org/10.1016/j.msec.2019.02.003

Cheng, Y., Li, C., Mu, R., Li, Y., Xing, T., Chen, B., & Huang, C. (2018). Dynamically long-term imaging of cellular RNA by fluorescent carbon dots with surface isoquinoline moieties and amines. *Analytical Chemistry, 90*(19). https://doi.org/10.1021/acs.analchem.8b02301

Das, P., Bose, M., Ganguly, S., Mondal, S., Das, A. K., Banerjee, S., & Das, N. C. (2017). Green approach to photoluminescent carbon dots for imaging of gram-negative bacteria *Escherichia coli. Nanotechnology, 28*(19). https://doi.org/10.1088/1361-6528/aa6714

Shuang, E., Mao, Q.-X., Wang, J.-H., & Chen, X.-W. (2021). Correction: Carbon dots with tunable dual emissions: From the mechanism to the specific imaging of endoplasmic reticulum polarity. *Nanoscale, 13*(5). https://doi.org/10.1039/d1nr90012a

Gao, G., Jiang, Y. W., Jia, H. R., Yang, J., & Wu, F. G. (2018). On-off-on fluorescent nanosensor for Fe^{3+} detection and cancer/normal cell differentiation via silicon-doped carbon quantum dots. *Carbon, 134*. https://doi.org/10.1016/j.carbon.2018.02.063

Gao, G., Jiang, Y. W., Yang, J., & Wu, F. G. (2017). Mitochondria-targetable carbon quantum dots for differentiating cancerous cells from normal cells. *Nanoscale, 9*(46). https://doi.org/10.1039/c7nr06764j

Geng, B., Yang, D., Pan, D., Wang, L., Zheng, F., Shen, W., Zhang, C., & Li, X. (2018). NIR-responsive carbon dots for efficient photothermal cancer therapy at low power densities. *Carbon, 134*, 153–162. https://doi.org/10.1016/j.carbon.2018.03.084

Guo, S., Sun, Y., Geng, X., Yang, R., Xiao, L., Qu, L., & Li, Z. (2020). Intrinsic lysosomal targeting fluorescent carbon dots with ultrastability for long-Term lysosome imaging. *Journal of Materials Chemistry B, 8*(4). https://doi.org/10.1039/c9tb02043h

Han, G., Zhao, J., Zhang, R., Tian, X., Liu, Z., Wang, A., Liu, R., Liu, B., Han, M. Y., Gao, X., & Zhang, Z. (2019). Membrane-Penetrating carbon quantum dots for imaging nucleic acid structures in live organisms. *Angewandte Chemie - International Edition, 58*(21). https://doi.org/10.1002/anie.201903005

He, D., Yang, X., He, X., Wang, K., Yang, X., He, X., & Zou, Z. (2015). A sensitive turn-on fluorescent probe for intracellular imaging of glutathione using single-layer MnO_2 nanosheet-quenched fluorescent carbon quantum dots. *Chemical Communications, 51*(79). https://doi.org/10.1039/c5cc05416h

Hua, X. W., Bao, Y. W., Chen, Z., & Wu, F. G. (2017). Carbon quantum dots with intrinsic mitochondrial targeting ability for mitochondria-based theranostics. *Nanoscale, 9*(30). https://doi.org/10.1039/c7nr03658b

Hua, X. W., Bao, Y. W., & Wu, F. G. (2018). Fluorescent carbon quantum dots with intrinsic nucleolus-targeting capability for nucleolus imaging and enhanced cytosolic and nuclear drug delivery. *ACS Applied Materials and Interfaces, 10*(13). https://doi.org/10.1021/acsami.7b19549

Jiang, Q., Liu, L., Li, Q., Cao, Y., Chen, D., Du, Q., Yang, X., Huang, D., Pei, R., Chen, X., & Huang, G. (2021). NIR-laser-triggered gadolinium-doped carbon dots for magnetic resonance imaging, drug delivery and combined photothermal chemotherapy for triple negative breast cancer. *Journal of Nanobiotechnology, 19*(1). https://doi.org/10.1186/s12951-021-00811-w

Jiang, X., Zong, S., Chen, C., Zhang, Y., Wang, Z., & Cui, Y. (2018). Gold-carbon dots for the intracellular imaging of cancer-derived exosomes. *Nanotechnology, 29*(17). https://doi.org/10.1088/1361-6528/aaaf14

Karakoçak, B. B., Laradji, A., Primeau, T., Berezin, M. Y., Li, S., & Ravi, N. (2021). Hyaluronan-conjugated carbon quantum dots for bioimaging use. *ACS Applied Materials and Interfaces, 13*(1). https://doi.org/10.1021/acsami.0c20088

Konar, S., Kumar, B. N. P., Mahto, M. K., Samanta, D., Shaik, M. A. S., Shaw, M., Mandal, M., & Pathak, A. (2019). N-doped carbon dot as fluorescent probe for detection of cysteamine and multicolor cell imaging. *Sensors and Actuators, B: Chemical, 286*. https://doi.org/10.1016/j.snb.2019.01.117

Kumari, A., Kumar, A., Sahu, S. K., & Kumar, S. (2018). Synthesis of green fluorescent carbon quantum dots using waste polyolefins residue for Cu2+ ion sensing and live cell imaging. *Sensors and Actuators, B: Chemical, 254*. https://doi.org/10.1016/j.snb.2017.07.075

Kundrotas, G., Karabanovas, V., Pleckaitis, M., Juraleviciute, M., Steponkiene, S., Gudleviciene, Z., & Rotomskis, R. (2019). Uptake and distribution of carboxylated quantum dots in human mesenchymal stem cells: Cell growing density matters. *Journal of Nanobiotechnology, 17*(1). https://doi.org/10.1186/s12951-019-0470-6

Li, S., Liu, Z., Ji, F., Xiao, Z., Wang, M., Peng, Y., Zhang, Y., Liu, L., Liang, Z., & Li, F. (2012). Delivery of quantum dot-siRNA nanoplexes in SK-N-SH cells for BACE1 gene silencing and intracellular imaging. *Molecular Therapy - Nucleic Acids, 1*(4). https://doi.org/10.1038/mtna.2012.11

Lin, Q., Li, Z., & Yuan, Q. (2019). Recent advances in autofluorescence-free biosensing and bioimaging based on persistent luminescence nanoparticles. *Chinese Chemical Letters, 30*(9). https://doi.org/10.1016/j.cclet.2019.06.016

Liu, H., Li, Z., Sun, Y., Geng, X., Hu, Y., Meng, H., Ge, J., & Qu, L. (2018). Synthesis of luminescent carbon dots with ultrahigh quantum yield and inherent folate receptor-positive cancer cell targetability. *Scientific Reports, 8*(1). https://doi.org/10.1038/s41598-018-19373-3

Liu, J. H., Li, R. S., Yuan, B., Wang, J., Li, Y. F., & Huang, C. Z. (2018). Mitochondria-targeting single-layered graphene quantum dots with dual recognition sites for ATP imaging in living cells. *Nanoscale, 10*(36). https://doi.org/10.1039/c8nr06061d

Liu, M. L., Chen, B. B., Li, C. M., & Huang, C. Z. (2019a). Carbon dots: Synthesis, formation mechanism, fluorescence origin and sensing applications. In *Green Chemistry, 21*(3). https://doi.org/10.1039/c8gc02736f

Liu, M. L., Chen, B. B., Li, C. M., & Huang, C. Z. (2019b). Carbon dots prepared for fluorescence and chemiluminescence sensing. In *Science China Chemistry, 62*(8). https://doi.org/10.1007/s11426-019-9449-y

Maghsoudinia, F., Tavakoli, M. B., Samani, R. K., Motaghi, H., Hejazi, S. H., & Mehrgardi, M. A. (2021). Bevacizumab and folic acid dual-targeted gadolinium-carbon dots for fluorescence/magnetic resonance imaging of hepatocellular carcinoma. *Journal of Drug Delivery Science and Technology, 61*. https://doi.org/10.1016/j.jddst.2020.102288

Matai, I., Sachdev, A., & Gopinath, P. (2015). Self-assembled hybrids of fluorescent carbon dots and PAMAM dendrimers for epirubicin delivery and intracellular imaging. *ACS Applied Materials and Interfaces, 7*(21). https://doi.org/10.1021/acsami.5b02095

Molkenova, A., Toleshova, A., Song, S. J., Kang, M. S., Abduraimova, A., Han, D. W., & Atabaev, T. S. (2020). Rapid synthesis of nontoxic and photostable carbon nanoparticles for bioimaging applications. *Materials Letters, 261*. https://doi.org/10.1016/j.matlet.2019.127012

Pan, T., Shen, M., Shi, J., Ning, J., Su, F., Liao, J., & Tian, Y. (2021). Intracellular potassium ion fluorescent nanoprobes for functional analysis of hERG channel via bioimaging. *Sensors and Actuators, B: Chemical, 345*. https://doi.org/10.1016/j.snb.2021.130450

Pandey, S., & Bodas, D. (2020). High-quality quantum dots for multiplexed bioimaging: A critical review. In *Advances in Colloid and Interface Science, 278*. https://doi.org/10.1016/j.cis.2020.102137

Phukan, K., Sarma, R. R., Dash, S., Devi, R., & Chowdhury, D. (2022). Carbon dot based nucleus targeted fluorescence imaging and detection of nuclear hydrogen peroxide in living cells. *Nanoscale Advances, 4*(1). https://doi.org/10.1039/d1na00617g

Qian, J., Quan, F., Zhao, F., Wu, C., Wang, Z., & Zhou, L. (2018). Aconitic acid derived carbon dots: Conjugated interaction for the detection of folic acid and fluorescence targeted imaging of folate receptor overexpressed cancer cells. *Sensors and Actuators, B: Chemical, 262.* https://doi.org/10.1016/j.snb.2018.01.227

Qin, H., Sun, Y., Geng, X., Zhao, K., Meng, H., Yang, R., Qu, L., & Li, Z. (2020). A wash-free lysosome targeting carbon dots for ultrafast imaging and monitoring cell apoptosis status. *Analytica Chimica Acta, 1106.* https://doi.org/10.1016/j.aca.2020.02.002

Ruan, S., Qian, J., Shen, S., Chen, J., Zhu, J., Jiang, X., He, Q., Yang, W., & Gao, H. (2014). Fluorescent carbonaceous nanodots for noninvasive glioma imaging after angiopep-2 decoration. *Bioconjugate Chemistry, 25*(12). https://doi.org/10.1021/bc500474p

Sarkar, P., Ghosh, S., & Sarkar, K. (2021). Folic acid based carbon dot functionalized stearic acid-g-polyethyleneimine amphiphilic nanomicelle: Targeted drug delivery and imaging for triple negative breast cancer. *Colloids and Surfaces B: Biointerfaces, 197.* https://doi.org/10.1016/j.colsurfb.2020.111382

Shivaji, K., Mani, S., Ponmurugan, P., De Castro, C. S., Lloyd Davies, M., Balasubramanian, M. G., & Pitchaimuthu, S. (2018). Green-synthesis-derived cds quantum dots using tea leaf extract: Antimicrobial, bioimaging, and therapeutic applications in lung cancer cells. *ACS Applied Nano Materials, 1*(4). https://doi.org/10.1021/acsanm.8b00147

Shuang, E., Mao, Q. X., Yuan, X. L., Kong, X. L., Chen, X. W., & Wang, J. H. (2018). Targeted imaging of the lysosome and endoplasmic reticulum and their pH monitoring with surface regulated carbon dots. *Nanoscale, 10*(26). https://doi.org/10.1039/c8nr03453b

Song, W., Duan, W., Liu, Y., Ye, Z., Chen, Y., Chen, H., Qi, S., Wu, J., Liu, D., Xiao, L., Ren, C., & Chen, X. (2017). Ratiometric detection of intracellular lysine and pH with one-pot synthesized dual emissive carbon dots. *Analytical Chemistry, 89*(24). https://doi.org/10.1021/acs.analchem.7b04211

Speranza, G. (2021). Carbon nanomaterials: Synthesis, functionalization and sensing applications. *Nanomaterials, 11*(4). https://doi.org/10.3390/nano11040967

Sun, S., Zhang, L., Jiang, K., Wu, A., & Lin, H. (2016). Toward high-efficient red emissive carbon dots: Facile preparation, unique properties, and applications as multifunctional theranostic agents. *Chemistry of Materials, 28*(23). https://doi.org/10.1021/acs.chemmater.6b03695

Tang, Z., Lin, Z., Li, G., & Hu, Y. (2017). Amino nitrogen quantum dots-based nanoprobe for fluorescence detection and imaging of cysteine in biological samples. *Analytical Chemistry, 89*(7). https://doi.org/10.1021/acs.analchem.7b00284

Vibhute, A., Nille, O., Kolekar, G., Rohiwal, S., Patil, S., Lee, S., & Tiwari, A. P. (2022). Fluorescent carbon quantum dots functionalized by Poly L-Lysine: Efficient material for antibacterial, bioimaging and antiangiogenesis applications. *Journal of Fluorescence, 32*(5). https://doi.org/10.1007/s10895-022-02977-4

Vibhute, A., Patil, T., Gambhir, R., & Tiwari, A. P. (2022). Fluorescent carbon quantum dots: Synthesis methods, functionalization and biomedical applications. *Applied Surface Science Advances, 11.* https://doi.org/10.1016/j.apsadv.2022.100311

Vibhute, A., Patil, T., Malavekar, D., Patil, S., Lee, S., & Tiwari, A. P. (2023). Green synthesis of fluorescent carbon dots from annona squamosa leaves: Optical and structural properties with bactericidal, anti-inflammatory, Anti-angiogenesis Applications. *Journal of Fluorescence, 0123456789.* https://doi.org/10.1007/s10895-023-03159-6

Wang, W. J., Xia, J. M., Feng, J., He, M. Q., Chen, M. L., & Wang, J. H. (2016). Green preparation of carbon dots for intracellular pH sensing and multicolor live cell imaging. *Journal of Materials Chemistry B, 4*(44). https://doi.org/10.1039/c6tb02071b

Wang, Y., Zhou, D., Huang, H., Wang, Y., Hu, Z., & Li, X. (2019). A yellow-emissive carbon nanodot-based ratiometric fluorescent nanosensor for visualization of exogenous and endogenous hydroxyl radicals in the mitochondria of live cells. *Journal of Materials Chemistry B, 7*(23). https://doi.org/10.1039/c9tb00289h

Wang, Z., Fu, B., Zou, S., Duan, B., Chang, C., Yang, B., Zhou, X., & Zhang, L. (2016). Facile construction of carbon dots via acid catalytic hydrothermal method and their application for target imaging of cancer cells. *Nano Research*, *9*(1). https://doi.org/10.1007/s12274-016-0992-2

Wei, Y., Gao, Y., Chen, L., Li, Q., Du, J., Wang, D., Ren, F., Liu, X., & Yang, Y. (2023). Carbon dots based on targeting unit inheritance strategy for Golgi apparatus-targeting imaging. *Frontiers of Materials Science*, *17*(1). https://doi.org/10.1007/s11706-023-0627-y

Wu, H., Pang, L. F., Wei, N., Guo, X. F., & Wang, H. (2021). Nucleus-targeted N-doped carbon dots via DNA-binding for imaging of hypochlorous in cells and zebrafish. *Sensors and Actuators, B: Chemical*, *333*. https://doi.org/10.1016/j.snb.2021.129626

Wu, X., Ma, L., Sun, S., Jiang, K., Zhang, L., Wang, Y., Zeng, H., & Lin, H. (2018). A versatile platform for the highly efficient preparation of graphene quantum dots: Photoluminescence emission and hydrophilicity-hydrophobicity regulation and organelle imaging. *Nanoscale*, *10*(3). https://doi.org/10.1039/c7nr08093j

Wu, X., Sun, S., Wang, Y., Zhu, J., Jiang, K., Leng, Y., Shu, Q., & Lin, H. (2017). A fluorescent carbon-dots-based mitochondria-targetable nanoprobe for peroxynitrite sensing in living cells. *Biosensors and Bioelectronics*, *90*. https://doi.org/10.1016/j.bios.2016.10.060

Yan, J., Hou, S., Yu, Y., Qiao, Y., Xiao, T., Mei, Y., Zhang, Z., Wang, B., Huang, C. C., Lin, C. H., & Suo, G. (2018). The effect of surface charge on the cytotoxity and uptake of carbon quantum dots in human umbilical cord derived mesenchymal stem cells. *Colloids and Surfaces B: Biointerfaces*, *171*. https://doi.org/10.1016/j.colsurfb.2018.07.034

Yang, L., Jiang, W., Qiu, L., Jiang, X., Zuo, D., Wang, D., & Yang, L. (2015). One pot synthesis of highly luminescent polyethylene glycol anchored carbon dots functionalized with a nuclear localization signal peptide for cell nucleus imaging. *Nanoscale*, *7*(14). https://doi.org/10.1039/c5nr01080b

Yin, X., Sun, Y., Yang, R., Qu, L., & Li, Z. (2020). RNA-responsive fluorescent carbon dots for fast and wash-free nucleolus imaging. *Spectrochimica Acta - Part A: Molecular and Biomolecular Spectroscopy*, *237*. https://doi.org/10.1016/j.saa.2020.118381

Yu, C., Jiang, X., Qin, D., Mo, G., Zheng, X., & Deng, B. (2019). Facile syntheses of S,N-Codoped carbon quantum dots and their applications to a novel Off-On nanoprobe for detection of 6-Thioguanine and its bioimaging. *ACS Sustainable Chemistry and Engineering*, *7*(19). https://doi.org/10.1021/acssuschemeng.9b02886

Yuan, F., Ding, L., Li, Y., Li, X., Fan, L., Zhou, S., Fang, D., & Yang, S. (2015). Multicolor fluorescent graphene quantum dots colorimetrically responsive to all-pH and a wide temperature range. *Nanoscale*, *7*(27). https://doi.org/10.1039/c5nr02007g

Yuan, M., Guo, Y., Wei, J., Li, J., Long, T., & Liu, Z. (2017). Optically active blue-emitting carbon dots to specifically target the Golgi apparatus. *RSC Advances*, *7*(79). https://doi.org/10.1039/c7ra09271g

Zhang, J., & Yu, S. H. (2016). Carbon dots: Large-scale synthesis, sensing and bioimaging. In *Materials Today*, *19*(7). https://doi.org/10.1016/j.mattod.2015.11.008

Zhang, Q. Q., Yang, T., Li, R. S., Zou, H. Y., Li, Y. F., Guo, J., Liu, X. D., & Huang, C. Z. (2018). A functional preservation strategy for the production of highly photoluminescent emerald carbon dots for lysosome targeting and lysosomal pH imaging. *Nanoscale*, *10*(30). https://doi.org/10.1039/c8nr03212b

Zhang, S., Ji, X., Liu, J., Wang, Q., & Jin, L. (2020). One-step synthesis of yellow-emissive carbon dots with a large Stokes shift and their application in fluorimetric imaging of intracellular pH. *Spectrochimica Acta - Part A: Molecular and Biomolecular Spectroscopy*, *227*. https://doi.org/10.1016/j.saa.2019.117677

Zhang, X., Chen, L., Wei, Y. Y., Du, J. L., Yu, S. P., Liu, X. G., Liu, W., Liu, Y. J., Yang, Y. Z., & Li, Q. (2022). Cyclooxygenase-2-targeting fluorescent carbon dots for the selective imaging of Golgi apparatus. *Dyes and Pigments*, *201*. https://doi.org/10.1016/j.dyepig.2022.110213

Zhang, Y., Shen, Y., Teng, X., Yan, M., Bi, H., & Morais, P. C. (2015). Mitochondria-targeting nanoplatform with fluorescent carbon dots for long time imaging and magnetic field-enhanced cellular uptake. *ACS Applied Materials and Interfaces*, *7*(19). https://doi.org/10.1021/acsami.5b00405

Zhi, B., Cui, Y., Wang, S., Frank, B. P., Williams, D. N., Brown, R. P., Melby, E. S., Hamers, R. J., Rosenzweig, Z., Fairbrother, D. H., Orr, G., & Haynes, C. L. (2018). Malic acid carbon dots: From super-resolution live-cell imaging to highly efficient separation. *ACS Nano*, *12*(6). https://doi.org/10.1021/acsnano.8b01619

Zhu, Z., Li, Q., Li, P., Xun, X., Zheng, L., Ning, D., & Su, M. (2019). Surface charge controlled nucleoli selective staining with nanoscale carbon dots. *PLoS ONE*, *14*(5). https://doi.org/10.1371/journal.pone.0216230

13 Cytotoxicity and Biocompatibility Analysis of Carbon Quantum Dots

Jincy Mathew, Bony K. John and Beena Mathew

13.1 INTRODUCTION

The growth of novel nanomaterials has resulted in revolutionary advancements in diverse scientific areas. CQDs are relatively new fluorescent nanoparticles of graphene having exceptional features such as good solubility, exceptional photobleaching resistance, excellent photoluminescence, good surface properties, effortless synthesis, outstanding biocompatibility, and low toxicity. The incomparable and promising properties of CQDs have elevated the attraction of CQDs among different research groups for diverse applications including theranostic, tissue engineering, bioimaging, biosensing, and drug administration [1–4]. CQDs with stimulating features can be used in various industrial areas in addition to biomedical applications [5–10]. However, before incorporating CQDs into biomedical applications, it is crucial to comprehensively evaluate their cytotoxicity and biocompatibility to ensure their safe use.

The widespread use of CQDs in novel photovoltaic, catalysis, and sensing applications has paved the way for the extensive appearance of CQDs in the environment [11]. Even though carbon as such is intrinsically nontoxic, carbon nanomaterials may result in hazardous effects on human health due to the explicit material and the structural arrangement. Therefore, it is essential to study the potential risks of CQDs to diverse living things [12, 13]. Cytotoxicity analysis evaluates the impact of CQDs on cell viability and cell function. Mainly, the cytotoxicity evaluation of CQDs has been done in limited human cell lines. So it is difficult to generalize the obtained results to other cell lines [6, 14]. Assessing the cytotoxicity of CQDs is a fundamental step in determining their safety for biological systems. Biocompatibility is a critical parameter for the translation of CQDs into clinical practice. Biocompatibility encompasses not only cytotoxicity but also the interaction of CQDs with biological systems at multiple levels, including cellular, tissue, and organismal responses.

DOI: 10.1201/9781003437857-15

Simple unicellular organisms such as eukaryotic model creatures resemble the cellular, biochemical, and molecular features of higher organisms and hence are mainly involved in the toxicity investigation study of various chemicals [8, 15]. CQDs derived from diverse precursor molecules have varied physicochemical properties and this turned out to be a challenge in their toxicity investigation [16]. The cellular level understanding of the toxicity mechanism of CQDs is a solution to overcome this problem [9, 10, 13]. The exterior chemistry and edge effect of CQDs suggest the resulting generation of reactive oxygen species (ROS) [8]. The study by Wang et al. showed that CQD-tempted release of ROS causes the damage of DNA in fibroblast cells (NIH/3T3) [9, 10]. A similar study by Jiang et al. reported the ROS generation in HeLa cells induced by hydrothermally synthesized CQDs [17]. The property of the specific CQD directly relates to the contribution of the generation of ROS to the CQD toxicity [16].

Understanding the synthesis methods is pivotal as it directly influences the properties and subsequent applications of CQDs. Various techniques, such as the top-down and bottom-up approaches, have been employed to synthesize CQDs with precise control over size, shape, and surface properties [18]. Moreover, advanced characterization techniques, including spectroscopy, microscopy, and surface analysis, are essential to determine the structural and chemical properties of CQDs, ensuring their reproducibility and reliability in biomedical applications. Despite being extensively researched for decades, CQDs are also a good substitute for semiconductor quantum dots because of their strong and controllable fluorescence properties, which allow for applications in the biomedical area. However, there are many disadvantages of semiconductor quantum dots, including severe toxicity due to the employment of heavy metals during their manufacture. While CQDs have low toxicity, hydrophilic surface, non-blinking fluorescence, photobleaching resistance, simple passivation, chemical stability, and good cellular compatibility, heavy metals are known to be extremely toxic even at lower levels, which makes them less suitable for clinical studies [19]. Due of biological and environmental safety issues, CQDs are leading the way in significant research efforts to provide environmentally acceptable, non-toxic replacements with desired qualities.

In this book chapter, we delve into the crucial aspects of cytotoxicity and biocompatibility analysis of carbon quantum dots (CQDs), exploring their potential in various biomedical applications. In recent years, the biomedical field has seen a surge in interest in CQDs, primarily due to their biocompatibility and low toxicity, which makes them promising candidates for various medical applications. However, before these nanostructures can be deployed in clinical settings, a comprehensive understanding of their cytotoxicity and biocompatibility is imperative. This book chapter aims to provide a comprehensive overview of the current state of research in this area, shedding light on the challenges and opportunities associated with the use of CQDs in biomedicine. By unraveling the intricate relationship between CQD properties and their interactions with biological systems, we hope to pave the way for the safe and effective utilization of these remarkable nanomaterials in a multitude of biomedical applications, ultimately enhancing healthcare and improving the quality of life for millions around the world.

13.2 CYTOTOXICITY AND BIOCOMPATIBILITY ASSESSMENT OF CQDs

13.2.1 RELEVANCE OF STUDYING CYTOTOXICITY AND BIOCOMPATIBILITY OF CQDs

The study of cytotoxicity and biocompatibility in the context of CQDs is of paramount importance for several reasons. CQDs have gained significant attention due to their potential applications in biomedicine, such as drug delivery, imaging, and diagnostics [2]. Before these applications can be realized, it is crucial to ensure that CQDs are safe for use in living systems. Studying cytotoxicity and biocompatibility helps determine whether CQDs have adverse effects on cells, tissues, or organisms and whether they can be employed in medical therapies.

CQDs are nanomaterials, and their small size and unique properties can lead to different interactions with biological systems compared to larger materials. Investigating cytotoxicity allows researchers to assess the impact of CQDs on cell viability, proliferation, and overall health. Understanding biocompatibility helps identify potential risks and safety concerns associated with CQD exposure [20]. Regulatory bodies, such as the Food and Drug Administration (FDA) in the United States, require thorough safety assessments of nanomaterials intended for medical use. Research on cytotoxicity and biocompatibility provides the data needed to comply with regulatory requirements and obtain approval for clinical trials and commercialization.

Different biomedical applications may require specific modifications of CQDs, such as surface functionalization or size adjustments. Studying biocompatibility helps researchers tailor CQDs to suit particular applications while ensuring they remain safe for use. Investigating cytotoxicity and biocompatibility provides insights into the mechanisms underlying CQD-cell interactions. This understanding is essential for designing safer nanomaterials and developing strategies to mitigate potential risks. Through the study of cytotoxicity and biocompatibility, researchers can also refine the design and synthesis of CQDs to enhance their biocompatibility. This may involve optimizing surface chemistry, size, shape, or other properties to minimize cytotoxic effects and maximize their utility in medicine [21–23].

Some biomedical applications, such as drug delivery systems, may require prolonged exposure of CQDs to living systems. Assessing biocompatibility over extended periods is vital to ensure that CQDs do not cause cumulative toxicity or other adverse effects over time. Importantly, ethical considerations are essential when developing new materials for biomedical applications. Ensuring the safety and biocompatibility of CQDs is not only a scientific responsibility but also an ethical obligation to protect the well-being of patients and the environment. The public's perception of nanotechnology and its applications in medicine is influenced by the safety record of nanomaterials. Demonstrating the biocompatibility and low cytotoxicity of CQDs contributes to building trust and acceptance of these technologies. These studies also extend to understanding the environmental impact of CQDs. As these materials may be used in various applications, including wastewater treatment, their effects on ecosystems must be evaluated to minimize environmental harm.

In summary, studying cytotoxicity and biocompatibility in the context of CQDs is critical for ensuring the safe and effective use of these nanomaterials in biomedical applications. These studies help assess potential risks, optimize CQD design, and pave the way for the development of innovative medical therapies and technologies while upholding ethical standards and regulatory compliance.

13.3 CYTOTOXICITY ASSESSMENT OF CQDs

In the discovery and advancement of therapeutics and medicines, cytotoxicity is the foremost concern. The use of drugs leads to serious side effects if they affect the normal cells instead of the disease-affected cells. This can be avoided by the introduction of targeted drug delivery and therapy. In this approach, nanoparticles such as quantum dots were often used as vehicles for drugs. The photoluminescence feature of quantum dots was also exploited for intracellular imaging. Later, quantum dots were replaced by CQDs because of the serious cytotoxic issues of quantum dots. Carbon materials are being looked into as potential eco-friendly, low cytotoxic materials for everyday usage. However, considering that they may enter the human body by injections, absorption through skin, breathing, and gastrointestinal digestion, it is important to evaluate the cytotoxic effects of CQDs on humans and animals [24]. To guarantee food packaging safety and for biomedical applications, it is therefore important to first consider CQD cytotoxicity. CQDs that may be produced using environmentally friendly processes from non-toxic raw materials have excellent biocompatibility in addition to antioxidant and antibacterial properties. Applications including biolabeling, antibacterial medication administration, food packaging, and cell imaging are made possible by CQDs' outstanding biocompatibility [25, 26]. CQDs are less toxic and extra biocompatible than conventional quantum dots. Therefore, diverse concentration levels of CQDs with or without surface functionalization were often studied for toxicity in various cell lines. The studies revealed the easy penetration of least cytotoxic CQDs into the cells [6, 27–29]. Some mice trials to assess the in vivo toxicity and immune response have been carried out to learn more about CQD cytotoxicity [30, 31]. For instance, upon injection with a high dose of CQDs, an enhancement in the Th1 and Tc lymphocyte levels was observed [30]. The surface properties of CQDs are directly related to their cytotoxicity. The cytotoxicity of CQDs depends on the charge and type of functionalities and not on the non-toxic carbon core [32]. Least toxic functional groups are neutral ones like polyethylene glycol (PEG), and the best results were obtained using CQD-PEG [16, 31, 33]. It has been shown that negatively charged functionalities, such as Pristine and CD-Pristine, can elicit oxidative stress, cell cycle arrest, and promoted proliferation. On the other hand, positively charged polyethyleneimine (PEI) and CQD-PEI like functional groups are known to trigger cell cycle halt during the G0 phase [16]. The toxicity of CQDs is mainly detected at higher concentrations greater than 50 µg/mL and are absent at concentrations less than 25 µg/mL. Previous studies have demonstrated that nanoparticles have a ROS-dependent effect on cellular morphology [34, 35]. Greater ROS generation leads to severe medical conditions like cancer, limitless proliferation, and even cell death [33, 34, 36]. Additionally, *in vivo* investigations on animals have demonstrated that CQD-PEG had no adverse effects when administered intravenously to mice for up to 28 days at doses of 8 to 40 mg/ kg of body weight. CQDs get clustered mainly in the liver and spleen, but they had no effect on how well these organs functioned. Furthermore, examinations of all physiological indicators at time intervals longer than those for the majority of in vivo imaging studies showed similarities between the control and various dosages of CQDs [37]. Both the *in vivo* and *in vitro* cytotoxicity studies have given promising outcomes [6, 27, 37]. However, before moving on to human investigations, it is still essential to identify the ideal passivating agent and the amount of CQDs in cultures of cells and various animal models, particularly with regard to the long-term consequences. The cytotoxic effects of food-derived CQDs in foods, such as coffee, barbeque, hamburgers, honey, cola, bread, and beer, among others, were documented in prior publications [38]. However, due to a potential application perspective, *in vivo* and *in vitro* cytotoxicity assessments of CQDs are essential in the food industry. The cytotoxicity of CQDs has thus far been studied on a number of occasions at the cellular level. In a study, Cailotto et al. examined the cytotoxicity of CQDs derived from fructose, ascorbic acid, and glucose against HeLa cell lines using a CellTiter-Glo® Luminescence assay [39]. They discovered that ascorbic acid-based CQDs demonstrated strong biocompatibility at low dosages (250 mg/mL), but glucose-based CQDs displayed great cell viability even at doses of 1000 mg/mL. Tan et al. found that even at a high dosage of 20 mg/mL, the CDs exhibited great biocompatibility and minimal cytotoxicity against mice osteoblast cells (MC3T3-E1) [21]. Human islet amyloid polypeptide (hIAPP) aggregation and cytotoxicity were tested in vitro using fluorinated graphene quantum dots (FGQDs), according to Yousaf et al. [40]. Since FGQDs have a lot of charge density and hydrophobic groups, they can attach to the hIAPP subunit and block the conformational change by delaying the time that hIAPP spends aggregating, which prevents the development of full fibrils. Red-fluorescent GQDs produced from *Mangifera indica* (mGQDs) were shown to be extremely biocompatible with the rat fibroblast cell type L929 at exceptionally high doses (0.1 mg/mL) after 24 h treatment [41]. Cytotoxicity analysis of CQDs based on gum tragacanth/chitosan and gum tragacanth alone was carried out by Mordi et al. As depicted in Figure 13.1, after 24 h exposure, both CQDs failed to induce cytotoxicity on normal HUVEC cell lines. According to Li et al., even though the concentration of spermidine-capped CQDs (Spd-CQDs) was 100-fold greater than the minimum inhibitory concentration (MIC) for bacteria, the hemolysis of human RBCs was minimal [42]. Jian at al. carried out another study and found that although there was a structural interaction between rabbit corneal keratocytes (RCK cells) and spermidine-derived CQDs (CQDspds), the treatment of CQDspds for bacterial keratitis had a negligible cytotoxic effect against RCK cells. Additionally, they confirmed that at doses of 100 mg/mL, CQDspds were safe for usage and did not impair human RBCs or induce hemagglutination or oxidative or genotoxic damage [43]. The in vivo and in vitro cytotoxicity of nitrogen-doped CQDs (N-CQDs) is determined by Zhao et al. Mammalian cells like PANC-1 and HeLa are examined in vitro using MTT assay for 24 hours after being subjected to a range of various N-CQD doses [44]. The mice used for the in vivo toxicity studies were exposed to a dose of 5 mg/mL of N-CQDs for 7 days, and the morphology of various organs was examined under an optical microscope. The collected data showed no pathological changes in any tissue

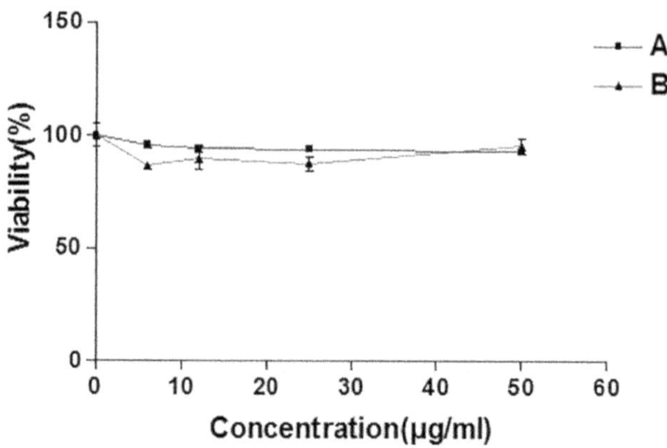

FIGURE 13.1   Cell viability effects of (A) gum tragacanth/chitosan and (B) gum tragacanth-based CQDs on the HUVEC cell line [20].

Copyright 2018. Reprinted with permission from Elsevier.

that had reacted with N-CQDs, which became clear by N-CQDs being digested into non-toxic components. The interaction of the CQDs with cells is a very complex phenomenon. Results vary depending on the cell system under investigation and the cytotoxicity test technique is employed. This interaction is also influenced by other factors, including shape and surface properties such as charge, coatings, and functional groups. However, the majority of the debate focused on cytotoxicity studies of CQDs, which showed that doses in the vicinity of 10–100 mg/mL were just slightly harmful to cells (10%–20%) and recommended to be safe for biomedical and food processing applications.

13.3.1   Various In Vitro and In Vivo Cytotoxicity Assays

The influence of CQDs on diverse cell lines is evaluated using *in vitro* and *in vivo* cytotoxicity assays, which are crucial techniques for gaining knowledge about the biocompatibility and potentially hazardous consequences of CQDs. Researchers can assess the reliability of CQDs for biological applications using these tests. Here are a few examples of frequently employed *in vitro* cytotoxicity tests for assessing CQDs.

The metabolic activity of cells is measured by the MTT assay (3-(4,5-dimethylthiazol-2-yl)-2,5-diphenyltetrazolium bromide assay) colorimetric test. MTT is a yellow tetrazolium salt that is reduced by living cells to produce purple formazan crystals. MTT test, which offers quantitative information on cell viability, is frequently used to evaluate the viability and proliferation of cells following prolonged exposure to CQDs [45, 46]. In MTT assay, the cell viability is calculated using the equation: Cell viability (%) = $Abs_{(s)}$ /$Abs_{(c)}$ * 100, where Abs(s) and Abs(c) are the sample absorbance with CQDs and of control, respectively.

Another cytotoxicity assessment method is the MTS assay (3-(4,5-dimethylthiazol-2-yl)-5-(3-carboxymethoxyphenyl)-2-(4- sulfophenyl) -2H-tetrazolium assay). The MTS assay examines the reduction of a tetrazolium salt to create a colored formazan product, just like the MTT assay does. MTS test is frequently used for high-throughput CQD cytotoxicity screening. Shorter incubation periods are a benefit of this test [47, 48].

When the cell membranes are disrupted or destroyed, in LDH release assay (lactate dehydrogenase assay), LDH gets released into the medium of the culture. This test counts the quantity of released LDH, which is indicative of cell damage. LDH release test is useful for determining membrane integrity and cell lysis during CQD-induced cytotoxicity [49]. Another commonly used method is the cell viability staining (e.g., Trypan Blue exclusion). Trypan Blue dye is taken up by non-viable cells but not by living cells. Calculating the number of stained and unstained cells gives an indication of cell viability. Cell viability following CQD exposure may be quickly and easily determined using Trypan Blue exclusion and comparable staining techniques [50].

Apoptosis/necrosis detection assays (e.g., Annexin V/PI staining) discriminate between necrotic and apoptotic cells using fluorescent markers. Propidium iodide (PI) designates necrotic cells, whereas Annexin V identifies apoptotic cells. They clarify whether apoptosis or necrosis is the method of cell death brought on by CQDs [51]. In reactive oxygen species (ROS) assays, oxidative stress is indicated by the formation of ROS. Intracellular ROS are measured by assays like DCFH-DA (2',7'-dichlorofluorescin diacetate). ROS tests can shed light on the possible oxidative harm triggered by CQDs [52].

Cell cycle analysis is another important study for cytotoxicity assessment. Propidium iodide DNA labeling and flow cytometry are used in cell cycle studies to map the cell distribution in various cell cycle stages (G0/G1, S, and G2/M). Cell cycle arrest can be a sign of cytotoxic effects brought on by CQDs, and this test aids in identifying it [53]. Mitochondrial membrane potential assay tracks variations in mitochondrial membrane potential, which can reveal apoptosis and dysfunctional mitochondria. It aids in determining how CQDs affect the health of mitochondria and the generation of energy [54]. In gene expression and proteomics analysis, by examining variations in gene expression and protein concentrations in response to CQD exposure, these molecular tests illuminate the underlying processes of cytotoxicity. A greater comprehension of how CQDs impact biological processes is provided through gene expression and proteomics investigations [55]. High-Content Screening (HCS) is another method that uses automated microscopy and image analysis to evaluate several cellular characteristics at once. In-depth, multiparametric examination of CQD-induced cytotoxicity is performed using HCS, enabling researchers to look at morphological modifications and subcellular effects [56]. CQD concentration, exposure time, and the particular cell type being treated are all important considerations when doing *in vitro* cytotoxicity tests using CQDs. Furthermore, using the right controls is essential for correctly interpreting the data. Together, these tests help us better understand the interaction of CQDs with cells and determine if they are safe for use in prospective biological applications.

The *in vivo* cytotoxicity studies involving animal models are essential for assessing the potential adverse effects of CQDs within complex biological systems. These studies provide valuable insights into how CQDs interact with living organisms, including their distribution, metabolism, and effects on various tissues and organs. An overview of *in vivo* cytotoxicity studies in animal models involving CQDs is as follows.

Researchers typically choose animal models that closely resemble the biological and physiological characteristics of humans. Commonly used animals include mice, rats, rabbits, and non-human primates [57]. The choice of species depends on the specific research objectives and the anticipated applications of CQDs in human medicine. CQDs can be administered to animals through various routes, including intravenous (IV), intraperitoneal (IP), intramuscular (IM), oral, and intratracheal (IT) routes. The administration route depends on the intended clinical application of CQDs and the desired target tissues or organs. Initial *in vivo* studies often focus on assessing acute toxicity. Animals are exposed to varying doses of CQDs, and their immediate responses are observed. Researchers monitor for signs of distress, changes in behavior, and acute physiological responses, such as changes in heart rate, blood pressure, and respiratory rate [58].

To assess chronic cytotoxicity and biocompatibility, animals are exposed to CQDs over an extended period, often ranging from weeks to several months [59]. These studies help identify any cumulative or delayed cytotoxic effects that may not be evident in acute toxicity assessments. Understanding the distribution of CQDs within the animal's body is crucial. Researchers use imaging techniques, such as positron emission tomography (PET), magnetic resonance imaging (MRI), and fluorescence imaging, to track the movement of CQDs. These studies reveal how CQDs are distributed among various tissues and organs over time. Tissue samples from various organs, especially those with high CQD accumulation, are collected for histopathological analysis. This involves examining tissue sections under a microscope to detect any structural abnormalities or damage. Histopathology provides insights into potential cytotoxic effects on specific organs [58]. Blood samples are collected to assess changes in hematological parameters (e.g., white blood cell count) and biochemical markers (e.g., liver enzymes) that could indicate systemic toxicity. Abnormalities in these parameters can indicate adverse effects of CQDs on blood and organ function. Studies may examine the immune response to CQDs, including assessments of cytokine levels and immune cell activation. This helps understand how CQDs interact with the immune system. Immune response data can also inform the potential use of CQDs in immunotherapy [60]. Investigating how CQDs are metabolized and excreted by the body is crucial for understanding their fate within living organisms. Studies may involve analyzing urine, feces, and other excretions to trace the elimination pathways [59]. Apart from these, *in vivo* studies involving animals must adhere to strict ethical guidelines and regulations to ensure the humane treatment of animals.

In vivo cytotoxicity studies in animal models provide crucial data for assessing the safety and biocompatibility of CQDs, offering insights into their potential for use in biomedical applications. These studies complement *in vitro* assessments and contribute to a comprehensive understanding of how CQDs interact with living organisms, helping to inform decisions about their clinical and environmental safety.

13.3.2 Factors Influencing Cytotoxicity of CQDs

The cytotoxicity of CQDs can be influenced by various factors, including concentration, exposure duration, and surface modifications. Understanding how these factors affect cytotoxicity is essential for assessing the safety of CQDs in biomedical applications and optimizing their use.

The main factors influencing the cytotoxicity of CQDs are concentration, exposure duration, surface modifications, aggregation state, cell or organism type, and surface contaminants. Higher concentrations of CQDs in cell cultures can lead to increased exposure levels, resulting in a more pronounced cytotoxic effect, particularly through elevated levels of reactive oxygen species. There is often a concentration threshold, a point above which cytotoxicity becomes more apparent, with the specific threshold varying based on CQD type, cell or organism type, and experimental conditions [61]. The dose-response relationship is a crucial aspect, with researchers studying concentration-dependent cytotoxicity profiles to establish safe exposure levels.

Additionally, the duration of CQD exposure plays a significant role, with short-term exposure to high concentrations causing immediate cell damage, while long-term exposure to lower concentrations may lead to chronic cytotoxicity affecting cell viability and function over time. Prolonged exposure can result in the accumulation of CQDs within cells or tissues. This accumulation may trigger cytotoxic responses, especially if CQDs are not efficiently metabolized or excreted. Surface modifications, including surface passivation, charge, functional groups, size, and shape, are also critical factors influencing CQD cytotoxicity. Surface passivation of CQDs involves coating their surfaces with biocompatible molecules, such as polymers or hydrophilic ligands. This can enhance their biocompatibility by reducing direct contact between CQDs and cells or tissues [62]. The surface charge of CQDs can affect their interaction with biological systems. Positively charged CQDs may exhibit higher cytotoxicity due to increased cellular uptake, while negatively charged CQDs may be less cytotoxic. The presence of specific functional groups on CQD surfaces can influence cytotoxicity. For instance, carboxyl-functionalized CQDs may exhibit different interactions with cells compared to amine-functionalized CQDs. While not strictly surface modifications, the size and shape of CQDs can influence their cytotoxicity. Smaller CQDs may have higher cellular uptake, potentially leading to increased cytotoxic effects. The shape of CQDs can also affect their cellular interactions [63].

The aggregation state of CQDs in biological media, cell, or organism type susceptibility, and the presence of surface contaminants are other key factors influencing cytotoxicity. The CQDs may aggregate in biological media due to factors like pH, ionic strength, and the presence of biomolecules. Aggregated CQDs can have different cytotoxicity profiles compared to well-dispersed CQDs. Aggregates may alter cellular uptake, ROS generation, and interactions with biomolecules. The cytotoxic response to CQDs can vary between different cell types, tissues, and organisms. Some cell types may be more susceptible to CQD-induced cytotoxicity due to differences in their internal environment, metabolic activity, or membrane characteristics [64]. CQD preparations may contain impurities or surface contaminants that contribute to cytotoxicity. Purification processes are essential to remove unwanted substances that could affect the biological response. The cytotoxicity of CQDs is a complex phenomenon influenced by various factors. Optimizing CQD properties and experimental conditions can lead to their safer and more effective use in biomedicine and other fields.

13.3.3 Underlying Mechanisms of CQD Cytotoxicity

Understanding the underlying mechanisms of cytotoxicity of CQDs is crucial for assessing their safety and developing strategies to mitigate associated risks. CQD cytotoxicity can be influenced by several mechanisms, and researchers have explored various strategies to enhance their biocompatibility. Some key mechanisms and mitigation strategies are as follows.

CQDs can generate reactive oxygen species (ROS) when exposed to biological environments. Excessive ROS production can lead to oxidative stress, damaging cellular components like DNA, proteins, and lipids. The physical interactions or membrane lipid peroxidation induced by ROS can cause membrane damage. The CQDs may disrupt cell membranes, compromising their integrity and leading to cell lysis. Cellular uptake of CQDs can be influenced by their size, surface chemistry, and charge. Internalization of CQDs may lead to intracellular accumulation and potential cytotoxic effects [16]. The CQDs can interfere with mitochondrial function, disrupting energy production and triggering apoptosis. Mitochondrial membrane potential can be affected, leading to the release of pro-apoptotic factors [65]. The CQD exposure may also trigger an immune response, leading to the release of pro-inflammatory cytokines. Prolonged inflammation can contribute to cytotoxicity and tissue damage. Genotoxicity assessments are crucial for evaluating long-term risks. The CQDs may induce DNA damage, which can lead to mutations and has the potential for carcinogenic effects [66].

The strategies to mitigate CQD cytotoxicity involves various methods. Modifying CQD surfaces with biocompatible molecules, such as polymers or hydrophilic ligands, can reduce direct contact with cells, mitigating membrane damage and ROS generation. Optimizing the size and shape of CQDs can influence their cellular uptake and toxicity. Smaller CQDs may exhibit reduced cytotoxicity. Surface passivation and antioxidant coatings can limit ROS production by CQDs [67]. These measures help prevent oxidative stress and its associated cytotoxic effects. Ensuring the use of non-toxic precursors and purification processes can minimize the presence of contaminants that contribute to cytotoxicity. Using lower CQD concentrations when possible, and minimizing exposure duration, can reduce cytotoxic effects. Establishing safe exposure thresholds is essential. Developing CQD formulations that selectively target specific cellular compartments or organelles can minimize overall cytotoxicity. Rigorous testing of CQDs *in vitro* and *in vivo* is essential for assessing their biocompatibility and identifying potential risks before clinical applications [61].

Tailoring CQD surface charges can influence cellular interactions. Neutral or negatively charged CQDs may exhibit reduced cytotoxicity compared to positively charged ones. Developing biodegradable CQD materials that can be metabolized and excreted from the body can mitigate long-term cytotoxicity risks associated with accumulation. Comprehensive characterization of CQD properties, including size, surface chemistry, and purity, is vital for ensuring reproducibility and minimizing cytotoxicity risks [68]. Adhering to regulatory guidelines and safety standards is essential for the safe development and commercialization of CQD-based products. Understanding the mechanisms of CQD cytotoxicity and implementing mitigation strategies are crucial steps in harnessing the potential of CQDs in various applications while ensuring their safety.

13.4   BIOCOMPATIBILITY ANALYSIS OF CQDs

Biocompatibility refers to the ability of a material or substance to interact with living organisms, such as cells, tissues, or organisms, in a way that does not produce harmful or adverse effects. In essence, a biocompatible material is one that is well-tolerated by biological systems and does not elicit detrimental reactions or responses when in contact with living matter. The CQDs will inescapably be released into the environment during the progressions of manufacturing, processing, labor, removal, and recuperation. The hydrophilic properties of CQDs have an effect on the ecosystem, especially on living things, food, and aquatic systems. Therefore, it is impossible to ignore the potential effects of CQDs on the environment. Recent investigations into the cytotoxic effects of CQDs on a variety of terrestrial creatures, including mice and rats, aquatic zebrafish, and particular cell bacteria, have demonstrated that they display high biocompatibility [69–72]. After being consumed by the living creature, CQDs did not significantly modify the pathology. They can exit an organism's body by typical metabolic pathways, for example, in the case of mice, rats, and zebrafish. On the other hand, multiple studies have shown that, when applied at the right concentration, CQDs have a favorable influence on plants, including their development and resilience to biotic and abiotic stress [73–76]. A sufficient amount of CQDs can support plant development by encouraging *Azotobacter* to fix nitrogen, assimilate nutrients, and speed up photosynthesis. During the development stages, it is crucial to accurately identify and assess the possible environmental concerns associated with the use of CQDs by determining their degrees of ecological effects and biological toxicity. The effects of CQDs on environments and biological occupants are also infrequently studied, which calls for careful evaluation in the future.

The biocompatibility study is of great importance in the context of CQDs because they have gained prominence for their potential applications in biomedicine, including drug delivery, bioimaging, and theranostics. To be used safely within the human body, CQDs must exhibit high biocompatibility to avoid adverse effects on cells, tissues, or organs. Poorly biocompatible CQDs can induce cytotoxic effects, such as cell damage, inflammation, or cell death. Ensuring biocompatibility is essential to minimize these adverse cellular responses. In many biomedical applications, CQDs are intended for prolonged or chronic use. Biocompatibility assessments help determine whether CQDs can be used safely over extended periods without causing cumulative toxicity or chronic health issues. Biocompatibility considerations extend to immune responses. Ideally, CQDs should not trigger significant immune reactions, as excessive immune responses can lead to inflammation, hypersensitivity, or autoimmune reactions. When CQDs are administered *in vivo*, they interact with the complex biological environment of living organisms. Ensuring biocompatibility is crucial to prevent adverse systemic responses and to promote the overall well-being of the organism [6, 77, 78].

Beyond biomedical applications, the biocompatibility of CQDs is relevant in environmental contexts. If CQDs are used in environmental remediation or monitoring, they should not introduce toxicity to ecosystems or aquatic life. Regulatory bodies, such as the FDA in the United States, require thorough assessments of biocompatibility for materials intended for use in medical devices or clinical applications. Compliance with these regulations is vital for commercialization. For medical applications involving patients, ensuring biocompatibility is a matter of patient safety and ethical responsibility. Patients should not be exposed to materials that could harm their health. Biocompatibility is a critical factor in the development and safe use of CQDs, especially in the context of their growing applications in biomedicine and environmental science. Evaluating and optimizing the biocompatibility of CQDs through rigorous testing and surface modifications are essential to harness their potential while ensuring safety for both biological systems and the environment.

13.4.1 THE IMPACT OF CQD PROPERTIES ON BIOCOMPATIBILITY

The properties of CQDs, including their size, shape, and surface chemistry, play a significant role in determining their biocompatibility. These properties can influence how CQDs interact with biological systems, impact cellular responses, and affect overall biocompatibility.

The size of CQDs can influence cellular uptake. Smaller CQDs typically have a greater surface area relative to their volume, making them more favorable for cellular internalization through processes like endocytosis or passive diffusion. Smaller CQDs may have an advantage in terms of tissue distribution. Their smaller size allows them to penetrate tissues more efficiently and reach target cells or organs. They may have a higher propensity to induce cytotoxic effects, especially when they accumulate within cellular compartments, as they can potentially interfere with cellular processes more effectively. In addition to this, the shape of CQDs can influence their interactions with cell membranes. Anisotropic shapes, such as rod-like or star-shaped CQDs, may have different membrane-penetrating abilities than spherical CQDs [79, 80]. The surface area of CQDs is directly related to their shape. Different shapes may offer varying amounts of surface area for interaction with biomolecules or cellular receptors. The shape of CQDs can also impact their distribution within tissues. Shapes that allow for greater cellular uptake may lead to different biodistribution profiles compared to shapes with less favorable cellular interactions.

The surface chemistry of CQDs is another important factor that influences its biocompatibility. The surface charge of CQDs can influence their interaction with cell membranes and cellular uptake. Positively charged CQDs may be more readily internalized, while negatively charged CQDs may exhibit reduced cellular uptake. Surface functionalization with specific chemical groups can enhance biocompatibility. For example, hydrophilic functional groups can improve CQD dispersibility in aqueous solutions and reduce aggregation. Surface chemistry can be tailored to attach targeting ligands, such as antibodies or peptides, which can enhance the specific binding of CQDs to target cells or tissues [81, 82]. This can improve the selectivity of CQDs for particular applications. Functionalization can also be used to reduce potential toxicity by passivating reactive surface sites that could generate reactive oxygen species (ROS) or lead to cellular damage.

13.4.2 Strategies for Enhancing the Biocompatibility of CQDs

Enhancing the biocompatibility of CQDs is crucial for their safe and effective use in various biomedical applications. Strategies for improving CQD biocompatibility can be tailored to specific applications and should address factors such as cytotoxicity, immunogenicity, and overall compatibility with biological systems. Here are some key strategies for enhancing the biocompatibility of CQDs for specific biomedical purposes:

CQDs with coating of biocompatible molecules, such as polymers or hydrophilic ligands, can reduce potential cytotoxicity by minimizing direct contact between CQDs and cells or tissues. The addition of polyethylene glycol (PEG) to CQD surfaces can improve their solubility and stability in aqueous environments, reduce non-specific interactions, and enhance circulation time *in vivo*. Functionalizing CQD surfaces with targeting ligands, such as antibodies, peptides, or aptamers, can enable specific binding to target cells or tissues, enhancing the selectivity of CQDs for biomedical applications like targeted drug delivery or cancer imaging. Modifying the size of CQDs to fall within a specific range can influence their cellular uptake and distribution within tissues, potentially reducing cytotoxicity and improving targeting efficiency [83, 84]. Tailoring the shape of CQDs, such as making them rod-shaped or star-shaped, can impact their cellular interactions and biodistribution, offering advantages for specific applications.

Adjusting the surface charge of CQDs can reduce non-specific interactions with cell membranes and minimize potential cytotoxicity. Negatively charged CQDs are often preferred for biocompatibility. Thorough purification processes are essential to remove unwanted impurities or byproducts generated during CQD synthesis, ensuring the purity and safety of the final CQD product. Developing CQD materials that are biodegradable and can be metabolized and excreted by the body can mitigate long-term cytotoxicity risks associated with accumulation. Incorporating antioxidant coatings on CQDs can help scavenge reactive oxygen species (ROS) produced by CQDs, reducing oxidative stress and potential cytotoxic effects [85].

Conduct rigorous *in vitro* biocompatibility assessments, including cell viability, ROS generation, and cytotoxicity assays, to identify potential issues and optimize CQD formulations. Perform thorough *in vivo* studies in animal models to evaluate the biodistribution, immunogenicity, and long-term effects of CQDs, simulating physiological conditions. Ensure that all research involving CQDs for biomedical applications adheres to ethical guidelines and regulatory requirements to protect the welfare of patients and research subjects. Comply with regulatory standards and seek necessary approvals for CQD-based medical devices, diagnostics, or therapies to ensure their safety and efficacy in clinical settings. Collaborate with multidisciplinary teams of researchers, including biologists, chemists, and clinicians, to leverage their expertise and collectively address biocompatibility challenges [86, 87].

Enhancing the biocompatibility of CQDs for specific biomedical applications is a multifaceted process that requires careful consideration of surface modifications, size, shape, and thorough testing. Tailoring CQDs to specific applications and optimizing their properties can lead to safer and more effective use in drug delivery, bioimaging, diagnostics, and other medical contexts.

13.5 BIOLOGICAL PROPERTIES OF CQDs

The past few years have witnessed great advancements in the fabrication of stable CQDs with strong photoluminescence properties and promising biological applications. However, the use of CQDs for further applications in living systems is being hindered by their biocompatibility concern. Over the last few years significant studies were carried out for evaluating the cytotoxicity in CQDs. For cytotoxicity evaluation, Yang et al. fabricated CQDs via arc discharge method with graphite rods refluxed in HNO_3 for a time period of 12h [88]. the CQDs were observed to be non-toxic till 0.4 mg/mL concentration. Zhao et al. carried out MTT assay of human kidney cell line using electrochemically synthesized CQDs from graphite [89]. The cell line was found to be undamaged, indicating the non-toxicity of CQDs. Studies were also done to test the cytotoxicity of PEG (polyethylene glycol) [88], PAA (polyacrylic acid) [90], and PEI (polyethyleneimine) [32] functionalized CQDs. The PEG functionalized CQDs were found to be non-toxic up to a higher concentration (greater than the required concentration for biological applications) [91, 92]. Work reported by Yang et al. evaluated the toxicity of PEG1500N passivated CQDs by injecting to mice for 28 days and the results proved the biocompatibility of passivated CQDs [91]. Cao et al. studied the toxicity effects of PEI, PEI-CQDs, and PPEI-EICQDs on the HT-29 cells using MTT assay. The results revealed the non-toxicity of PEI on the cells even at greater concentrations. Compared to PPEI-EICQDs, PEI-CQDs were found to be more toxic due to the presence of more EI units in it [93]. Some studies suggested the detrimental effects of free PAA in non-aqueous solution to cells even at low concentrations. Both free PAA and PAA-CQDs were found to be deadly to cells when exposed for 24 h and less harmful when exposed for 4 h at the same concentrations [32]. To sum up, CQDs functionalization using PEG and PPEI-EI can find application in *in vivo* bioimaging and biosensing even at high concentrations.

High toxicity molecules such as PAA can still be utilized for CQD functionalization provided that their concentration and incubation time are sufficiently lowered. The cell viability assay was used to evaluate the cellular toxicity of N-doped CQDs (N-CQDs). HepG2 cells were cultured with N-CQDs and CQDs at varying doses for a duration of 24 h. Compared to CQDs, N-CQDs were less hazardous. The outcomes demonstrated that the cell viability maintained at high concentrations, indicating the superior cellular compatibility and lack of toxicity of N-CQDs lead to their promising applications in cell imaging [94].

13.6 BIOMEDICAL APPLICATIONS OF CQDs

The optical and physicochemical characteristics of CQDs make them a great option for use in biological applications. Their fluorescent feature enables them to be monitored throughout the body through biosensing, bioimaging, and medication administration due to their tiny size and cellular compatibility. Due to the aforementioned characteristics of CQDs, including low toxicity, aqueous solubility, chemical inertness, non-blinking, and excitation- and size-dependent fluorescence emission, they can be used in a variety of biomedical applications, including gene delivery, electrochemical biosensing, pharmaceutical formulations, photodynamic and photothermal therapy, and the treatment of bacterial infections and inflammations.

13.6.1 Bioimaging

Quantum dots, or QDs, have been the subject of much research in the last several decades for both *in vivo* and *in vitro* bioimaging. Because of their remarkable properties, such as strong fluorescence, durability, and resistance to metabolic degradation, traditional QDs are frequently preferred over organic dyes and fluorophores in a variety of applications [95]. Notwithstanding these benefits, heavy metal toxicity and temperature sensitivity have shown to be drawbacks. Interestingly, at 4°C, QDs did not internalize. QDs were able to enter cells by endocytosis, but they were still unable to penetrate the nucleus. As a result, the use of CQDs in biological labelling and bioimaging has gained a great deal of attention. The current discovery that CQDs can emit photoluminescence in the near-infrared (NIR) spectral region holds particular significance for *in vivo* nanotechnology. This is attributed to the transparency of body tissues in the NIR window, emphasizing the potential of CQDs in advancing bioimaging techniques.

Yang et al. synthesized CQDs from nitric acid treatment of carbon soot and functionalized it using PEG1500 [91]. The cytotoxicity and biocompatibility of the same was compared with commercial CdSe/ZnS QDs semiconductor. The CQDs with a 20 % quantum yield and size less than 10 nm was found to be more fluorescent and biocompatible than QDs with size more than 20 nm. The CQDs with small size can be therefore applied as probes for biological sensing and in *in vivo* administrations. In an experiment, poly(propionyl ethylenimine-coethylenimine) was used by Cao and colleagues to make surface passivated CQDs, which resulted in high luminescence intensity in the NIR spectrum when excited by two photons [94]. The power of a pulsed infrared laser determined the brightness. The semiconductor QDs described in the literature were contrasted with the passivated CQDs. Following an incubation period with human breast cancer cells, these water-soluble CQDs with size less than 5 nm were stimulated with 800 nm laser pulses, and pictures were captured. The cytoplasm and cell membrane were marked by CQDs, but they were unable to enter the nucleus. In order to identify the nucleus, CQDs paired with TAT, a protein generated from the human immune deficiency virus, which enables CQDs to build up inside cells and make their way to the nucleus.

For the purpose of bioimaging, surface passivation enables CQDs to alter their optical characteristics. In the work by Shereema et al., passivated CQDs were created by heating maltose in a microwave [96]. Even after 24 h of incubation, CQDs were still able to penetrate the cells and produce green fluorescence, and cell viability was unaffected (Figure 13.2). Moreover, CQDs with a size of less than 10 nm were created utilizing a straightforward hydrothermal process with alkali lignin, citric acid, and ethylenediamine of various molar ratios. Even after 24 h, they showed 90 % cell viability when incubated with HeLa cells at a dosage of 0.62 mg mL^{-1}. Through the process of endocytosis, a significant number of CQDs were seen to enter the cells and emitted fluorescence. They mostly gathered in the cytoplasm, and the nucleus was shown to emit modest emissions. These CQDs released multicolor fluorescence when stimulated at various wavelengths. CQDs have significant potential in the domains of bioimaging and biolabeling because of their low toxicity, biocompatibility, and inherent capacity to emit multicolor fluorescence [97]. Moradi et al. studied the cell cytotoxicity of hydrothermally synthesized CQDs from Gum Tragacanth and

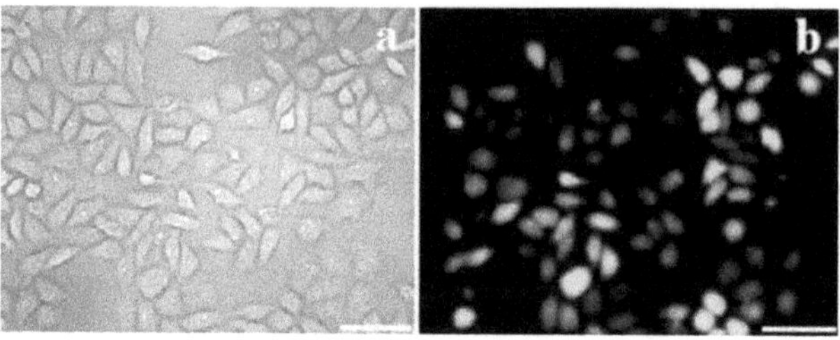

FIGURE 13.2 (a) Transmitted light image and (b) fluorescence image of 24 h CQDs incubated HeLa cells showing the cell labelling applications. [96].

Copyright 2015. Reprinted with permission from Elsevier.

chitosan based bio-polymers for bioimaging applications [20]. The fluorescence microscope images illustrating the distribution of Gum Tragacanth/chitosan and Gum Tragacanth-based CQDs within the HUVEC cell line is given in Figure 13.3. Hydrothermally generated CQDs have also been used in *in vivo* investigations for optical bioimaging. CQDs with a size range of 2 to 6 nm were effectively created utilizing glucose and xylose, byproducts of biorefineries, which were amino-passivated using urea. In order to determine if as-prepared CQDs are suitable for bioimaging, their photophysical characteristics were examined. When excited at a wavelength of 365 nm, it exhibited stable fluorescence behavior in comparison to the commercial fluorophore 4′,6-diamidino-2-phenylindole (DAPI), even when exposed to temperature changes of 4°C to 60°C and photobleaching treatment. L929 fibro-blasts were cultured on CQDs, and up to 400 mg/mL, their cell viability was still higher than 90 %. For *in vivo* optical imaging investigation, tumor cells were injected into a naked mouse via the tail vein, and CQDs were injected intravenously. It was noted that CQDs had excellent bioimaging performance, minimal toxicity, and anti-oxidant action in both *in vitro* and *in vivo* imaging assays [98].

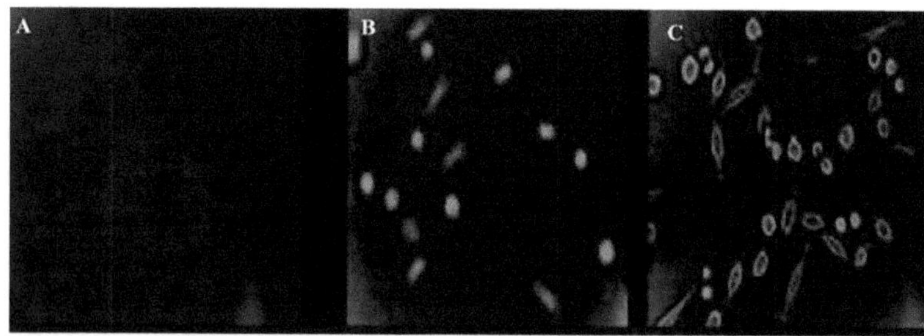

FIGURE 13.3 Fluorescence microscopy images illustrating the distribution of gum traga-canth/chitosan and gum tragacanth-based CQDs within the HUVEC cell line. (A) Image of control cells incubated without the compound. (B) and (C) Images of cells exposed to 50 µg/mL of gum tragacanth/chitosan and gum tragacanth-based CQDs, respectively, for a duration of 4 hours [20].

Copyright 2018. Reprinted with permission from Elsevier.

13.6.2 DIAGNOSIS

Diagnostics is a significant area in which CQDs are used in biomedicine. Disease diagnosis in vivo has been accomplished by semiconductive quantum dots [99, 100]. Comparing quantum dot-based nanoprobes to other current technologies, they are quick and affordable. CQDs are preferred for in vivo labeling due to their reduced toxicity as compared to conventional semiconductive quantum dots [59]. Cl-CQDs were created by functionalizing CQDs made from MWCNTs (multiwalled carbon nanotubes) with –COCl by acid and $SOCl_2$ treatment [101]. To detect the protein desmin, Cl-CQDs were then conjugated with anti-desmin. Patients with colorectal cancer have elevated levels of desmin in their serum [101, 102]. With great specificity and sensitivity, our CQD-based nanoprobes may be utilized to identify desmin in patient blood samples [101]. This finding should pave the way for further study into the creation of an affordable, precise, and sensitive diagnostic platform utilizing CQDs. Peroxynitrite (ONOO-), a reactive oxygen species generated in mitochondria, has recently been detected using CQD-based nanoprobes (Figure 13.4) [103]. Reactive oxygen/nitrogen species (ROS/RNS) are created during the ATP generation process and are crucial for cell signaling. However, given that peroxynitrites are often seen in a wide range of illnesses, it is thought that increased synthesis of these compounds may be the cause of some ailments [104]. Additionally, there is

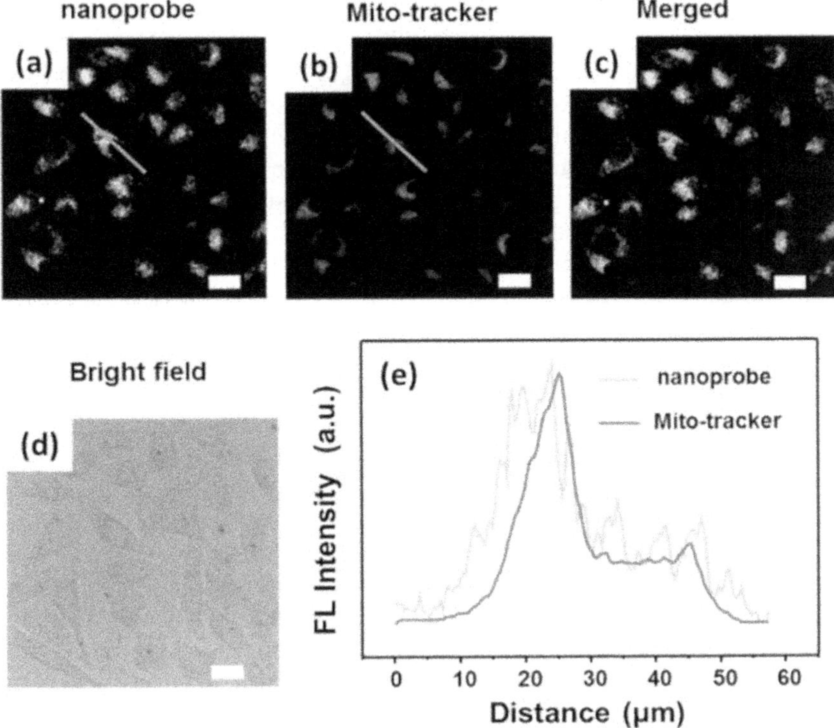

FIGURE 13.4 Confocal fluorescence images showing the mitochondria targeting ability of CQD-based nanoprobes [103].

a correlation between high ROS/RNS and mitochondria-induced programmed cell death. Thus, the accurate diagnosis of various medical diseases depends greatly on the intracellular detection of peroxynitrite. O-phenylenediamine, which was likewise able to detect peroxynitrite with great sensitivity (detection limit of 13.5 nM) and selectivity in live cells, was also used to construct mitochondria directing TPP (triphenylphosphonium)-modified CQDs (CQD-TPP) [103]. These on-off fluorescence nanoprobes based on CQDs have demonstrated tremendous promise for the advancement of mitochondria targeted in living cells for treatments and diagnostics.

It was recently discovered that CQDs might distinguish between malignant and normal cells according to their redox potential [95]. The solvothermal treatment of glycerol and N-(3-(trimethoxysilyl)propyl) ethylenediamine produced silicon and N-doped CQDs, which demonstrated sensitivity for Fe^{3+} ions with a detection limit of 16nM and an on-off fluorescence mechanism. Because the reductive environment of malignant cells lowered Fe^{3+} ions and caused the CQDs' fluorescence to revive, these CQDs with Fe^{3+} ions ($CQDs/Fe^{3+}$) may detect cancer cells using an on-off-on process [105]. Carbon quantum dots-apatamer conjugates and additional FA-CQDs were able to identify cancer cells with specificity [106, 107].

13.6.3 Biosensing

CQDs can be employed as biosensors because of their good water solubility, non-toxicity, outstanding cellular compatibility, excitation-dependent multicolor emission, permeability to cells, strong photostability, and low toxicity. Visual monitoring of glucose [108], cellular iron [109], phosphate [110], nucleic acid [111], potassium iron, and pH [112] is possible using CQD-based biosensors. CQDs are a great fluorescent assay for single-base mismatch-specific nucleic acid detection. Single-stranded DNA (ssDNA) probes are labeled by CQDs through p-p interactions. Fluorescence is quenched and hybridized to the target to form double-stranded DNA (dsDNA). This process results in the desorption of dsDNA from the CQD surface with more recovered fluorescence, thereby probing the target DNA [111]. Reactive oxygen species (ROS) are significant indicators for several illnesses, such as cancer, inflammatory or infectious diseases, DNA damage, rheumatoid arthritis, neurological illnesses, and drug screening for chemotherapy. One way to selectively destroy cancer cells is to manipulate reactive oxygen species (ROS) with oxidation-reduction active chemicals. ROS sensors, which use ascorbic acid hydrogel-based encapsulated CQDs, have been created to detect reactive oxygen species (ROS) (Figure 13.5). Measuring ROS levels following the administration of chemotherapeutic drugs is how they are used to assess the drug's effectiveness [113]. The one-pot pyrolysis process yields N-doped CQDs with a high QY of around 49.5% and strong photoluminescence, which are utilized for the inner filter effect (IFE)-based β-glucuronidase (GLU) inhibitor activity measurement (Figure 13.6). Because GLU has the potential to alter the fluorescence intensity of N-doped CQDs and prevent the growth of cancer cells, it is a highly valuable biomarker for the diagnosis of early-stage cancer and many physiological illnesses [114].

Thus far, several investigations have demonstrated that CQDs made using simple techniques are capable of detecting a wide range of ions, metals, and compounds

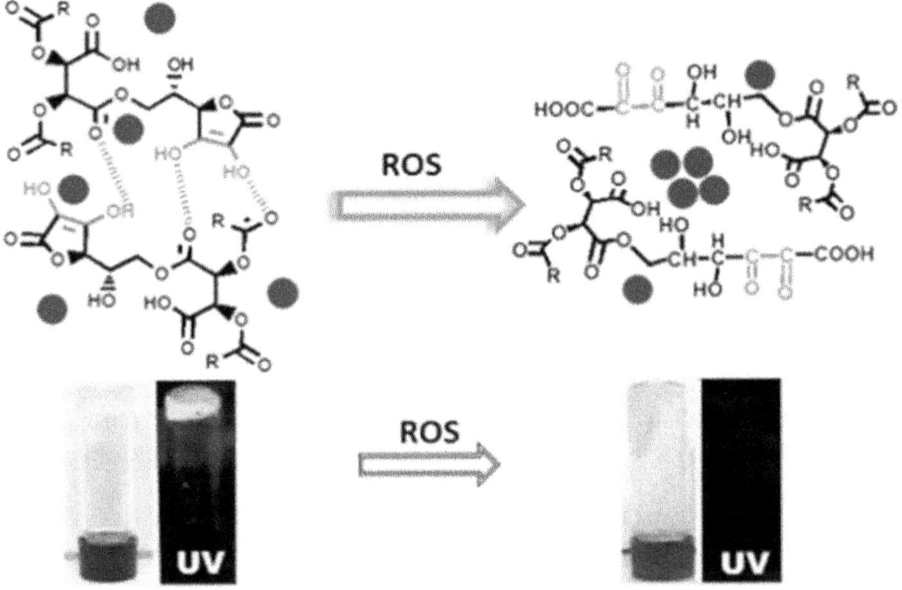

FIGURE 13.5   Ascorbic acid-based hydrogel CQDs for ROS sensing as a result of CQD aggregation and its fluorescence quenching [113].

Copyright 2017. Reprinted with permission from American Chemical Society.

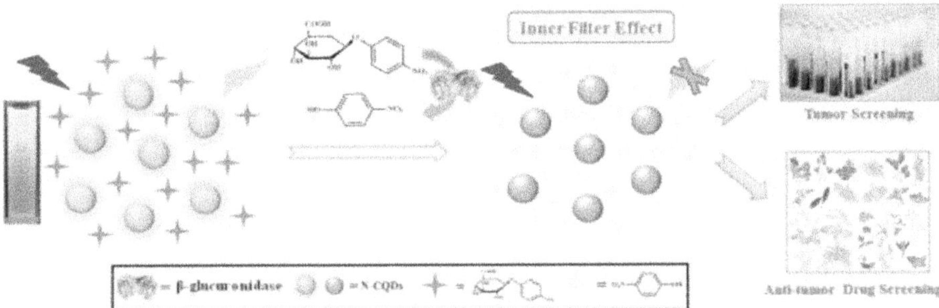

FIGURE 13.6   N-CQDs fluorescent sensor for β-glucuronidase based on inner filter effect [114].

Copyright 2017. Reprinted with permission from Elsevier.

with high sensitivity and selectivity. Biological and chemical situations will inevitably use CQDs for sensing applications because of their inherent capacity to detect metal ions. This is caused by the metal ions' attraction to the aromatic residues found on the surface of CQDs. CQDs are a useful tool for metal sensing because, even at low concentrations, metal binding to them causes fluorescence quenching. In a study, N-(β-aminoethyl)-γ-aminopropyl methoxysilane (AEAPMS) was used to synthesize CQDs. The residues of ethylenediamine and methoxysilane groups were coated on rhodamine B-doped silica nanoparticles, allowing them to detect Cu^{2+} ions [115]. Rhodamine B emitted red fluorescence while CQDs released blue fluorescence when excited at a single wavelength. Without influencing rhodamine B, CQDs quenched fluorescence when they came into contact with Cu^{2+} ions. The purpose of the *in vitro* experiment was to determine if dual emission nanoparticles could be produced by incubating them with MCF-7 cells. Fluorescence images were captured when blue and red wavelengths were emitted. The intensity of blue fluorescence reduced more than that of red fluorescence upon the addition of Cu^{2+} ions. All of these results point to the possibility that CQDs might serve as affordable, sensitive, non-invasive detectors that enhance human health.

13.6.4 ELECTROCHEMICAL BIOSENSING

CQDs show tremendous promise for application in biosensing, optical sensing, photovoltaics, chemical sensors, nanomedicine, and electrocatalysis due to their high stability, surface functionalization, and strong electrical conductivity [116, 117]. Due to their electrocatalytic properties, CQDs have garnered significant interest in the development of electrochemical biosensors for the detection of biomolecules such as glucose and dopamine, DNA, hemoglobin, cholesterol, glucose, L-cysteine, ascorbic acid, histene, and human carcinoembryonic antigen. They are also involved in the detection and reduction of H_2O_2. It has also been observed that CQDs containing polymers may detect hemoglobin with enhanced selectivity and sensitivity [118, 119]. As of now, there is a report of an instance of CQDs being utilized as an electrode modifier in the fabrication of a DNA sensor to identify changes in single genes [120]. CQD nano-composites (PtNPsCQDs/IL-GO) have been shown to be employed for H_2O_2 detection in one study (Figure 13.7). Because of their distinct chemical structure, they offer several active sites for electrochemical oxidation and reduction processes in addition to improved H_2O_2 catalysis. As demonstrated by the findings of the investigation, these electrochemical sensors (PtNPs-CDs/ILGO) have a low detection limit of 0.1 µM and a large selectivity ranging from 1 to 900 µM

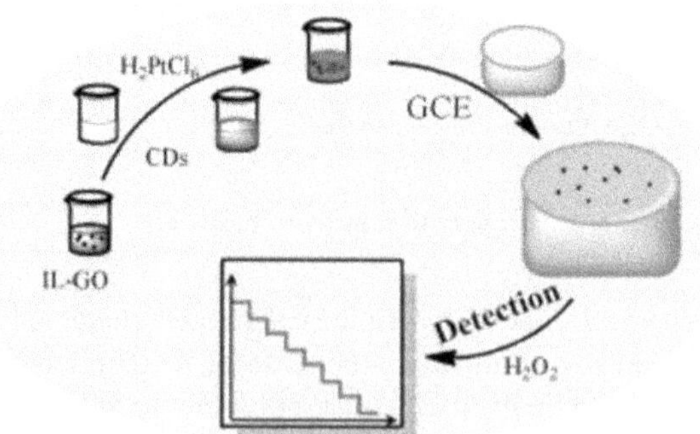

FIGURE 13.7   PtNPsCQDs/IL-GO based electrochemical detection of H_2O_2 [121].

Copyright 2018. Reprinted with permission from Elsevier.

with regard to the reduction of H_2O_2, which are qualities of high conductivity and electrocatalytic activity [121]. According to another study, CQDs may be combined with N-doped GQDs to create electrochemical biosensors by encasing them in Pt nanocrystals. Good catalytic activity is demonstrated by this nanocomposite in the electrochemical biosensing of damaged DNA markers. With the use of carbon-based ceramic electrodes, glucose oxidase, and GQDs, another electrochemical biosensor has been created to detect glucose. These graphene-based CQDs are attractive for electrochemical biosensors because of their excellent biocompatibility, hydrophobic carbon frame, hydrophilic edges, and increased enzyme uptake on electrodes [122].

13.6.5 DETECTION OF FOOD TOXINS

The special optical qualities of CQDs can be utilized to identify infections, heavy metals, and harmful compounds in food [98]. CQDs can be made from natural food items, and they are used to identify food toxins. For example, CQDs synthesized from apple juice are used to identify *P. aeruginosa* and *M. tuberculosis* bacteria as well as *M. oryzae* fungal cells [123]. The presence of toxic metals in soil is a serious problem since they are hazardous to people, cannot be broken down by microbes, may be consumed by plants, and can find their way into food products. According to Fan et al., CQDs composed of honey, maize flour, spoilt milk, and chine grass are employed as fluorescent detectors for the imaging of various heavy metal ions [124]. *Citrus sinensis* and *Citrus limon* skins were utilized to prepare two different kinds of CQDs via the one-pot synthesis technique. The as-synthesized CQDs had many of the same features, but they differed in a few key particular aspects. Because of their robust fluorescence qualities and the oxygen and nitrogen functional groups they have on their surface, CQDs may be used in a variety of ways. Fe^{3+} and tartrazine were detected using synthesized CQDs as chemosensors as shown in Figure 13.8. [125]. In a different study, a sensing technology for the detection of food additives was created based on the fluorescence properties of CQDs. *Flamboyant mirim* (FM), a leguminous plant, was used to create CQDs since it is an inexpensive and sustainable precursor. Following spectroscopy evaluation, the fluorescence response of CQDs was assessed using LDA in the presence of various compounds used in food product formulation. FM-CQDs are then employed as imaging probes to identify additives in pickled olives [126]. Thus, it may be said that CQDs made from natural sources may be employed to identify food poisons such as food pathogens, heavy metal ions, and other poisonous chemicals.

13.6.6 DRUG DELIVERY

In recent advancements of nanomedicine, significant progress has been made in developing drug delivery systems that enable precise targeting and delivery of drugs to specific areas within the body. These delivery systems are often combined with fluorescent nanomaterials for imaging purposes. Quantum dots, characterized by their small sizes, diverse surface chemistry, and fluorescence properties, have emerged as effective vehicles for drug delivery in therapeutic applications. The localization of these nanovehicles can be achieved through *in vitro* or *in vivo* methods,

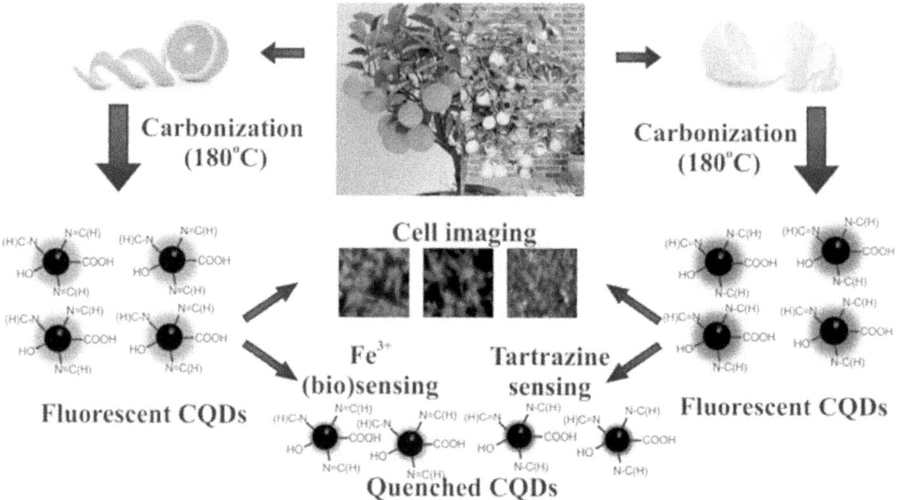

FIGURE 13.8 *Citrus sinensis* and *Citrus limon* peel-derived CQD-based detection of Fe^{3+} and tartrazine in food samples [125].

Copyright 2017. Reprinted with permission from Elsevier.

including high-performance liquid chromatography (HPLC) and the fluorescence emission properties of certain drugs, although these methods are time-consuming [127]. Over the past few years, QDs have played a key role in the creation of various drug delivery systems [128–131]. Additionally, CQDs, primarily composed of carbon, nitrogen, oxygen, and hydrogen atoms, have demonstrated their suitability as drug delivery systems. CQDs, with sizes less than 10 nm, have garnered attention due to their outstanding properties, including fluorescence emission, straightforward preparation, easy passivation, biocompatibility, aqueous solubility, lack of toxicity, and chemical inertness. This makes them highly promising candidates for advancing drug delivery systems [132].

One of the most frequently used model anticancer drugs in drug delivery systems, doxorubicin (DOX) has also been loaded on CQDs for drug delivery. One possible mechanism for DOX loading on the CQDs is the presence of functional groups that form a bond with the DOX; on the other hand, the main hypothesized mechanisms for the observed enhanced drug loading on the CQDs are the electrostatic attraction between DOX with positive charge and CQDs with negative charge, as well as the hydrophilicity of the CQDs, which encourages hydrogen bonding between DOX and CQDs [133]. The drug delivery process for CQDs-DOX involves many phases, such as: a) entering the cell by endocytosis and producing vesicles; b) moving the vesicles into the lysosomes; and c) releasing the protonated DOX into the acidic environment of the lysosomes and entering the cell nucleus [134]. A pH-sensitive CQDs-heparin-DOX nanovehicle for administering drugs was created by loading DOX onto CQDs that were fixed onto heparin (an auxiliary medication) via electrostatic interactions [135]. Hydrogen bonding can also be used to load mitomycin drugs onto CQDs, which can then be released when the connection breaks under tumor acidic conditions [136]. Active and deceased cancer cells can be distinguished by tracking the fluorescence of the CQDs in the delivery systems and examining the emission's position with respect to the cell nucleus. To be taken up by A549 cells, CQDs were added to hydrogels either with or without the anticancer medication 5-fluorouracil. Using an excitation wavelength of 360 nm, fluorescence microscopy observations showed blue emission from Hoechst 33342, a cell staining dye, and green emission from CQDs. As the concentration of CQDs in the gel grew, so did their green emission, which was concentration dependent. The nucleus of living cells may be distinguished by its lack of fluorescence. On the other hand, it was noted that a reduction in cell size causes the fluorescence to move from the cytoplasm to the nucleus [137]. Compared to using the medication alone, when CQDs are applied to drug delivery systems, the application may produce greater localization of medication-loaded CQDs in tumor cells. To deliver DOX to cancer cells, hydrothermally produced CQDs from milk were used. The adenoid cystic carcinoma cell line (ACC-2) was shown to be more hazardous to DOX-loaded CQDs than the mouse fibroblast cell line (L929). The drug delivery method of DOX-loaded CQDs became more localized in the tumor lines nucleus with a higher rate of death in the ACC-2 cells, according to fluorescence imaging, as compared to DOX alone (Figure 13.9). [133]. In an additional *in vivo* experiment, the suppression of cancer cell proliferation by DOX-linked CQDs demonstrated superior results when compared to the injection of free DOX. These delivery systems were treated with HepG2 and MCF-7 cancer cell lines to examine their pharmacological and imaging properties, and to confirm the DOX-linked CQDs activity in the body. The MTT cell proliferation experiment demonstrated that DOX-attached CQDs are more cytotoxic to cancer cells than they are to normal cells. Using a two-photon laser confocal microscope, the DOX-linked CQDs were stimulated at a wavelength of 380 nm. HepG2 cells showed almost minimal background fluorescence. Following a 24-hour incubation period using HepG2 cells, the free CQDs moved into the nucleus, whereas the luminescence of DOX-coupled CQDs was observed in the cytoplasm. This has been explained by the fact that free CQDs are smaller than DOX-conjugated ones. The bare CQDs demonstrated minimal cytotoxicity and excellent photostability even after 240 hours in aqueous circumstances [138]. Deng et al. reported a versatile NO-delivery platform by covalently bonding ruthenium nitrosyl and folic acid to CQDs, allowing targeted, light-controlled NO release and fluorescence tracking for specific cancer cell recognition [139]. In a distinct study, a nanogel matrix for drug loading, combined with CQDs for real-time fluorescence imaging, demonstrated controlled, folate receptor-targeted release within cancer cells, showcasing its superior capability for monitored drug delivery [140]. Hollow CQDs, synthesized at 6.8 nm diameter with a quantum yield of 7%, served as a pH-responsive drug delivery system for DOX, demonstrating stable, non-aggregating behavior and controlled release at pH 7.4 and pH 5.0, mimicking extracellular and lysosomal environments, respectively, with successful internalization and nucleus targeting in A549 cells [134]. As a drug delivery platform, CQDs integrated into polymer dendrimers with a three-dimensional structure and functional groups on the outside were utilized. They confirmed apoptosis induction in breast cancer (MCF-7) cells and showed enhanced fluorescence in close proximity

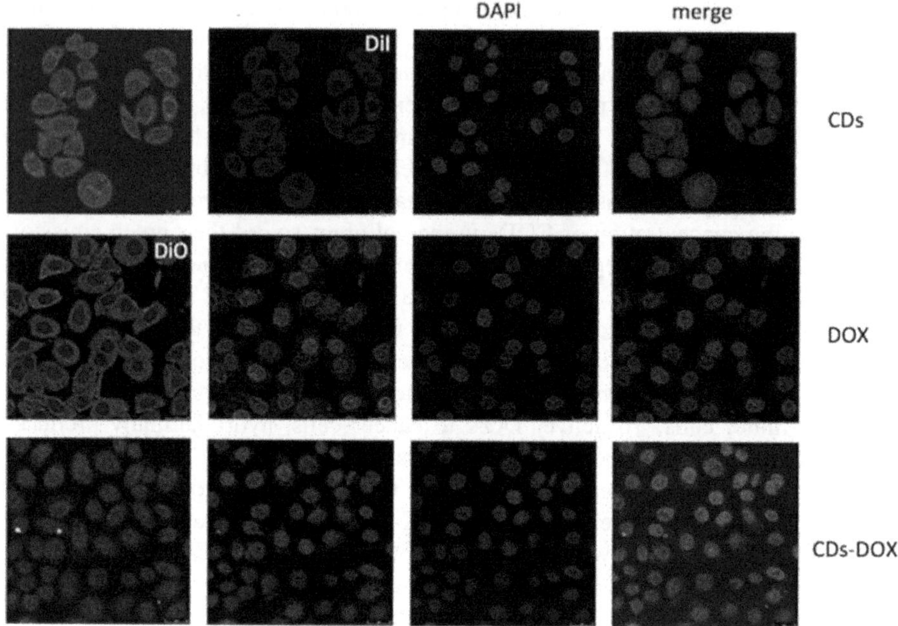

FIGURE 13.9 Fluorescence images of CQDs, DOX, and CQDs-DOX mixed ACC-2 cells for 4 h [133].

Copyright 2017. Reprinted with permission from Elsevier.

to dendrimer amine groups for tracking and cytotoxicity assessment [141]. CQDs were utilized for controlled in vitro release of dopamine hydrochloride (DA), an inotropic vasopressor agent for neurological diseases, demonstrating biocompatibility with neuro 2A cells, enhanced penetration into blood capillaries, improved drug permeability, and no observed toxic effects on mice weight over a 45-day observation period [142].

13.6.7 Gene Delivery

Fluorescent nanomaterials are employed in gene delivery, with non-viral vectors such as cationic polymers and liposomes offering safer alternatives to viral vectors, providing high transfection efficiency and simultaneous imaging, although lacking inherent self-tracking ability. Multifunctional vectors are having improved transfection efficiency, simultaneous imaging capability, and reduced toxicity and this can lead to a more reliable gene delivery therapy [143]. CQDs are interesting choice for multifunctional vectors because they can be used to deliver genes using fluorescence imaging. The CQDs/pDNA complex transfection investigations showed that transfection efficiency comparable to Lipofectamine2000 (positive control) performance and significantly higher than other positive controls (such as semiconductor QDs) could be obtained. The CQDs were also chosen for gene delivery over the cationic transfection reagent, PEI, because of their reduced toxicity. Condensation impacts on pDNA prevent pDNA enzymolysis during transport, increasing the produced CQDs' transfection effectiveness [144]. Using microwave pyrolysis, citric acid and PEI were combined to create cationic CQDs, which were then utilized to introduce small interfering RNA (siRNA) to several cell lines. The CQDs' transfection effectiveness and cytotoxicity were compared to those of the PEI, the precursor used in their synthesis. When delivering siRNA to the cells, the CQDs worked well. It was possible to accomplish 85% gene knockdown for weight ratios of 50-100 and 55% targeted gene knockdown CQDs/siRNA weight ratio of 12 [145]. While PEI, as a polymer gene carrier, binds to the cells readily and has a high transfection effectiveness, the cationic CQDs/gene plasmid SOX9 (pSOX9) nanomaterials demonstrated superior transfection efficiency than the PEI-CQDs/pDNA complexes. The use of cytotoxic-free, fine-particle-sized CQDs may help enhance the adhesion of pDNA to the cell membrane [143]. Das et al. explored environmentally friendly RNA interference technology for insect control by comparing CQDs, chitosan, and silica nanoparticles as carriers for double-stranded RNA targeting mosquito genes, revealing that CQDs were more efficient in retaining, delivering, and inducing gene silencing and mortality in *Aedes aegypti* larvae compared to chitosan and silica nanoparticles [146].

The CQDs, when paired with quencher nanoparticles, function as a fluorescent tool to monitor the association and dissociation of polyplexes in the cytoplasm. Kim et al. demonstrated this by using CQDs to track the formation and breakdown of a delivery complex involving CQDs and gold nanoparticles modified with cationic polymer PEI during transfection, revealing fluorescence changes indicative of complex formation and dissociation facilitated by pDNA and salt-induced disruption of charge interactions [147]. The PEI molecule has the ability to both passivate the CQDs' surface and function as a polyelectrolyte that condense DNA. Intense multi-color fluorescence and improved photostability were displayed using CQD-PEI. High-efficiency CQD-PEI-driven transfection of genes was observed in COS-7 and HepG2 cells [148]. Hu et al. employed branched PEI-based CQDs (PCD) having a QY of 54.3% for gene delivery in order to observe gene expression (Figure 13.10.) [1]. The DNA/PCD complexes were generated by mixing and had varying DNA/PCD weight ratios. The intensity of the fluorescence grew as the ratio of DNA to PCD weight dropped. The PCD fluorescence was shown to be an appropriate labeling tool for gene delivery. Nevertheless, the reporter gene of enhanced green fluorescent protein (EGFP) fluorescence does not superimpose with the fluorescence of some PCDs. This occurrence happens as a result of the CQDs' broken PEI chains, which prevent them from serving as gene carriers.

13.6.8 CROSSING BLOOD-BRAIN BARRIER

Over the past several years, research on nanoparticles have shifted to concentrate increasingly on creating medicine delivery systems. These carriers have been studied in the field of nanomedicine; they aid in the formulation of drugs and enable sustained drug release at the intended locations. These nanoparticles are coupled with diagnostic probes and made to target hard-to-reach locations for improved medication delivery [149]. Nanoparticles like CQDs play a crucial role in biomedical applications due to their small size, facilitating drug delivery across the blood-brain

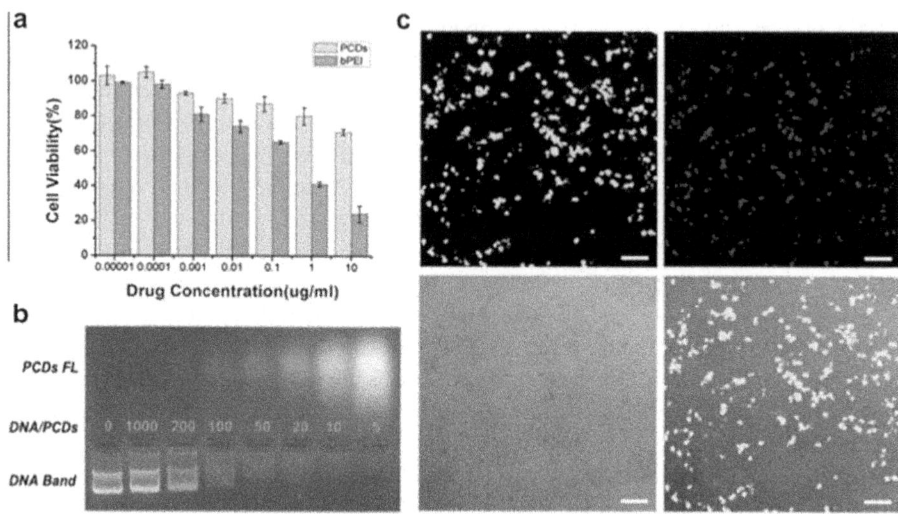

FIGURE 13.10 Biocompatibility and cell cytotoxicity study of polyethyleneimine-based CQDs and its gene delivery applications [1].

Copyright 2014. Reprinted with permission from Elsevier.

barrier, especially for substances like proteins and peptides; however, it is vital to ensure that the nanoparticle sizes are smaller than capillaries to prevent blockages and facilitate elimination by the body's reticuloendothelial system. Delivering imaging probes to brain tumors is challenging due to the blood-brain barrier, with success depending on the size and topography of the imaging probe. Li et al. reported that six hours after injection, CQDs were seen in several mouse organs and displayed bright fluorescence. A few of them are also seen in the brain, suggesting that CQDs have the capacity to penetrate the blood-brain barrier and reach the brain [150]. For *in vivo* imaging application, polymer-coated nitrogen-doped CQDs can enter glioma cells, aided by their hydrophilic polymer coating, enhancing blood circulation, targeting cancerous areas, and suggesting improved blood-brain barrier crossing for glioma fluorescence imaging [151]. A study by Mintz et al. shows the synthesis of tryptophan-based CQDs [152]. The CQDs, prepared with tryptophan and specific nitrogen dopants, demonstrate excitation wavelength-dependent emission, low toxicity, and successful entry into the central nervous system of zebrafish, suggesting a promising avenue for drug delivery and imaging in the brain. Confocal microscopy images depicting the same are given in Figure 13.11.

13.6.9 Photodynamic Therapy/Photothermal Therapy

When treating non-cancerous issues, photodynamic therapy (PDT) is particularly effective since it is non-invasive and has less adverse effects than other treatments for cancer. Photothermal coupling agents are necessary for effective PDT implementation [153]. A novel therapeutic agent, combining DOX, sgc8c aptamer, and SWCNTs-PEG-Fe$_3$O$_4$@CQDs, demonstrates multifunctionality and targeted killing of cancer

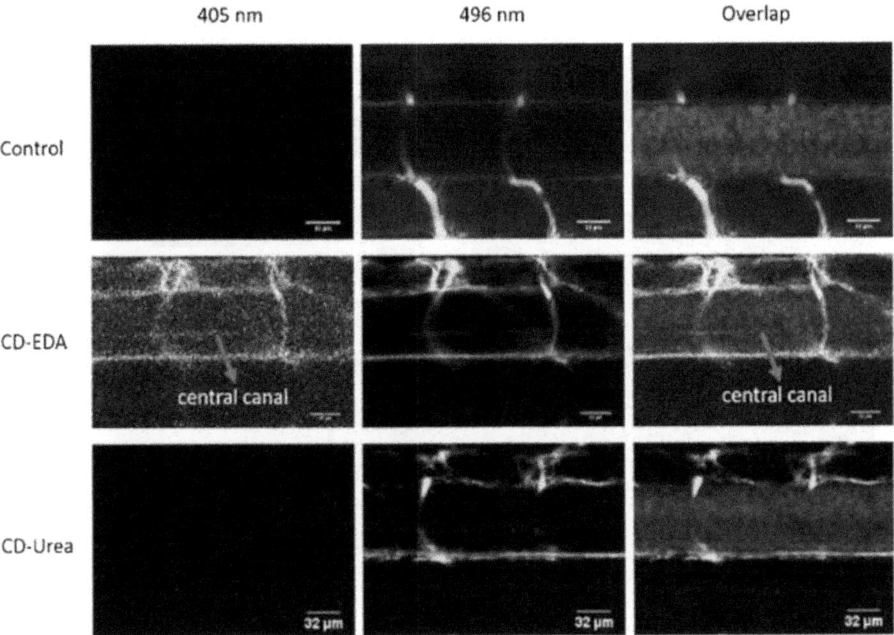

FIGURE 13.11 Confocal microscopy images showing the blood-brain barrier crossing ability of tryptophan CQDs injected into zebrafish [152].

Copyright 2019. Reprinted with permission from Elsevier.

cells through photodynamic or photothermal drug release. These nano-carriers are biocompatible, hydrophilic, and stable, with magnetic properties suitable for magnetic resonance imaging and precise drug delivery, making them favorable for treating cervical cancer and other diseases [154]. A CQD nano-composite, designed for effective cancer cell treatment, is made with folic acid and riboflavin, allowing it to deliver chemotherapy drugs with enhanced efficiency. This composite, when exposed to near-infrared light, releases the drugs, leading to increased drug accumulation in cells and improved effectiveness in killing cancer cells as depicted in Figure 13.12. [155]. CQDs and C60 fullerenes are proposed as photosensitizer medications that, when photoexcited, trigger an autophagic response, facilitating the detection of photodynamic cytotoxicity and allowing easy entry into target cells [153].

13.6.10 PHARMACEUTICAL FORMULATIONS/MEDICINAL COMBINATIONS

CQDs are increasingly used in various biological applications as a safer alternative to toxic nanoparticles, yet limited research exists on their impact on peptide and protein fibrillation. In a study, CQDs with a diameter of around 4 nm were found to effectively prevent insulin fibrillation, with a concentration of 40 µg/mL inhibiting fibrillation for 5 days at 65°C, compared to insulin denaturation within 3 hours in the absence of CQDs (Figure 13.13). This fibrillation-preventing effect arises from the reaction between CQDs and insulin components, making CQDs potential

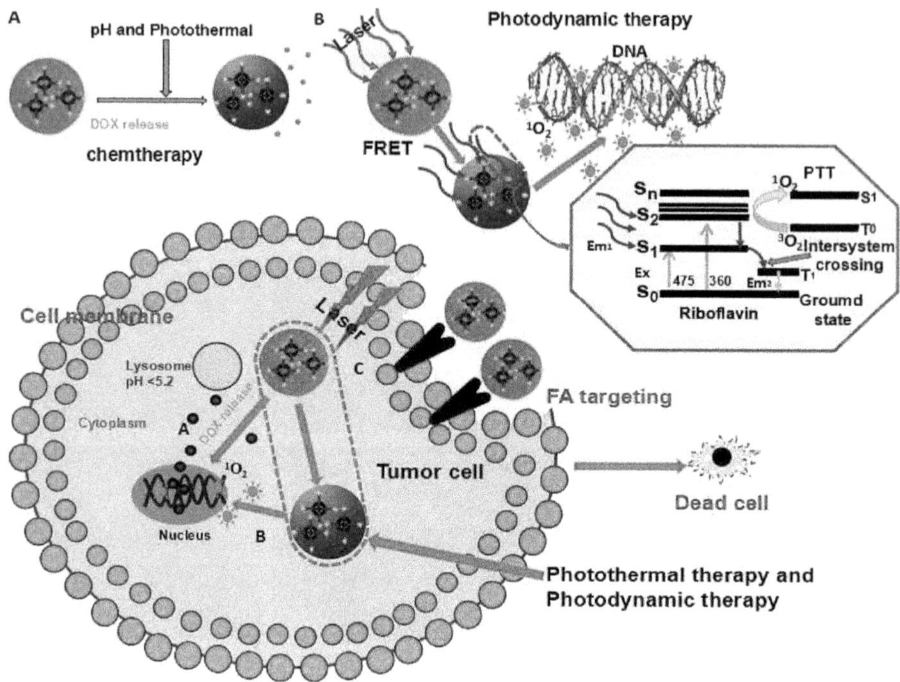

FIGURE 13.12　Schematic illustration of DOX release using CQDs and the possible cancer photodynamic therapy mechanism [155].

Copyright 2017. Reprinted with permission from Elsevier.

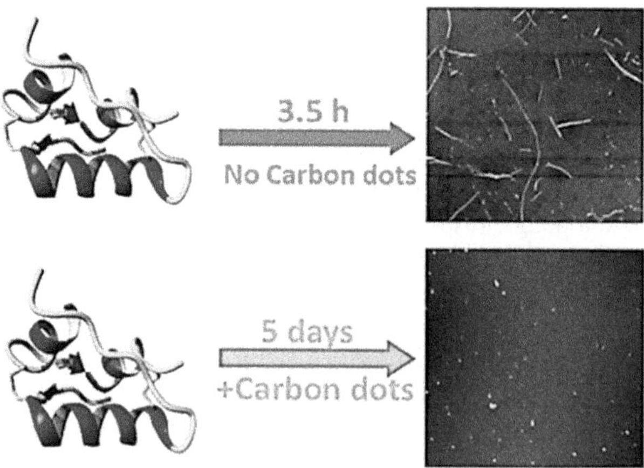

FIGURE 13.13　Scheme for the inhibitory effect of human insulin fibrillation of CQDs [156].

Copyright 2015. Reprinted with permission from American Chemical Society.

candidates for use in biological and pharmaceutical applications, particularly in insulin formulation [156]. In a different study, three gel formulations containing N-hydroxyphthalimide CQDs (NHF-CDs) were created, and their rheological analysis demonstrated that NHF-CD-loaded gels have the potential to significantly impact cell size, organization, spheroid number, as well as the multiplication and aggregation of tumor cells [157].

13.6.11 ANTIBACTERIAL EFFECT

Polyamine-derived carbon quantum dot polyamines (CQDPAs) with strong antibacterial activity have been developed for treating bacterial keratitis, demonstrating potential for clinical applications in treating eye infections and other bacteria-induced infections [43]. Quaternary ammonium CQDs, synthesized using a green method, exhibit effective antimicrobial activity against gram-positive bacteria, with promising results in treating pneumonia in mice, demonstrating their potential as encouraging agents for the treatment of gram-positive bacterial infections (Figure 13.14). To combat drug-resistant bacteria, particularly *Staphylococcus* and MRSA, N-doped CQDs synthesized using a one-step strategy exhibit antibacterial activity by destroying their cell structures through specific interactions, mimicking the effects of vancomycin in treating MRSA-induced wound infections, while showing no effectiveness against *E. coli* [158]. CQDs derived from curcumin exhibit antiviral activity against

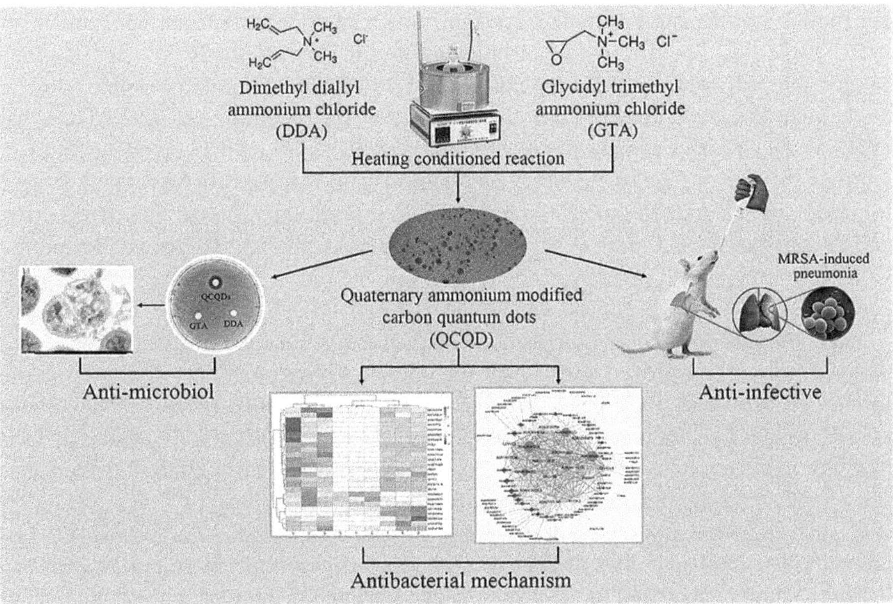

FIGURE 13.14 Schematic representation of the anti-microbial, anti-bacterial, and anti-infective activity of quaternary ammonium CQDs [158].

enterovirus, with their effectiveness depending on the synthesis heating temperature, demonstrating high biocompatibility and substantial inhibitory efficacy against viral infections in RD cells [159].

13.7 CONCLUSIONS

The chapter provides a comprehensive assessment of the current understanding of the cytotoxicity and biocompatibility of CQDs in various biomedical applications. CQDs have emerged as a promising nanomaterial with unique optical properties and versatile applications in bioimaging, drug delivery, biosensing, and therapeutics. However, a thorough evaluation of their safety profile is necessary to ensure their successful translation into clinical practice. This chapter also highlights the increasing interest in CQDs because of their many uses in the environmental and health domains. The biomedical area uses CQDs for biomarkers, bioimaging, biosensing, and nanomedicine because of its adjustable photoluminescence property, low toxicity, chemical stability, and hydrophilic nature. While semiconductor quantum dots are less commonly used as direct labels or tags, CQDs are used as carriers and provide a safer option. Despite their potential, there are now obstacles to their practical application, including poor quantum yield, repeatability, and preparation-related problems. Future study is expected to concentrate on adjusting the sizes, forms, repeatability, and specificity of CQDs in order to improve their functionality and overcome current constraints.

CQDs have special characteristics, and one of the most important factors influencing these characteristics is their size. Their low toxicity makes them very useful for use in biological activities, since it is favorable for a variety of *in vivo* applications. In an attempt to address the poor quantum yield of CQD nanocomposites, attempts are being undertaken to synthesize them using surface functionalization and bandgap engineering, which expands their potential uses. Even though it can be difficult to regulate the size of CQDs, current research highlights the need for better manufacturing methods in order to obtain the appropriate morphology, better size distribution, and flawless surfaces for the best possible biological activities. To assess and contrast CQDs, scientists are investigating a range of synthesis techniques from diverse sources.

This chapter provides a comprehensive overview of various cytotoxicity assessment techniques employed to evaluate the potential adverse effects of CQDs on different cell lines and organisms. It explores in vitro methods, such as cell viability assays, reactive oxygen species (ROS) generation, apoptosis assays, and cell morphology analysis, as well as *in vivo* studies utilizing animal models. Furthermore, this chapter investigates the factors influencing the cytotoxicity of CQDs, including size, surface chemistry, concentration, and exposure duration. Additionally, the biocompatibility analysis of CQDs is explored, considering their interactions with biological systems, including blood components, immune responses, and organ-specific toxicity. The impact of CQDs on the behavior and functionality of various cell types, such as stem cells and neuronal cells, is also discussed. The chapter emphasizes the importance of biocompatibility assessments to determine the suitability of CQDs for specific biomedical applications.

In conclusion, this chapter provides a comprehensive analysis of the cytotoxicity and biocompatibility of CQDs. It serves as a valuable resource for researchers, scientists, and biomedical engineers involved in the development and application of CQDs in various biomedical fields, including drug delivery, bioimaging, and therapeutics. The findings presented herein will aid in the safe and effective utilization of CQDs for future biomedical applications. While recent research has shed light on the biocompatibility of CQDs, several challenges remain. Achieving standardized protocols for cytotoxicity and biocompatibility assessment is essential for comparing results across studies. Additionally, long-term safety assessments and rigorous toxicological studies are needed to ensure the safe clinical translation of CQD-based therapies. Moreover, the potential environmental impact of CQD disposal should not be overlooked. Overall, thorough cytotoxicity and biocompatibility analyses are crucial for assessing the safety and potential applications of CQDs in biomedical settings. These evaluations help ensure that CQDs are compatible with biological systems and minimize any potential risks associated with their use.

REFERENCES

[1] Hu, L., Sun, Y., Li, S., Wang, X., Hu, K., Wang, L., … Wu, Y. (2014). Multifunctional carbon dots with high quantum yield for imaging and gene delivery. *Carbon, 67*, 508–513. https://doi.org/10.1016/j.carbon.2013.10.023.

[2] Ostadhossein, F., & Pan, D. (2017). Functional carbon nanodots for multiscale imaging and therapy. *Wiley Interdisciplinary Reviews: Nanomedicine and Nanobiotechnology, 9*(3), e1436. https://doi.org/10.1002/wnan.1436.

[3] Zheng, X. T., Ananthanarayanan, A., Luo, -K. Q., & Chen, P. (2015). Glowing graphene quantum dots and carbon dots: Properties, syntheses, and biological applications. *Small, 11*(14), 1620–1636. https://doi.org/10.1002/smll.201402648

[4] Zhu, S., Song, Y., Zhao, X., Shao, J., Zhang, J., & Yang, B. (2015). The photoluminescence mechanism in carbon dots (graphene quantum dots, carbon nanodots, and polymer dots): Current state and future perspective. *Nano Research, 8*(2), 355–381. https://doi.org/10.1007/s12274-014-0644-3.

[5] Cayuela, A., Soriano, M. L., Carrillo-Carrión, C., & Valcárcel, M. (2016). Semiconductor and carbon-based fluorescent nanodots: The need for consistency. *Chemical Communications, 52*(7), 1311–1326. https://doi.org/10.1039/c5cc07754k.

[6] Holá, K., Zhang, Y., Wang, Y., Giannelis, E. P., Zbořil, R., & Rogach, A. L. (2014). Carbon dots-Emerging light emitters for bioimaging, cancer therapy and optoelectronics. *Nano Today, 9*(5), 590–603. https://doi.org/10.1016/j.nantod.2014.09.004.

[7] Shen, J., Zhu, Y., Yang, X., & Li, C. (2012). Graphene quantum dots: Emergent nanolights for bioimaging, sensors, catalysis and photovoltaic devices. *Chemical Communications, 48*(31), 3686. https://doi.org/10.1039/c2cc00110a.

[8] Wang, S. J., Cole, I., Zhao, D., & Li, Q. (2016). The dual roles of functional groups in the photoluminescence of graphene quantum dots. *Nanoscale, 8*(14), 7449–7458. https://doi.org/10.1039/c5nr07042b.

[9] Wang, D., Zhu, L., Chen, J., & Dai, L. (2015). Can graphene quantum dots cause DNA damage in cells? *Nanoscale, 7*(21), 9894–9901. https://doi.org/10.1039/c5nr01734c.

[10] Wang, Z., Zeng, H., & Sun, L. (2015). Graphene quantum dots: Versatile photoluminescence for energy, biomedical, and environmental applications. *Journal of Materials Chemistry C, 3*(6), 1157–1165. https://doi.org/10.1039/c4tc02536a.

[11] Wang, X., Sun, G., Li, N., & Chen, P. (2016). Quantum dots derived from two-dimensional materials and their applications for catalysis and energy. *Chemical Society Reviews*, *45*(8), 2239–2262. https://doi.org/10.1039/c5cs00811e.

[12] Feng, L., & Liu, Z. (2011). Graphene in biomedicine: Opportunities and challenges. *Nanomedicine*, *6*(2), 317–324. https://doi.org/10.2217/nnm.10.158.

[13] Seabra, A. B., Paula, A. J., De Lima, R., Alves, O. L., & Durán, N. (2014). Nanotoxicity of graphene and graphene oxide. *Chemical Research in Toxicology*, *27*(2), 159–168. https://doi.org/10.1021/tx400385x.

[14] Dhawan, A., & Sharma, V. (2010). Toxicity assessment of nanomaterials: Methods and challenges. *Analytical and Bioanalytical Chemistry*, *398*(2), 589–605. https://doi.org/10.1007/s00216-010-3996-x.

[15] Willaert, R., Kasas, S., Devreese, B., & Dietler, G. (2016). Yeast NanoBiotechnology. *Fermentation*, *2*(4), 18. https://doi.org/10.3390/fermentation2040018.

[16] Havrdová, M., Holá, K., Skopalík, J., Tománková, K., Petr, M., Čépe, K., Polakova, K., Tucek, J., Bourlinos, A.B., & Zbořil, R. (2016). Toxicity of carbon dots - Effect of surface functionalization on the cell viability, reactive oxygen species generation and cell cycle. *Carbon*, *99*, 238–248. https://doi.org/10.1016/j.carbon.2015.12.027.

[17] Jiang, D. Y., Chen, Y., Li, N., Li, W., Wang, Z., Zhu, J., Zhang, H., Liu, B., & Xu, S. (2015). Synthesis of luminescent graphene quantum dots with high quantum yield and their toxicity study. *PLOS ONE*, *10*(12), e0144906. https://doi.org/10.1371/journal.pone.0144906.

[18] Liu, J., Li, R., & Yang, B. (2020). Carbon dots: A new type of carbon-based nanomaterial with wide applications. *ACS Central Science*, *6*(12), 2179–2195. https://doi.org/10.1021/acscentsci.0c01306.

[19] Yang, S., Sun, J., Li, X., Zhou, W., Wang, Z., He, P., … Jiang, M. (2014). Large-scale fabrication of heavy doped carbon quantum dots with tunable-photoluminescence and sensitive fluorescence detection. *Journal of Materials Chemistry. A, Materials for Energy and Sustainability*, *2*(23), 8660–8667. https://doi.org/10.1039/c4ta00860j.

[20] Moradi, S., Sadrjavadi, K., Farhadian, N., Hosseinzadeh, L., & Shahlaei, M. (2018). Easy synthesis, characterization and cell cytotoxicity of green nano carbon dots using hydrothermal carbonization of Gum Tragacanth and chitosan bio-polymers for bioimaging. *Journal of Molecular Liquids*, *259*, 284–290. https://doi.org/10.1016/j.molliq.2018.03.054.

[21] Bi, J., Li, Y., Wang, H., Song, Y., Cong, S., Li, D., … Tan, M. (2017). Physicochemical properties and cytotoxicity of carbon dots in grilled fish. *New Journal of Chemistry*, *41*(16), 8490–8496. https://doi.org/10.1039/c7nj02163a.

[22] Su, W., Wu, H., Xu, H., Zhang, Y., Li, Y., Li, X., & Fan, L. (2020). Carbon dots: A booming material for biomedical applications. *Materials Chemistry Frontiers*, *4*(3), 821–836. https://doi.org/10.1039/c9qm00658c.

[23] Nocito, G., Calabrese, G., Forte, S., Petralia, S., Puglisi, C., Campolo, M., … Conoci, S. (2021). Carbon dots as promising tools for cancer diagnosis and therapy. *Cancers*, *13*(9), 1991. https://doi.org/10.3390/cancers13091991.

[24] Volkov, Y., McIntyre, J., & Prina-Mello, A. (2017). Graphene toxicity as a double-edged sword of risks and exploitable opportunities: A critical analysis of the most recent trends and developments. *2D Materials*, *4*(2), 022001. https://doi.org/10.1088/2053-1583/aa5476.

[25] Roy, S., Ezati, P., & Rhim, J. (2021). Gelatin/carrageenan-based functional films with carbon dots from enoki mushroom for active food packaging applications. *ACS Applied Polymer Materials*, *3*(12), 6437–6445. https://doi.org/10.1021/acsapm.1c01175.

[26] Namdari, P., Negahdari, B., & Eatemadi, A. (2017). Synthesis, properties and biomedical applications of carbon-based quantum dots: An updated review. *Biomedicine & Pharmacotherapy*, *87*, 209–222. https://doi.org/10.1016/j.biopha.2016.12.108.

[27] Holá, K., Bourlinos, A. B., Kozák, O., Berka, K., Šišková, K., Havrdová, M., … Zbořil, R. (2014). Photoluminescence effects of graphitic core size and surface functional groups in carbon dots: COO- induced red-shift emission. *Carbon, 70*, 279–286. https://doi.org/10.1016/j.carbon.2014.01.008.

[28] Li, N., Liang, X., Wang, L., Li, Z., Li, P., Zhu, Y., & Jiang, S. (2012). Biodistribution study of carbogenic dots in cells and in vivo for optical imaging. *Journal of Nanoparticle Research, 14*(10). https://doi.org/10.1007/s11051-012-1177-x.

[29] Ray, S. C., Saha, A., Jana, N. R., & Sarkar, R. (2009). Fluorescent carbon nanoparticles: Synthesis, characterization, and bioimaging application. *The Journal of Physical Chemistry C, 113*(43), 18546–18551. https://doi.org/10.1021/jp905912n.

[30] Gao, Z., Shen, G., Zhao, X., Dong, N., Jia, P., Wu, J., … Wang, Y. (2013). Carbon dots: A safe nanoscale substance for the immunologic system of mice. *Nanoscale Research Letters, 8*(1), 276. https://doi.org/10.1186/1556-276x-8-276.

[31] Wang, K., Gao, Z., Gao, G., Yan, W., Wang, Y., Shen, G., & Cui, D. (2013). Systematic safety evaluation on photoluminescent carbon dots. *Nanoscale Research Letters, 8*(1), 122. https://doi.org/10.1186/1556-276x-8-122.

[32] Wang, Y., Anilkumar, P., Cao, L., Liu, J., Luo, P. G., Tackett, K. N., … Sun, Y. (2011). Carbon dots of different composition and surface functionalization: Cytotoxicity issues relevant to fluorescence cell imaging. *Experimental Biology and Medicine, 236*(11), 1231–1238. https://doi.org/10.1258/ebm.2011.011132.

[33] Li, J., Zhang, G., Zhang, C., Sun, L., Jiang, Y., Yan, C., … Yang, J. (2013). Quantum dot-related genotoxicity perturbation can be attenuated by PEG encapsulation. *Mutation Research/Genetic Toxicology and Environmental Mutagenesis, 753*(1), 54–64. https://doi.org/10.1016/j.mrgentox.2013.01.006.

[34] Buyukhatipoglu, K., & Clyne, A. M. (2011). Superparamagnetic iron oxide nanoparticles change endothelial cell morphology and mechanics via reactive oxygen species formation. *Journal of Biomedical Materials Research Part A, 96A*(1), 186–195. https://doi.org/10.1002/jbm.a.32972.

[35] Soenen, S. J., Manshian, B. B., Himmelreich, U., Demeester, J., Braeckmans, K., & De Smedt, S. C. (2014). The performance of gradient alloy quantum dots in cell labeling. *Biomaterials, 35*(26), 7249–7258. https://doi.org/10.1016/j.biomaterials.2014.05.023.

[36] Liu, Y., Wang, W., Yang, J., Zhou, C., & Sun, J. (2013). pH-sensitive polymeric micelles triggered drug release for extracellular and intracellular drug targeting delivery. *Asian Journal of Pharmaceutical Sciences, 8*(3), 159–167. https://doi.org/10.1016/j.ajps.2013.07.021.

[37] Yang, S., Wang, X., Wang, H., Lu, F., Luo, P. G., Cao, L., … Sun, Y. (2009). Carbon dots as nontoxic and high-performance fluorescence imaging Agents. *The Journal of Physical Chemistry C, 113*(42), 18110–18114. https://doi.org/10.1021/jp9085969.

[38] Wang, H., Su, W., & Tan, M. (2020). Endogenous fluorescence carbon dots derived from food items. *The Innovation, 1*(1), 100009. https://doi.org/10.1016/j.xinn.2020.04.009.

[39] Cailotto, S., Amadio, E., Facchin, M., Selva, M., Pontoglio, E., Rizzolio, F., … Perosa, A. (2018). Carbon dots from sugars and ascorbic acid: Role of the precursors on morphology, properties, toxicity, and drug uptake. *ACS Medicinal Chemistry Letters, 9*(8), 832–837. https://doi.org/10.1021/acsmedchemlett.8b00240.

[40] Yousaf, M., Huang, H., Li, P., Wang, C., & Yang, Y. (2017). Fluorine functionalized graphene quantum dots as inhibitor against hIAPP amyloid aggregation. *ACS Chemical Neuroscience, 8*(6), 1368–1377. https://doi.org/10.1021/acschemneuro.7b00015.

[41] Kumawat, M. K., Thakur, M., Gurung, R. B., & Srivastava, R. (2017). Graphene quantum dots from *mangifera indica*: Application in near-infrared bioimaging and intracellular nanothermometry. *ACS Sustainable Chemistry & Engineering, 5*(2), 1382–1391. https://doi.org/10.1021/acssuschemeng.6b01893.

[42] Li, Y., Harroun, S. G., Su, Y., Huang, C., Unnikrishnan, B., Lin, H., … Huang, C. (2016). Synthesis of self-assembled spermidine-carbon quantum dots effective against multidrug-resistant bacteria. *Advanced Healthcare Materials*, 5(19), 2545–2554. https:// doi.org/10.1002/adhm.201600297.

[43] Jian, H., Wu, R., Lin, T., Li, Y., Lin, H., Harroun, S. G., … Huang, C. (2017). Super-cationic carbon quantum dots synthesized from spermidine as an eye drop formulation for topical treatment of bacterial keratitis. *ACS Nano, 11*(7), 6703–6716. https://doi. org/10.1021/acsnano.7b01023.

[44] Zhao, C., Wang, X., Wu, L., Wen, W., Zheng, Y., Lin, L., … Lin, X. (2019). Nitrogen-doped carbon quantum dots as an antimicrobial agent against *Staphylococcus* for the treatment of infected wounds. *Colloids and Surfaces B: Biointerfaces, 179*, 17–27. https://doi.org/10.1016/j.colsurfb.2019.03.042.

[45] D'souza, S. L., Deshmukh, B., Bhamore, J. R., Rawat, K. A., Lenka, N., & Kailasa, S. K. (2016). Synthesis of fluorescent nitrogen-doped carbon dots from dried shrimps for cell imaging and boldine drug delivery system. *RSC Advances, 6*(15), 12169–12179. https:// doi.org/10.1039/c5ra24621k.

[46] Arul, V., Edison, T. N. J. I., Lee, Y. R., & Sethuraman, M. G. (2017). Biological and cata-lytic applications of green synthesized fluorescent N-doped carbon dots using *Hylocereus undatus. Journal of Photochemistry and Photobiology B: Biology, 168*, 142–148. https:// doi.org/10.1016/j.jphotobiol.2017.02.007.

[47] Sun, Y., Zheng, S., Liu, L., Kong, Y., Zhang, A., Xu, K., & Han, C. (2020). The cost-effective preparation of green fluorescent carbon dots for bioimaging and enhanced intra-cellular drug delivery. *Nanoscale Research Letters, 15*(1), 1–9. https://doi.org/10.1186/ s11671-020-3288-0.

[48] Wang, B., Yang, B., Liu, L., Yan, G., Yan, H., Feng, J., … Sun, H. (2019). Osteogenic potential of Zn^{2+}-passivated carbon dots for bone regeneration *in vivo. Biomaterials Science, 7*(12), 5414–5423. https://doi.org/10.1039/c9bm01181a.

[49] Esfandiari, N., Bagheri, Z., Ehtesabi, H., Fatahi, Z., Tavana, H., & Latifi, H. (2019). Effect of carbonization degree of carbon dots on cytotoxicity and photo-induced toxicity to cells. *Heliyon, 5*(12), e02940. https://doi.org/10.1016/j.heliyon.2019.e02940.

[50] Jin, L., Ren, K., Xu, Q., Hong, T., Wu, S., Zhang, Y., & Wang, Z. (2018). Multifunctional carbon dots for live cell staining and tissue engineering applications. *Polymer Composites, 39*(1), 73–80. https://doi.org/10.1002/pc.23903.

[51] Sangeetha, V., Sri, S., Solanki, P. R., & Mohanan, P. (2021). Mechanism of action and cellular responses of HEK293 cells on challenge with zwitterionic carbon dots. *Colloids and Surfaces B: Biointerfaces, 202*, 111698. https://doi.org/10.10/16/j.colsurfb.2021. 111698.

[52] Das, B., Pal, P., Dadhich, P., Dutta, J., & Dhara, S. (2018). In vivo cell tracking, reactive oxygen species scavenging, and antioxidative gene down regulation by long-term expo-sure of biomass-derived carbon dots. *ACS Biomaterials Science & Engineering, 5*(1), 346–356. https://doi.org/10.1021/acsbiomaterials.8b01101.

[53] Şimşek, S., Şüküroğlu, A. A., Yetkin, D., Özbek, B., Battal, D., & Genç, R. (2020). DNA-damage and cell cycle arrest initiated anti-cancer potency of super tiny carbon dots on MCF7 cell line. *Scientific Reports, 10*(1), 13880. https://doi.org/10.1038/s41598-020-70796-3.

[54] Guo, S., Sun, Y., Wu, Z., Yang, R., Qu, L., & Li, Z. (2022). Simultaneous monitor-ing of mitochondrial viscosity and membrane potential based on fluorescence changing and location switching of carbon dots in livingcells. *Carbon, 195*, 112–122. https://doi. org/10.1016/j.carbon.2022.04.006.

[55] Tong, T., Hu, H., Zhou, J., Deng, S., Zhang, X., Tang, W., … Liang, J. (2020). Glycyrrhizic-acid-based carbon dots with high antiviral activity by multisite inhibition mechanisms. *Small, 16*(13), 1906206. https://doi.org/10.1002/smll.201906206.

[56] Hua, Y., Li, J., Song, Y., Zhao, H., Wei, Z., Li, X., ... Jiang, J. (2018). Synthesis of ginsenoside Re-based carbon dots applied for bioimaging and effective inhibition of cancer cells. *International Journal of Nanomedicine, 13*, 6249–6264. https://doi.org/10.2147/ijn.s176176.

[57] Ge, J., Jia, Q., Liu, W., Guo, L., Liu, Q., Lan, M., ... Wang, P. (2015). Red-Emissive carbon dots for fluorescent, photoacoustic, and thermal theranostics in living mice. *Advanced Materials, 27*(28), 4169–4177. https://doi.org/10.1002/adma.201500323.

[58] Wang, K., Gao, Z., Gao, G., Yan, W., Wang, Y., Shen, G., & Cui, D. (2013). Systematic safety evaluation on photoluminescent carbon dots. *Nanoscale Research Letters, 8*(1), 1–9. https://doi.org/10.1186/1556-276x-8-122.

[59] Tao, H., Yang, K., Ma, Z., Wan, J., Zhang, Y., Kang, Z., & Liu, Z. (2011). In vivo NIR fluorescence imaging, biodistribution, and toxicology of photoluminescent carbon dots produced from carbon nanotubes and graphite. *Small, 8*(2), 281–290. https://doi.org/10.1002/smll.201101706.

[60] Huang, S., Li, B., Ashraf, U., Li, Q., Lu, X., Gao, X., ... Cao, S. (2020). Quaternized cationic carbon dots as antigen delivery systems for improving humoral and cellular immune responses. *ACS Applied Nano Materials, 3*(9), 9449–9461. https://doi.org/10.1021/acsanm.0c02062.

[61] Anand, A., Unnikrishnan, B., Wei, S., Chou, C. P., Zhang, L., & Huang, C. (2019). Graphene oxide and carbon dots as broad-spectrum antimicrobial agents: A minireview. *Nanoscale Horizons, 4*(1), 117–137. https://doi.org/10.1039/c8nh00174j.

[62] Fan, J., Claudel, M., Ronzani, C., Arezki, Y., Lebeau, L., & Pons, F. (2019). Physicochemical characteristics that affect carbon dot safety: Lessons from a comprehensive study on a nanoparticle library. *International Journal of Pharmaceutics, 569*, 118521. https://doi.org/10.1016/j.ijpharm.2019.118521.

[63] Yan, J., Hou, S., Yu, Y., Qiao, Y., Xiao, T., Yan, M., ... Suo, G. (2018). The effect of surface charge on the cytotoxicity and uptake of carbon quantum dots in human umbilical cord derived mesenchymal stem cells. *Colloids and Surfaces B: Biointerfaces, 171*, 241–249. https://doi.org/10.1016/j.colsurfb.2018.07.034.

[64] Liu, Y., Sun, Z., Liu, J., Zhang, Q., Liu, Y., Cao, A., ... Wang, H. (2022). On the cellular uptake and exocytosis of carbon dots-significant cell type dependence and effects of cell division. *ACS Applied Bio Materials, 5*(9), 4378–4389. https://doi.org/10.1021/acsabm.2c00542.

[65] Ben-Zichri, S., Rajendran, S., Bhunia, S. K., & Jelinek, R. (2022). Resveratrol carbon dots disrupt mitochondrial function in cancer cells. *Bioconjugate Chemistry, 33*(9), 1663–1671. https://doi.org/10.1021/acs.bioconjchem.2c00282.

[66] Havrdová, M., Urbančič, I., Tománková, K., Malina, L., Štrancar, J., & Bourlinos, A. B. (2021). Self-targeting of carbon dots into the cell nucleus: Diverse mechanisms of toxicity in NIH/3T3 and L929 Cells. *International Journal of Molecular Sciences, 22*(11), 5608. https://doi.org/10.3390/ijms22115608.

[67] Wareing, T. C., Gentile, P., & Phan, A. N. (2021). Biomass-based carbon dots: Current development and future perspectives. *ACS Nano, 15*(10), 15471–15501. https://doi.org/10.1021/acsnano.1c03886.

[68] Ramachandran, P., Lee, C. Y., Doong, R., Oon, C. E., Thanh, N. T. K., & Lee, H. L. (2020). A titanium dioxide/nitrogen-doped graphene quantum dot nanocomposite to mitigate cytotoxicity: Synthesis, characterisation, and cell viability evaluation. *RSC Advances, 10*(37), 21795–21805. https://doi.org/10.1039/d0ra02907f.

[69] Biswas, A., Khandelwal, P., Das, R., Salunke, G., Alam, A., Ghorai, S., ... Poddar, P. (2017). Oxidant mediated one-step complete conversion of multi-walled carbon nanotubes to graphene quantum dots and their bioactivity against mammalian and bacterial cells. *Journal of Materials Chemistry B, 5*(4), 785796. https://doi.org/10.1039/c6tb02446g.

[70] Licciardello, N., Hunoldt, S., Bergmann, R., Singh, G., Mamat, C., Faramus, A., … Stephan, H. (2018). Biodistribution studies of ultrasmall silicon nanoparticles and carbon dots in experimental rats and tumor mice. *Nanoscale, 10*(21), 9880–9891. https://doi.org/10.1039/c8nr01063c.

[71] Zhang, M., Wang, H., Song, Y., Huang, H., Shao, M., Liu, Y., & Li, H. (2018). Pristine carbon dots boost the growth of *Chlorella vulgaris* by enhancing photosynthesis. *ACS Applied Bio Materials, 1*(3), 894–902. https://doi.org/10.1021/acsabm.8b00319.

[72] Wei, X., Li, L., Liu, J., Yu, L., Li, H., Cheng, F., … Li, B. (2019). Green synthesis of fluorescent carbon dots from gynostemma for bioimaging and antioxidant in zebrafish. *ACS Applied Materials & Interfaces, 11*(10), 9832–9840. https://doi.org/10.1021/acsami.9b00074.

[73] Li, J., Lian, X., Cheng, Y., Cheng, Y., Wang, Y., Wang, X., & Ding, L. (2019). Applications of carbon quantum dots to alleviate Cd^{2+} phytotoxicity in *Citrus maxima* seedlings. *Chemosphere, 236*, 124385. https://doi.org/10.1016/j.chemosphere.2019.124385.

[74] Lian, X., Guo, H., Wang, S., Li, J., Wang, Y., & Xing, B. (2019). Carbon dots alleviate the toxicity of cadmium ions (Cd^{2+}) toward wheat seedlings. *Environmental Science. Nano, 6*(5), 1493–1506. https://doi.org/10.1039/c9en00235a.

[75] Wang, H., Li, H., Zhang, M., Song, Y., Huang, J., Huang, H., … Kang, Z. (2018). Carbon dots enhance the nitrogen fixation activity of *Azotobacter chroococcum*. *ACS Applied Materials & Interfaces, 10*(19), 16308–16314. https://doi.org/10.1021/acsami.8b03758.

[76] Wang, H., Zhang, M., Song, Y., Li, H., Huang, H., Shao, M., & Liu, Y. (2018). Carbon dots promote the growth and photosynthesis of mung bean sprouts. *Carbon, 136*, 94–102. https://doi.org/10.1016/j.carbon.2018.04.051.

[77] Emam, A. N., Loutfy, S. A., Mostafa, A., Awad, H. M., & Mohamed, M. (2017). Cytotoxicity, biocompatibility and cellular response of carbon dots-plasmonic based nanohybrids for bioimaging. *RSC Advances, 7*(38), 23502–23514. https://doi.org/10.1039/c7ra01423f.

[78] Li, S., Guo, Z., Zhang, Y., Wang, X., & Liu, Z. (2015). Blood compatibility evaluations of fluorescent carbon dots. *ACS Applied Materials & Interfaces, 7*(34), 19153–19162. https://doi.org/10.1021/acsami.5b04866.

[79] Tian, X., Zeng, A., Liu, Z., Zheng, C., Wei, Y., Yang, P., … Xie, F. (2020). Carbon quantum dots: In vitro and in vivo studies on biocompatibility and biointeractions for optical imaging. *International Journal of Nanomedicine, 15*, 6519–6529. https://doi.org/10.2147/ijn.s257645.

[80] Tungare, K., Bhori, M., Racherla, K. S., & Sawant, S. (2020). Synthesis, characterization and biocompatibility studies of carbon quantum dots from *Phoenix dactylifera. 3 Biotech, 10*(12), 540. https://doi.org/10.1007/s13205-020-02518-5.

[81] Malmir, S., Karbalaei, A., Pourmadadi, M., Hamedi, J., Yazdian, F., & Navaee, M. (2020). Antibacterial properties of a bacterial cellulose CQD-TiO_2 nanocomposite. *Carbohydrate Polymers, 234*, 115835. https://doi.org/10.1016/j.carbpol.2020.115835.

[82] Gogoi, S., Kumar, M., Mandal, B. B., & Karak, N. (2015). High performance luminescent thermosetting waterborne hyperbranched polyurethane/carbon quantum dot nanocomposite with in vitro cytocompatibility. *Composites Science and Technology, 118*, 39–46. https://doi.org/10.1016/j.compscitech.2015.08.010.

[83] Hu, X., Sun, A., Kang, W., & Zhou, Q. (2017). Strategies and knowledge gaps for improving nanomaterial biocompatibility. *Environment International, 102*, 177–189. https://doi.org/10.1016/j.envint.2017.03.001.

[84] Alaghmandfard, A., Sedighi, O., Rezaei, N. T., Abedini, A., Khachatourian, A. M., Toprak, M. S., & Seifalian, A. M. (2021). Recent advances in the modification of carbon-based quantum dots for biomedical applications. *Materials Science and Engineering: C, 120*, 111756. https://doi.org/10.1016/j.msec.2020.111756.

[85] Molaei, M. J. (2019). Carbon quantum dots and their biomedical and therapeutic applications: A review. *RSC Advances*, *9*(12), 6460–6481. https://doi.org/10.1039/c8ra08088g.

[86] Khan, A., Ezati, P., Kim, J., & Rhim, J. (2023). Biocompatible carbon quantum dots for intelligent sensing in food safety applications: Opportunities and sustainability. *Materials Today Sustainability*, *21*, 100306. https://doi.org/10.1016/j.mtsust.2022.100306.

[87] Shen, L. (2011). Biocompatible polymer/quantum dots hybrid materials: Current status and future developments. *Journal of Functional Biomaterials*, *2*(4), 355–372. https://doi.org/10.3390/jfb2040355.

[88] Yang, S., Cao, L., Luo, P. G., Lu, F., Wang, X., Wang, H., … Sun, Y. (2009). Carbon dots for optical imaging in vivo. *Journal of the American Chemical Society*, *131*(32), 11308–11309. https://doi.org/10.1021/ja904843x.

[89] Zhao, Q., Zhang, Z., Huang, B., Peng, J., Zhang, M., & Pang, D. (2008). Facile preparation of low cytotoxicity fluorescent carbon nanocrystals by electrooxidation of graphite. *Chemical Communications*, *7*(41), 5116–5118. https://doi.org/10.1039/b812420e.

[90] Wang, Y., Bao, L., Liu, Z., & Pang, D. (2011). Aptamer biosensor based on fluorescence resonance energy transfer from upconverting phosphors to carbon nanoparticles for thrombin detection in human plasma. *Analytical Chemistry*, *83*(21), 8130–8137. https://doi.org/10.1021/ac201631b.

[91] Yang, S., Wang, X., Wang, H., Lu, F., Luo, P. G., Cao, L., … Sun, Y. (2009). Carbon dots as nontoxic and high-performance fluorescence imaging agents. *The Journal of Physical Chemistry C*, *113*(42), 18110–18114. https://doi.org/10.1021/jp9085969.

[92] Wang, X., Cao, L., Yang, S., Lu, F., Meziani, M. J., Tian, L., … Sun, Y. (2010). Bandgap-like strong fluorescence in functionalized carbon nanoparticles. *Angewandte Chemie International Edition*, *49*(31), 5310–5314. https://doi.org/10.1002/anie.201000982.

[93] Cao, L., Wang, X., Meziani, M. J., Lu, F., Wang, H., Luo, P. G., … Sun, Y. (2007). Carbon dots for multiphoton bioimaging. *Journal of the American Chemical Society*, *129*(37), 11318–11319. https://doi.org/10.1021/ja073527l.

[94] Qi, H., Teng, M., Liu, M., Liu, S., Li, J., Yu, H., … Guo, Z. (2019). Biomass-derived nitrogen-doped carbon quantum dots: Highly selective fluorescent probe for detecting Fe3+ ions and tetracyclines. *Journal of Colloid and Interface Science*, *539*, 332–341. https://doi.org/10.1016/j.jcis.2018.12.047.

[95] Zheng, X. T., Ananthanarayanan, A., Luo, K. Q., & Chen, P. (2014b). Glowing graphene quantum dots and carbon dots: Properties, syntheses, and biological applications. *Small*, *11*(14), 1620–1636. https://doi.org/10.1002/smll.201402648.

[96] Shereema, R. M., Sankar, V., Raghu, K. G., Rao, T. P., & Shankar, S. S. (2015). One step green synthesis of carbon quantum dots and its application towards the bioelectroanalytical and biolabeling studies. *Electrochimica Acta*, *182*, 588–595. https://doi.org/10.1016/j.electacta.2015.09.145.

[97] Xue, B., Yang, Y., Sun, Y., Fan, J., Li, X., & Zhang, Z. (2019). Photoluminescent lignin hybridized carbon quantum dots composites for bioimaging applications. *International Journal of Biological Macromolecules*, *122*, 954–961. https://doi.org/10.1016/j.ijbiomac.2018.11.018.

[98] Huang, C., Hung, Y., Weng, Y., Chen, W., & Lai, Y. (2019). Sustainable development of carbon nanodots technology: Natural products as a carbon source and applications to food safety. *Trends in Food Science and Technology*, *86*, 144–152. https://doi.org/10.1016/j.tifs.2019.02.016.

[99] Larson, D. R., Zipfel, W. R., Williams, R. M., Clark, S. W., Bruchez, M. P., Wise, F. W., & Webb, W. W. (2003). Water-Soluble quantum dots for multiphoton fluorescence imaging in vivo. *Science*, *300*(5624), 1434–1436. https://doi.org/10.1126/science.1083780.

[100] Zheng, Y., Gao, S., & Ying, J. Y. (2007). Synthesis and cell-imaging applications of glutathione-capped CdTe quantum dots. *Advanced Materials*, *19*(3), 376–380. https://doi.org/10.1002/adma.200600342.

[101] Li, C., Yan, Z., Chen, L., Jin, J., & Li, D. (2017). Desmin detection by facile prepared carbon quantum dots for early screening of colorectal cancer. *Medicine*, *96*(5), e 5521. https://doi.org/10.1097/md.0000000000005521.

[102] Ma, Y., Peng, J., Liu, W., Zhang, P., Huang, L., Gao, B., … Qin, H. (2009). Proteomics identification of desmin as a potential oncofetal diagnostic and prognostic biomarker in colorectal cancer. *Molecular & Cellular Proteomics*, *8*(8), 1878–1890. https://doi.org/10.1074/mcp.m800541-mcp200.

[103] Wu, X., Sun, S., Wang, Y., Zhu, J., Jiang, K., Leng, Y., … Lin, H. (2017). A fluorescent carbon-dots-based mitochondria-targetable nanoprobe for peroxynitrite sensing in living cells. *Biosensors and Bioelectronics*, *90*, 501–507. https://doi.org/10.1016/j.bios.2016.10.060.

[104] Kawanishi, S., & Inoue, S. (1997). Damage to DNA by reactive oxygen and nitrogen species. *PubMed*, *69*(8), 1014–1017. Retrieved from https://pubmed.ncbi.nlm.nih.gov/9301323.

[105] Gao, G., Jiang, Y., Jia, H., Yang, J., & Wu, F. (2018). On-off-on fluorescent nanosensor for Fe^{3+} detection and cancer/normal cell differentiation via silicon-doped carbon quantum dots. *Carbon*, *134*, 232–243. https://doi.org/10.1016/j.carbon.2018.02.063.

[106] Liu, H., Li, Z., Sun, Y., Geng, X., Hu, Y., Meng, H., … Qu, L. (2018). Synthesis of luminescent carbon dots with ultrahigh quantum yield and inherent folate receptor-positive cancer cell targetability. *Scientific Reports*, *8*(1), 1086. https://doi.org/10.1038/s41598-018-19373-3.

[107] Motaghi, H., Mehrgardi, M. A., & Bouvet, P. (2017). Carbon dots-AS1411 aptamer nanoconjugate for ultrasensitive spectrofluorometric detection of cancer cells. *Scientific Reports*, *7*(1), 10513. https://doi.org/10.1038/s41598-017-11087-2.

[108] Shi, W., Wang, Q., Long, Y., Cheng, Z., Chen, S., Zheng, H., & Huang, Y. (2011). Carbon nanodots as peroxidase mimetics and their applications to glucose detection. *Chemical Communications*, *47*(23), 6695–6697. https://doi.org/10.1039/c1cc11943e.

[109] Zhu, A., Qu, Q., Shao, X., Kong, B., & Tian, Y. (2012). Carbon-dot-based dual-emission nanohybrid produces a ratiometric fluorescent sensor for in vivo imaging of cellular copper ions. *Angewandte Chemie International Edition*, *51*(29), 7185–7189. https://doi.org/10.1002/anie.201109089.

[110] Zhao, H., Liu, L. Q., De Liu, Z., Wang, Y., Zhao, X., & Huang, C. (2011). Highly selective detection of phosphate in very complicated matrixes with an off-on fluorescent probe of europium-adjusted carbon dots. *Chemical Communications*, *47*(9), 2604–2606. https://doi.org/10.1039/c0cc04399k.

[111] Li, H., Zhang, Y., Wang, L., Tian, J., & Sun, X. (2011). Nucleic acid detection using carbon nanoparticles as a fluorescent sensing platform. *Chemical Communications*, *47*(3), 961–963. https://doi.org/10.1039/c0cc04326e.

[112] Wei, W., Xu, C., Ren, J., Xu, B., & Qu, X. (2012). Sensing metal ions with ion selectivity of a crown ether and fluorescence resonance energy transfer between carbon dots and graphene. *Chemical Communications*, *48*(9), 1284–1286. https://doi.org/10.1039/c2cc16481g.

[113] Bhattacharya, S., Sarkar, R., Nandi, S., Porgador, A., & Jelinek, R. (2016). Detection of reactive oxygen species by a carbon-dot-ascorbic acid hydrogel. *Analytical Chemistry*, *89*(1), 830–836. https://doi.org/10.1021/acs.analchem.6b03749.

[114] Lu, S., Li, G., Lv, Z., Qiu, N., Kong, W., Gong, P., … Wu, Y. (2016). Facile and ultrasensitive fluorescence sensor platform for tumor invasive biomaker β-glucuronidase detection and inhibitor evaluation with carbon quantum dots based on inner-filter effect. *Biosensors and Bioelectronics*, *85*, 358–362. https://doi.org/10.1016/j.bios.2016.05.021.

[115] Liu, X., Zhang, N., Bing, T., & Shangguan, D. (2014). Carbon dots based dual-emission silica nanoparticles as a ratiometric nanosensor for Cu^{2+}. *Analytical Chemistry*, *86*(5), 2289–2296. https://doi.org/10.1021/ac404236y.

[116] Li, W., Wei, Z., Wang, B., Liu, Y., Song, H., Tang, Z., ... Lu, S. (2020). Carbon quantum dots enhanced the activity for the hydrogen evolution reaction in ruthenium-based electrocatalysts. *Materials Chemistry Frontiers, 4*(1), 277–284. https://doi.org/10.1039/c9qm00618d.

[117] Wang, D. M., Lin, K., & Huang, C. (2018). Carbon dots-involved chemiluminescence: Recent advances and developments. *Luminescence, 34*(1), 4–22. https://doi.org/10.1002/bio.3570.

[118] Barati, A., Shamsipur, M., & Abdollahi, H. (2015). Hemoglobin detection using carbon dots as a fluorescence probe. *Biosensors and Bioelectronics, 71*, 470–475. https://doi.org/10.1016/j.bios.2015.04.073.

[119] Kour, R., Arya, S., Young, S., Gupta, V., Bandhoria, P., & Khosla, A. (2020). Review-recent advances in carbon nanomaterials as electrochemical biosensors. *Journal of the Electrochemical Society, 167*(3), 037555. https://doi.org/10.1149/1945-7111/ab6bc4.

[120] Campuzano, S., Yáñez-Sedeño, P., & Pingarrón, J. M. (2019). Carbon dots and graphene quantum dots in electrochemical biosensing. *Nanomaterials, 9*(4), 634. https://doi.org/10.3390/nano9040634.

[121] Chen, D., Zhuang, X., Zhai, J., Zheng, Y., Lu, H., & Chen, L. (2018). Preparation of highly sensitive Pt nanoparticles-carbon quantum dots/ionic liquid functionalized graphene oxide nanocomposites and application for H_2O_2 detection. *Sensors and Actuators B: Chemical, 255*, 1500–1506. https://doi.org/10.1016/j.snb.2017.08.156.

[122] Hoang, V. C., Dave, K., & Gomes, V. G. (2019). Carbon quantum dot-based composites for energy storage and electrocatalysis: Mechanism, applications and future prospects. *Nano Energy, 66*, 104093. https://doi.org/10.1016/j.nanoen.2019.104093.

[123] Mehta, V. N., Jha, S., Basu, H., Singhal, R. K., & Kailasa, S. K. (2015). One-step hydrothermal approach to fabricate carbon dots from apple juice for imaging of mycobacterium and fungal cells. *Sensors and Actuators B: Chemical, 213*, 434–443. https://doi.org/10.1016/j.snb.2015.02.104.

[124] Fan, H., Zhang, M., Bhandari, B., & Yang, C. (2020). Food waste as a carbon source in carbon quantum dots technology and their applications in food safety detection. *Trends in Food Science and Technology, 95*, 86–96. https://doi.org/10.1016/j.tifs.2019.11.008.

[125] Chatzimitakos, T., Kasouni, A., Sygellou, L., Avgeropoulos, A., Troganis, A. N., & Stalikas, C. D. (2017). Two of a kind but different: Luminescent carbon quantum dots from Citrus peels for iron and tartrazine sensing and cell imaging. *Talanta, 175*, 305–312. https://doi.org/10.1016/j.talanta.2017.07.053.

[126] Carneiro, S. V., Holanda, M., Cunha, H., Oliveira, J.A., Pontes, S. M. A., Cruz, A., ... Fechine, P. B. A. (2021). Highly sensitive sensing of food additives based on fluorescent carbon quantum dots. *Journal of Photochemistry and Photobiology A: Chemistry, 411*, 113198. https://doi.org/10.1016/j.jphotochem.2021.113198.

[127] Probst, C., Zrazhevskiy, P., Bagalkot, V., & Gao, X. (2013). Quantum dots as a platform for nanoparticle drug delivery vehicle design. *Advanced Drug Delivery Reviews, 65*(5), 703–718. https://doi.org/10.1016/j.addr.2012.09.036.

[128] Iannazzo, D., Pistone, A., Salamò, M., Galvagno, S., Romeo, R., Giofrè, S. V., ... Di Pietro, A. (2017). Graphene quantum dots for cancer targeted drug delivery. *International Journal of Pharmaceutics, 518*(1–2), 185–192. https://doi.org/10.1016/j.ijpharm.2016.12.060.

[129] Ding, H., Fan, Z., Zhao, C., Lv, Y., Ma, G., Wei, W., & Zhang, T. (2017). Beyond a carrier: Graphene quantum dots as a probe for programmatically monitoring anti-cancer drug delivery, release, and response. *ACS Applied Materials & Interfaces, 9*(33), 27396–27401. https://doi.org/10.1021/acsami.7b08824.

[130] Pardo, J., Peng, Z., & Leblanc, R. M. (2018). Cancer targeting and drug delivery using carbon-based quantum dots and nanotubes. *Molecules, 23*(2), 378. https://doi.org/10.3390/molecules23020378.

[131] Liao, W., Zhang, L., Zhong, Y., Shen, Y., Li, C., & An, N. (2018). Fabrication of ultrasmall WS2 quantum dots-coated periodic mesoporous organosilica nanoparticles for intra-cellular drug delivery and synergistic chemo-photothermal therapy. *Onco Targets and Therapy*, 1949-1960. https://doaj.org/article/ba06e4f61fe942ffa6c6392d8374cef7.

[132] Li, W. Q., Wang, Z., Hao, S., Sun, L., Nisic, M., Cheng, G., ... Zheng, S. (2018). Mitochondria-based aircraft carrier enhances in vivo imaging of carbon quantum dots and delivery of anticancer drug. *Nanoscale*, *10*(8), 3744–3752. https://doi.org/10.1039/c7nr08816g.

[133] Yuan, Y., Guo, B., Hao, L., Liu, N., Lin, Y., Guo, W., ... Gu, B. (2017). Doxorubicin-loaded environmentally friendly carbon dots as a novel drug delivery system for nucleus targeted cancer therapy. *Colloids and Surfaces B: Biointerfaces*, *159*, 349–359. https://doi.org/10.1016/j.colsurfb.2017.07.030.

[134] Wang, Q., Huang, X., Long, Y., Wang, X., Zhang, H., Zhu, R., ... Zheng, H. (2013). Hollow luminescent carbon dots for drug delivery. *Carbon*, *59*, 192–199. https://doi.org/10.1016/j.carbon.2013.03.009.

[135] Zhang, M., Yuan, P., Zhou, N., Su, Y., Shao, M., & Chi, C. (2017). pH-Sensitive N-doped carbon dots-heparin and doxorubicin drug delivery system: preparation and anticancer research. *RSC Advances*, *7*(15), 9347–9356. https://doi.org/10.1039/c6ra28345d.

[136] D'souza, S. L., Chettiar, S. S., Koduru, J. R., & Kailasa, S. K. (2018). Synthesis of fluorescent carbon dots using *Daucus carota subsp. sativus* roots for mitomycin drug delivery. *Optik*, *158*, 893–900. https://doi.org/10.1016/j.ijleo.2017.12.200.

[137] Sachdev, A., Matai, I., & Gopinath, P. (2016). Carbon dots incorporated polymeric hydro-gels as multifunctional platform for imaging and induction of apoptosis in lung cancer cells. *Colloids and Surfaces B: Biointerfaces*, *141*, 242–252. https://doi.org/10.1016/j.colsurfb.2016.01.043.

[138] Lee, H. U., Park, S. Y., Park, E. S., Son, B., Lee, S. C., Lee, J. W., ... Lee, J. Y. (2014). Photoluminescent carbon nanotags from harmful cyanobacteria for drug delivery and imaging in cancer cells. *Scientific Reports*, *4*(1), 4665. https://doi.org/10.1038/srep04665.

[139] Deng, Q., Xiang, H., Tang, W., An, L., Yang, S., Zhang, Q., & Liu, J. (2016). Ruthenium nitrosyl grafted carbon dots as a fluorescence-trackable nanoplatform for visible light-controlled nitric oxide release and targeted intracellular delivery. *Journal of Inorganic Biochemistry*, *165*, 152–158. https://doi.org/10.1016/j.jinorgbio.2016.06.011.

[140] Li, W., Liu, Q., Zhang, P., & Liu, L. (2016). Zwitterionic nanogels crosslinked by fluorescent carbon dots for targeted drug delivery and simultaneous bioimaging. *Acta Biomaterialia*, *40*, 254–262. https://doi.org/10.1016/j.actbio.2016.04.006.

[141] Matai, I., Sachdev, A., & Gopinath, P. (2015). Self-Assembled hybrids of fluorescent carbon dots and PAMAM dendrimers for epirubicin delivery and intracellular imag-ing. *ACS Applied Materials & Interfaces*, *7*(21), 11423–11435. https://doi.org/10.1021/acsami.5b02095.

[142] Khan, M. S., Pandey, S., Talib, A., Bhaisare, M. L., & Wu, H. (2015). Controlled delivery of dopamine hydrochloride using surface modified carbon dots for neuro diseases. *Colloids and Surfaces B: Biointerfaces*, *134*, 140–146. https://doi.org/10.1016/j.colsurfb.2015.06.006.

[143] Cao, X., Wang, J., Deng, W., Chen, J., Wang, Y., Zhou, J., ... Xu, X. (2018). Photoluminescent cationic carbon dots as efficient non-viral delivery of plasmid SOX9 and chondrogenesis of fibroblasts. *Scientific Reports*, *8*(1), 7057. https://doi.org/10.1038/s41598-018-25330-x.

[144] Zhou, J., Deng, W., Wang, Y., Cao, X., Chen, J., Wang, Q., ... Xu, X. (2016). Cationic carbon quantum dots derived from alginate for gene delivery: One-step synthesis and cellular uptake. *Acta Biomaterialia*, *42*, 209–219. https://doi.org/10.1016/j.actbio.2016.06.021.

[145] Pierrat, P., Wang, R., Kereselidze, D., Lux, M., Didier, P., Kichler, A., ... Lebeau, L. (2015). Efficient in vitro and in vivo pulmonary delivery of nucleic acid by carbon dot-based nanocarriers. *Biomaterials, 51*, 290–302. https://doi.org/10.1016/j.biomaterials.2015.02.017.

[146] Das, S., Debnath, N., Cui, Y., Unrine, J. M., & Palli, S. R. (2015). Chitosan, carbon quantum dot, and silica nanoparticle mediated dsRNA delivery for gene silencing in *Aedes aegypti*: A comparative analysis. *ACS Applied Materials & Interfaces, 7*(35), 19530–19535. https://doi.org/10.1021/acsami.5b05232.

[147] Kim, J., Park, J., Kim, H. W., Singha, K., & Kim, W. J. (2013). Transfection and intracellular trafficking properties of carbon dot-gold nanoparticle molecular assembly conjugated with PEI-pDNA. *Biomaterials, 34*(29), 7168–7180. https://doi.org/10.1016/j.biomaterials.2013.05.072.

[148] Liu, C., Zhang, P., Zhai, X., Tian, F., Li, W., Yang, J., ... Liu, W. (2012). Nanocarrier for gene delivery and bioimaging based on carbon dots with PEI-passivation enhanced fluorescence. *Biomaterials, 33*(13), 3604–3613. https://doi.org/10.1016/j.biomaterials.2012.01.052.

[149] Xu, G., Mahajan, S. D., Roy, I., & Yong, K. (2013). Theranostic quantum dots for crossing blood-brain barrier in vitro and providing therapy of HIV-associated encephalopathy. *Frontiers in Pharmacology, 4*, 140. https://doi.org/10.3389/fphar.2013.00140.

[150] Li, N., Liang, X., Wang, L., Li, Z., Li, P., Zhu, Y., & Jiang, S. (2012b). Biodistribution study of carbogenic dots in cells and in vivo for optical imaging. *Journal of Nanoparticle Research, 14*(10), 1177. https://doi.org/10.1007/s11051-012-1177-x.

[151] Wang, Y., Meng, Y., Wang, S., Li, C., Shi, W., Chen, J., ... Huang, R. (2015). Direct solvent-derived polymer-coated nitrogen-doped carbon nanodots with high water solubility for targeted fluorescence imaging of Glioma. *Small, 11*(29), 3575–3581. https://doi.org/10.1002/smll.201403718.

[152] Mintz, K. J., Mercado, G., Zhou, Y., Ji, Y., Hettiarachchi, S. D., Liyanage, P. Y., ... Dallman, J. E. (2019). Tryptophan carbon dots and their ability to cross the blood-brain barrier. *Colloids and Surfaces B: Biointerfaces, 176*, 488–493. https://doi.org/10.1016/j.colsurfb.2019.01.031.

[153] Marković, Z. M., Ristić, B., Arsikin, K., Klisic, D., Harhaji-Trajković, L., Marković, B. M. T., ... Trajković, V. (2012). Graphene quantum dots as autophagy-inducing photodynamic agents. *Biomaterials, 33*(29), 7084–7092. https://doi.org/10.1016/j.biomaterials.2012.06.060.

[154] Zhang, M., Wang, W., Cui, Y., Chu, X., Sun, B., Zhou, N., & Shen, J. (2018). Magnetofluorescent Fe_3O_4/carbon quantum dots coated single-walled carbon nanotubes as dual-modal targeted imaging and chemo/photodynamic/photothermal triple-modal therapeutic agents. *Chemical Engineering Journal, 338*, 526–538. https://doi.org/10.1016/j.cej.2018.01.081.

[155] Zhang, M., Wang, W., Zhou, N., Yuan, P., Su, Y., Shao, M., ... Pan, F. (2017). Near-infrared light triggered photo-therapy, in combination with chemotherapy using magnetofluorescent carbon quantum dots for effective cancer treating. *Carbon, 118*, 752–764. https://doi.org/10.1016/j.carbon.2017.03.085.

[156] Li, S., Wang, L., Chusuei, C. C., Suarez, V. M., Blackwelder, P., Mićić, M., ... Leblanc, R. M. (2015). Nontoxic carbon dots potently inhibit human insulin fibrillation. *Chemistry of Materials, 27*(5), 1764–1771. https://doi.org/10.1021/cm504572b.

[157] Logigan, C., Tiron, C., Carasevici, E., Stan, C. S., Ibanescu, S. A., Simionescu, B. C., & Peptu, C. A. (2019). Entrapment of N-Hydroxyphthalimide carbon dots in different topical gel formulations: New composites with anticancer activity. *Pharmaceutics, 11*(7), 303. https://doi.org/10.3390/pharmaceutics11070303.

[158] Zhao, C., Wu, L., Wang, X., Weng, S., Ruan, Z., Liu, Q., … Lin, X. (2020). Quaternary ammonium carbon quantum dots as an antimicrobial agent against gram-positive bacteria for the treatment of MRSA-infected pneumonia in mice. *Carbon*, *163*, 70–84. https://doi.org/10.1016/j.carbon.2020.03.009.

[159] Lin, C., Chang, L., Chu, H., Lin, H., Chang, P. C., Wang, C. H., … Huang, C. (2019). High amplification of the antiviral activity of curcumin through transformation into carbon quantum dots. *Small*, *15*(41), 1902641. https://doi.org/10.1002/smll.201902641.

14 Application of Carbon Quantum Dots in Dye Removal and Wastewater Treatment

Chirantan Kar and Pradip Kumar Sukul

14.1 INTRODUCTION TO DYE REMOVAL AND WASTEWATER TREATMENT

Industrial wastewater pollution is a serious problem that affects human health and the environment. According to Ryder (2017), industrial waste effluents account for 56% of the global freshwater discharge, which is about 2212 km^3 per year [1]. The dye industry is one of the major sources of industrial wastewater pollution, contributing to 17%–20% of the total [2]. The textile dyes are harmful because they contain dangerous chemicals (such as heavy metals, sulphur, nitrates, and soaps) that are toxic and carcinogenic. They also make the water coloured and turbid, which produces a bad smell and reduces the light penetration. This affects the aquatic life by lowering the oxygen level in the water [3].

Organic dyes are main effluent discharges from textile and related industry. They are highly toxic due to their organic structure, very well known to cause several health issues like irritation to eyes, gastrointestinal tract and respiratory tract [4]. The treatment of the industrial dye containing wastewater cannot be done by simply treated by conventional wastewater treatment plants. Several technologies have been developed to reduce the amount of dye contamination from water. Traditional techniques are based on the physical interaction such as adsorption, ultrafiltration, reverse osmosis and activated carbon filtration. These processes simply transfer the dye molecules from one medium to another one which finally produces solid wastes. Further treatment processes of such solid wastes are more expensive. Chemical processes have been developed to overcome these issues of solid wastes, which include chlorination, chemical oxidation, ozonation, etc. One such important process is the advanced oxidation processes (AOPs) which is a great solution. In this process, highly reactive oxygen species (ROS) are used to completely break down the structure of the organic dye into harmless small fragments. The ROS was produced by following the method of photocatalysis, electrochemistry and heterogeneous/homogeneous catalysis [5]. In certain industries, Fenton process is applied to remove organic dyes where hydroxyl radicals were the species to convert the dyes into harmless molecules [6]. But Fenton process was not much effective due to the limitations of unstable reagents for transport and storage. Moreover, this process produces huge amounts of iron sludge for post-treatment which was industrially not acceptable.

Researchers are trying to find new strategies to solve the issue which could be cost-effective and easy to handle. Among many strategies, catalytic approach which involves simultaneous removal and degradation of the dyes finds attraction to the industries. The ideal approach should include the environmentally friendly process of synthesis of catalytic materials, low-cost reagents and easy protocols.

Photocatalysis is an emerging tool for degrading waste dyes from both atmospheric and aquatic contaminants. Semiconductor-based photocatalysts accelerate the destruction of the organic dye/contaminants in the presence of sunlight. Although photocatalytic materials are attractive towards dye degradation, two major issues hindered their application in commercial scale. These two major issues are the fast charge recombination and restricted light absorption properties of the photocatalytic materials.

A new type of zero-dimensional material, called carbon quantum dots (CQDs), has emerged as a promising candidate for photocatalytic applications. CQDs are small, round particles with a size of 2–10 nm [7]. They have a mixed structure of amorphous and nanocrystalline carbon, with some parts resembling graphite (sp2 carbon) or graphene oxide sheets and some parts having diamond-like sp3 carbon bonds [8]. CQDs have many potential uses in various fields, such as bioimaging, drug delivery, photodynamic therapy, chemical sensing, biosensing, electrocatalysis and photocatalysis. The advantageous properties of CQDs compared to conventional semiconductor quantum dots are their unique chemical composition, bright and tunable photoluminescence, facile functionalization and excellent physicochemical and photochemical stability, low toxicity and less cost. CQDs have shown excellent absorption of UV-Vis light due to the Sp^2 C = C double bond's tendency to undergo π-π* transition in the inner core (HOMO-LUMO) when exposed to sunlight. The outer layer of CQDs could be modified with varieties of functional groups to tune their physical and chemical properties. From the circular economy perspective, CQDs are particularly attractive as they could be synthesized from a variety of precursors obtained from the natural sources, such as orange peel [9], tea [10], olive pit [11], egg white [12], alginate [13], glucose [14], chitosan [15], fructose [16], ascorbic acid [17] and citric acid [18], which can be easily recovered from food and organic waste.

CQDs exhibit quantum confinement effect typically not visible in the case of general semiconductor quantum dots, which causes the increase of the bandgap with decreasing size. Most of the photocatalysts absorb UV light when exposed to sunlight which is not beneficial for real applications as majority of solar energy is concentrated in the visible region. The surface of the CQDs could easily be modified with nitrogen to tune their absorption in the visible region to NIR region. Pyrrolic nitrogen was inserted to the surface of CQDs by Permatasari et al., to produce a red-shift in absorbance from 550 to 650 nm [19]. Geng et al. created CQDs which absorb NIR-II light by adding 4.3% graphitic nitrogen to CQDs [20]. CQDs can show outstanding photocatalytic dye degradation without the need for heteroatom doping.

14.2 METHYLENE BLUE DYE REMOVAL

Vassalini et. al. have explored the alginate solution-induced ionotropic gelation of oxide powders to prepare a pollutant capturing macrobeads as an efficient photocatalyst for the removal of methylene blue (MB) dye from water [21]. They have prepared a complex blend of a mixture of depolymerized alginate, organic acids, and CQDs. This multifunctional blend results in adsorption/photodegradation performances which cannot be achieved by functionalizing the beads with the same components taken when alone. The active composite consists of a complex mixture of depolymerized alginate, organic acids, and CQDs. The synthetic route reduces synthesis time, purification steps and energy consumption compared to previously reported procedures for the preparation of CQDs. They have prepared TiO_2 macrobeads which strongly improves the adsorption of pollutants and enables fast water decontamination. The decomposition of the dye was not only observed under UV illumination, but they also showed potential degradation under direct solar irradiation. They have prepared three different metal oxide-based CQD macrobeads (TiO_2, Al_2O_3 and yttria-stabilized ZrO_2) through ionotropic gelation. The corresponding commercial oxide powders were combined with alginate to form beads of an average diameter of 0.6 mm for Al_2O_3, 0.9 mm for TiO_2 and 0.8 mm for YSZ. For the synthesis of the macrobeads, first 400 mg of sodium alginate and 100 mg of sodium citrate were dissolved in 50 mL of Milli-Q water. The mixture was vigorously agitated for 15 min to make the alginate aggregates soluble and subsequently 8.5 g of TiO_2 nanopowder was added to the mixture. The dispersed solution was homogenized by using a ultrasonicator bath for 30 min. The prepared homogeneous solution was added dropwise into the crosslinking solution which was previously prepared by dissolving 2.94 g of $CaCl_2 \cdot 2H_2O$ in 200 mL of water/ethanol (80/20 vol%) mixture. The crosslinking was allowed to complete for 24 h to provide TiO_2 beads. Then, the beads were washed several times with Milli-Q water so that excessive Ca^{2+} ions can be removed. Finally, the beads were dried at room temperature. The same procedure was followed for the synthesis of Al_2O_3 and YSZ ZrO_2 beads. The *Alginate-Derived Active Blend* was then prepared by dissolving 45 mg of sodium alginate in 50 mL of Milli-Q water and treated the solution in a microwave digestion system.

The adsorption and photocatalytic degradation were determined using a methylene blue (MB) solution (6.5×10^{-6} M solution). Functionalization with the alginate-derived blend successfully enhanced the adsorption capability of all the oxide beads. It was observed that the functionalization had increased the adsorption of the MB dye in dark after 90 minutes. The enhancement of the adsorption was from 20% to 77% in the case of Al_2O_3, from 27% to 74% in the case of YSZ, and from 23% to 82% for TiO_2. In case of all the beads, the MB adsorption followed through a pseudo-second-order isotherm, indicating that the blend did not follow the modified MB adsorption mechanism. The mechanism involved chemical and electrostatic forces between the surface of oxide beads, which had negative groups attached to it, and the solution's MB^+ molecules, which had a positive charge. TiO_2 beads showed additional improvement of the dye decontamination which was due to the photocatalytic degradation activity and hence reduced the time for complete removal of MB from 75 to 30 min. This very short time complete degradation of MB dye was possible only due to the presence of CQDs in the blend.

Chai et. al. have created nitrogen-doped CQDs decorated with 2D graphitic carbon nitride (g-C_3N_4) for photocatalytic degradation of MB dye [22]. They have systematically investigated the effect of the synthetic route towards the catalytic degradation efficiencies. They have taken inexpensive precursors (citric acid and urea) to produce the CQDs and g-C_3N_4. The methods for the synthesis of the CQDs were mechanical mixing, thermal polymerization and the hydrothermal approach. It was found that the hydrothermal approach is the most effective method to produce the most efficient CQDs as photocatalysts.

CQD-based photocatalysts were prepared stepwise by preparing first nitrogen-doped CQDs (NCQD) and graphitic C_3N_4 and then the composite NCQD/g-C_3N_4 by mixing in different techniques. The details of the synthesis are given below.

For the synthesis of NCQDs, a specific amount of citric acid and urea was taken in 15 ml of distilled water and dissolved. Then, the mixture was transferred to a Teflon-sealed autoclave reactor which was operated at 150°C for 4 h. Then the tube was allowed to cool to room temperature. The solution obtained was dark brown in colour which was centrifuged at 12,000 rpm for 20 min to eliminate larger particles and the supernatant was collected. Finally, the supernatant was dried in an oven, yielding dark brown NCQD powder. g-C_3N_4 was synthesized by taking urea in a porcelain and then heated in a furnace to 550°C with a ramping rate of 5°C/min for 3h. Then the porcelain was cooled to give g-C_3N_4 as beige-coloured powder.

The CQDs/g-C_3N_4 composite was prepared by three different techniques. The first technique was mechanical mixing where NCQDs were mixed with g-C_3N_4 using a pestle and mortar and labelled as NCQD/g-C_3N_4 (Mech). In thermal polymerization technique, NCQDs were dissolved in water and ultrasonicated to create homogeneous dispersion. Then urea was mixed with the dispersed NCQDs and stirred. The solution was then vaporized at 90°C to get semi-solid materials. The semi-solid materials were then transferred into porcelain and heated to 550°C in a furnace with a ramping rate of 15°C/min for 2h. It was cooled to room temperature to give NCQD/g-C_3N_4 (Poly). In hydrothermal synthesis method, first C_3N_4 was exfoliated by ultrasonication in water and mixed with NCQDs. The mixture was stirred, and hydrothermal reaction was done in a sealed Teflon-coated autoclave at 120°C for 4 h to give a filter cake-like product (Figure 14.1). The obtained product was dried at 70°C overnight to give NCQD/g-C_3N_4.

The photocatalytic efficiencies of the composite of CQDs were studied in the degradation of methylene blue (MB) under LED light irradiation. It was reported that NCQD/g-C_3N_4 (Mech) exhibited a rate constant, k of 1.478×10^{-3} min^{-1}, which was just 1.12 times higher than that of pure g-C_3N_4. Therefore, the mechanical mixing method showed negligible improvement in the photocatalytic activity, which could be the reason of loosely connected heterojunctions [23]. In comparison to mechanically mixed composites, the NCQD/g-C_3N_4 hybrid prepared via the thermal polymerization route exhibited a slight increase in photocatalytic activity. The sample showed a rate constant of 2.445×10^{-3} min^{-1}, which was 1.86-fold higher compared to pure g-C_3N_4. In the thermal polymerization route, less activity was observed due to the decarboxylation of functional groups at higher temperatures and aggregation of CQDs. The hydrothermal route was found to be the most effective method to perform the dye degradation. As can be seen from Figure 14.2, the hybrid composite

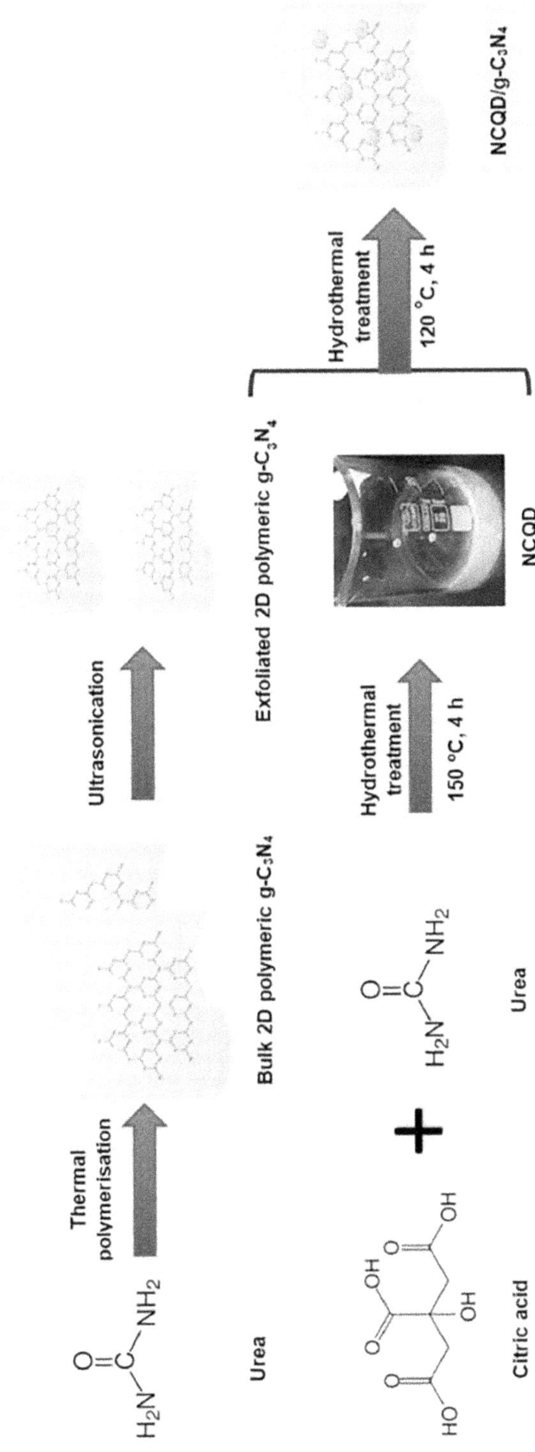

FIGURE 14.1 Schematic representation of the hydrothermal route for the synthesis of NCQD/g-C$_3$N$_4$ composite. Reproduced with permission from [22], copyright 2020, Elsevier.

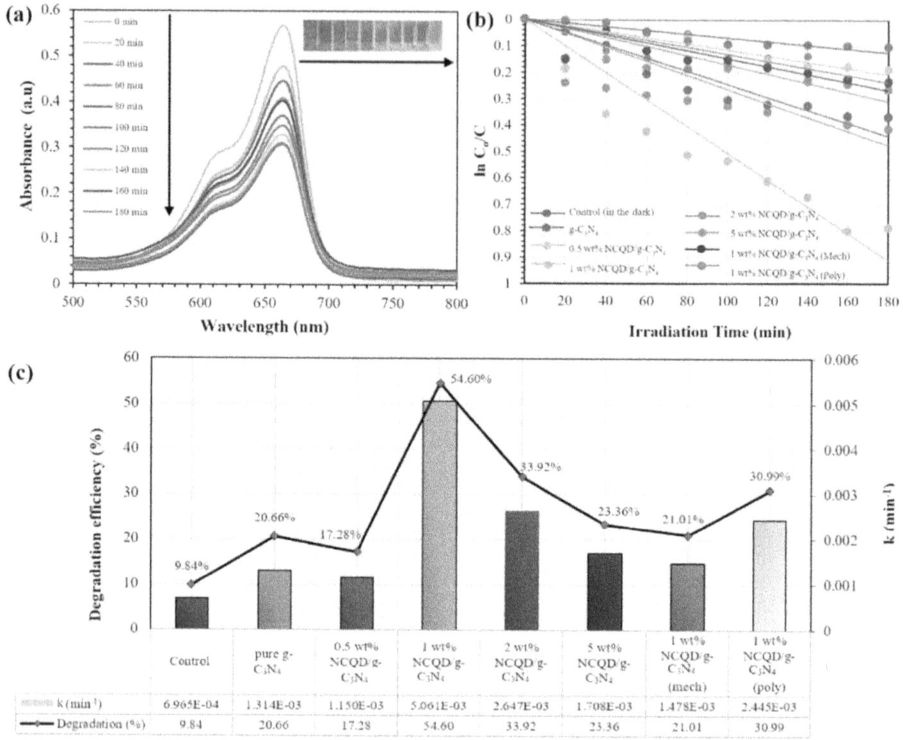

FIGURE 14.2 (a) Time dependent UV-Vis spectra of 1 wt% NCQD/g-C$_3$N$_4$. (b) Plot of NCQD mass dependent photocatalytic MB dye degradation over pure g-C$_3$N$_4$ and NCQD/g-C$_3$N$_4$. (c) Comparison of dye degradation efficiency of all samples under LED light irradiation. Inset picture shows the gradual change in the colour of MB with irradiation time.

Reproduced with permission from [22], copyright 2020, Elsevier.

displayed a significantly higher rate constant of 5.061×10^{-3} min^{-1}, which was 3.85 times higher than that of pure sample.

The mechanism of the dye degradation is as shown in Figure 14.3. Upon light irradiation, electrons were excited from the valence band (VB) to the conduction band (CB) of g-C$_3$N$_4$ which creates holes on the VB. The photoinduced electrons rapidly migrate from the surface of g-C$_3$N$_4$ to the NCQDs as the energy level of the NCQD is lower than the CB of the g-C$_3$N$_4$. The high electron storage capacitance and electron conductivity enabled the efficient separation of electron-hole pairs as confirmed by EIS analysis which hinders charge recombination and improves the photocatalytic performance. It was reported that the adsorption of MB was improved on the surface of the composite due to the π-π interactions. Next, superoxide anion radicals were formed due to the reaction of the electrons of the CB with molecular oxygen. The as-formed superoxide radicals react with MB to oxidize it. Furthermore, the hole produced in the VB of the g-C$_3$N$_4$ migrates to the surface and reacts with the hydroxyl species to form active hydroxyl radicals. This was plausible due to the presence of more positive VB position of the composite than the OH-/OH radical. These

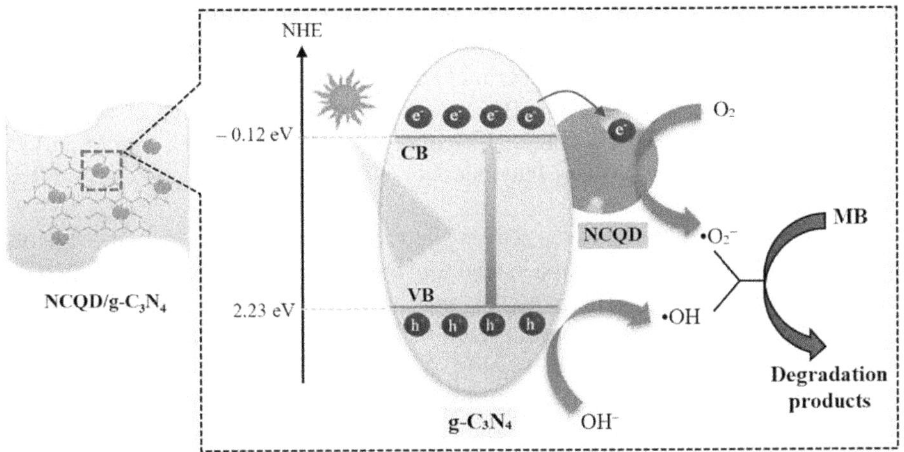

FIGURE 14.3 Mechanism of photocatalytic dye degradation of MB dye over NCQD/g-C$_3$N$_4$ catalyst.

Reproduced with permission from [22], copyright 2020, Elsevier.

reactive species present on the surface of the as-synthesized photocatalyst composite react with the MB molecule to form degradation products.

Sonkar et al. developed red emitting Mg-N-embedded carbon dots for sunlight-induced photocatalytic degradation of pollutant dyes [24]. Green synthesis technique was used to fabricate the "red emitting magnesium-nitrogen embedded carbon dots" (r-Mg-N-CD) from the leaves extract of Bougainvillea plant as a natural source of carbon. The extraction of fragrances and essential oils from the flowers and leaves of Bougainvillea plant were used to synthesize CQDs by carbonizing in a simple domestic microwave. The young leaves of the plant were washed with distilled water and chopped into 1-cm-sized pieces and blended to mix with ethanol/water (1:1) mixture. The solution was kept at 40°C for 10 min under sonication. Then it was carbonized for 15 minutes 90% power (1400 W) in a domestic microwave oven. The produced particles were centrifuged to give red colour-emitting graphitic carbon dots (r-Mg-N-CD) having the quantitative yield of ~ 70 % (with respect to the as-prepared bulk sample).

The r-Mg-N-CD was a potential photocatalyst material for the degradation of pollutant dyes (methylene blue) in the presence of sunlight.

Typically, a stock solution of MB dye was prepared in deionized water and the r-Mg-N-CD was added to it under constant stirring for 30 minutes. The mixture of the solution was used to determine the concentration of MB dye using UV-Vis absorbance spectroscopy at a wavelength of 664 nm. The significant efficiency under sunlight was compared with artificial light (100 W tungsten bulb). The continuous decrease in the concentration of MB was monitored by the r-Mg-N-CD when exposed to different sources of light. The sunlight irradiation exhibited highest photocatalytic activity (99.1 %) compared to the artificial light source (100 W tungsten bulb).

The plausible degradation mechanism was established by applying trapping experiment. In general, a photocatalyst generates three types of reactive species as superoxide, holes and hydroxyl radicals under sunlight irradiation, which catalysed the photodegradation of the organic dyes. The specific roles of these reactive species were monitored by the trapping experiment using three different types of scavengers such as the para-benzoquinone (p-BZQ) as a scavenger for the trap of superoxide (O^{2-}), disodium ethylene diamminetetraacetate (Na_2-EDTA) for the trap of surface generated holes (h^+) and tertiary butyl alcohol (t-BA) for the trap of hydroxyl (OH·) radicals, respectively.

The molar concentration of the scavengers varied from low to high in the aqueous system of MB-r-Mg-N-CD to understand the influence of the reactive species on the photodegradation of dye. The photodegradation efficiency was reduced by approx. 55% in the presence of low concentration of BZQ. The efficiency was reduced by approx. 25% in the presence of Na_2-EDTA and t-BA. The results of the trapping experiment indicate that the holes and hydroxyl radicals also participated with the superoxide for the MB degradation. The breakdown of the MB dye was not only by the superoxide radicals but also by holes and the hydroxide radicals.

Qureshi et. al. developed perovskite-based carbon dots-$BaZrO_{3-\delta}$ (CD-BZO) composite for improved photocatalytic MB dye degradation [25]. The CD-BZO composite was synthesized by hybridizing the pre-synthesized CDs and BZOs in ethanol. The carbon dots were synthesized via hydrothermal method. Citric acid was taken as the precursor in water in a Teflon-coated reactor. The solution in the Teflon-coated tube was made homogeneous and kept inside a stainless-steel jacket of an oven at 200°C for 5 h. After cooling to room temperature, the formed brownish red solution was filtered and dialyzed. Finally, the dialyzed solution was dried to give the carbon dots. BZO was prepared as hollow spheres by following hydrothermal method. A stoichiometric amount of $BaCl_2 \cdot 2H_2O$ and $ZrOCl_2 \cdot 8H_2O$ was mixed in a 20 M KOH aqueous solution inside a Teflon-coated stainless-steel autoclave. It was kept inside an oven at 200°C for 24 hours. After cooling down, the precipitate of BZO was washed with water, dilute acetic acid and ethanol. Then, the washed BZO was dried. The photocatalyst, hybrid of CDs and BZO, was prepared by mixing CDs and BZO in a specific amount in ethanol and then dried using a rotary evaporator.

The photocatalytic dye degradation was performed by taking MB dye solution in a round bottom flask by illuminating with a 300-W tungsten-halogen lamp. Aqueous NH_3 solution was added to the dye solution to adjust the pH at 13. The hybrid catalyst, CD-BZO, exhibited 90% efficiency within 1 h. The enhancement in dye degradation efficiency of CD-BZO nanohybrids compared to bare BZO could be explained by the enhanced light absorptivity and superior charge-transfer capability of the CDs.

The mechanism of the dye degradation followed several steps as described below. In the first step, CDs and BZO absorb suitable energy light. This absorbed light promotes electrons to their respective conduction bands (CBs), creating holes in the valence bands. As CDs have superior charge-transfer property, there was enhanced transfer of the photogenerated electrons from the conduction band of BZO. This enhancement reduces the probability of carrier recombination between electrons and holes in BZO. In addition, CDs have unique upconversion PL property which also photoexcite BZO and increase the carrier density. In the next step, O_2 reacts with the above electrons generated in the conduction bands of BZO and CDs to form superoxide radical anions in the solution. Similarly, photogenerated holes can react with water and produce hydroxyl radicals. Later, hydrogen peroxide was formed due to the recombination of these hydroxyl radicals. Finally, these hydroxyl radicals oxidize the dye molecules and hydrogen peroxide regenerates hydroxyl radicals in the solution by reacting with superoxide radical anions.

14.3　RHODAMINE B DYE REMOVAL

Jayamurugan et. al. created nanohybrid catalysts as sonocatalysts for the degradation of Rhodamine B (RhB) dye in aqueous medium [26]. They have developed amido-amine-functionalized carbon dot (CD)-polymer matrix anchored with palladium (Pd) nanoparticles. The nanohybrid catalyst exhibited the synergistic effect of CDs and Pd nanoparticles.

The synthesis of the nanohybrid catalysts was done by following two steps. First, the amide-linked polymers (CD-CONH and BTC-CONH) were synthesized by the reaction between CDs and benzene 1,3,5-tricarboxylic acid (BTC). Subsequently, the product was treated with benzene 1,4-diamine to give amide-linked polymers. In the second step, the PdCl2 was refluxed with amide-linked polymers in ethanol to produce nanohybrid catalysts (Pd@CD-CONH and Pd@BTC-CONH).

The sonocatalytic degradation of the RhB organic dye was tested by taking nanohybrid catalysts (Pd@CD-CONH and Pd@BTC-CONH) the aqueous solution of the RhB organic dye under sonication in the dark. The degradation efficiency was 99.9% within 5 min, as indicated by the disappearance of the absorption band λmax (554 nm) of RhB in the dark under sonication. Surprisingly, the catalyst did not exhibit superior performance in the presence of room visible light, probably due to the poor absorption in the visible region, as indicated by the UV−vis spectrum.

The proposed mechanistic steps for the sonocatalytic dye degradation are described as follows:

Based on these results, the following equations are proposed for the mechanistic steps involved in the thermal catalysis process under dark ambient conditions.

$$\text{dye} + \text{catalyst} + \text{US} \rightarrow \text{catalyst}\left(\text{dye.ads}\right) \tag{14.1}$$

$$\text{catalyst}\left(\text{dye.ads}\right) + \text{US} \rightarrow h_{VB}^{+} + e_{CB}^{-} \tag{14.2}$$

$$H_2O + h_{VB}^{+} \rightarrow {}^{\bullet}OH + H^{+} \tag{14.3}$$

$$e_{CB}^{-} + O_2\left(\text{dissolved}\right) \rightarrow O_2^{\bullet -} \tag{14.4}$$

$$O_2^{\bullet -} + H \rightarrow HO_2^{\bullet} \tag{14.5}$$

$$2HO_2^{\bullet} \rightarrow O_2 + H_2O_2 \tag{14.6}$$

$$H_2O_2 + e^{-} + US \rightarrow {}^{\bullet}OH + OH^{-} \tag{14.7}$$

$$O_2^{\bullet -} / {}^{\bullet}OH / HO_2^{\bullet} + \text{dye} / \text{dye}^{+} \rightarrow \rightarrow \text{sono-degraded small organic product} \tag{14.8}$$

Fluorescent CQDs with high quantum yield (QY) using aqua mesophase pitch (AMP) as the carbon source has been reported by Jiao et al. [27]. using the hydrothermal method. The dye degradation efficiency for RhB organic dye was 97% after 4h under sunlight and this method also exhibited the maintenance of 93% efficiency after 5 times recycled. First, the AMP was prepared by oxidizing coal tar pitch, alkali re-dissolving and precipitation. Then, CQDs were synthesized by taking AMP in deionized water and keeping it in an autoclave with PTFE lining tubes maintaining the temperature of 180°C for 48 h. Finally, the solution was cooled down and centrifuged to give CQDs which was preserved under dark conditions. The surface of the as-synthesized CQDs was modified by ammonia to produce N-CQDs. The UV-Vis spectra of Rh B solution in the range of 480–600 nm reduced significantly after adding N-CQDs. The intensity of the adsorption band decreased obviously after adding N-CQDs, indicating the effect of the N-CQDs on the structure of Rh B molecules which undergoes degradation.

14.4 CRYSTAL VIOLET DYE REMOVAL

Das et. al. developed polyvinylpyrrolidone (PVP)-based polymeric hydrogel crosslinked by CQDs for the adsorption and photocatalytic degradation of Crystal Violet (CV) dyes [28]. The monolayer adsorption of CV dye was facilitated by hydrogen bonding, inductive effect, and π-π interaction with the polymer backbone as well as the CQDs. The dye degradation strategy was based on the unique Reactive Oxygen Species (ROS) generating ability of the CD embedded in the hydrogel matrix upon exposure to sunlight.

The hydrogel-CQD composite displayed adsorption and photocatalytic degradation of dyes with an additional advantage of antibacterial activity (Figure 14.4). The method of the formation of the composite was inexpensive. First CQDs were synthesized from lemon juice and cysteamine which have $-NH_2$, -OH, -SH and –COOH functional groups on their surface. These functional groups were responsible for dye sorption that play a significant role in dye adsorption. The hydrogel was formed due to the crosslinking of CQDs with the dangling carboxylic acid groups produced by the ring-opening of PVP. The N/S-doped blue fluorescence CQDs were synthesized by using aminoethanol and cysteamine as the source of N/S. Carboxylated PVP was conjugated with the CQDs using EDC/NHS as the mediator which created an amide bond. The CQDs present in the composite matrix were able to generate ROS efficiently upon exposure to light. This ROS was responsible to degrade the adsorbed CV dye within 30 minutes exposure to sun light. CQDs help to retard the recombination of the photogenerated electron-hole pair and facilitate the production of ROS which oxidizes the dye molecules and thus decomposition occurs. The degradation efficiency was greater than 90%. The mechanism of the degradation was established by trapping experiment of the ROS where radical scavengers were used. The surface-generated holes (h^+) were trapped by Na_2EDTA, superoxide (O^{2-}) was trapped by parabenzoquinone (p-BZQ) and hydroxyl radical was trapped by methanol (MeOH). The decrease in the photodegradation process was the result of the radical scavengers in dye degradation (Figure 14.5).

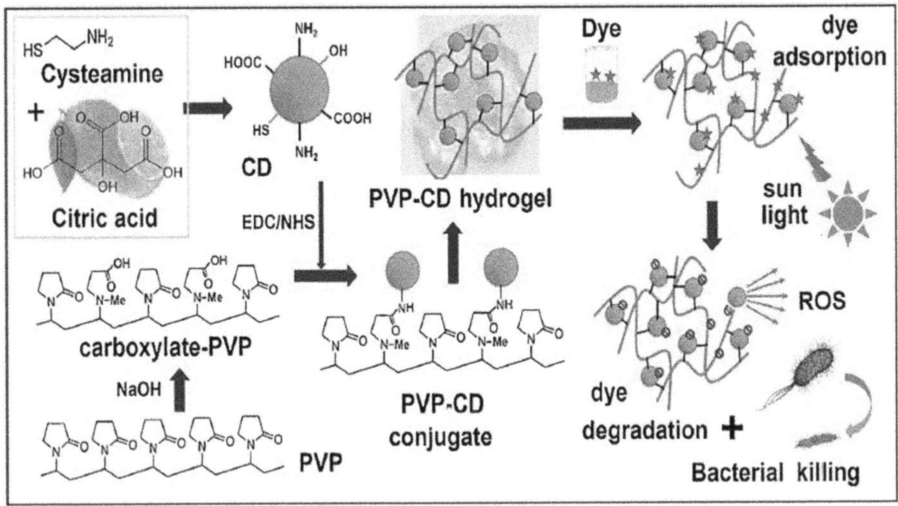

FIGURE 14.4 Schematic representation of preparation of PVP-CD hybrid hydrogel from carboxylated-PVP and CQDs for adsorption and photodegradation of CV dye along with killing of bacteria.

Reproduced with permission from [28], copyright 2020, Elsevier.

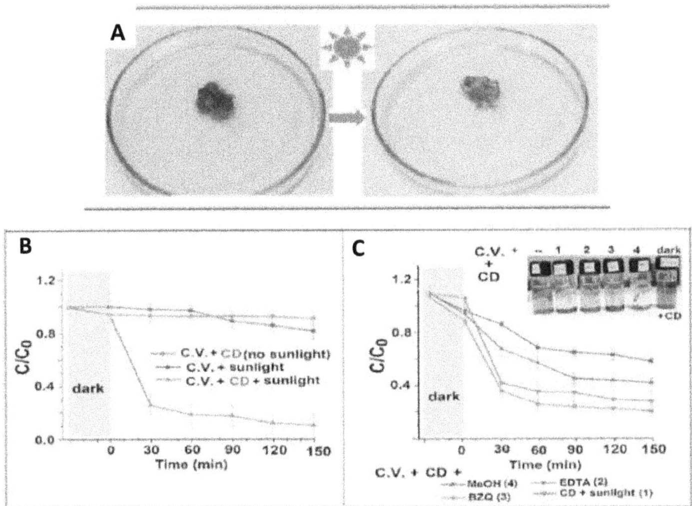

FIGURE 14.5 (A) Photodegradation Crystal Violet (C.V.) by CQDs in PVP-CD hydrogel exposed to sunlight for 30 min. B and C. Plot of (C/C_0) vs. time for C.V. exposed to sunlight in the presence of CD and ROS quenchers, respectively. Inset images C.V. co-incubated with ROS quenchers and exposed to sunlight, respectively.

Reproduced with permission from [28], copyright 2020, Elsevier.

14.5   METHYL ORANGE DYE

Jamila et. al. created nitrogen-doped carbon quantum dots (NCQDs)/graphene oxide/ WO_3 ternary catalyst for the photocatalytic degradation of methyl orange (MO) dye [29]. The ternary photocatalyst was synthesized by forming the composite of N-doped CQDs with GO-modified WO_3 nanosheets (Figure 14.6). NCQDs were used to modify the morphological and the optical properties of the WO_3 nanosheets. The addition of the NCQDs exhibited the reduction of the bandgap of WO_3 nanosheets and tremendously decreased the PL intensity which suppressed the recombination rate of the electron and hole pair. This enhanced the photochemical dye degradation efficiency. Pure WO_3 sheets showed only 23% dye degradation efficiency, whereas it exhibited 47% degradation efficiency when mixed with GO. Two factors are responsible for such enhancement of the efficiencies; first, GO increases the surface area

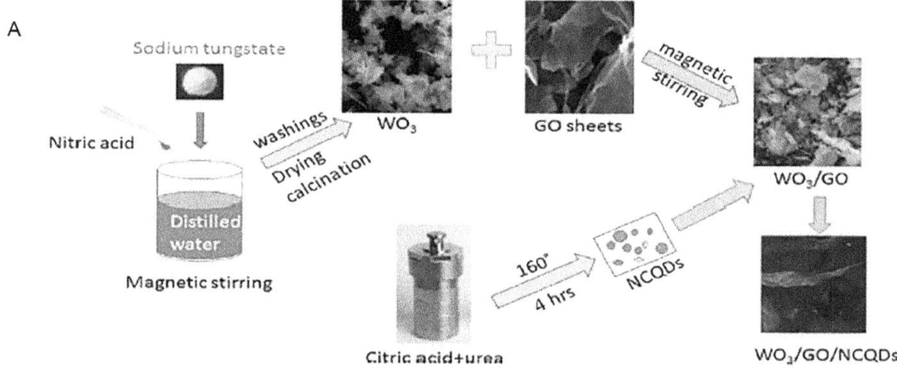

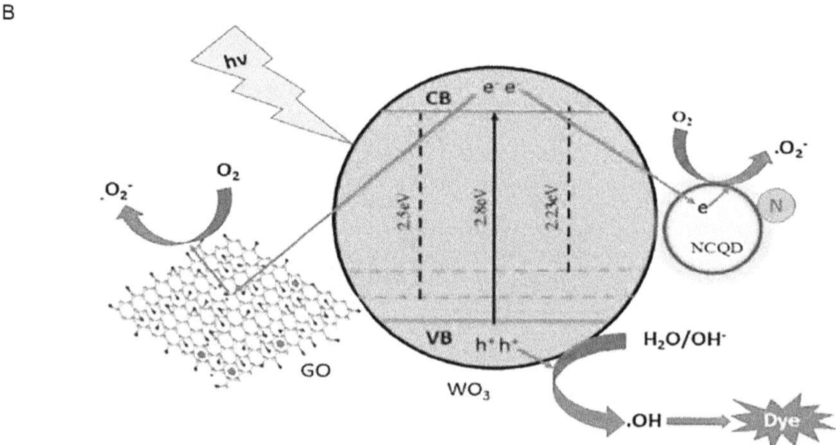

FIGURE 14.6   (A) Synthetic scheme for the production of photocatalyst, WO_3/GO/NCQDs. (B) Proposed mechanism for the methyl orange dye degradation using the composite of WO_3/GO/NCQDs as photocatalyst.

and second one was that GO reduced the band gap of WO_3 from 2.8 to 2.5 eV. The ternary photocatalyst, which was the composite of $NCQDs/GO/WO_3$, dramatically enhanced the efficiency by 86%.

14.6 APPLICATION OF CQDs FOR DETECTION OF METAL IONS AND ORGANIC MATTERS IN WASTEWATER

CQDs have great optical and luminescence properties that make them suitable as a fluorescent probe for various metal ions [30]. In a recent report, Pourreza N. *et al* have reported the fluorescence sensing of Hg (II) in an aqueous sample using CQDs as a probe [31]. In this study, CQDs work as a switch ON sensor for metal ions. Multiple samples containing various concentrations of Hg (II) ions are prepared my dissolving a certain amount of Hg (II) salts in aqueous solution. Water samples are treated with various amounts of CQDs, and it was observed that the Hg (II) ion concentration as low as 1.26 ng/mL can be detected from observable changes in the emission intensity of the CQDs. It is suggested that Hg (II) ions could bind with oxygen-containing functional groups of CQD surfaces. The mechanism behind the quenching process is the formation of a non-radiative species due to the electron transfer from the oxygen-containing groups of CQDs to the Hg(II) ions. Apart from Hg(II) ions, several CQD-based sensors for detecting Cu(II) ions are also known [32]. It has been found that the fluorescence intensity of CQDs gradually decreases with the increasing concentration of the metal ion. The reason behind the quenching is the proposed chelation of the Cu (II) by the carboxyl and carbonyl groups on the CQD surfaces.

Another application of CQDs is to detect Cr^{6+} ions. The presence of Cr^{6+} can be measured by the changes in the emission wavelengths of the CQDs. The isolated CQDs show an emission peak at 425 nm [34]. But in the presence of an increasing amount of Cr^{6+}, the fluorescence intensity of CQDs quenches gradually. The reason behind the quenching is attributed to the Cr^{6+}-induced inner filter effect (IFE) which leads to the shielding of the excitation and emission intensities of the CQDs, i.e., the quencher (Cr^{6+}) absorbs some of the light that excites or comes from the CQDs. Another reason behind this phenomenon is upon excitation, the electrons go from a low to a high energy level and then come back down. When they do, they don't release the energy as light but combine with holes instead to form non-radiative recombination [33]. This process reduces the fluorescence of CQDs [35]. Another reason for the fluorescence reduction is the inner filter effect. This happens when the quencher (Cr^{6+}) absorbs some of the light that excites or comes from the CQDs. So, the CQDs get less excited and produce less fluorescence light that can be easily quenched by Cr^{6+} [36].

CQDs also displays excellent emission intensity within a broad pH range from 2 to 11 (but the intensity significantly decreases at a pH below 2 or over 11) as shown in Figure 14.7. This characteristic property makes it a suitable candidate for detecting metal ions in the wastewater sample coming from various sources at different pH values.

CQDs co-doped with elements like nitrogen and phosphorus are also known and applied for fluorescence sensing of metal ions [37, 38]. Doping effectively helps in tuning the fluorescence characteristic of the probe. It has been reported that doping

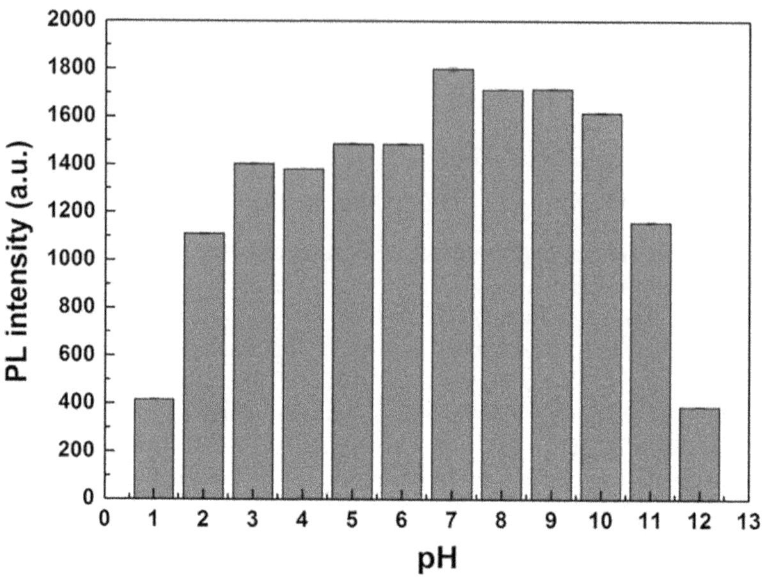

FIGURE 14.7   pH-dependent fluorescence intensity of CQDs.

Reproduced with permission from [33], copyright 2018, Elsevier.

helps in the creation of new electronic state and enhances the emission intensity and quantum yield by more than 20%. In a recent study by Guo et al, it has been reported that nitrogen and phosphorus-doped CQDs [39] can generate a bright blueish green emission with excellent photostability. They have applied the co-doped CQDs to detect Fe^{3+} selectively in aqueous solution in the presence of other interfering cations.

In a similar work, Deng et al have also reported the use of nitrogen-doped CQDs as a fluorescent probe for sensitive detection of Fe^{3+} ions [40]. The CQDs reported were synthesized from hydrothermal treatment of inexpensive and easily available biomass tar and ethylenediamine solution. This nitrogen co-doped CQDs show significant quenching of emission intensity on the addition of different amounts of Fe^{3+}. Quenching occurs when the electron donating functional groups of the nitrogen-doped CQDs form a non-radiative chelation complex with the metal ions. Generally, the oxygen containing functionalities on the CQDs behave as the chelator for selective binding of the metal ions. As shown in Figure 14.8, the selective quenching of the fluorescence spectra of nitrogen-doped CQDs depends on the strong electrostatic interaction between the Fe^{3+} ions and the quantum dot surface. When CQDs are excited by external radiation, the electrons from the ground state jump to the excited state, but later they undergo a radiation-less transfer to the empty 3d orbital of the bound Fe^{3+} ions, which also proves that the quenching mechanism is dynamic in nature. The presence of various electron donor functionalities like hydroxyl, phenolic, carboxylic and amine groups present on the CQD surface helps them to strongly bind to the Fe^{3+} metal ions.

CQDs are also used in detecting organic compounds mixed with wastewater. Recently, Liang et al. [41] have reported on the determination of hematin by using

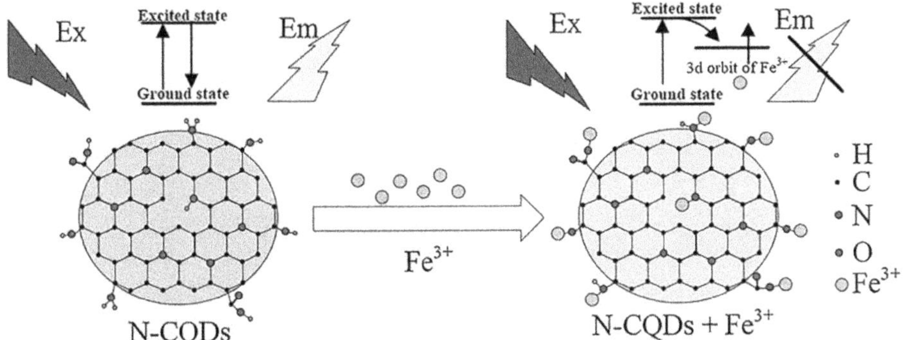

FIGURE 14.8 Iron (III)-dependent fluorescence quenching mechanism of N-CQDs.
Reproduced with permission from [40], copyright 2018, Elsevier.

CQDs, one of the major by-products formed due to the oxidation of haemoglobin and is considered to be poisonous. The CQDs they have fabricated for this purpose have a quantum yield of 43.9% and show excellent stability within a broad pH range of 7.00 to 11.00. It has been found that the bright emission of the CQDs at 505 nm gradually decreased in the presence of the increasing amount of the hematin. They have also tried to detect the analyte hematin using the UV-Vis spectrometry method, although the changes in the absorption spectra of the CQDs are directly proportional to the increasing concentration of hematin, but the detection limit is beyond the fluorescence method. The study revealed that the detection limit for hematin using fluorescence method is 0.1 μL. The study is significant because it can lead to further research in the application of CQDs for detecting other poisonous organic matter in wastewater.

14.7 APPLICATION OF CQDs FOR ADSORPTION OF INORGANIC MATTERS IN WASTEWATER

Adsorption treatment can use CQDs to remove both organic and inorganic pollutants. Research has shown that CQDs can be modified to N-CQDs (nitrogen-doped-CQDs), and their surface activity can be tested by adsorbing Cd^{2+} and Pb^{2+} ions from wastewater [42]. N-CQDs have a large surface area, adjustable surface chemistry and non-toxic property, which make them effective in adsorbing Cd^{2+} and Pb^{2+} ions from water through surface adsorption method. The surfaces or edges of CQDs can enhance the possibility of interaction (chemical and physical interactions) among particles [43]. Moreover, it can also change the energy band gap of quantum dots and improve the adsorption capability [44].

The N-CQDs have the ability to adsorb 37% of Cd^{2+} and 75% of Pb^{2+} from the water sample, as shown in Figure 14.9. The N-CQDs have a large specific surface area that can facilitate the adsorption of heavy metal ions from water [45]. Generally, the particle sizes of N-CQDs are near 10 nm, which can provide a large surface area for high adsorption capability of heavy metals from water. In addition, the electron

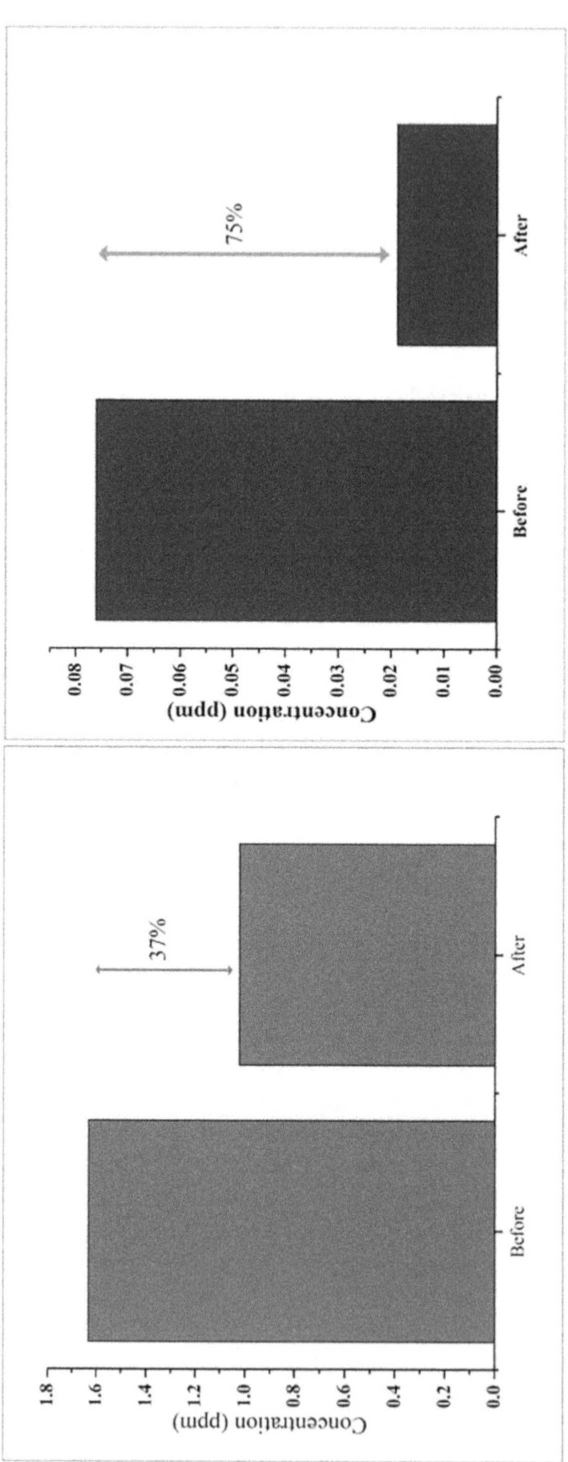

FIGURE 14.9   The red bar plot [at left] represents removal of Cd^{2+} and the blue bar plot [at right] represents removal of Pb^{2+} using nitrogen-doped-CQDs. Reproduced with permission from [42], copyright 2019, Elsevier.

dense nitrogen atoms and oxygenated-functional groups on the N-CQDs surfaces can act as effective sites for adsorption of metal ions [46].

CQDs have various polar moieties and large amounts of functional groups on their surfaces, which makes them an effective adsorbent for removing toxic substances from wastewater. The metal ions can bind to the active sites of different functional groups, such as amine and carboxyl groups; the force acting between the CQDs and the metal ions is either due to electrostatic attraction or π-π stacking interactions. A nanocomposite (PECQDs/MnFe$_2$O$_4$) adsorbent was fabricated by combining the polyethyleneimine-functionalized CQDs with the magnetic materials (MnFe$_2$O$_4$) [47]. This nanocomposite had a high adsorption capacity and a strong magnetic field that can be applied efficiently in the exclusion of uranium.

Although at lower pH, there is a strong electrostatic repulsion between the positively charged surface of the adsorbent and uranium (UO$_2^{2+}$), but with increasing pH, the adsorption rate increases to a maximum of 91%. The rate of adsorption again starts to reduce at a pH over 7.5, which is also because of the electrostatic repulsion; at higher pH, the nanocomposite (PECQDs/MnFe$_2$O$_4$) surface develops a negative charge due to deprotonation and UO$_2^{2+}$ transform into negatively charged species (UO$_2$)$_3$(OH)$_7^-$ and UO$_2$(OH)$_3^-$. However, the uranium adsorption was improved by the interactions between uranium ions and several functional groups, such as NH$_2$, OH and COOH, on the adsorbent [48]. In addition, the hydrophilicity of the adsorbent was enhanced by the oxygenated-functional groups on the CQD surfaces, which also increased the adsorption activity [49]. However, without CQDs, MnFe2O4 as adsorbent could only achieve 25% of uranium adsorption.

The solution pH greatly affects the adsorption capacity. The adsorption capacity is weaker when the solution pH is lower [50]. In a solution with low pH, hydrogen ions and metal ions compete for the adsorption sites. The metal ions cannot adsorb well onto the adsorbent because they are repelled by the high concentration of hydrogen ions in the acidic solution [51, 52]. At a higher pH, the surface of the adsorbing material becomes negatively charged due to the loss of protons to an alkaline environment.

The attractive forces between the adsorbent and metal ions are increased by the deprotonation process [53]. Therefore, electrostatic interactions can help the sorbent and adsorbent to combine, which improves the adsorption. Generally, the adsorption process depends on two main factors: surface area and polarity of the adsorbent materials. The surface area of CQDs can reach up to 1690 m^2/gm, which makes it ideal for use in the adsorption study [54]. The Brunauer-Emmett-Teller (BET) surface area and pore volume measurements can be used to study the surface area and textural properties of CQDs. Researchers have studied the adsorption capacity of three different kinds of adsorbents (Fe$_3$O$_4$, C11-Fe$_3$O$_4$ and CQDs/C11-Fe$_3$O$_4$) to remove benzo[a]pyrene (BaP) from wastewater samples [55]. They have also compared the surface area of these absorbents using BET measurements; the surface areas for Fe$_3$O$_4$, C11-Fe3O4 and CQDs/C11-Fe$_3$O$_4$ were found to be 88.2, 163.5 and 289.8 m^2 g^{-1}, respectively. This confirms that presence of CQDs is related to a higher BET surface area. Hence, nanocomposites of CQDs with iron oxide can offer a larger adsorption area for almost 93.9% adsorption of BaP.

In a different report, a group of scientists has done comparative BET measurement between bismuth oxychloride (BiOCl) and BiOCl/NCQDs [56]. The BET surface area found for (BiOCl) and BiOCl/NCQDs was 33.1 m²/gm and 60.0 m²/gm, respectively. It was also found that the pore volume of BiOCl is 0.168 cm³/gm and the pore volume of BiOCl/NCQDs is 0.239 cm³/gm. Similar to a previous study, here also the increased BET surface area had resulted in higher adsorption capacity of the composite material towards metal ions from wastewater.

Different studies have been conducted to further understand the properties of various CQD nanocomposites. FTIR studies with CQDs and aluminium oxide (Al_2O_3) nanocomposite indicated that Al-O bond might be formed between the carboxylic acid functionalities of the CQDs and the aluminium oxide. DFT studies on the same system are also used to further understand the chemical and physical interactions between CQDs and alumina [57].

Nitrogen-doped CQDs (NCQDs) are reported to be prepared from various sources, one of such sources is citric acid materials. These NCQDs are combined with iron oxide to form $NCQDs/Fe_2O_3$ nanocomposites and are used for adsorbing lead from wastewater. The incorporation of nitrogen atom in the structure of NCQDs has enhanced the possibility of donation of nitrogen lone pair to the empty d orbital of lead metal ions; this interaction has further increased the adsorption capacity of the material. The amine groups on the NCQDs work as the binding site for improving the adsorption ability of the NCQDs [58].

14.8 APPLICATION OF CQD NANOCOMPOSITE AS NANO FILTERS

CQDs are very tiny particles that can be mixed with water and used to make thin layers of material (Thin Film Nanocomposite or TFN membranes) which can filter out unwanted substances. CQDs are good at attracting water molecules and letting them pass through the membrane easily. This is because they are very small and have a positive or negative charge that helps them move water along. The CQDs also make the membrane more water-friendly [59], which means that water can flow through it faster and more smoothly.

Researchers have found a way to add CQDs to thin layers of material (polyamide layer membranes) that can filter out unwanted substances. They did this by using a method called interfacial polymerization [60]. They used three kinds of CQDs that had different functionalities added to them (carboxyl, amino and sulphur) to see how they affected the performance of antifouling. Antifouling means preventing the build-up of dirt and other substances on the membrane. They measured the antifouling performance by using two indicators: flux recovery ratio (FRR) and total fouling ration (R_t). These are shown in Figure 14.10. All the membranes that had CQDs added to them had better FRR and lower R_t than the ones that did not. This means that the CQDs helped the membranes to resist fouling better. The researchers said that this was because the CQDs were water-friendly and could reduce the sticking of water-hating dirt and help remove dirt [60].

Researchers have tested how well CQD membranes can remove selenium and arsenic from water [61]. These are two harmful elements that can cause health problems. They found that CQD membranes were good at letting water pass through and filtering out these elements. This was because the CQDs were water-friendly and had

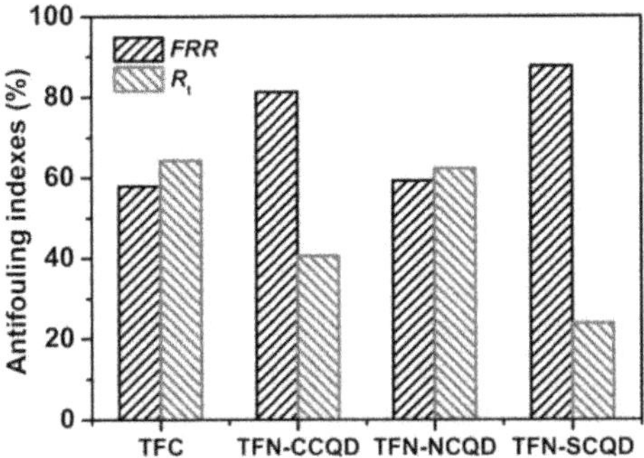

FIGURE 14.10 Flux recovery ratio (FRR) and total fouling ration (R$_t$) of anti-fouling thin-film composites and CQD-based thin film nanocomposites.

Reproduced with permission from [60], copyright 2018, Elsevier.

very small holes on their surface. The CQDs also mixed well with the thin layer of material (polyamide) that was used to make the membrane. The CQDs had polar groups or atoms on their surface that could bond with the polyamide through hydrogen bonding interactions and non-specific interaction. This also made the polyamide more hydrophilic and less likely to undergo crosslinking reaction between their monomers [62].

It is also found that thin layers of materials (TFN membranes) that have CQDs added to them have very good filtering ability with impressive water permeability and has a very high rejection rate (99%) for harmful elements [63]. The CQDs make the TFN membranes more efficient and powerful. The TFN membranes with CQDs also keep their performance even when they are exposed to dirty water [64]. They can purify about four times more water than the TFN membranes without CQDs.

These thin layers of material (TFN membranes) that have CQDs added to them are hydrophilic and have more negative charges on their surface than the polymer layer because of the carboxylic acid groups from the CQDs, the amount of this charges may increase with the increasing number of carboxylic acid groups in the CQDs. This makes them better at filtering out elements that have a negative charge from the water [65]. The TFN membranes with CQDs also resist negatively charged substances better because the substance of the same type of charge is pushed away by the membrane surface [63]. Additionally, TFN membranes with CQDs can purify more water because they have a large surface area, have more space between the layers and have more oxygen groups in the thin layer of materials [66].

Adding CQDs to membranes can make them better at filtering different types of liquids (organic, polar and non-polar). CQDs are hydrophilic and have groups of atoms that can attract water. This can reduce the sticking of unwanted substances through non-specific interaction. CQDs can also help water-like liquids pass through the membrane by giving them places to bond with. The membrane with CQDs can show up to 54.3% enhancement of solvent flux and 40.5% enhancement of solvent uptake. The membrane with CQDs can also block liquids that are not hydrophilic, which makes it more selective.

Researchers have found a way to add CQDs to thin layers of material (TFN membranes) that can filter out unwanted substances from water. They said that this membrane is very good for reverse osmosis, which is a process that can make salty water drinkable. The membrane can let water pass through easily and keep it clean. The CQDs make the membrane more hydrophilic with smaller pores. This helps the membrane to remove harmful elements such as selenium and arsenic from water [61]. The CQDs on the TFN membrane can also help to purify brackish water [66].

In addition, sodium-ion-modified CQDs (Na-CQDs) were used to enhance the TFN membranes for selenium and arsenic removal in a previous study [65]. The membranes were coated with different amounts of Na-CQDs (0.02, 0.05, 0.08 and 0.12 wt%). The best performance was achieved by the TFN membrane with 0.05 wt% of Na-CQDs, which had a water flux of 10.4 LMH/bar and an ions rejection of 98%. The membrane also showed excellent antifouling property. The reason for this result is the strong interactions between the hydroxyl and carboxyl groups of Na-CQDs and the polyamide selective layer. The CQDs had hydrophilic groups that formed continuous ionic channels for easy proton transport [67] and improved the surface wettability and anti-fouling performance of the membrane [68].

14.9 APPLICATION OF CQD NANOCOMPOSITES AS A DISINFECTING AGENT FOR WASTEWATER

In our previous section, we have already discussed various applications of CQDs in wastewater treatment and monitoring. For instance, they can detect harmful substances in industrial waste [69] and extract uranium from water [70]. Moreover, CQDs can act as adsorbents to remove Cd (II) [71] and benzopyrene from environmental water samples [72].

CQDs have also been used as an antimicrobial agent to degrade bacteria. A study showed that CQDs and TiO2 formed a composite with a new chemical bond (Ti-O-C) that had lasting antibacterial properties [73]. Another study tested the antibacterial activity of CQDs, TiO_2 and $CQDs-TiO_2$ against *E. coli* and *S. aureus* [74]. They added suspensions of these materials to tubes with bacteria samples and incubated them at 37 °C under visible light for 24 h.

The results showed that CQDs-TiO2 retained 82% of its antibacterial property, which was sufficient to effectively inhibit bacterial growth. On the other hand, pure TiO_2 exhibited almost no antibacterial activity due to the formation of clusters, which reduced its antibacterial efficiency. Therefore, $CQDs-TiO_2$ can be used as a potent antibacterial agent that can enhance the degradation of bacteria.

The mechanism of photocatalytic degradation of *E. coli* by $CQDs-TiO_2$ as a photocatalyst is illustrated in Figure 14.11. The photocatalytic degradation of *E. coli* is initiated by the photogeneration of electron-hole pairs on the surface of CQDs. The electrons can undergo a reductive process with oxygen molecules to produce superoxide anion, and the holes that are formed can oxidize water molecules to generate reactive hydroxyl radicals [75]. CQDs are suitable as an effective photocatalyst because they are water-dispersible, photosensitive materials that have a high antibacterial activity against bacteria. Moreover, CQDs are resistant to photobleaching [76].

The viability loss of bacteria samples is presented in Fig. 14.12. The result indicates that $CQDs-TiO_2$ had an antibacterial property of almost 90% under visible

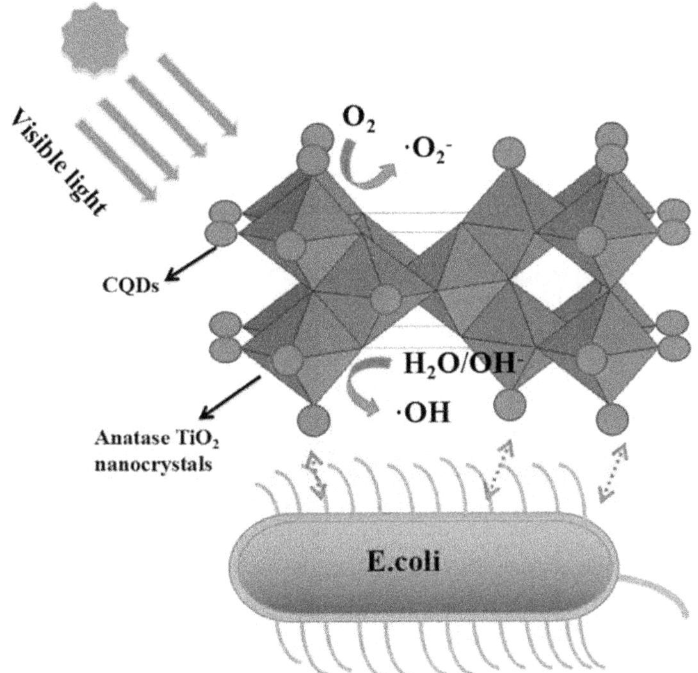

FIGURE 14.11 Light-catalysed antibacterial function of CQDs-TiO$_2$.

Reproduced with permission from [74], copyright 2019, Elsevier.

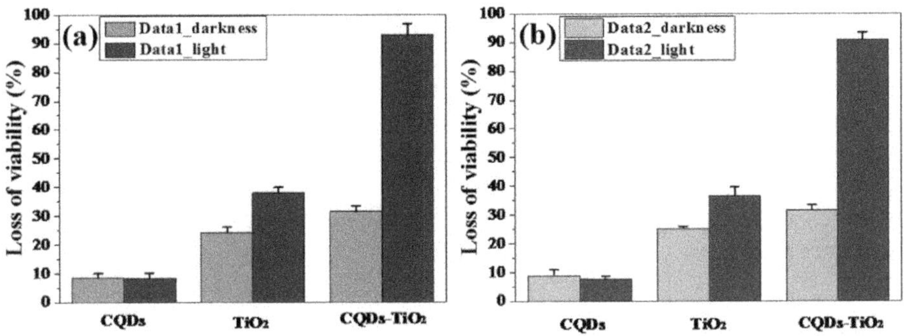

FIGURE 14.12 Cytotoxicity study of (a) *E. coli* (a) and (b) *S. aureus* after exposure for 24 h in the presence of CQDs, TiO$_2$ and CQDs-TiO$_2$.

Reproduced with permission from [74], copyright 2019, Elsevier.

light, which was higher than TiO$_2$ and CQDs alone. CQDs-TiO$_2$ composites had stronger antibacterial activity because they could generate more free radicals. These free radicals would attack the bacteria and cause the decomposition of organic materials in the bacterial cells as well as their cell membrane [74].

CQDs are a promising material for developing antibacterial agents due to their controlled size, water dispersibility and good antimicrobial properties. Therefore,

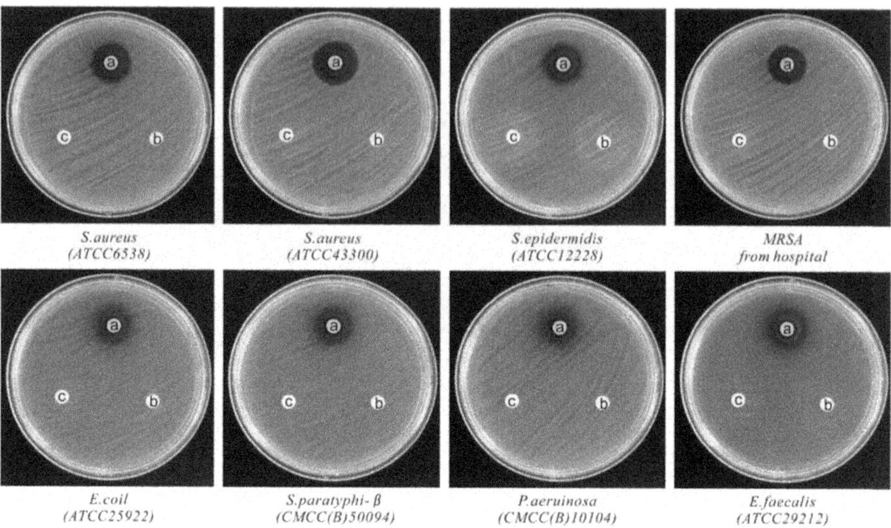

FIGURE 14.13   Glass dishes showing antibacterial activity of NCQDs, glucose and DETA against different species of bacteria.

Reproduced with permission from [77], copyright 2019, Elsevier.

NCQDs were synthesized to investigate their antimicrobial activity against *Staphylococcus* [77]. Eight different species of bacteria are shown in Figure 14.13, the agar plates contain NCQDs (disk a), glucose (disk b) and diethylenetriamine (DETA) (disc c).

According to the findings, only Gram-positive *Staphylococcus* was affected by the specific antibacterial activity of the NCQDs. The disks that contained glucose and DETA did not show any antibacterial effect, because the NCQDs could damage the cell structure of the bacteria. The NCQDs first interacted with the bacteria that had a negative charge. Then, they attached themselves to certain sites on the *Staphylococcus* surfaces and killed the bacteria cells. The CQDs showed more antibacterial activity when exposed to UV light, because of their fluorescence and photobleaching resistance [78].

14.10   CONCLUSION

The advantages of using CQDs as a photocatalyst for wastewater treatment are the simple, cheaper, and efficient routes of their synthesis. Whereas the synthesis of other semiconductor-based fluorescent nanomaterials is expensive and required highly skilled laboratory techniques. The unique photochemical properties, high fluorescence properties, tunable band gaps, upconversion photoluminescence properties and chemical stabilities are the key factors for choosing CQDs as the photocatalytic materials for dye degradation in wastewater. CQDs have a wide range of harvesting light from UV-Vis to NIR, which makes them perfect for photocatalytic applications. They have been chosen for photodegradation of dye contaminants from wastewater due to their chemically inert characteristics and non-metallic nature. The most interesting thing about CQDs are their simple way to synthesize from naturally occurring materials and easy modifications of the surface. CQDs can form composites with almost all types of semiconductors to tune their band gaps so that the recombination of the electron and hole pair can be stopped which control the efficiency of the photocatalysts. Although CQDs are perfect candidates for wastewater treatment as photocatalysts, unfortunately, CQDs with high quantum yields still remain rare. Future research should focus on increasing the quantum yields of CQDs. The UCPL mechanism of CQDs is still not understood properly. So, future research goal could be to understand the photogenerated electron transfer route in the UCPL process.

REFERENCES

[1] Environment, U. N. (2017, August 4). *2017 UN World Water Development Report, Wastewater: The Untapped Resource.* UNEP - UN Environment Programme. https://www.unep.org/resources/publication/2017-un-world-water-development-report-wastewater-untapped-resource#:~:text=The%202017%20edition%20of%20the

[2] Akpan, U. G., & Hameed, B. H. (2009). Parameters affecting the photocatalytic degradation of dyes using TiO2-based photocatalysts: A review. *Journal of Hazardous Materials, 170*(2-3), 520–529. https://doi.org/10.1016/j.jhazmat.2009.05.039

[3] Kant, R. (2012). Textile dyeing industry an environmental hazard. *Natural Science, 04*(01), 22–26. https://doi.org/10.4236/ns.2012.41004

[4] Kanagamani, K., Muthukrishnan, P., Shankar, K., Kathiresan, A., Barabadi, H., & Saravanan, M. (2019). Antimicrobial, cytotoxicity and photocatalytic degradation of norfloxacin using *Kleinia grandiflora* mediated silver nanoparticles. *Journal of Cluster Science, 30*(6), 1415–1424. https://doi.org/10.1007/s10876-019-01583-y

[5] Pera-Titus, M., Garcia-Molina, V., Baños, M. A., Giménez, J., & Esplugas, S. (2004). Degradation of chlorophenols by means of advanced oxidation processes: A general review. *Applied Catalysis B: Environmental, 47*(4), 219–256. https://doi.org/10.1016/j.apcatb.2003.09.010

[6] He, J., Yang, X., Men, B., & Wang, D. (2016). Interfacial mechanisms of heterogeneous Fenton reactions catalyzed by iron-based materials: A review. *Journal of Environmental Sciences, 39*, 97–109. https://doi.org/10.1016/j.jes.2015.12.003

[7] Ying Lim, S., Shen, W., & Gao, Z. (2015). Carbon quantum dots and their applications. *Chemical Society Reviews, 44*(1), 362–381. https://doi.org/10.1039/C4CS00269E

[8] Reckmeier, C. J., Schneider, J., Xiong, Y., Häusler, J., Kasák, P., Schnick, W., & Rogach, A. L. (2017). Aggregated molecular fluorophores in the ammonothermal synthesis of carbon dots. *Chemistry of Materials, 29*(24), 10352–10361. https://doi.org/10.1021/acs.chemmater.7b03344

[9] Prasannan, A., & Imae, T. (2013). One-pot synthesis of fluorescent carbon dots from orange waste peels. *Industrial & Engineering Chemistry Research, 52*(44), 15673–15678. https://doi.org/10.1021/ie402421s

[10] Achyut Konwar, Upama Baruah, Deka, M. J., Hussain, A. A., Haque, R., Arup Kumar Pal, & Chowdhury, D. (2017). Tea-carbon dots-reduced graphene oxide: An efficient conducting coating material for fabrication of an E-Textile. *ACS Sustainable Chemistry & Engineering, 5*(12), 11645–11651. https://doi.org/10.1021/acssuschemeng.7b03021

[11] Guo, J., Li, H., Ling, L., Li, G., Cheng, R., Lu, X., Xie, A.-Q., Li, Q. X., Wang, C.-F., & Chen, S. (2020). Green synthesis of carbon dots toward anti-counterfeiting. *8*(3), 1566–1572. https://doi.org/10.1021/acssuschemeng.9b06267

[12] Zhang, Z., Sun, W., & Wu, P. (2015). Highly photoluminescent carbon dots derived from egg white: Facile and green synthesis, photoluminescence properties, and multiple applications. *ACS Sustainable Chemistry & Engineering, 3*(7), 1412–1418. https://doi.org/10.1021/acssuschemeng.5b00156

[13] Atienzar, P., Primo, A., Lavorato, C., Molinari, R., & García, H. (2013). Preparation of graphene quantum dots from pyrolyzed alginate. *Langmuir, 29*(20), 6141–6146. https://doi.org/10.1021/la400618s

[14] Das, R. K., Kar, J. P., & Mohapatra, S. (2016). Enhanced photodegradation of organic pollutants by Carbon Quantum Dot (CQD) Deposited Fe3O4@mTiO2 Nano-Pom-Pom Balls. *Industrial & Engineering Chemistry Research, 55*(20), 5902–5910. https://doi.org/10.1021/acs.iecr.6b00792

[15] Majumdar, S., Gargee, K., Neelam, G., Thakur, D., & Chowdhury, D. (2016). Carbon-Dot-Coated alginate beads as a smart stimuli-responsive drug delivery system. *ACS Applied Materials & Interfaces, 8*(50), 34179–34184. https://doi.org/10.1021/acsami.6b10914

[16] Hakima, B., Wang, Q., Barras, A., Li, M., Toufik, H., Szunerits, S., & Rabah, B. (2016). Green chemistry approach for the synthesis of ZnO–carbon dots nanocomposites with good photocatalytic properties under visible light. *Journal of Colloid and Interface Science, 465*, 286–294. https://doi.org/10.1016/j.jcis.2015.12.001

[17] Miao, R., Luo, Z., Zhong, W., Chen, S., Jiang, T., Dutta, B., Youmna Nasr, Zhang, Y., & Suib, S. L. (2016). Mesoporous TiO2 modified with carbon quantum dots as a high-performance visible light photocatalyst. *Applied Catalysis B-Environmental, 189*, 26–38. https://doi.org/10.1016/j.apcatb.2016.01.070

[18] Safardoust-Hojaghan, H., & Salavati-Niasari, M. (2017). Degradation of methylene blue as a pollutant with N-doped graphene quantum dot/titanium dioxide nanocomposite. *Journal of Cleaner Production, 148*, 31–36. https://doi.org/10.1016/j.jclepro.2017.01.169

[19] Permatasari, F. A., Fukazawa, H., Ogi, T., Iskandar, F., & Okuyama, K. (2018). Design of Pyrrolic-N-Rich carbon dots with absorption in the first near-infrared window for photothermal therapy. *ACS Applied Nano Materials, 1*(5), 2368–2375. https://doi.org/10.1021/acsanm.8b00497

[20] Gengan, S., Ananda Murthy, H. C., Sillanpää, M., & Nhat, T. (2022). Carbon dots and their application as photocatalyst in dye degradation studies- Mini review. *Results in Chemistry, 4*, 100674. https://doi.org/10.1016/j.rechem.2022.100674

[21] Vassalini, I., Gjipalaj, J., Crespi, S., Gianoncelli, A., Mella, M., Ferroni, M., & Alessandri, I. (2020). Alginate-derived active blend enhances adsorption and photocatalytic removal of organic pollutants in water. *4*(7), 1900112. https://doi.org/10.1002/adsu.201900112

[22] Seng, R. X., Tan, L.-L., Lee, W. P. C., Ong, W.-J., & Chai, S.-P. (2020). Nitrogen-doped carbon quantum dots-decorated 2D graphitic carbon nitride as a promising photocatalyst for environmental remediation: A study on the importance of hybridization approach. *Journal of Environmental Management, 255*, 109936. https://doi.org/10.1016/j.jenvman.2019.109936

[23] Ong, W.-J., Putri, L. K., Tan, Y.-C., Tan, L.-L., Li, N., Ng, Y. H., Wen, X., & Chai, S.-P. (2017). Unravelling charge carrier dynamics in protonated g-C3N4 interfaced with carbon nanodots as co-catalysts toward enhanced photocatalytic CO2 reduction: A combined experimental and first-principles DFT study. *Nano Research, 10*(5), 1673–1696. https://doi.org/10.1007/s12274-016-1391-4

[24] Bhati, A., Anand, S. R., Gunture, Garg, A., Khare, P., & Sonkar, S. K. (2018). Sunlight-induced photocatalytic degradation of pollutant dye by highly fluorescent red-emitting Mg-N-Embedded carbon dots. *6*(7), 9246–9256. https://doi.org/10.1021/acssuschemeng.8b01559

[25] Patra, A. S., Gogoi, G., & Qureshi, M. (2018). Ordered–disordered $BaZrO_{3-\delta}$ hollow nanosphere/carbon dot hybrid nanocomposite: A new visible-light-driven efficient composite photocatalyst for hydrogen production and dye degradation. *ACS Omega*, *3*(9), 10980–10991. https://doi.org/10.1021/acsomega.8b01577

[26] Selim, A., Kaur, S., Dar, A. B., Sartaliya, S. & Jayamurugan, G. (2020). Synergistic effects of carbon dots and palladium nanoparticles enhance the sonocatalytic performance for rhodamine B *Degradation in the Absence of Light*, *5*(35), 22603–22613. https://doi.org/10.1021/acsomega.0c03312

[27] Cheng, Y., Bai, M., Su, J., Fang, C., Li, H., Chen, J. M., & Jiao, J. (2019). Synthesis of fluorescent carbon quantum dots from aqua mesophase pitch and their photocatalytic degradation activity of organic dyes. *35*(8), 1515–1522. https://doi.org/10.1016/j.jmst.2019.03.039

[28] Nayak, S., Prasad, S., Mandal, D., & Das, P. (2020). Carbon dot cross-linked polyvinylpyrrolidone hybrid hydrogel for simultaneous dye adsorption, photodegradation and bacterial elimination from waste water. *392*, 122287–122287. https://doi.org/10.1016/j.jhazmat.2020.122287

[29] Jamila, G. S., Sajjad, S., Leghari, S. A. K., & Long, M. (2020). Nitrogen doped carbon quantum dots and GO modified WO3 nanosheets combination as an effective visible photo catalyst. *Journal of Hazardous Materials*, *382*, 121087. https://doi.org/10.1016/j.jhazmat.2019.121087

[30] Devi, P., Thakur, A., Chopra, S., Kaur, N., Kumar, P., Singh, N., Kumar, M., Shivaprasad, S. M., & Nayak, M. K. (2017). Ultrasensitive and selective sensing of selenium using nitrogen-rich ligand interfaced carbon quantum dots. *ACS Applied Materials & Interfaces*, *9*(15), 13448–13456. https://doi.org/10.1021/acsami.7b00991

[31] Nahid, P., & Matineh, G. (2019). Green synthesized carbon quantum dots from Prosopis juliflora leaves as a dual off-on fluorescence probe for sensing mercury (II) and chemet drug. *Materials Science and Engineering: C*, *98*, 887–896. https://doi.org/10.1016/j.msec.2018.12.141

[32] Murugan, N., Prakash, M., Jayakumar, M., Sundaramurthy, A. & Sundramoorthy, A. K. (2019). Green synthesis of fluorescent carbon quantum dots from Eleusine coracana and their application as a fluorescence "turn-off" sensor probe for selective detection of Cu2+. *476*, 468–480. https://doi.org/10.1016/j.apsusc.2019.01.090

[33] Li, Y., Liu, Y., Shang, X., Chao, D., Zhou, L., & Zhang, H. (2018). Highly sensitive and selective detection of Fe3+ by utilizing carbon quantum dots as fluorescent probes. *Chemical Physics Letters*, *705*, 1–6. https://doi.org/10.1016/j.cplett.2018.05.048

[34] Athika, M., Prasath, A., Duraisamy, E., Sankar Devi, V., Selva Sharma, A., & Elumalai, P. (2019). Carbon-quantum dots derived from denatured milk for efficient chromium-ion sensing and supercapacitor applications. *Materials Letters*, *241*, 156–159. https://doi.org/10.1016/j.matlet.2019.01.064

[35] Xu, X., He, L., Long, Y., Pan, S., Liu, H., Yang, J., & Hu, X. (2019). S-doped carbon dots capped ZnCdTe quantum dots for ratiometric fluorescence sensing of guanine. *Sensors and Actuators B: Chemical*, *279*, 44–52. https://doi.org/10.1016/j.snb.2018.09.102

[36] Feng, S., Gao, Z., Liu, H., Huang, J., Li, X., & Yang, Y. (2019). Feasibility of detection valence speciation of Cr(III) and Cr(VI) in environmental samples by spectrofluorimetric method with fluorescent carbon quantum dots. *Spectrochimica Acta Part A: Molecular and Biomolecular Spectroscopy*, *212*, 286–292. https://doi.org/10.1016/j.saa.2018.12.055

[37] Omer, K. M., Tofiq, D. I., & Ghafoor, D. D. (2019). Highly photoluminescent label free probe for Chromium (II) ions using carbon quantum dots co-doped with nitrogen and phosphorous. *Journal of Luminescence*, *206*, 540–546. https://doi.org/10.1016/j.jlumin.2018.10.100

[38] Datta, B. K., Thiyagarajan, D., Kar, C., Ramesh, A., & Das, G. (2015). A near-infrared emissive Al3+ sensing platform for specific detection in solution, cells and probing DNase activity. *Analytica Chimica Acta*, *882*, 76–82. https://doi.org/10.1016/j.aca.2015.04.032

[39] Guo, Y., Cao, F., & Li, Y. (2018). Solid phase synthesis of nitrogen and phosphor co-doped carbon quantum dots for sensing Fe3+ and the enhanced photocatalytic degradation of dyes. *Sensors and Actuators B: Chemical, 255*, 1105–1111. https://doi.org/10.1016/j.snb.2017.08.104

[40] Deng, X., Feng, Y., Li, H., Du, Z., Teng, Q., & Wang, H. (2018). N-doped carbon quantum dots as fluorescent probes for highly selective and sensitive detection of Fe3+ ions. *Particuology, 41*, 94–100. https://doi.org/10.1016/j.partic.2017.12.009

[41] Liang, J. Y., Han, L., Liu, S. G., Ju, Y. J., Gao, X., Li, N. B., & Luo, H. Q. (2019). Green fluorescent carbon quantum dots as a label-free probe for rapid and sensitive detection of hematin. *Spectrochimica Acta Part A: Molecular and Biomolecular Spectroscopy, 212*, 167–172. https://doi.org/10.1016/j.saa.2019.01.001

[42] Sabet, M., & Mahdavi, K. (2019). Green synthesis of high photoluminescence nitrogen-doped carbon quantum dots from grass via a simple hydrothermal method for removing organic and inorganic water pollutions. *Applied Surface Science, 463*, 283–291. https://doi.org/10.1016/j.apsusc.2018.08.223

[43] Agarwal, S., Sadeghi, N., Tyagi, I., Gupta, V. K. & Fakhri, A. (2016). Adsorption of toxic carbamate pesticide oxamyl from liquid phase by newly synthesized and characterized graphene quantum dots nanomaterials. *478*, 430–438. https://doi.org/10.1016/j.jcis.2016.06.029

[44] Abdelsalam, H., Teleb, N. H., Yahia, I. S., Zahran, H. Y., Elhaes, H., & Ibrahim, M. A. (2019). First principles study of the adsorption of hydrated heavy metals on graphene quantum dots. *Journal of Physics and Chemistry of Solids, 130*, 32–40. https://doi.org/10.1016/j.jpcs.2019.02.014

[45] Azimi, A., Azari, A., Rezakazemi, M., & Ansarpour, M. (2017). Removal of heavy metals from industrial wastewaters: A review. *ChemBioEng Reviews, 4*(1), 37–59. https://doi.org/10.1002/cben.201600010

[46] Dou, J., Gan, D., Huang, Q., Liu, M., Chen, J., Deng, F., Zhu, X., Wen, Y., Zhang, X., & Wei, Y. (2019). Functionalization of carbon nanotubes with chitosan based on MALI multicomponent reaction for Cu2+ removal. *International Journal of Biological Macromolecules, 136*, 476–485. https://doi.org/10.1016/j.ijbiomac.2019.06.112

[47] Huang, S., Jiang, S., Pang, H., Wen, T., Asiri, A. M., Alamry, K. A., Alsaedi, A., Wang, X., & Wang, S. (2019). Dual functional nanocomposites of magnetic MnFe2O4 and fluorescent carbon dots for efficient U(VI) removal. *Chemical Engineering Journal, 368*, 941–950. https://doi.org/10.1016/j.cej.2019.03.015

[48] Gan, D., Liu, M., Huang, H., Chen, J., Dou, J., Wen, Y., Huang, Q., Yang, Z., Zhang, X., & Wei, Y. (2018). Facile preparation of functionalized carbon nanotubes with tannins through mussel-inspired chemistry and their application in removal of methylene blue. *Journal of Molecular Liquids, 271*, 246–253. https://doi.org/10.1016/j.molliq.2018.08.079

[49] Liu, Y., Huang, H., Gan, D., Guo, L., Liu, M., Chen, J., Deng, F., Zhou, N., Zhang, X., & Wei, Y. (2018). A facile strategy for preparation of magnetic graphene oxide composites and their potential for environmental adsorption. *Ceramics International, 44*(15), 18571–18577. https://doi.org/10.1016/j.ceramint.2018.07.081

[50] Zhang, X., Ceccarelli, M., Liu, M., Tian, J., Zeng, G., Li, Z., Wang, K., Zhang, Q., Wan, Q., Deng, F., & Wei, Y. (2015). Preparation of amine functionalized carbon nanotubes via a bioinspired strategy and their application in Cu2+ removal. *343*, 19–27. https://doi.org/10.1016/j.apsusc.2015.03.081

[51] Lei, Y., Cui, Y., Huang, Q., Dou, J., Gan, D., Deng, F., Liu, M., Li, X., Zhang, X., & Wei, Y. (2019). Facile preparation of sulfonic groups functionalized Mxenes for efficient removal of methylene blue. *Ceramics International, 45*(14), 17653–17661. https://doi.org/10.1016/j.ceramint.2019.05.331

[52] Pradhan, K., Das, G., Kar, C., Mukherjee, N., Khan, J., Mahata, T., Barman, S., & Ghosh, S. (2020). Rhodamine-based metal chelator: A potent inhibitor of metal-catalyzed amyloid toxicity. *ACS Omega*, *5*(30), 18958–18967. https://doi.org/10.1021/acsomega.0c02235

[53] Chaudhry, S. A., Khan, T. A., & Ali, I. (2016). Adsorptive removal of Pb(II) and Zn(II) from water onto manganese oxide-coated sand: Isotherm, thermodynamic and kinetic studies. *Egyptian Journal of Basic and Applied Sciences*, *3*(3), 287–300. https://doi.org/10.1016/j.ejbas.2016.06.002

[54] Ren, X., Zhang, F., Guo, B., Gao, N., & Zhang, X. (2019). Synthesis of N-Doped micropore carbon quantum dots with high quantum yield and dual-wavelength photoluminescence emission from biomass for cellular imaging. *Nanomaterials*, *9*(4), 495. https://doi.org/10.3390/nano9040495

[55] Yang, D., Tammina, S. K., Li, X., & Yang, Y. (2019). Enhanced removal and detection of benzo[a]pyrene in environmental water samples using carbon dots-modified magnetic nanocomposites. *Ecotoxicology and Environmental Safety*, *170*, 383–390. https://doi.org/10.1016/j.ecoenv.2018.11.138

[56] Mou, Z., Zhang, H., Liu, Z., Sun, J., & Zhu, M. (2019). Ultrathin BiOCl/nitrogen-doped graphene quantum dots composites with strong adsorption and effective photocatalytic activity for the degradation of antibiotic ciprofloxacin. *Applied Surface Science*, *496*, 143655. https://doi.org/10.1016/j.apsusc.2019.143655

[57] Liu, X., Li, J., Wu, X., Zeng, Z., Wang, X., Hayat, T., & Zhang, X. (2017). Adsorption of carbon dots onto Al2O3 in aqueous: Experimental and theoretical studies. *Environmental Pollution*, *227*, 31–38. https://doi.org/10.1016/j.envpol.2017.04.041

[58] Ceccarelli, M., Zhao, J., Liu, M., Chen, J., Zhu, X., Wu, T., Tian, J., Wen, Y., Zhang, X., & Wei, Y. (2018). Preparation of polyethylene polyamine@tannic acid encapsulated MgAl-layered double hydroxide for the efficient removal of copper (II) ions from aqueous solution. *82*, 92–101. https://doi.org/10.1016/j.jtice.2017.10.019

[59] Zeng, Z., Yu, D., He, Z., Liu, J., Xiao, F.-X., Zhang, Y., Wang, R., Bhattacharyya, D., & Tan, T. T. Y. (2016). Graphene oxide quantum dots covalently functionalized PVDF membrane with significantly-enhanced bactericidal and antibiofouling performances. *Scientific Reports*, *6*(1). https://doi.org/10.1038/srep20142

[60] Sun, H., & Wu, P. (2018). Tuning the functional groups of carbon quantum dots in thin film nanocomposite membranes for nanofiltration. *Journal of Membrane Science*, *564*, 394–403. https://doi.org/10.1016/j.memsci.2018.07.044

[61] He, M., Guo, X., Huang, J., Shen, H., Zeng, Q., & Wang, L. (2018). Mass production of tunable multicolor graphene quantum dots from an energy resource of coke by a one-step electrochemical exfoliation. *Carbon*, *140*, 508–520. https://doi.org/10.1016/j.carbon.2018.08.067

[62] Gai, W., Zhao, D. L., & Chung, T.-S. (2018). Novel thin film composite hollow fiber membranes incorporated with carbon quantum dots for osmotic power generation. *Journal of Membrane Science*, *551*, 94–102. https://doi.org/10.1016/j.memsci.2018.01.034

[63] Zhao, D. L., & Chung, T.-S. (2018). Applications of carbon quantum dots (CQDs) in membrane technologies: A review. *Water Research*, *147*, 43–49. https://doi.org/10.1016/j.watres.2018.09.040

[64] Bi, R., Zhang, Q., Zhang, R., Su, Y., & Jiang, Z. (2018). Thin film nanocomposite membranes incorporated with graphene quantum dots for high flux and antifouling property. *Journal of Membrane Science*, *553*, 17–24. https://doi.org/10.1016/j.memsci.2018.02.010

[65] He, Y., Zhao, D. L., & Chung, T.-S. (2018). Na+ functionalized carbon quantum dot incorporated thin-film nanocomposite membranes for selenium and arsenic removal. *Journal of Membrane Science*, *564*, 483–491. https://doi.org/10.1016/j.memsci.2018.07.031

[66] Gai, W., Zhao, D. L., & Chung, T.-S. (2019). Thin film nanocomposite hollow fiber membranes comprising Na+-functionalized carbon quantum dots for brackish water desalination. *Water Research*, *154*, 54–61. https://doi.org/10.1016/j.watres.2019.01.043

[67] Parthiban, V., Panda, S. K., & Sahu, A. K. (2018). Highly fluorescent carbon quantum dots-Nafion as proton selective hybrid membrane for direct methanol fuel cells. *Electrochimica Acta*, *292*, 855–864. https://doi.org/10.1016/j.electacta.2018.09.193

[68] Ng, L. Y., Ng, C. Y., Mahmoudi, E., Ong, C. B., & Mohammad, A. W. (2018). A review of the management of inflow water, wastewater and water reuse by membrane technology for a sustainable production in shrimp farming. *Journal of Water Process Engineering*, *23*, 27–44. https://doi.org/10.1016/j.jwpe.2018.02.020

[69] Li, H.-Y., Li, D., Guo, Y., Yang, Y., Wei, W., & Xie, B. (2018). On-site chemosensing and quantification of Cr(VI) in industrial wastewater using one-step synthesized fluorescent carbon quantum dots. *Sensors and Actuators B: Chemical*, *277*, 30–38. https://doi.org/10.1016/j.snb.2018.08.157

[70] Huang, S., Jiang, S., Pang, H., Wen, T., Asiri, A. M., Alamry, K. A., Alsaedi, A., Wang, X., & Wang, S. (2019). Dual functional nanocomposites of magnetic MnFe2O4 and fluorescent carbon dots for efficient U(VI) removal. *Chemical Engineering Journal*, *368*, 941–950. https://doi.org/10.1016/j.cej.2019.03.015

[71] Rahmanian, O., Dinari, M., & Abdolmaleki, M. K. (2018). Carbon quantum dots/layered double hydroxide hybrid for fast and efficient decontamination of Cd(II): The adsorption kinetics and isotherms. *Applied Surface Science*, *428*, 272–279. https://doi.org/10.1016/j.apsusc.2017.09.152

[72] Yang, D., Tammina, S. K., Li, X., & Yang, Y. (2019). Enhanced removal and detection of benzo[a]pyrene in environmental water samples using carbon dots-modified magnetic nanocomposites. *Ecotoxicology and Environmental Safety*, *170*, 383–390. https://doi.org/10.1016/j.ecoenv.2018.11.138

[73] Yu, H., Zhao, Y., Zhou, C., Shang, L., Peng, Y., Cao, Y., Wu, L.-Z., Tung, C.-H., & Zhang, T. (2014). Carbon quantum dots/TiO2 composites for efficient photocatalytic hydrogen evolution. *Journal of Materials Chemistry A*, *2*(10), 3344. https://doi.org/10.1039/c3ta14108j

[74] Yan, Y., Kuang, W., Shi, L., Ye, X., Yang, Y., Xie, X., Shi, Q., & Tan, S. (2019). Carbon quantum dot-decorated TiO2 for fast and sustainable antibacterial properties under visible-light. *Journal of Alloys and Compounds*, *777*, 234–243. https://doi.org/10.1016/j.jallcom.2018.10.191

[75] Moradlou, O., Rabiei, Z., & Delavari, N. (2019). Antibacterial effects of carbon quantum dots@hematite nanostructures deposited on titanium against Gram-positive and Gram-negative bacteria. *Journal of Photochemistry and Photobiology A: Chemistry*, *379*, 144–149. https://doi.org/10.1016/j.jphotochem.2019.04.047

[76] Marković, Z. Kováčová, M., Humpolíček, P., Budimir, M. D., Vajďák, J., Kubát, P., Mičušík, M., Švajdlenková, H., Danko, M., Capáková, Z., Lehocký, M., Marković, B., & Špitalský, Z. (2019). Antibacterial photodynamic activity of carbon quantum dots/ polydimethylsiloxane nanocomposites against Staphylococcus aureus, Escherichia coli and Klebsiella pneumoniae. *26*, 342–349. https://doi.org/10.1016/j.pdpdt.2019.04.019

[77] Zhao, C., Wang, X., Wu, L., Wu, W., Zheng, Y., Lin, L., Weng, S., & Lin, X. (2019). Nitrogen-doped carbon quantum dots as an antimicrobial agent against Staphylococcus for the treatment of infected wounds. *179*, 17–27. https://doi.org/10.1016/j.colsurfb.2019.03.042

[78] Marković, Z., Kováčová, M., Humpolíček, P., Budimir, M. D., Vajďák, J., Kubát, P., Mičušík, M., Švajdlenková, H., Danko, M., Capáková, Z., Lehocký, M., Marković, B., & Špitalský, Z. (2019). Antibacterial photodynamic activity of carbon quantum dots/ polydimethylsiloxane nanocomposites against Staphylococcus aureus, Escherichia coli and Klebsiella pneumoniae. *26*, 342–349. https://doi.org/10.1016/j.pdpdt.2019.04.019

15 Application of Carbon Quantum Dots in Energy and Electronic Applications

M. K. Bera

15.1 INTRODUCTION

Global green energy and green electronics require greener energy solutions to accomplish their goals. Energy storage and electrical technology help to make better use of natural energy sources. They also aid in the mitigation of the drawbacks of intermittent energy sources and electrical components. CQDs are a family of carbonaceous nanomaterials that have received a lot of attention due to their enhanced surface and optoelectronic capabilities. Particularly, luminous CQDs, which are typically semiconductor nanocrystals with a quantum confinement effect, have found extensive use in several electric and sustainable energy conversion applications (*Carbon Quantum Dots for Sustainable Energy and Optoelectronics*, 2023; Sikiru et al., 2023).

CQDs are often utilized in electrode materials as a supplement or derivative, utilizing their unique electrical characteristics and simplicity of operation to boost the supercapacitors' energy density. In addition, CQDs and their composites provide an economical, secure, and eco-friendly way to enhance the functionality of different energy conversion, electrical, and optoelectronic devices, such as luminescent solar concentrators, photovoltaics, photodiodes, hydrogen or oxygen evolution reaction in primary and secondary batteries, memory devices, lasers, down-conversion or electroluminescent white and multicolor light emitting diodes with intriguing tunable optical and fluorescence properties (Chaudhary et al., 2023; T. Yuan et al., 2023).

This chapter focuses on several types of CQDs and their nanocomposites produced by various green synthesis routes or synthetic processes in order to harness their fascinating features for application in energy and electronics as schematically presented in Figure 15.1. Additionally, prospective applications of CQDs as standalone materials as well as in organic and inorganic composites are discussed. Commercial applications of CQDs, however, are still in their early stages and confront two key challenges: the first is how to develop facile, economical and ecologically sustainable large-scale synthesis methods and the second is to widen the application fields. A large variety of electrode materials are needed for the industrial production of energy storage systems as well as other electronics and optoelectronic

DOI: 10.1201/9781003437857-17

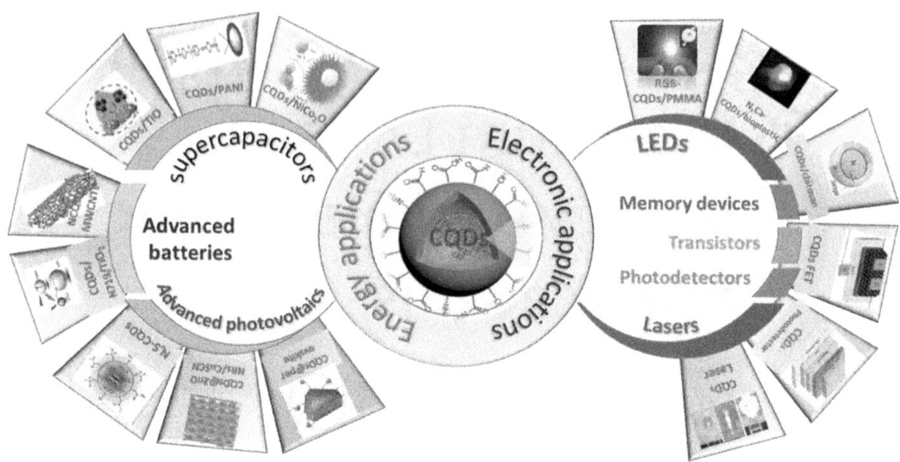

FIGURE 15.1 Graphic illustration of the various energy and electronic applications of CQDs and their nanocomposites.

devices; therefore, the processes must be repeatable, controlled, and overall economically and environmentally sustainable. CQDs have demonstrated significant potential for next-generation energy and electrical applications, although being far from being completely implemented.

15.2 APPLICATION OF CQD COMPOSITES IN SUPERCAPACITORS

Renewable and sustainable sources of energy storage are being sought relentlessly, owing to the global economy's fast expanding demand and the worrying amount of fossil fuel depletion. The growing reliance on internet of things (IoT), internet of medical things (IoMT), hybrid electric vehicles, portable electronic gadgets, memory backup systems, etc. necessitates the development of smart and efficient energy storage and conversion technologies to meet some of the enormous energy difficulties at a reasonable cost with a minimal negative impact on the environment. In this respect, supercapacitors (SCs) have a greater energy and power density (>10 kWkg^{-1}) than batteries, as well as a longer lifespan ($>10^5$ cycles) than a conventional capacitor (Inayat et al., 2023; Kaur et al., 2023).

Supercapacitors may be divided into two groups based on how they store energy. There are two different kinds of capacitors: the electrical double layer capacitor (EDLC), which uses electrolyte ions to store charges close to the electrode interface, and the pseudocapacitor, which has a greater specific capacitance (C_s) and energy density (E_s) due to reversible Faradaic processes. In addition, hybrid ion capacitors (HICs) and asymmetric capacitors (ACs) have both been proven.

The Ragone plot, illustrated in Figure 15.2, is used to evaluate the merits of storage devices for energy and shows that supercapacitors perform similarly to regular capacitors and batteries.

In order to improve device performance, most publications on CQD-based SCs combine CQDs with traditional electrode materials including activated carbons,

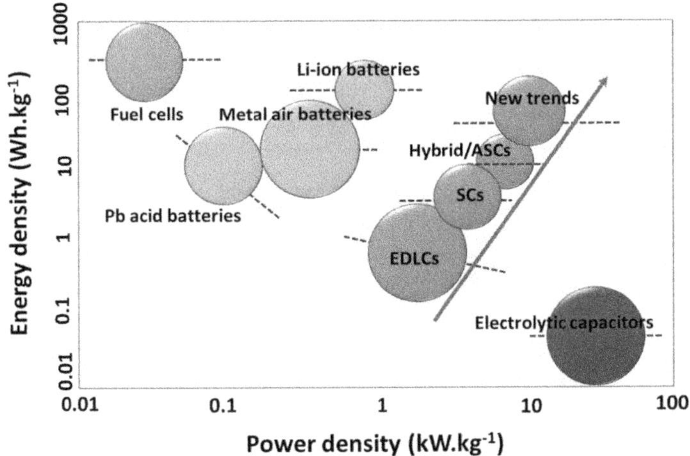

FIGURE 15.2 Ragone's plot for comparing the performance of various energy storage and conversion systems, demonstrating the development of energy-power density of various types of SCs and the position that future devices are predicted to achieve.

metal oxides, metal-organic frameworks, polymer semiconductor materials, etc. Figure 15.3 illustrates various CQD composites for supercapacitor applications. Since CQDs often include hydrophilic functional groups on their surfaces, they can improve electrode waterproofing, as demonstrated by their use with $NiCo_2O_4$ nanowires as shown in Figure 15.4a (J. Wang et al., 2019b). Additionally, because the CDs/$NiCo_2O_4$ electrode receives electrolyte ions more readily and performs electrochemically better than a bare $NiCo_2O_4$ electrode, electrical conductivity may be changed. As shown in Figure 15.4a, the C_s of CQDs/$NiCo_2O_4$ as compared to $NiCo_2O_4$ alone increased significantly from 699 to 2202 F.g⁻¹.

Another attractive material that is easily manufactured using a hydrothermal process is CQD composites with transition metal sulfides. It has been claimed that

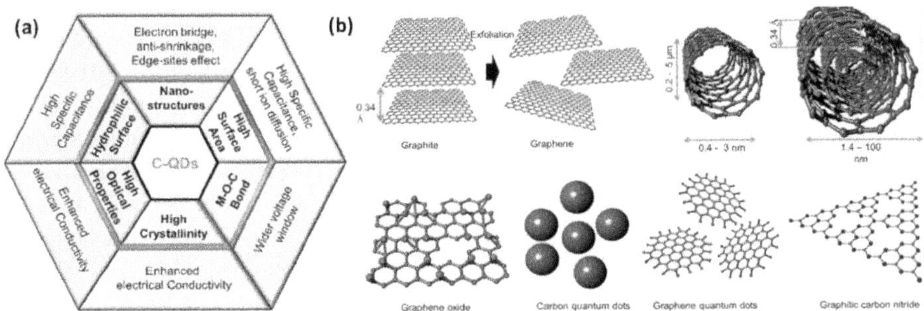

FIGURE 15.3 (a) Aa diagram highlighting the advantages of CQD nanocomposites for application in supercapacitors, and (b) schematics of graphene and carbon quantum dot porous dot-sheet structure (Permatasari et al., 2021).

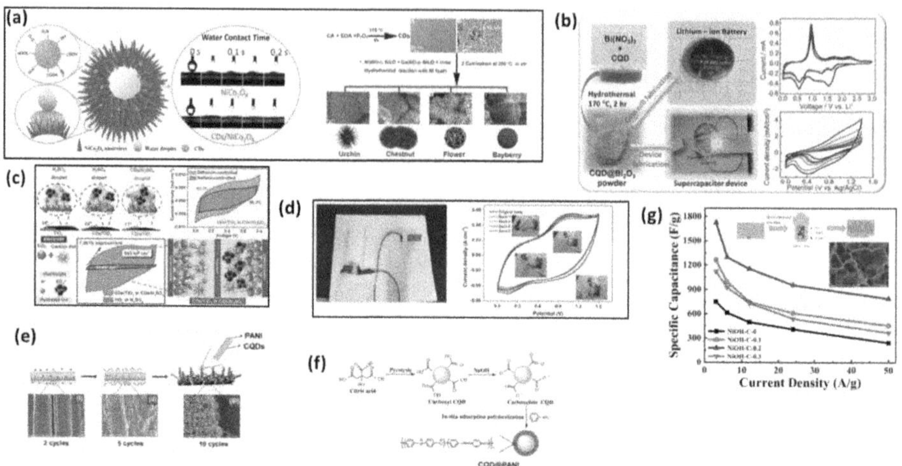

FIGURE 15.4   (a) An illustrated diagram of the CQD influence on the hydrophilicity characteristics of $NiCo_2O_4$ and different morphologies of CQD/ $NiCo_2O_4$ composites (J. Wang et al., 2019b). (b) CQD-anchored bismuth oxide composites (Prasath et al., 2019). (c) CQD/ TiO_2 nanocomposite SC. (d) ASC based on CQD/NiCoLDH-3@CC drives a digital clock. CV curves in a bending condition. (e)–(f) Core shells CQDs@PANI and concerning SEM images of CQDs-PANI/CFs(Li) are depicted schematically. (g) Schematic of specific capacitance obtained from self-sufficient arrays of the α-Ni(OH)$_2$ nanosheet reformed with CQDs.

(a) Reproduced under CC-BY License, (b) Reproduced under CC-BY License., (c) Reproduced with permission (Pholauyphon et al., 2022). Copyright 2022, Elsevier, (d) Reproduced with permission (W. Chen et al., 2023). Copyright 2023, Elsevier, (e–f) Reprinted (adapted) with permission from (Lingyun Li et al., 2019b; Z. Zhao & Xie, 2017). Copyright 2019, American Chemical Society, (g) Reproduced with permission (W. Sun & Lu, 2023). Copyright 2023, Elsevier.

CQDs/NiS composites can withstand 2000 cycles of the charging and discharging process with a specific capacity of up to 880 F/g (Kandra & Bajpai, 2020). The charge transfer procedure was made better by including the CQD into this NiS matrix. Likewise, utilizing spoilt milk-derived CQDs, Prasath et al. have synthesized CQD-Bi_2O_3 nanocomposites by hydrothermal technique (Prasath et al., 2019). The CQD-Bi_2O_3 nanocomposites demonstrated strong electrochemical activity with a capacity of discharge around 1500 mA.h g^{-1} (@ 0.2 C). This nanocomposite electrode-based supercapacitor demonstrated strong reversal and a large specific capacity of 343 C/g @ 0.5 Ag^{-1} in 3M KOH (see Figure 15.4b). The asymmetric device made of reduced graphene oxide and CQD-Bi_2O_3 nanocomposite, however, was able to attain E_s of 88 Wh.kg^{-1} for a given power density value of 2799 W kg^{-1}, whereas the electrical power density attained a maximum value of 8400 W kg^{-1} with an E_s value of 32 W.h kg^{-1}.

Furthermore, the structures of transition metal oxide and metal chalcogenides may be considerably changed by the presence of CQDs. Ji et al. discovered a floral pattern in NiO/CDs after mixing NiO with CDs. The synthesis procedure also creates the porous structure, which enhances the electrolyte's ability to penetrate the electrode

(Ji et al., 2020c). Others have claimed that the materials' structures are also altered by the carbon present during the synthesis process when CD-containing composites are produced (Ji et al., 2020a; Narayanan, 2017). CQDs are claimed to not only improve metal oxide supercapacitor performance but also to act as a structural guiding agent in $NiCo_2O_4$ composites (J.-S. Wei et al., 2016). The nanostructure morphology of $NiCo_2O_4$ varies dramatically when the concentration of CQDs is changed. These various morphologies produce a diverging sort of particular surface area, resulting in distinct C_s values and cycle durability for each composite. Additionally, with the addition of CQDs, the resistance of NiS/CQD materials drops from 150 W to just 75 W. Another instance of composite work using CoS, a different transition metal sulfide, was described by Ji et al. CoS/N-doped CQDs have a greater specific area than CoS alone. However, they discovered that severe nitrogen doping in CQDs may restrict contact among the electrode and the electrolyte, helping to resolve a separate issue by lowering C_s (Ji, Li, et al., 2020b). Recently, CQD/TiO_2 nanocomposite electrode-based SC in the presence of 1 M H_2SO_4 electrolyte showed an increment of C_s by 237% in comparison to intrinsic TiO_2 as illustrated in Figure 15.4c (Pholauyphon et al., 2022). The inclusion of CQDs to the electrolyte or electrode resulted in an overall performance improvement of 1261% due to the positive synergistic benefits of enhancing ion transport routes, lowering series resistance, and other variables.

In recent times, a flexible symmetric supercapacitor built of MCQDs and MnO_2 composite maintained its 85.6 % capacitance with a density of current value of 2 mA.cm^{-2} after 10,000 charging and discharge cycles (G. Yang & Park, 2023). Additionally, the device was also capable of producing highest power density value of ~4.8 W.cm^{-2} (@E_s value of 2.3 mWh cm^{-2}), while it was also produced a peak E_s value of 11.16 mW h cm^{-2} (@ power density of 311.6 mW.cm^{-2}) (G. Yang & Park, 2023). The same one-step electrodeposition process was utilized to synthesize CQD-modified ε-MnO_2 nanosheets having an abundance of oxygen vacancies and poor crystallinity on carbon fabric. The CQDs/ε-MnO_2 electrode produced good mechanical characteristics and electrochemical activity, with a large C_s of 334.5 F.g^{-1} at 1 A.g^{-1}, which was much superior to the pristine ε-MnO_2 electrode (Quan et al., 2023). The flexible SC in Figure 15.4d showed a high C_s of 1587.1 F.g^{-1} at 1 A.g^{-1} along with reasonable good cycle stability and a capacitance retention of 60.1% due to NiCoLDH (nickel cobalt layered double hydroxides) nanosheet arrays embedded with CQDs (W. Chen et al., 2023).

On the other hand, polymer semiconductors are other interesting electrode materials that have been utilized with CQDs. It was shown that the non-covalent approach between CQDs and a conductive polymer such as electrostatic contact, π-π stacking interaction or van der Waals interaction, is responsible for the increased SC performances of CQD/conducting polymer electrodes (Lingyun Li et al., 2019b; Z. Zhao & Xie, 2017). Essentially, the core-shell structure of CQDs covered with the polyaniline (PANI) polymer was recently produced by pyrolysis. One of the crucial factors for displaying the highest C_s with this composite was determined to be the ratio of aniline to CQDs. Figure 15.4e shows that the CQDs@PANI electrode preserves capacity better than bare CQDs or bare PANI electrodes after 500 cycles, retaining 87.7% of its initial capacity (Lingyun Li et al., 2019b). Additionally, as demonstrated in Figure 15.4f, the CQD-PANI composite and the employed electrolyte have improved contact conformation as a result of production of CQD nanocomposites using photoassisted cyclic voltammetry (Z. Zhao & Xie, 2017). Additionally, it has been found that CQDs may significantly affect the development of a porous framework in CQDs/PPy composites once a conductive polymer is being produced, leading to the generation of larger nanoislands with electrodeposition time (Jian et al., 2017). The hydroxyl groups also act as strong electron donors and reductants on CQD surfaces (Essner & Baker, 2017; Privitera et al., 2016). Even after being composited with CQDs, the cycling ability of PPy as a conductive polymer remains low.

Green synthesis of CQDs has become a popular and environmentally benign technique for SC. In this scenario, Inayat et al. have reported that tea leaves biomass-derived CQD-based supercapacitors showed an exceptional C_s of 302.0 F.g^{-1} (@0.5 A.g^{-1}), a good cyclability (5000 cycles) of 144.4 F.g^{-1} (@ 20 A.g^{-1}), and decent rate performance (186.4 Fg^{-1} @ 20 Ag^{-1}). The CQD electrodes further demonstrated improved energy as well as power density values of 41.9 Wh g^{-1} and 250 Wg^{-1}, respectively, at a current flow of 0.5 A.g^{-1} (Inayat et al., 2023). Baslak et al. (2023) employed a hydrothermal technique for synthesizing CQDs from *S. vuralii* plant extract, yielding rechargeable symmetrical capacitor characteristics with charging and discharging capacities of 10.42 F.g^{-1} and 8.26 F.g^{-1}, respectively.

It was recently discovered that a mixture of graphene nanoplatelets (GNP), polypyrrole, and carbon quantum dots may produce both EDLC and pseudocapacitance. CQDs and GNPs were utilized to change the outer layer of the eggshell membrane in the aforementioned device, resulting in a greater surface area. Based on this GNP-CD-PPy, it was observed that CQDs helped increase capacitance to levels more than 80% of the initial performance requirement (Moreno Araújo Pinheiro Lima & de Oliveira, 2020; Xiang Zhang et al., 2017). Again, the ability of composite CQDs with conductive polymers to make flexible SCs is unique and warrants more investigation. Table 15.1 highlights the reported CQD composite electrode materials' present state of the art.

CQDs derived from green algae (*Halimeda opuntia*) recently demonstrated a C_s of 311 F g^{-1} (Al-Ghamdi et al., 2023). Two nanosheet arrays decorated with carbon quantum dots (CQDs/α-Ni(OH)$_2$) were created using a one-step hydrothermal synthesis. In comparison to the 750.7 Fg^{-1} of bare α-Ni(OH)$_2$ shown in Figure 15.4g, the best electrode exhibited a high C_s value of 1724.0 F/g at 3 Ag^{-1} (W. Sun & Lu, 2023).

15.3 APPLICATION OF CQD NANOCOMPOSITES IN ADVANCED BATTERIES

Recently, the application of carbon quantum dots in next-generation batteries has shown enormous potential. CQDs have been effectively used as electrode materials, separators, or electrolytes in several high-tech metal-ion batteries, notably Li, Na, K-ion batteries, as well as Li-S or metal (Al, Zn, Fe etc.)-air batteries.

15.3.1 CQD NANOCOMPOSITES AS CATHODE MATERIALS

Electrode materials have a major impact on the electrochemical efficiency of rechargeable batteries. Numerous high-capacity anode material types have been

TABLE 15.1

List of Various Carbon Quantum Dot Composites Used in Supercapacitors

Electrode Materials	Electrolyte	Specific Capacitance $(F \cdot g^{-1}$ @ $A \cdot g^{-1})$	Rate Capability $(F \cdot g^{-1}$ @ $A \cdot g^{-1})$	Voltage Window (V)	References
CQDs derived from spent tea leaves	4 M H_2SO_4	302.0 @ 0.5	186.4 @ 20	–	Inayat et al. (2023)
CQDs derived from *Sideritis vuralii* leaves	3 M KOH	10.42 @ 0.5	–	–	Başlak et al. (2023)
CQDs/ε-MnO$_2$ nanosheet	0.1 M Mn(CH$_3$CO$_2$)$_2$ + 0.1 M anhydrous Na$_2$SO$_4$	334.5 @ 1	–	–	Quan et al. (2023)
CQD/NiCoLDH-3@CC	6 M KOH	1587.1 @ 1	1281.2 @ 20	0–1.5	C.-J. Lee et al. (2017)
CQDs/GCE	6 M KOH	311 @ 1	–	–0.4–0.4	Al-Ghamdi et al. (2023)
CQDs/α-Ni(OH)2) nanosheet	6 M KOH	1724.0 @ 3	–	–	W. Sun & Lu (2023)
CQDs/Bi$_2$O$_3$	3 M KOH	343 @ 0.5	343–61 @ 0.5–1.6	0–0.8	Prasath et al. (2019)
CQDs/MoS$_2$/ZnS	6 M KOH	2899.5 @ 5–20	2899.5–1400 @ 5–20	0–0.5	J. Zheng et al. (2019)
NPO-CQDs/HPC	4 M H_2SO_4	510 @ 1	510–408 @ 1–10	–0.4–0.6	Ji-Shi Wei et al. (2018)
CoS/N-CQDs	3 M KOH	697 @ 1	697–485 @ 1–20	0–0.6	Ji Li et al. (2020)
CQDs/GF/NiCo$_2$S$_4$	1 M H_2SO_4	1348 @ 0.5	1348–877 @ 0.5–10	0–0.6	L. Xu et al. (2019)
CNT/Bi$_2$O$_3$/GO/CQDs	6 M KOH	1.90 mAh.cm^{-2} @ 1 mA·cm^{-2}	1.57 mAh.cm^{-2} @ 200 mA·cm^{-2}	–1.05–0	W. Wang et al. (2019c)
N-CQDs/PANI	1 M H_2SO_4	498 @ 1	498–348 @ 1–10	–0.2–0.8	Q. Wang et al. (2017a)
Mn/PANI/N-CQDs	1 M LiPF$_6$	595 @1	–	–2.5–2.5	Alaş et al. (2019)
CQDs/NiCo$_2$O$_4$ nanowire	3M HCl	2202 @ 1	–	–0.2–0.8	J. Wang et al. (2019b)
CQDs/RuO$_2$	1 M H_2SO_4	594 @ 1	–	0–1.0	Y. Zhu et al. (2013)
CQDs/TiO$_2$	1 M H_2SO_4	643 mF.cm^{-2}	–	0–0.8	Pholauyphon et al. (2022)
CQDs/NiS	2 M KOH	880 @ 1	–	–0.1–0.25	Sahoo et al. (2018)
CQDs/Polypyrrole	1 M KCl	424.6 @ 1	–	0–0.8	Jian et al. (2017)

investigated, among which are carbon and titanium (such as $Li_4Ti_5O_{12}$, TiO_2) materials based on alloys (Sb, Si, Si, NiSb, etc.), materials containing metal oxides or sulfides (Mn_3O_4, MoS_2, Sb_2S_3), and others (J. Chen et al., 2015; Hou et al., 2014; Yonggang Wang et al., 2009; J. Zhou et al., 2015). On the other hand, CQDs have mostly been employed as surface coatings in cathode material applications.

For the purpose of surface engineering, Balogun et al. synthesized VO_2 nanowires that were subsequently grown on 3D-carbon fabric (Balogun et al., 2016). CQDs facilitate faster transport, operate as a sensitizer, and prevent agglomeration, providing structural integrity to VO_2 nanowires (see Figure 15.5a). When applied to Li-ion batteries, the cathode has an acceptable capacity of discharge value of 402 mAh g^{-1} (@ 0.3 C) and can produce as high as 168 mAh g^{-1} even @ 60 C.

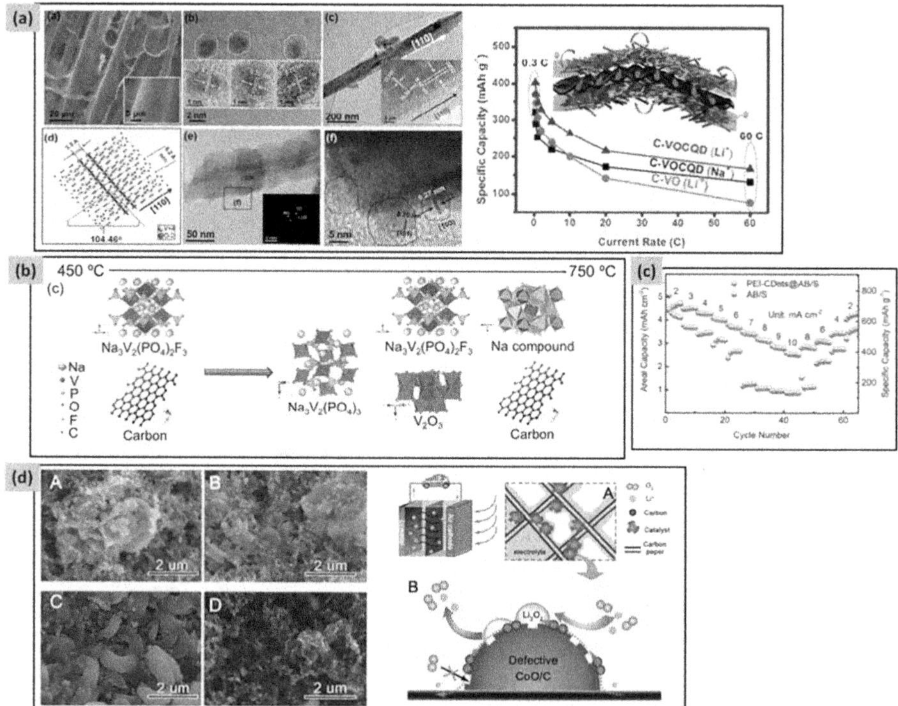

FIGURE 15.5 (a) Morphology of CQDs and C-VOCQD nanowire. Schematic illustration of the C-VOCQD-based electrode made of interlaced nanowires. (b) Structure evolution of NVPF@CQD as the cathode electrode. (c) Comparison of the rate performance between the AB/S and PEI-CDots@AB/S cathodes. (d) CoO/C-based cathodes captured using SEM in various charge-discharge stages. Carbon and oxygen vacancies interact synergistically in CoO/C.

(a) Reprinted (adapted) with permission from (Balogun et al., 2016). Copyright 2016. American Chemical Society, (b) Reproduced with permission (Z. Yang et al., 2020). Copyright 2020, Elsevier, (c) Reproduced with permission (Hu et al., 2019). Copyright 2019, Wiley-VCH, (d) Reprinted (adapted) with permission from Gao et al. (2016). Copyright 2016. American Chemical Society.

The performance of CQD-modified sodium vanadium fluorophosphate ($Na_3V_2O_{2x}$ $(PO_4)_2F_{3-2x}$ ($0 \le x \le 1$) nanocomposites being used as a cathodic material for sodium-ion batteries (SIBs) has been reported to be outstanding. As illustrated in Figure 15.5b, the CQDs@NVPF electrode show excellent rate performances when employed as the cathode in SIBs, with values of 126.6 and 84.7 mAh g^{-1} @ 0.2 and @ 50 C, respectively, while exhibiting good cycle stability (S. Liu et al., 2020b; Z. Yang et al., 2020).

Hu et al. synthesized CQDs functionalized with polyethyleneimine (PEI-CQDs) to enhance the efficiency of lithium-sulfur batteries with heavy sulfur load as well as their ability to run at high current densities (2019). The PEI-CQDs@AB/S cathode was prepared by mixing PEI-CQDs with sulfur, polyvinylidene fluoride and acetylene black.

The Li-S batteries modified with PEI-CQDs displayed an incredible spatial capacity of 3.3 mAhcm^{-1} when subjected to a considerable sulfur loading (~6.60 mg) and a high density of current (8 mA cm^{-2}); even following 400 cycles, the capacity degradation was just 0.07% per cycle (see Figure 15.5c). The study demonstrates how PEI-CQDs may enhance Li$^+$ conductivity at the solid-electrolyte interfaces and how their amine groups might offer a wide range of adsorption sites, inhibiting the dissolution of polysulfides.

Besides, CQDs have also been used in metal-air batteries. Gao et al. propose a novel technique for improving CoO catalytic activity by integrating CQDs and oxygen vacancies (Gao et al., 2016). They were able to synthesize CoO/C composite by mixing CoO with CQDs and oxygen vacancy defects and calcinating the source made by modifying cobalt(II) acetate with ethanol (see Figure 15.5d). The CoO/C cathode demonstrated improved rate performance, capacity, and cyclic stability when compared to pure CoO containing oxygen vacancies. This is likely because CQDs and oxygen vacancies have a synergistic impact on the oxygen reduction reaction or oxygen evolution reaction.

15.3.2 CQD NANOCOMPOSITES AS ANODE MATERIALS

Graphite continues to be the dominant anode material for commercial batteries due to its plentiful supplies, inexpensive, and superior conductivity. In the beginning, Javed et al. employed CQDs in a carbon-based anode material derived from glucose for Li-ion batteries (Javed et al., 2019). CQD-based anode exhibits high stable cyclic permanence and Li/Na storing capability, confirming the promise of CQDs for Li-ion batteries. When employed as an anode in Li-ion batteries, they can achieve a high capacity of 864.9 mAhg^{-1} @ 0.5 C after 500 cycles, as well as a capacity of 340.2 mAhg^{-1} at a high rate of 20 C even after 500 cycles (see Figure 15.6a). An environmentally safe and sustainable method of synthesizing N-doped CQDs derived from egg yolk was developed by Wang et al. (S. Wang et al., 2018). These CQDs have good stability and fluorescence properties. They have outstanding electrochemical performance when utilized as anodes of LIBs following carbonization (Figure 15.6b).

The remarkable cycle stability, security, and barely volume expansion of titanium-based materials have also piqued the scientific community's attention. The most practicable anode material for LIBs has been considered to be lithium titanate (LTO,

$Li_4Ti_5O_{12}$). It has been observed that adding Al and Mn co-doped CQDs to the LTO nanocomposite increases its electrical properties (Figure 15.6c) (Lin Li et al., 2019a; Nan et al., 2019). The LIB capacity and charge and discharge rates were successfully enhanced by the nanocomposites. LIB showed a specific capacity value of 296.50 mAh g^{-1} during initial cycle at 0.1 C, a reduced impedance of 16.8Ω, and a capacity that remained constant after 100 cycles of use was 236 mAh g^{-1}.

(a)

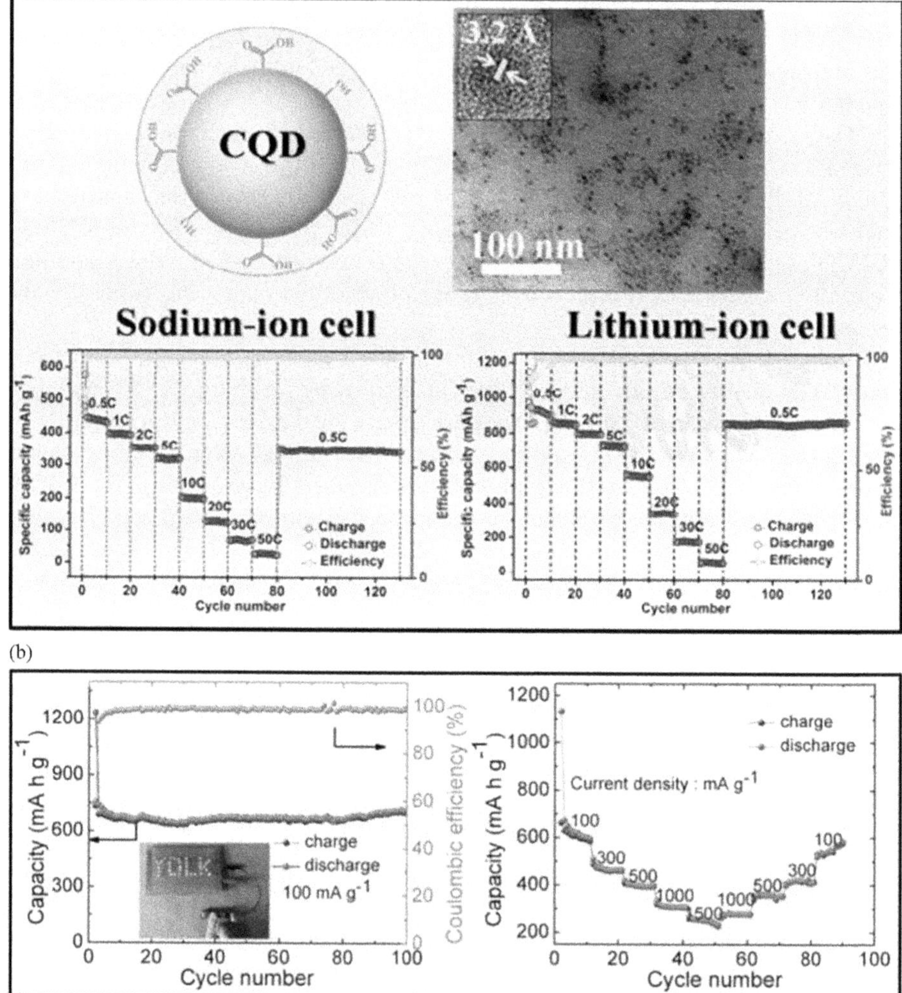

(b)

FIGURE 15.6 (a) HRTEM image of CQDs derived from glucose oxidation. At various current densities in Li-ion and Na-ion batteries, the CQD electrode's rate performance and associated Coulombic efficiencies were examined. (b) Cyclic Coulombic efficiencies and rate performances of egg yolk-derived CQD nanocomposite electrodes in LIBs.

(a) Reproduced with permission (Javed et al., 2019). Copyright 2019, Elsevier, (b) Reproduced with permission (S. Wang et al., 2018). Copyright 2018, Elsevier.

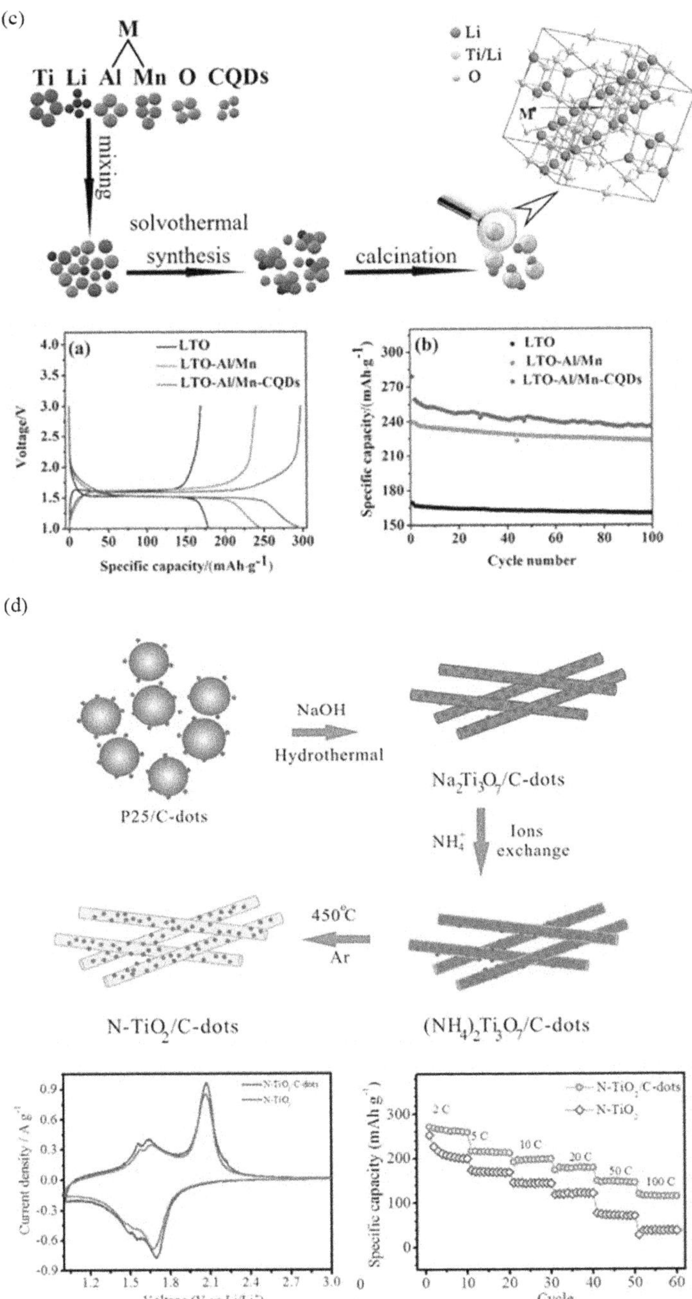

FIGURE 15.6 (c) Schematic of a CQD-modified LTO electrode. Charge/discharge along with the specific capacity curve (Nan et al., 2019). (d) Schematic of N-TiO$_2$/CQDs nanocomposite formation and the corresponding CV plot and rate performance of LIBs (Y. Yang et al., 2015).

Another TiO_2-based anode that uses TiO_2-nanorods coated with N-CQDs has been studied (Y. Yang et al., 2015). The galvanostatic charging and discharging curves along with cyclic performance of LIBs are illustrated in Figure 15.6d, which shows approx. 91.6% capacity retention after 1000 cycles despite high rate of 10 C. However, in sodium-ion batteries, carbon-coupled TiO_2 composites showed significant reversal specific capacities (264.10 mAh g^{-1} @ 0.1 C), and even following two thousands cycles, a capacity retention of 94.7% was achieved to a value of around 108.20 mAh g^{-1} @10 C (J. Chen et al., 2016; M. Wu et al., 2020).

Anode materials based on metal compounds have also been the focus of CQD research. The manganese oxide (Mn_3O_4) nanocomposite materials modified with CQDs were initially demonstrated using a green electrochemical technique (Jing et al., 2015). The initial coulombic efficiency of Mn_3O_4/CQDs electrodes was found to be better than that of pristine Mn_3O_4, most likely due to the octahedral Mn_3O_4 in the Mn_3O_4/CQDs composites being of substantial value to reduce the resistance of charge transfer via exchange of Mn or O atomic layers. Furthermore, even after 50 cycles, the capacity of discharge of Mn_3O_4/CQDs composites was about 934 mAh g^{-1} @ 100 mA g^{-1}, which exceeded the value of that without CQDs by almost five times, demonstrating superior stability in cyclic behavior. Similarly, the high safety and structural stability of Nb_2O_5 has also made it a preferred choice for LIB anodes. In fact, the as-prepared Nb_2O_5/carbon nanocomposite demonstrated greater specific capacity, decent rate capability, and enhanced stability during cycles in comparison to pristine Nb_2O_5 (J. Lin et al., 2018). Likewise, bismuth oxide (Bi_2O_3)/ carbon nanocomposite has emerged as an intriguing anode material for LIBs that demonstrated high electrochemical activity, delivering a primary capacity of discharge value of 1500 mAh g^{-1} (@ 0.2 C) and maintaining ~1200 mAh g^{-1} for the following three cycles. This was more than the previously stated value for Bi_2O_3 alone, Bi_2O_3/rGO nanocomposite, and 3D ordered macroporous β-Bi_2O_3 anode materials (Deng et al., 2017; Zhen Li et al., 2016; Prasath et al., 2019).

Conversely, several metal anodes, including as Ge, Sn, Sb, and others, have been recommended for SIBs because of their strong mass/volume capacities. The Sb@ CQD nanocomposites were successfully synthesized by Liu et al. at room temperature, and they showed it to have a substantial specific capacity of 635 and 334 mAh g^{-1}@0.1 and 2 A g^{-1}, respectively (F. Liu et al., 2020a). CQD-modified anode materials were also successfully utilized in potassium-ion batteries by developing a porous nanostructured N-doped carbon materials (Hong et al., 2019). When used as PIB anodes, they produced a specific capacity value of 254 (@ 0.1 A g^{-1}) and 160 mAh g^{-1} (@ 1.0 A g^{-1}), respectively in the 100 cycles followed by 800 cycles.

15.3.3   CQD Nnanocomposites as Separators

The development of an easy and cost-effective technology for separators, particularly in Li-S batteries, is crucial since inserting sulfur in separators has been demonstrated to inhibit cyclic performance. In this regard, functionalization of separators with carbon materials have shown promise. CQD-modified new separators were developed by coating multiwalled carbon nanotubes with N-doped CQDs (MWCNTs/NCQDs) in Li-S batteries as shown in Figure 15.7a (Pang et al., 2018). There is evidence to support that the MWCNTs/N-CQD coating inhibits polysulfide shuttle by physical shielding and chemisorption.

By virtue of the synergistic effects of MWCNTs and N-CQDs, Li-S batteries exhibit exceptional cycle performance and a comparatively high early discharge rate of 1330.8 mAhg^{-1}.

15.3.4 CQDs in Electrolytes

The production of lithium dendrites, induced by a dispersion imbalance of lithium ions and an electric field at the electrode-electrolyte interface, is one of the most critical issues with lithium ion batteries (Shen et al., 2019). Nitrogen-doped carbon dots have been used in Li-S batteries as electrolyte additives to reduce translocation and for dissolving lithium polysulfide (LiPS) by forming a polysulfide barrier coating that may be maintained to avoid sulfur loss (Fu et al., 2020). It has been shown that a solidification layer of LiPS/N-CQDs forms immediately after mixing Li$_2$S$_6$ solution and N-CQDs (0.3 wt%) into the electrolyte, thereby preventing Li$_2$S$_6$ from diffusing into the electrolyte (see Figure 15.7b).

In summary, CQDs have demonstrated intriguing applications in many advanced batteries. However, further studies on large-scale manufacturing techniques and rigorous regulations are necessary before CQDs can be widely used in energy storage systems.

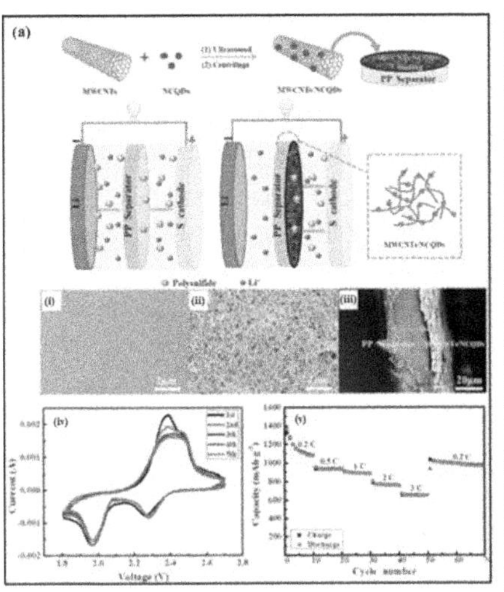
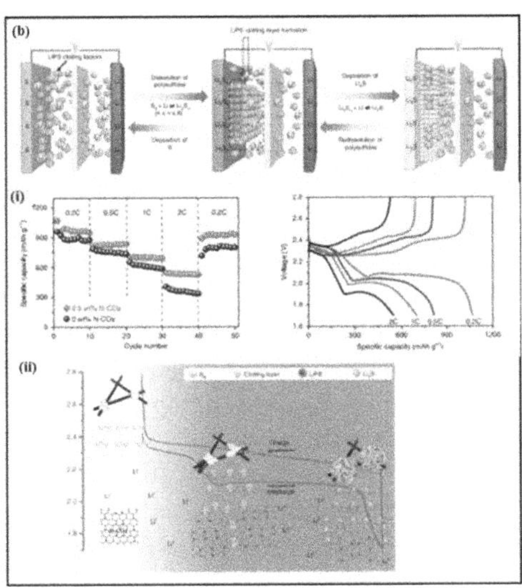

FIGURE 15.7 (a) A diagram illustrating the application of MWCNTs/N-doped CQD composite-coated separator in Li-S battery. (i)–(iii) Corresponding SEM images of MWCNTs/N-doped CQD composite-coated separator and (iv)–(v) cyclic voltammograms and rate performances. (b) Schematic showing lithium polysulfide (LiPS) clotting mechanisms. (i) Rate performance and voltage profile of Li-S cell with electrolyte containing 0.5 wt% N-CQDs. (ii) Proposed clotting mechanism during charging and discharging cycles (Fu et al., 2020).

15.4 APPLICATION OF CARBON QUANTUM DOTS IN ADVANCED PHOTOVOLTAICS

Photovoltaic technologies, both present and future, are critical components of renewable energy resources. When compared to alternative power generation technologies, photovoltaic is typically the most cost-effective approach for fulfilling the predicted spike in global energy demand over the next several decades. This section has gone through how to use CQDs in a variety of solar cell types, including dye-sensitized solar cells, solid-state solar cells, organic solar cells, and perovskite solar cells of varying capacities. A variety of low-cost CQDs produced from natural extracts have been used to fabricate photovoltaic devices.

15.4.1 CQDs in Dye and Quantum Dot-Sensitized Solar Cells

CQDs have been effectively used to modify photoanodes, counter electrodes (CE) or dye/QDs sensitizers either in dye and or quantum dot-sensitized solar cells (DSSCs/QDSSCs). Meng et al. have reported all-weather solar cell architecture by modifying mesoscopic titanium dioxide/long-persistence phosphor-based photoanodes and employing soybean-derived CQDs as a sensitizer (Y. Meng et al., 2017). The device attained an efficiency of up to 7.97% while providing consistent electrical supply for several hours. In a similar manner, it was reported that DSSCs composed of photoanodes made of ZnO nanoparticles and sensitized by N-doped CQDs had an enhanced efficiency of 1.18% compared to ZnO alone (0.88%) (Chava et al., 2017). It is proposed that N-CQDs can act as a donor material, extend the absorption spectrum, and play an essential role in charge transfer kinetics. Another study found that the conversion efficiency of DSSC made using ZnO@CQDs/N719, where CQDs were synthesized from ethylenediamine/citric acid, was 5.9% as illustrated in Figure 15.8a (Efa & Imae, 2019). Furthermore, by integrating fluorescent CQDs into the dye sensitizer, N719-TiO$_2$ photoanode-based DSSC efficiency was demonstrated to improve 21%, from 7.25% to 8.7%, presumably because CQDs may operate as both a light-harvesting agent and an electron-transport channel in a dye-sensitized film (N719-TiO$_2$) as shown in Figure 15.8b (Shi et al., 2016). Various heteroatom-doped CQDs were also proven to improve the photovoltaic performances. Liu et al. proved that applying energy-graded configurations of CQDs doped with heteroatoms is a potential technique for fabricating absorbers free of defects for DSSCs. They were successful in fabricating graded energy levels by S- and N-doped CQDs from lotus root powder with efficiency as high as 9.04% (L. Liu et al., 2019). In addition to the previously mentioned sensitizers and photoanode substitutions, it has been shown that using CQDs to alter the photophysical and electrical properties of the counter electrode material is a successful method for enhancing device performance. The high efficiency of 7.01% of the bifacial DSSCs constructed using CQD-containing CoSe CEs was attained by improved optical transmission and broad absorption of CEs (W. Zhu et al., 2017). Recently, N-doped CQD-modified multiwalled carbon nanotubes (MWCNTs) used as a counter electrode in DSSCs were shown to boost efficiency by up to 9.28% above pristine MWCNTs CE (6.17%, see Figure 15.8c) (Ali et al., 2021).

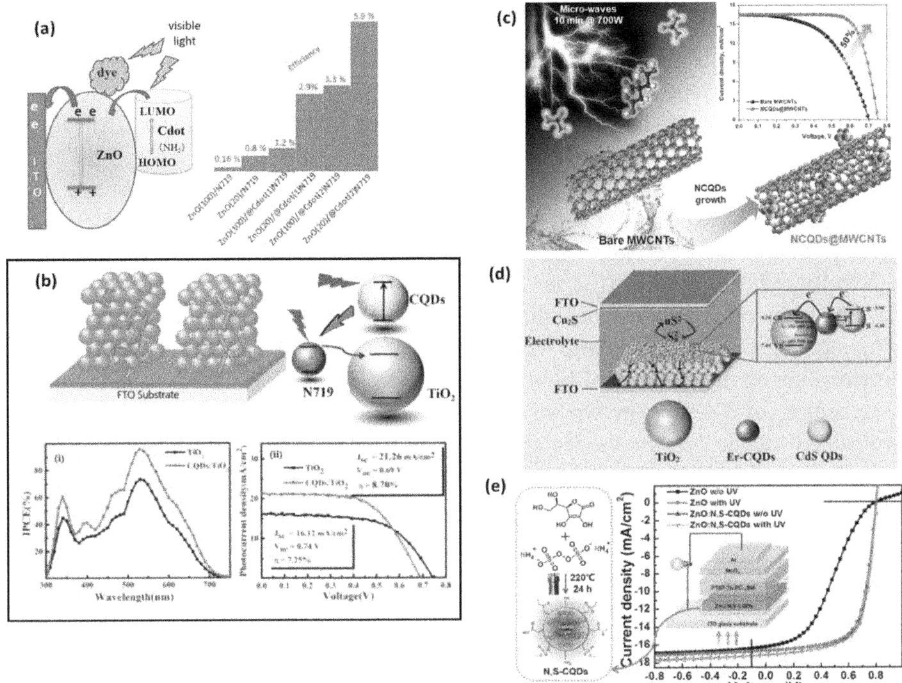

FIGURE 15.8   (a) Influence of CQDs on ZnO-nanoparticle-based DSSCs. (b) Fluorescent CQDs in the TiO$_2$ photoanode of DSSCs with N719 sensitization. (i)-(ii) Corresponding incident photon-to-current efficiency and current-voltage plot for the pure TiO$_2$ and CQDs/TiO$_2$-based DSSCs. (c) Nitrogen-doped CQD-modified multiwalled CNT exhibits 50% higher photovoltaic performance. (d) Impact of Er-doped CQD-sensitized photoanode in CdS-based QDSSCs. (e) ZnO ETL decorated with N, S co-doped-CQDs shows increased power conversion efficiency.

(a) Reproduced with permission (Efa & Imae, 2019). Copyright 2019, Elsevier, (b) Reproduced with permission (Shi et al., 2016). Copyright 2016, Wiley-VCH, (c) Reproduced with permission (Ali et al., 2021). Copyright 2021, Elsevier, (d) Reproduced with permission (C. Zhao et al., 2018). Copyright 2018, Elsevier, (e) Reprinted (adapted) with permission from (Yaling Wang et al., 2019d). Copyright 2019. American Chemical Society.

CQDs were utilized in QDSSCs as a sensitizer to improve photovoltaic performance, much as DSSCs as seen in Figure 15.8d, the power conversion efficiency of CdS-based QDSSCs was demonstrated to increase with an Er-doped CQD-sensitized photoanode (C. Zhao et al., 2018). Likewise, N-doped CQDs were also reported to improve the efficiency in CdS-QDSSC from 0.430% to 0.606% (Huang et al., 2020). This is attributable to the integration of CQDs, which may increase the absorption range, reduce charge recombination at the photoanode/electrolyte contact significantly, and perhaps generate type I band alignments between QDs and CQDs.

15.4.2 CQDs in Organic Solar Cells

Polymer solar cells, often referred to as bulk heterojunction organic photovoltaics, have lately gained popularity due to their appealing features, including economical, flexible, and large-scale mass manufacturing of large-area devices via roll-to-roll processing. In order to fabricate these devices, two materials: conjugated polymers that are predominantly p-type and fullerene derivatives of the n-type—that take electrons must be stacked. The most widely used naturally nanostructured material is a mixture of fullerene derivative (6,6-phenylC61 butyric acid methyl ester) and poly-3-hexylthiophene (P3HT) (Essner & Baker, 2017). The limited carrier mobility of organic semiconductors restricts the thickness of these devices, which leads to undesired charge recombination and has a detrimental effect on the efficiency of power conversion and the quantity of light that can be collected. CQDs have been employed as acceptors of electrons in two ways to promote greener replacements: (i) the CQDs are mixed together in the device's active layer and (ii) the substitute for the fullerene derivative is CQD. The photoluminescence quenching effect generated by the presence of CQDs when paired with the P3HT film can be seen from the fact that CQDs take electrons from P3HT that has been photoexcited, inhibiting radiation-induced electron-hole recombination (Xiaoting Feng et al., 2015). On the other hand, Privitera and colleagues showed that organosoluble CQDs doped with N and functionalized with thiophene were effective electron donors for PCBM in both liquid and solid mixtures. The thiophene moiety employed was shown to affect more durable charge pair states, leading to increased recombination of charges and a decrease in the amount of photoinduced free-of-charge carriers (Privitera et al., 2016).

Inverted OPVs, on the other hand, are gaining popularity because of their improved device stability and manufacturing capacity over bulk heterojunction OPVs. Because of the design of the device, buffer layers, sometimes referred to as electron transport layers (ETL), must be used between the polymer film and the cathode (such as glass coated with ITO) in order to minimize the cathode work function and maintain a disconnected and consequent removal of charge carriers. The most often used ETLs are metal oxides like ZnO or TiO_2; however, Cs_2CO_3 is also becoming more and more popular due to its excellent electron injection and simplicity of manufacture. CQDs doped with nitrogen and sulfur (N,S-CQDs) are demonstrated in Figure 15.8e to be excellent surface modifiers for ZnO and light-soaking free in inverted OPVs, with better efficiencies up to 9.31% (Yaling Wang et al., 2019d). Furthermore, CQD composites were used as ETLs. CQDs@polyethyleneimine composite-based device exhibits reduced dark current and better electron removal in the presence of light, having a maximum efficiency of 9.53%, V_{oc} of 0.73 volts, J_{sc} of 18.37 milliampere-cm^{-2}, and FF of 71.1% (Zhiqi Li et al., 2018). In a further study, CQDs@polyethyleneimine ethoxylate composite as an ETL was used in inverted OPVs with an efficiency of power conversion value of 8.35% (Lim et al., 2018).

15.4.3 CQDs in Solid-state Nanostructured Solar Cells

Solid-state photovoltaics have historically provided unmatched photovoltaic efficiencies owing to the materials and manufacturing process used; yet, they are still constrained by excessive cost-to-power output ratios and the usage of potentially dangerous chemicals to the environment. In this context, CQDs provide a realistic exploration for appropriate, affordable, and non-toxic substitutes for sensitizers, charge transfer media, and energy downshifting layers in solar cells using solid-state nanostructures. Briscoe at al. have demonstrated that biomass-derived (glucose, chitin, and chitosan) CQDs can be effectively used as sensitizers in ZnO nanorods and copper thiocyanide (CuSCN)-based solid-state solar cells as shown in Figure 15.9a (Briscoe et al., 2015). Given its high series resistance and low efficiency (0.017%), the device with glucose-CQD sensitization had the least short circuit current. Contrarily, the reduced covering density of chitin-derived-CQDs was insufficient to prevent interfacial recombination, causing lower efficiency (0.032%). However, among the three types of CQDs, chitosan-derived-CQDs generated the device with the best performance, with a PCE of 0.061%. Additionally, in a variety of solid-state nanostructured solar cells, including semiconductor QDs, crystalline Si, and cells made of silicon nanowires, CQDs have been employed either as an effective separator a blocking layer of charge carriers (Narayanan et al., 2013; Xie et al., 2014). According to Narayanan et al., the use of glucose-derived CQDs as the transfer of

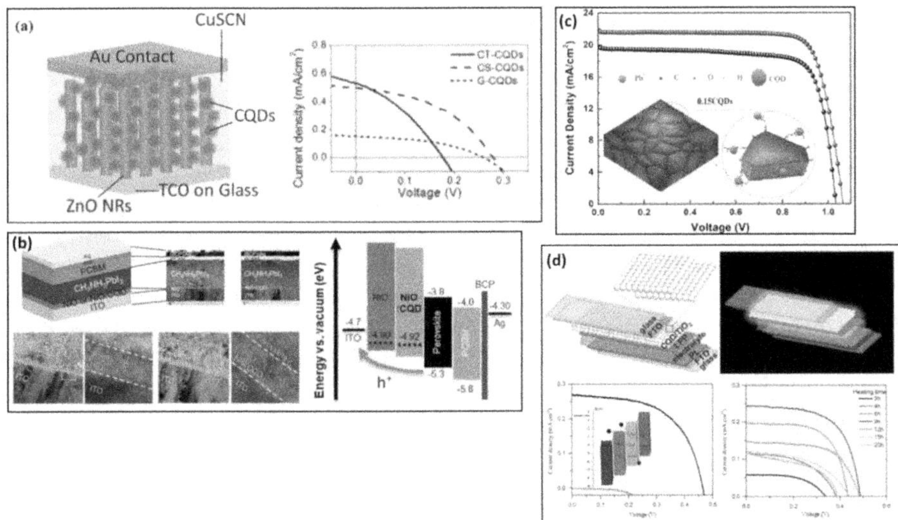

FIGURE 15.9 (a) Schematic of nanostructured solar cell based on CQD-coated ZnO nanorods along with current-voltage characteristics. (b) Schematic sketch, SEM images, and the corresponding energy band alignment of a perovskite solar cell. (c) Current-voltage characteristics of an inverted PSC following grain boundary passivation using CQDs. (d) Schematic structure, photoluminescence diagram, and current-voltage characteristics of an all-weather CQD solar cell.

(a) Reproduced with permission (Briscoe et al., 2015). Copyright 2015, Wiley-VCH, (b) Reproduced with permission (Kim et al., 2020). Copyright 2020, Elsevier, (c) Reprinted (adapted) with permission from Ma et al. (2019). Copyright 2019. American Chemical Society, (d) Reproduced with permission (J. Yang et al., 2017). Copyright 2017, Royal Society of Chemistry.

charge layer in a solid-state battery composed of copper phthalocyanine molecules that are submerged in a sulfide ion-dependent gel electrolyte that are acting as acceptors and ZnS monolayer enclosed CdS QDs as donors led to improved photovoltaic parameters (Narayanan et al., 2013). Similarly, Xie et al. showed that when electrochemically produced CQDs were used in a hierarchical Si nanowire array, the photovoltaic parameters were discovered to be influenced by Si functionality, CQD coating extent, and individual CQD size (Xie et al., 2014). Another important aspect has been explored by implementing energy down-shifting layers (EDSLs). Since higher energy photons like UV have a better likelihood of being absorbed and do not result in inefficient energy losses from electron thermalization, one should convert these photons to energies that are more closely related with the bandgap like the visible region. CQDs are great candidates for EDSLs in this aspect due to their high luminescence, excitation wavelength reliant emission, tunable bandgaps according to their sizes, and ease of synthesis. Pelayo et al. used commercial Si solar cells to apply CQDs (Pelayo et al., 2016). The downshifting effect resulted to improvements in PCE over devices that do not have an EDSL having a value of 2%–5%, depending on the current applied in the electrochemical synthesis of CQDs.

15.4.4 CQDs in Perovskite Solar Cells

Perovskite solar cells (PSCs) are quickly establishing themselves as a new paradigm in photovoltaic energy conversion. It has been reported that CQDs may be used in PSCs as a hole transport material (HTM) and to control charge recombination by modifying the interfacial properties. In 2016, Paulo et al. proposed their preliminary study on CQDs as an HTM (Paulo et al., 2016). With the use of a hydrothermal procedure, they synthesized solution-processed CQDs from citric acid, which they subsequently mixed with methylammonium lead iodide (MAPI) perovskite. The tunable bandgap of the CQDs efficiently aided in hole migration and stopped the perovskite from leaking electrons into the CQDs. Similar to this, Benetti et al. showed extremely stable and efficient PSCs by introducing CQDs into graphene oxide where the work function of graphene oxide could be pushed down. This accelerates the pace of hole injection and inhibits the kinetics of recombination between electrons and holes. As a consequence, the efficiency with CQDs is higher (16.2%) than without (14.7%) (Benetti et al., 2019). Another study by Kim et al. showed how the surfaces of the CQDs that are rich in oxygen and nitrogen enhanced the electronic characteristics of the NiO and properly matched with the perovskite and conducting glass workfunctions to form p-i-n-type PSCs, which showed increased solar efficiencies of 15.66% to 17.02% (see Figure 15.9b) (Kim et al., 2020). Additionally, CQDs aid in preventing ambient moisture and slowing the formation of holes in perovskite films. Similarly, to increase light absorption and passivate the borders of perovskite film grains, CQDs with surface-enhanced properties have been used. According to Ma et al., the addition of CQDs enhanced the absorbance while also diminishing intrinsic defects in perovskites as shown in Figure 15.9c (Ma et al., 2019). Similarly, Xu et al. reported that various surface functional groups of CQDs modify the size of grains, crystalline properties and superior hydrophobic properties of perovskite films (T. Xu et al., 2021). Wen et al. discovered that CQDs enhanced the efficiency and stability of the MAPI film, which they attributed to the MAPI film's increased crystallization and grain size, as well as the reduced carrier recombination (Wen et al., 2020). In addition, Han et al. employed CQDs as an interface modifier layer, which not only increases hole transmission to the electrode but also reduces the state of defects in the perovskite layer, improving solar performance by up to 13.3% (Han et al., 2019).

15.4.5 CQDs in All-Weather Solar Cells

Realizing consistent power production with great efficiency under cloudy, rainy, hazy, and nighttime situations is still a difficult task. The actual demonstration of all-weather solar cells' feasibility opens the way for a future revolution in photovoltaic technology. Leveraging the CQDs' prominent photoelectron excitation activities and their light-emitting/storing capabilities of long perseverance phosphors, Yang et al. developed all-weather solar cells with an optimal dark efficiency of 14.8% along with outstanding enduring stability, as shown in Figure 15.9d (J. Yang et al., 2017). Finally, various solar cell device performance parameters are shown in Table 15.2.

15.5 OPTOELECTRONICS APPLICATIONS OF CARBON QUANTUM DOTS

The use of CQDs in optoelectronics is increasingly gaining popularity and they have excellent prospects. Aside from the well-known benefits of CQDs as inexpensive, non-toxic, and ecologically benign materials, a wide range of accessible synthetic and post-synthetic processes allows for the production of CQDs with the appropriate optical and electrical characteristics. CQD applications in LEDs are usually classified into two categories: down-conversion and electroluminescent. The first category of LEDs can be produced quickly by depositing CQDs on a commercially available UV-LED that serves as a source of excitation; these LEDs, which are white LEDs (WLEDs) with varying color temperatures, are extensively addressed in the literature as a type of demonstrative devices with variable emission throughout a wide spectrum range. CQDs, on the other hand, are utilized as an active layer in the second category of LEDs, where electroluminescence is generated by injecting charges while being illuminated.

15.5.1 Down-Conversion CQD-based LEDs

The process of down-conversion used to produce white light depends on the absorption of ultraviolet or blue light produced by commercial LED chips consisting of InGaN, GaN, and other materials. This results in the emission of longer wavelength light like green and red again, as illustrated in Figure 15.10a. He et al. demonstrated WLEDs by coating commercial UV-LED chips with white light emitting phosphor composites based on CQDs embedded in the zinc borate matrix (He et al., 2020). They have shown that the temperature of white light may be adjusted by varying the ratio of CQDs to zinc borate. In another study, CQD composites were made by embedding them in phthalimide crystals and then utilized to make WLEDs, as illustrated in Figure 15.10b (Y. Zheng et al., 2020). The WLEDs have CIE coordinates of

TABLE 15.2

A Comparison of Various Device Performance Parameters of CQD Nanocomposite-Based Solar Cells

Precursor	Role of CQD	Solar Cell Stack	J_{sc} (mA.cm^{-2})	V_{oc} (V)	η (%)	References
γ-butyrolactone	sen*	FTO-glass/TiO$_2$ NPs/CQDs/I$_3^-$:I$^-$/Pt-metal	0.53	0.38	0.13	Mirtchev et al. (2012)
Melamine, glycerol	sen*	FTO-glass/TiO$_2$ NPs/CQDs/I$_3^-$:I$^-$/ Pt-metal	0.8	0.57	0.13	C. Wang et al. (2012)
Graphite rods	sen*	Ti-foil/TiO$_2$ NTs/CQDs/I$_3^-$:I$^-$/ Pt-metal	0.02	0.58	0.004	M. Sun et al. (2014)
Monkey grass	sen*	FTO-glass/TiO$_2$ NPs/CQDs/I$_3^-$:I$^-$/ Pt-metal	1.93	0.49	0.53	Verma et al. (2021)
Citric acid, urea, formic acid	sen*	FTO-glass/TiO$_2$ NPs/CQDs/I$_3^-$:I$^-$/ Pt-metal	0.99	0.49	0.50	Margraf et al. (2016)
Strawberry powder	sen*	FTO-glass/m-TiO$_2$/CQDs/LPP/I$_3^-$:I$^-$/ Pt-metal	0.059	0.228	0.011	J. Yang et al. (2017)
Carbon soot (from polystyrene foam)	PD/co-sen*	FTO-glass/TiO$_2$:CQD-grafted graphene/ CdS:CdSe/Na$_2$S:S/Cu$_2$S	11.65	0.56	4.04	Y. Zhang et al. (2016b)
L-ascorbic acid	ED/co-sen*	FTO-glass/TiO$_2$NPs/PbSe:CdS:CQDs/Na$_2$S/ MWCNTs	17.07	0.69	4.84	Kokal et al. (2015)
Citric acid	CED	FTO-glass/TiO$_2$ NPs/N719/I$_3^-$:I$^-$/PANI:CQDs	10.3	0.76	5.71	K. Lee et al. (2015)
Citric acid, oleylamine	EA	ITO-glass/PEDOT:PSS/P3HT:CQDs/Al metal	0.29	1.59	0.23	Kwon et al. (2014)
D-glucose, Octadecylamine	EA	ITO-glass/PEDOT:PSS/PFO-DBT:CQDs (or ZnO@CQDs)/Al metal	6.0	0.80	1.5	R. Sharma et al. (2015)
Polystyrene-co-maleic anhydride, Ethylenediamine	a-D	ITO-glass/TiO$_2$/PCDTBT:PC71BM:CQDs/MoO$_3$/ Ag metal	12.28	0.86	5.98	C. Liu et al. (2014)
Citric acid, urea	BL/HEL	ITO-glass/TiO$_2$/PCDTBT:PC71BM/CQDs/MoO$_3$/ Ag metal	13.70	0.86	6.51	Xinyuan Zhang et al. (2016a)
Acetylene	BL	ITO-glass/PEDOT:PSS/P3HT:PC61BM(or PTB7: PC61BM, PTB7-Th:PC71BM)/CQDs/Al metal	9.44	0.63	2.97	Ding et al. (2017)
CA, p-phenylenediamine	HEL	FTO-glass/TiO$_2$/CH3NH3PbI3/CQDs/Au metal	7.83	0.515	2.07	Paulo et al. (2016)
Graphite Rods	HEL	In:Ga/n-Si/Si NWs/CQDs/Au metal	17.6	0.34	2.6	Xie et al. (2014)

sen*: sensitizer, PD/co-sen*: photoanode dopant/co-sensitizer, ED/co-sen*: electron donor/co-sensitizer, CED: counter electrode dopant, EA: electron acceptor, a-D: active layer dopant, BL/HEL: buffer layer/hole extraction layer, BL: buffer layer, HEL: hole extraction layer

(0.3352, 0.3145), a color rendering index, a CRI of 82, and a color temperature of 5340 K. By doping CQDs to an extremely opaque substrate made of methyltriethoxysilane and 3-triethoxysilylpropylamine, Yuan et al. developed CQDs/gel glasses nanocomposites with up to 80% quantum yield (B. Yuan et al., 2018a). The fabricated WLEDs showed a CRI and luminous efficiency value of 92.9 and of 71.75 lm W^{-1}, respectively, as shown in Figure 15.10c. Li et al. used a solvothermal approach to produce RGB color emitting CQDs with o-phenylenediamine and tris(hydroxymethyl)aminomethane buffer, and then fabricated WLEDs by

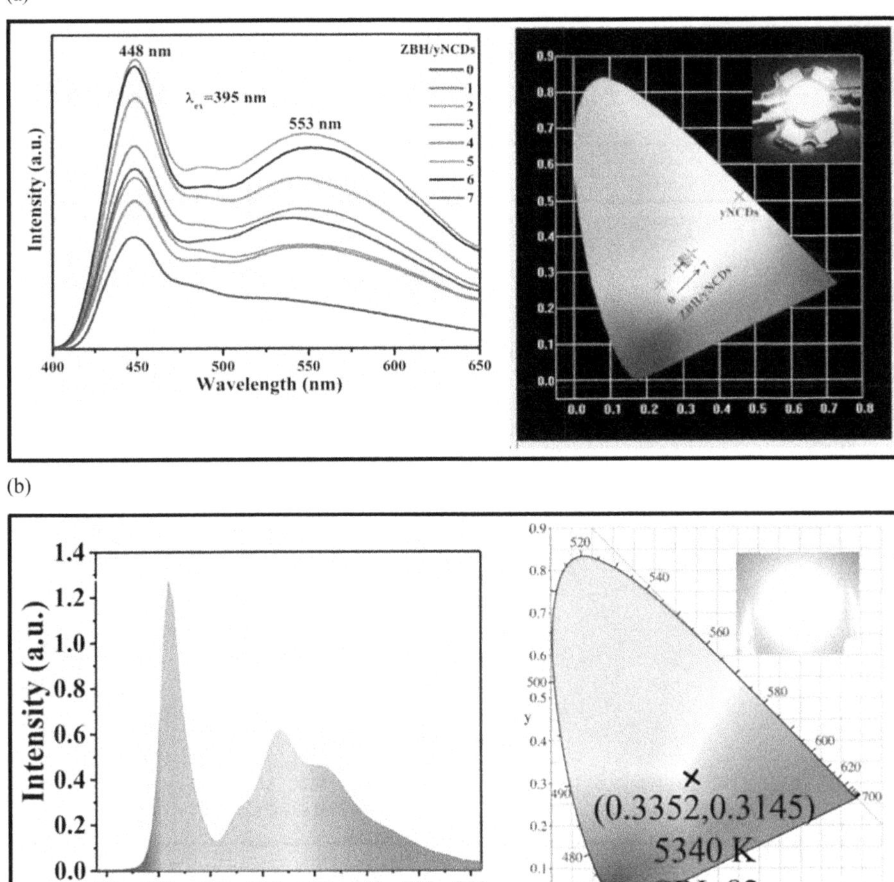

FIGURE 15.10 (a) PL emission spectra and CIE chromaticity diagram of zinc borate/carbon dot composite phosphor-based LEDs (He et al., 2020). (b) Luminescence spectra and CIE diagram of CQDs and phthalimide composite phosphor-based WLEDs (Y. Zheng et al., 2020).

(a) Reproduced under CC-BY License, (b) Reproduced under CC-BY License.

(Continued)

(c)

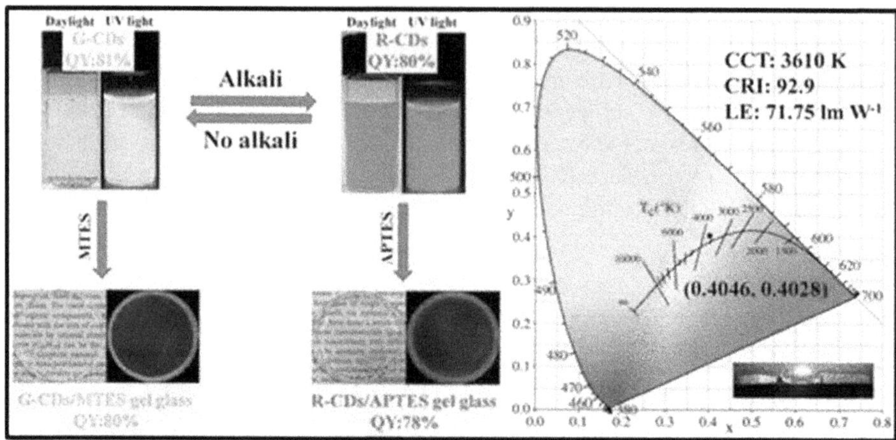

(d)

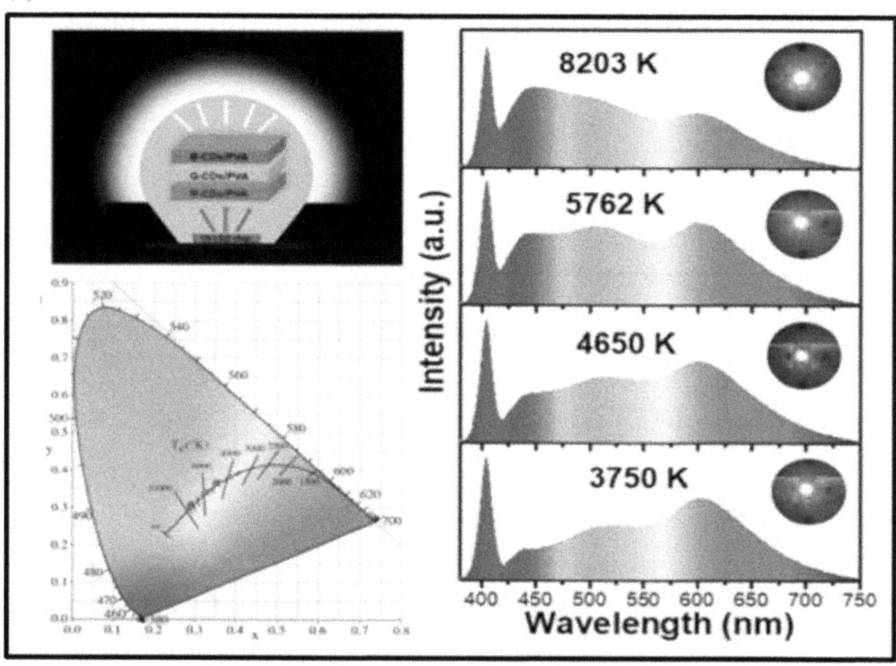

FIGURE 15.10 (CONTINUED) (c) Reversibly switchable green-red emissive CQD composites for WLEDs. (d) CIE coordinates, CCT, and emission spectra of WLEDs based on CQDs produced from o-phenylenediamine are shown in the image of a multilayered trichromatic WLED.

(c) Reprinted (adapted) with permission from (B. Yuan et al., 2018a). Copyright 2018. American Chemical Society (d) Reproduced with permission (X. Li et al., 2020). Copyright 2020, Royal Society of Chemistry.

(Continued)

(e)

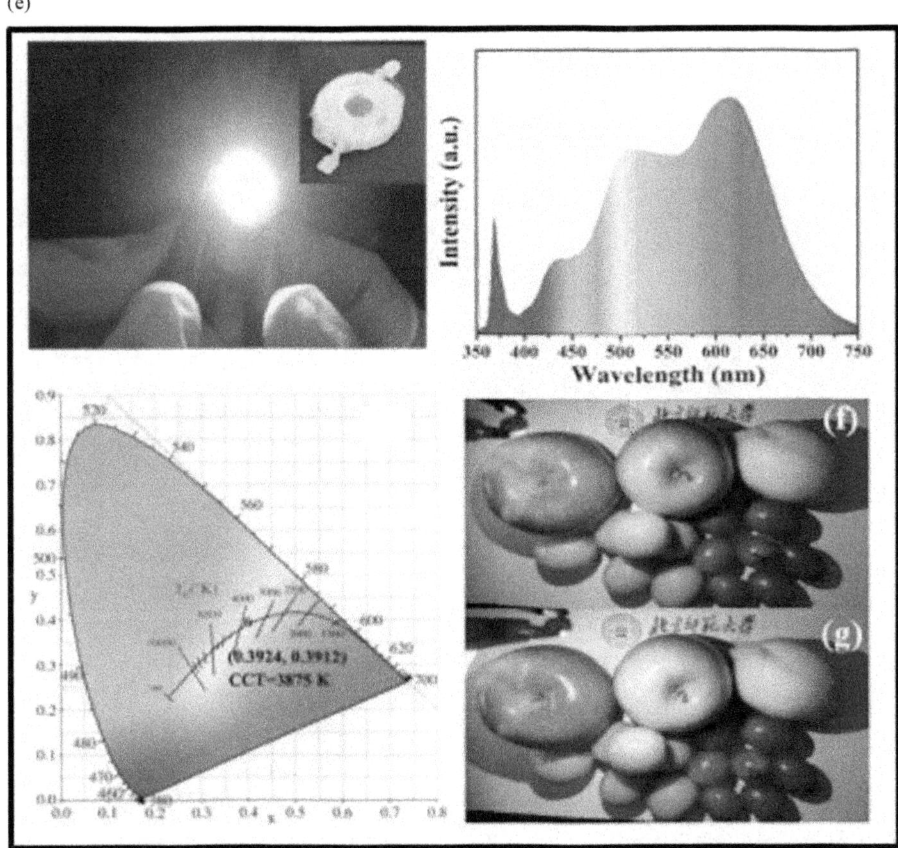

FIGURE 15.10 (CONTINUED)   (e) Illustrations of the warm WLED, CIE coordinates, EL spectra, and fruit color taken under commercial WLED and fabricated WLED.

(e) Reproduced with permission (Z. Wang et al., 2017b). Copyright 2017, Wiley-VCH.

(Continued)

combining Tri-color CQDs films with an ultraviolet LED chip which exhibited a CIE of (0.362, 0.370) and a CRI of 96.5 as shown in Figure 15.10d (X. Li et al., 2020). Another study developed WLEDs using green and orange emissive starch/ CQD phosphors with a 21% photoluminescence quantum yield (CIE: (0.41, 0.45), CCT: 3708 K) (Qu et al., 2016). Wang et al. demonstrated the fabrication of WLEDs employing RGB-CQD/PMMA composite phosphors by integrating them on a UV-LED chip, and they demonstrated good warm white light properties (CIE:0.3924, 0.3912, CCT:3875 K, CRI:97, luminous efficiency:31.3 lm .W^{-1}) as shown in Figure 15.10e (Z. Wang et al., 2017b). In a separate experiment, sodium silicate and polydimethylsiloxane were combined with colorful CQDs made from urea and citric acid in three distinct solvents (water, glycerol, and dimethylformamide) (Tian et al., 2017). Thereafter, WLEDs were fabricated on blue-emitting InGaN

(f)

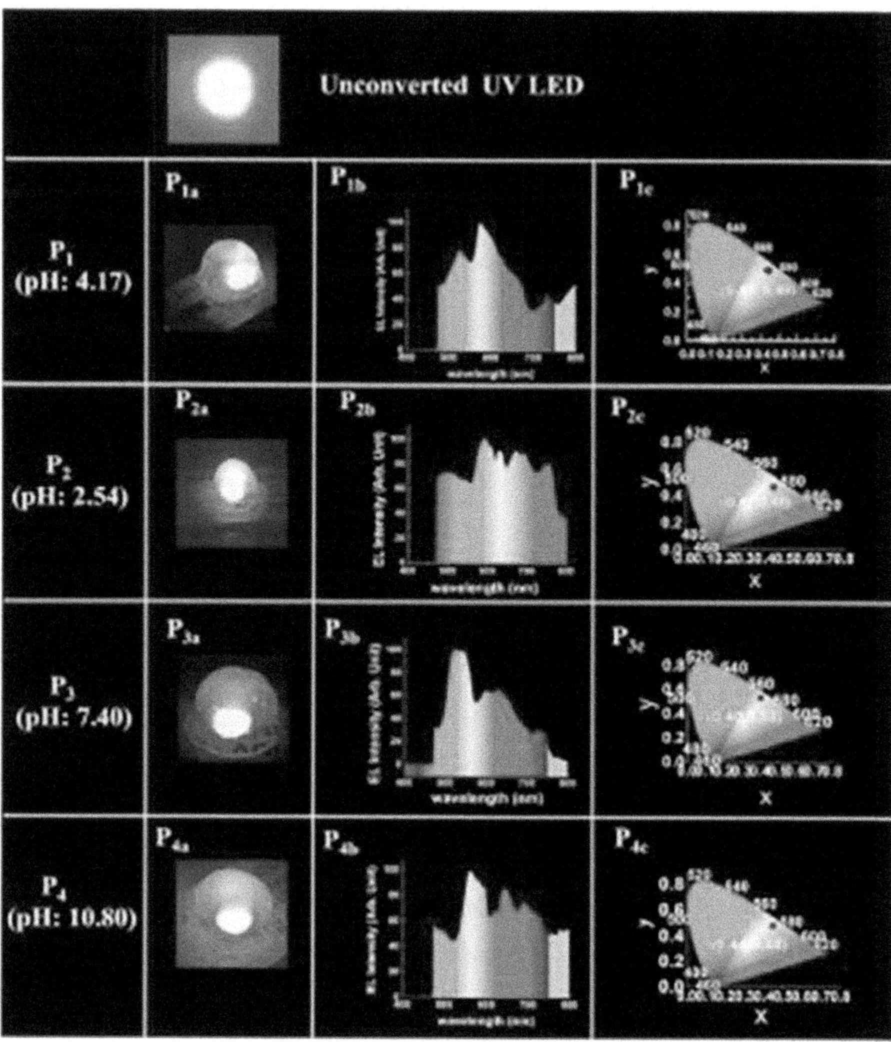

FIGURE 15.10 (CONTINUED)   (f) pH-sensitive EL spectra and related CIE chromaticity coordinates of LEDs developed through fusing a UV-LED chip with a composite phosphor built of *Brassica juncea* flower-derived N, Ca-co-doped CQDs.

(f) Reproduced with permission (Varun Dutt Sharma et al., 2023). Copyright 2023, Elsevier.

chips which achieved CIE, CCT, CRI, and luminous efficiency of (0.34, 0.31), 5048 K, 82.4, and 8.34 lmW^{-1}, respectively. Another WLED based on CQDs exhibited CIE coordinates, CCT, and CRI of (0.33, 0.34), 5129 K, and 79, respectively, when hydrogen peroxide treatment enhanced the optical transitions resulting from surface states (Z. Zhou et al., 2018). A composite phosphor made of CQDs and graphitic carbon nitride (g-C$_3$N$_4$) was synthesized on a big scale from citric acid and aqueous urea solution using a green microwave-aided in situ heating method (L. Meng et al., 2020). The manufactured WLEDs demonstrated a power efficiency of up to 42 lmW^{-1}. Sharma et al. recently demonstrated how a biodegradable bioplastic synthesized from maize starch was utilized to develop a N, Ca-co-doped CQDs@bioplastic composite phosphor that can be used to make colorful LEDs and optical displays (Varun Dutt Sharma et al., 2023). The effects of *Brassica*-derived CQD concentrations and pH sensitivity were further studied. As illustrated in Figure 15.10f, the CIE chromatic coordinates were observed to shift slightly from (0.44, 0.49) to (0.44, 0.48) as the pH value rises from acid to base (from pH: 2.54 vs. 10.8). In another work, they demonstrated the conversion of UV-LED into yellowish-green LED using a phosphor based on *Cissus quadrangularis*-derived N-doped CQDs embedded in epoxy resin (V.D. Sharma et al., 2022).

15.5.2 ELECTROLUMINESCENT CQD-BASED LEDS

A WLED with the highest external quantum yield of 0.083% and a CRI of 82 was reported in one of the early publications on CQD-based electroluminescent LEDs (F. Wang et al., 2011). Significant progress in the area has been made in recent years, with the efficiency of such devices increasing to 4% with the brightest luminosity of 5,240 cd.m^{-2} as shown in Figure 15.11a (F. Yuan et al., 2020). Later, by modifying the design of the device and injecting current density (through regulating the applied voltage), multicolor emission (white, blue, magenta or cyan) was made possible from the same CQD-based LEDs. The device showed highest luminosity of 24 cd.m^{-2} for blue emission, while it was 90 cd.m^{-2} for white emission, as illustrated in Figure 15.11b (Xiaoyu Zhang et al., 2013). Yuan et al. developed highly efficient monochromatic CQD-based LEDs with various emission colors (blue to red) as can be seen from Figure 15.11c. Furthermore, they created WLEDs that are nearly pure white light, with CIE coordinates of (0.30, 0.33). These WLEDs have a maximum brightness of 2050 cd.m^{-2} and a current efficiency value of 1.1 cd.A^{-1} (F. Yuan et al., 2017). In another study, multicolored narrow bandwidth emission from triangular CQDs with a quantum yield of up to 54%–72% has been demonstrated by Yuan et al (2018b). These CQDs may produce multicolored light-emitting diodes with the highest luminance of 1882–4762 cd m^{-2} and current efficiencies of 1.22–5.11 cdA^{-1} (Figure 15.11d). Do et al. investigated the effect of electronic states caused by direct doping on the electroluminescence of N- and S-doped CQDs in LEDs (Do et al., 2016). These LEDs provide wide electroluminescence that spans the visible light spectrum from 500 to 700 nm, providing brilliant, pure white light with the CIE coordinate (0.2894, 0.3351). These LEDs showed maximum brightness of around 80 cd.m^{-2} and quantum efficiency around 0.6%. By combining blue emissive CQDs, green-yellow emissive ZnO nanowires, and a thin PMMA polymer layer to produce organic/inorganic hybrid heterojunction LEDs using PEDOT:PSS/ZnO nanowires, Qi et al. showed yet another innovative method for constructing electroluminescent WLEDs (C. Qi et al., 2020). The structure also has an isolating PMMA layer to prevent the recombination of charges at the anode and to restrict injection of electrons from the CQD-covering active layer to that of hole transport layer. PMMA caused a

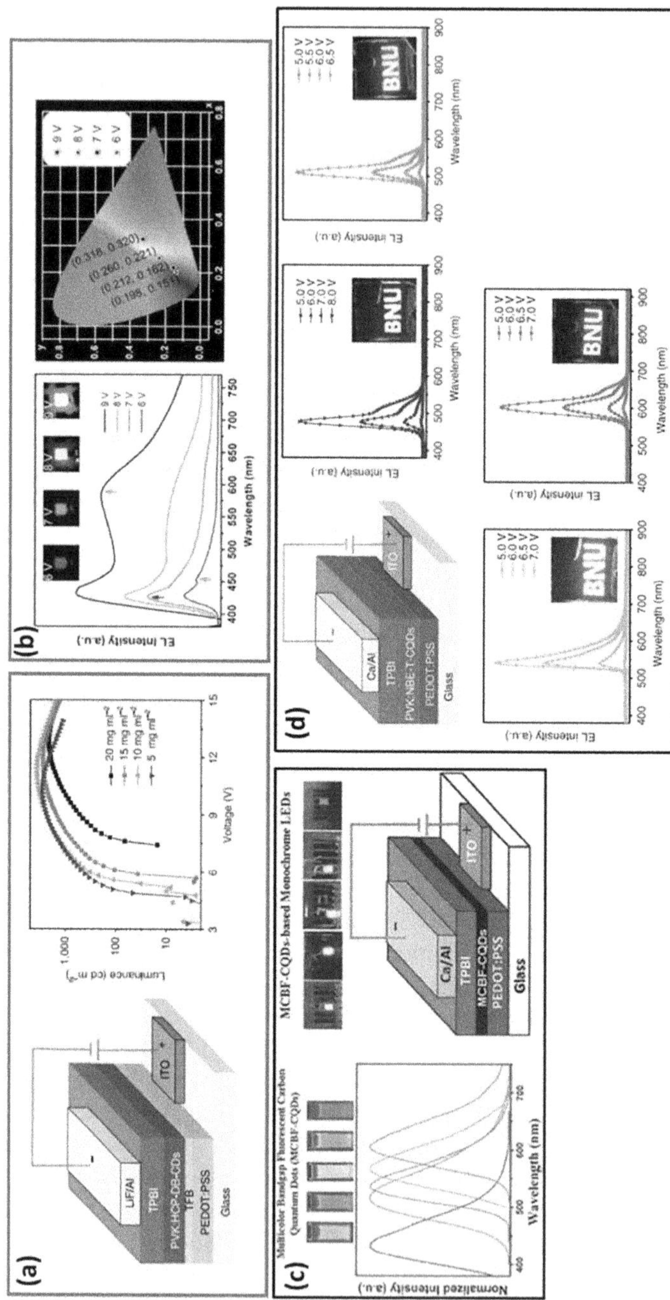

FIGURE 15.11 (a) Device structure and luminescence–voltage characteristics of CQD-containing deep blue LEDs with outstanding color purity. (b) Electroluminescence spectra and CIE 1931 coordinates of blue, cyan, magenta, and white emissions. (c) Typical device structure and normalized PL spectra of multicolor bandgap fluorescent CQD-based LEDs. (d) LED structure and electroluminescence spectra of multicolor (red, green, blue, yellow) broadband emission of triangular CQD-containing LEDs (F. Yuan et al., 2018b).

change in the color of CQD emission from green-yellow to white by increasing the blue emission of CQDs. Finally, Table 15.3 summarizes this section by presenting the most recent literature data on CQD-based WLEDs.

15.6 NANOELECTRONIC APPLICATIONS OF CARBON QUANTUM DOTS

CQDs is of tremendous interest because, like other carbon allotropes, it is abundant in nature, easy to deal with, and has the same electrical properties as an intrinsic semiconductor. Hence, in this chapter, we want to understand the role of CQDs in the realm of nanoelectronics.

15.6.1 CQDs in Memory Devices

Raeis-Hosseini et al. in 2023 have demonstrated biomemristor device performances utilizing CQD-chitosan nanocomposites as a solid polymer electrolyte layer on top of coplanar asymmetric nanogap Al-Au electrodes as shown in Figure 15.12a (Raeis-Hosseini et al., 2023). The biomemristor device demonstrated a high on/off ratio of more than 10^6, low durability of 160 cycles, retention of more than 10^4 seconds, and reliable and dependable bipolar resistive switching properties. In another work, Qi et al. exhibited improved low resistance state preservation in CQD-graphene oxide nanocomposite-based resistive random access memory (RRAM) devices (M. Qi et al., 2018). Despite the relatively small compliance current of 100 µA, consistent resistive switching characteristics with high retention were achieved rather than unpredictable switching.

15.6.2 CQDs in Field-Effect Transistors

Kwon et al. have demonstrated electrical characteristics of field-effect transistors (FETs) by implementing CQDs as a channel (Kwon et al., 2013). To explore the ligand length dependency on field-effect mobility, a variety of primary amines with different ligand lengths were utilized to synthesize colloidal CQDs and exchange them. The devices demonstrated ambipolar conductivity, with electron mobility as high as 8.49×10^{-5} cm^2 V^{-1}s^{-1} and maximum hole mobility of 3.88×10^{-5} cm^2 V^{-1}s^{-1} (see Figure 15.12b for further details).

15.6.3 CQDs in Photodetectors

CQDs have also been employed in photodetector applications. CQDs' strong absorbance peak transition at roughly 250 nm, caused by the π-π^*, makes it ideal for deep-UV photoluminescence and photodetection applications. Wu et al. have demonstrated an all-carbon-based ultraviolet photodetector based on N-CQDs/graphene hybrid composites that displays considerable negative photoconductivity (X. Wu et al., 2019). The device exhibited a negative responsivity value up to 2.5 10^4 AW^{-1} in the UV zone, which was ascribed to two conflicting processes (see Figure 15.12c for

TABLE 15.3

Various metrics of CQD-based LEDs

CQD Precursors (synthesis process)	Composite Matrix	CIE Chromaticity Coordinates	CRI	CCT (K)	Luminous Efficiency of LED's (lm W^{-1})	References
CA, urea, NaOH (Hydrothermal)	Epoxy resin	(0.366, 0.366)	93.5	4333	52.3	Jian-Yong Wei et al. (2020)
3,4,9,10-Tetranitroperylene, NaOH; ethanol (Solvothermal)	MTES and APTES	(0.4046, 0.4028)	92.9	3610	71.75	B. Yuan et al. (2018a)
CA and EDA (Hydrothermal)	PMMA	(0.32, 0.33)	91		15.1	H. Lin et al. (2020)
p-PD, ethanol, NaOH and IPTS (Solvothermal)	PMMA/ APTES–Gel and PS	(0.397, 0.428);(0.385, 0.345)	70; 85	3949; 4494	15.88; 22	Ren et al. (2018)
CA, urea aqueous solution (microwave-assisted)	TEOS, PDMS	(0.33, 0.34)	79	5603	28	D. Zhou et al. (2017)
CA and 1-hexadecylamine; dimethylbenzene (Solvothermal)	PDMS	(0.335, 0.332), (0.331, 0.328)	>89	6000	–	Cheng et al. (2020)
o-PD or p-PD; dimethylformamide (Solvothermal)	PVB	(0.3943, 0.3869)	83	3722	66.17	S. Lin et al. (2017)
CA and PAN; ethanol (Solvothermal)	Epoxy resin	(0.29, 0.31)	82.4		–	Yan et al. (2020)
CA and urea, water (Microwave-assisted)	Graphitic carbon nitride (g-C$_3$N$_4$), epoxy resin	(0.29, 0.33)		7557	42	L. Meng et al. (2020)
o-PD and Tris, H$_2$SO$_4$ and water (Solvothermal)	PVA	(0.362, 0.370)	96.5	4650	–	X. Li et al. (2020)
1,3-dihydroxynaphthalene and KIO$_4$, ethanol (Solvothermal)	Silicone or PMMA	(0.3924, 0.3912)	97	3875	31.3	Z. Wang et al. (2017b)

CA and urea dissolved in either water, glycerol or DMF (Hydro/Solvothermal)	Sodium silicate; PDMS	(0.34,0.31)	82.4	5048	8.34	Tian et al. (2017)
CA, ammonia water, followed by H_2O_2-treatment (Microwave-assisted)	PDMS	(0.34, 0.37)	79	5240	–	Z. Zhou et al. (2018)
CA and urea, dissolved in either water, glycerol or DMF (Hydro/Solvothermal)	Sodium silicate, PDMS	(0.27, 0.31); (0.32, 0.33); (0.41, 0.41)	85; 88; 86	9927; 6109; 3510	7.8; 6.3; 5.2	Tian et al. (2019)
l-Aspartic acid, NH_3-solution (Hydrothermal)	Epoxy resin	(0.30, 0.35)	83	6987	1.281	Xiangyu Feng et al. (2019)
CA and urea; NH_3-solution, water (Hydrothermal)	Zr-MOF, thermal-curable silicone resin	(0.31, 0.34)	82		1.7	A. Wang et al. (2019a)
urea and CA; water (Hydrothermal)	PMMA	(0.30, 0.36)			–	C. Qi et al. (2020)
CA and urea, dimethylformamide (Solvothermal)	Starch	(0.41, 0.45)		3708	–	Qu et al. (2016)
phthalic acid, formamide and glycerol (Solvothermal)	Phthalimide crystals	(0.3352, 0.3145)	82	5430	–	Y. Zheng et al. (2020)
Brassica flower extract (Hydrothermal)	Bioplastic	(0.44, 0.49) to (0.44, 0.48) pH:2.54 to 10.8	–	–	–	Varun Dutt Sharma et al. (2023)

Abbreviations: CA: citric acid, **EDA**: ethylenediamine, **PD**: phenylenediamine, **IPTS**: 3-isocyanatopropyltriethoxysilane, **Tris**: tris(hydroxymethyl)aminomethane, **PDMS**: polydimethylsiloxane, **DMF**: Dimethylformamide, **PAN**: (2-pyridylazo)-2-naphthol, **PVA**: poly(vinyl alcohol), **PMMA**: poly(methyl methacrylate), **MTES**: methyltriethoxysilane, **PS**: polystyrene, **PVB**: polyvinyl butyral, **DAN**: diaminonaphthalene, **PVK**: poly(N-vinyl carbazole), **MOF**: metal–organic framework, **PDMS**: polydimethylsiloxane, **TEOS**: tetraethyl orthosilicate, **APTES**: 3-triethoxysilylpropylamine.

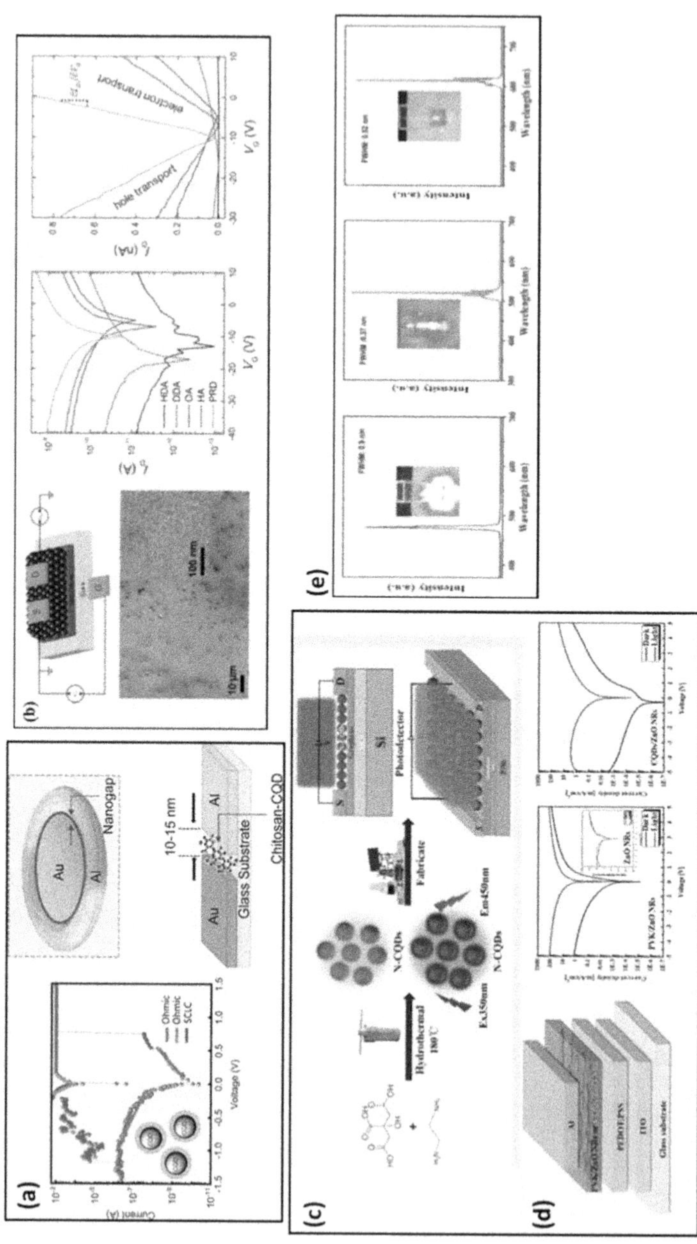

FIGURE 15.12   (a) Schematic diagram of the electrical performance of a biomemristor made of CQD-chitosan nanocomposite with coplanar nanogap electrodes (Raeis-Hosseini et al., 2023). (b) Schematic and transfer characteristics of CQD-channel FET. (c) Hydrothermally synthesized nitrogen-doped CQDs for photodetector application. (d) Schematic and J-V characteristics of CQD-based hybrid UV photodetector. (e) Blue, green, and red random lasing from triangular-CQDs/Au–Ag bimetallic porous nanowire composites.

(a) Reproduced under CC-BY License, (b) Reprinted (adapted) with permission from (Kwon et al., 2013). Copyright 2013. American Chemical Society, (c) Reprinted (adapted) with permission from (X. Wu et al., 2019). Copyright 2019. American Chemical Society, (d) Reproduced with permission (S.-W. Lee et al., 2016). Copyright 2016, Elsevier, (e) Reproduced with permission (F. Yuan et al., 2019). Copyright 2019, Wiley-VCH.

detail). The first is caused by oxygen adsorption and photodesorption, and the second by surface defects in N-CQDs. In a different work, Sarkar et al. showed how CQDs made from organic waste might be used as a possible broad-spectrum photodetector in an organic-inorganic hybrid heterostructure using a Si-compatible process-line (Sarkar et al., 2019). Silver nanoparticles, AgNPs and reduced graphene oxide, rGO were incorporated into the CQDs to further enhance the broadband photoresponse. Due to effective carrier movement, optimal incorporation of rGO enhanced photoresponse, but localized surface plasmon resonance in AgNPs increased optical absorption. The device demonstrated maximum responsiveness and detectivity values of $\sim$1 A W^{-1} and 2×10^{12} Jones, respectively. In another work, a UV photodetector was designed by utilizing hybrid CQDs and ZnO nanorod composite (S.-W. Lee et al., 2016). The UV photodetector displayed a high selectivity of 8.33×10^{12} Jones under an irradiation of 365 nm UV radiation with a power of 1 mW/cm^2, which is greater than that of poly-n-vinyl carbazole (PVK)/ZnO nanorod-based composite as can be seen from Figure 15.12d. Sahatiya et al. exhibited device characteristics of a 2D MoS$_2$-CQDs-based flexible broadband photodetector in which hydrothermal growth of MoS$_2$ on cellulose paper and CQD was synthesized via a simple, low-cost pyrolysis technique utilizing chia seeds (Sahatiya et al., 2018). The wide-band absorption of MoS$_2$ in the visible and near-infrared wavelengths, along with the UV absorption of CQD, deepens the absorbance range. In the UV, NIR, and visible regions, the developed sensor's responsiveness was measured to be around 8.40, 2.62, and 18.12 mA.W^{-1}, respectively.

15.6.4 CQDs in Laser

Extensive research has been dedicated to the development of low-threshold random lasers with strong monochromaticity in anticipation of a wide range of applications, notably military armament and clinical operations. Yuan et al. have developed consistent and random lasing emissions with a low threshold that span from blue to red using the narrow bandwidth emission of triangular shaped-CQDs (F. Yuan et al., 2019). They demonstrated powerful multicolor fluorescent CQD-based random full-color lasing with thresholds ranging from 2.1 to 5.8 mJ.cm^{-2} in blue, green, red, and white emission, as illustrated in Figure 15.12e. However, the vast full width at half maxima and Stokes shifts over 80 nm undoubtedly impede maintaining population inversion and exciton energy dissipation throughout the pumping operation, demanding more research in the near future to solve these issues.

15.7 CONCLUSIONS AND FUTURE PERSPECTIVES OF CARBON QUANTUM DOTS IN ENERGY AND ELECTRONICS APPLICATIONS

Luminescent carbon quantum dots are fascinating newcomers to the field of nanomaterials in a variety of energy and electronics applications. This chapter discusses a viewpoint on the present and emerging uses of CQDs, as well as a critical examination of a few particular sectors that are projected to affect our day-to-day perspectives. Future energy storage and conversion technologies will greatly benefit from the utilization of CQDs due to their distinct and intrinsic properties. The necessity for utilizing more energy and changing it in an ecologically acceptable manner is becoming increasingly apparent to scientists and researchers. Consequently, research into the utilization of CQDs or nanomaterials that have been modified by CQDs have increased dramatically in recent years. Fortunately, it is possible for CQDs to have different electrical and chemical structures depending on their dimension, shape, heteroatom doping or surface functional groups. CQDs are being added into nanomaterials to enhance their capacity to harvest solar cells and raise their efficiency due to their remarkable optoelectronic properties that can distinguish charge carriers having a small band gap and minimal light absorption. CQDs are often utilized in solar systems as sensitizers and co-sensitizers, energy downshifting layers, electron transporting layers, or hole transport materials because of their substantial surface area, excellent electron mobility, and rapid charge transfer. This enables them to take in light across a broad range. CQDs also have unknown properties that restrict their employment in energy-storage devices by keeping the details of their nanoscale chemical and physical makeup a secret. The fast expansion of their raw material sources is a key barrier to CQD industrialization and synthesis.

Aside from that, the ability to reduce CQD production costs lacks homogeneity, which is now preventing their broad application and commercialization. However, the ultimate goal is to integrate cost-effective, non- or low-toxic, sustainable, and efficient production processes. There are still certain areas where further effort may be accomplished to advance the progress made in this synthesis. When it comes to green chemical combinations and low-cost production techniques, this sort of study presents an abundance of alternatives. Taking into account the benefits and constraints discussed in this chapter, future research into the development of affordable and sustainable nanocomposites employing CQDs for energy-storage applications is envisaged. Although it has been demonstrated that CQDs are useful in energy applications, certain critical problems and hurdles must still be overcome in order to gain a deep knowledge of the underlying process and method, as well as key information regarding the electrochemical performance. Similarly, the optical properties of CQDs are still unknown, necessitating more research to offer credible evidence from experiments for their characterization (for instance, the impact of size, doping, surface chemistry etc.).

Furthermore, a thorough investigation is required to comprehend the interaction of the most often employed hybrid structure alongside its functional substitutes. Because of non-radiation-induced recombination and bonding with nearby atoms, organic moieties on CQD surfaces pose significant problems in electronic applications such as photodetectors and electronic sensors. Fluorescence intensity is critical for detecting objects using a luminescence-based sensor. CQDs with high quantum yields remain a challenge to date with a few exceptions. Therefore, future study should focus on the synthesis process that produces high photoluminescence, quantum yield, chemical and photostability in the context of top-down approach. Additionally, surface defects must be avoided since recombination would otherwise negate the benefits. It is envisaged that more affordable, straightforward, and innovative synthesis procedures with novel promising applications in the energy and electronics sectors will be developed in the near future in order to further utilize the potential of these increasingly important carbon nanomaterials.

REFERENCES

Al-Ghamdi, S. A., Darwish, A. A. A., Hamdalla, T. A., Pasha, A., Elnair, M. E., Al-Atawi, A., & Khasim, S. (2023). Biological synthesis of novel carbon quantum dots using Halimeda opuntia green algae with improved optical properties and electrochemical performance for possible energy storage applications. *International Journal of Electrochemical Science*, *18*(5), 100102. https://doi.org/10.1016/j.ijoes.2023.100102

Alaş, M. Ö., Güngör, A., Genç, R., & Erdem, E. (2019). Feeling the power: robust supercapacitors from nanostructured conductive polymers fostered with Mn 2+ and carbon dots. *Nanoscale*, *11*(27), 12804–12816. https://doi.org/10.1039/C9NR03544C

Ali, M., Riaz, R., Anjum, A. S., Sun, K. C., Li, H., Ahn, S., Jeong, S. H., & Ko, M. J. (2021). Microwave-assisted ultrafast in-situ growth of N-doped carbon quantum dots on multiwalled carbon nanotubes as an efficient electrocatalyst for photovoltaics. *Journal of Colloid and Interface Science*, *586*, 349–361. https://doi.org/10.1016/j.jcis.2020.10.098

Balogun, M.-S., Luo, Y., Lyu, F., Wang, F., Yang, H., Li, H., Liang, C., Huang, M., Huang, Y., & Tong, Y. (2016). Carbon quantum dot surface-engineered VO 2 interwoven nanowires: A flexible cathode material for lithium and sodium ion batteries. *ACS Applied Materials & Interfaces*, *8*(15), 9733–9744. https://doi.org/10.1021/acsami.6b01305

Başlak, C., Öztürk, G., Demirel, S., Kocyigit, A., Doğu, S., & Yıldırım, M. (2023). Green synthesis of carbon quantum dots from Sideritis vuralii and its application in supercapacitors. *Inorganic Chemistry Communications*, *153*, 110845. https://doi.org/10.1016/j.inoche.2023.110845

Benetti, D., Jokar, E., Yu, C.-H., Fathi, A., Zhao, H., Vomiero, A., Wei-Guang Diau, E., & Rosei, F. (2019). Hole-extraction and photostability enhancement in highly efficient inverted perovskite solar cells through carbon dot-based hybrid material. *Nano Energy*, *62*, 781–790. https://doi.org/10.1016/j.nanoen.2019.05.084

Briscoe, J., Marinovic, A., Sevilla, M., Dunn, S., & Titirici, M. (2015). Biomass-derived carbon quantum dot sensitizers for solid-state nanostructured solar cells. *Angewandte Chemie International Edition*, *54*(15), 4463–4468. https://doi.org/10.1002/anie.201409290

Carbon Quantum Dots for Sustainable Energy and Optoelectronics. (2023). Elsevier. https://doi.org/10.1016/C2020-0-03426-2

Chaudhary, M., Xin, C., Hu, Z., Zhang, D., Radtke, G., Xu, X., Billot, L., Tripon-Canseliet, C., & Chen, Z. (2023). Nitrogen-doped carbon quantum dots on graphene for field-effect transistor optoelectronic memories. *Advanced Electronic Materials*. https://doi.org/10.1002/aelm.202300159

Chava, R. K., Im, Y., & Kang, M. (2017). Nitrogen doped carbon quantum dots as a green luminescent sensitizer to functionalize ZnO nanoparticles for enhanced photovoltaic conversion devices. *Materials Research Bulletin*, *94*, 399–407. https://doi.org/10.1016/j.materresbull.2017.06.040

Chen, J., Hou, H., Yang, Y., Song, W., Zhang, Y., Yang, X., Lan, Q., & Ji, X. (2015). An electrochemically anodic study of anatase TiO2 tuned through carbon-coating for high-performance lithium-ion battery. *Electrochimica Acta*, *164*, 330–336. https://doi.org/10.1016/j.electacta.2015.02.202

Chen, J., Zou, G., Hou, H., Zhang, Y., Huang, Z., & Ji, X. (2016). Pinecone-like hierarchical anatase TiO 2 bonded with carbon enabling ultrahigh cycling rates for sodium storage. *Journal of Materials Chemistry A*, *4*(32), 12591–12601. https://doi.org/10.1039/C6TA03505A

Chen, W., Quan, H., & Chen, D. (2023). Carbon quantum dots boosted structure stability of nickel cobalt layered double hydroxides nanosheets electrodeposited on carbon cloth for energy storage. *Surfaces and Interfaces*, *36*, 102498. https://doi.org/10.1016/j.surfin.2022.102498

Cheng, S., Ye, T., Mao, H., Wu, Y., Jiang, W., Ban, C., Yin, Y., Liu, J., Xiu, F., & Huang, W. (2020). Electrostatically assembled carbon dots/boron nitride nanosheet hybrid nanostructures for thermal quenching-resistant white phosphors. *Nanoscale*, *12*(2), 524–529. https://doi.org/10.1039/C9NR07785E

Deng, Z., Liu, T., Chen, T., Jiang, J., Yang, W., Guo, J., Zhao, J., Wang, H., & Gao, L. (2017). Enhanced electrochemical performances of Bi 2 O 3/rGO nanocomposite via chemical bonding as anode materials for lithium ion batteries. *ACS Applied Materials & Interfaces*, *9*(14), 12469–12477. https://doi.org/10.1021/acsami.7b00996

Ding, Y., Zhang, F., Xu, J., Miao, Y., Yang, Y., Liu, X., & Xu, B. (2017). Synthesis of short-chain passivated carbon quantum dots as the light emitting layer towards electroluminescence. *RSC Advances*, *7*(46), 28754–28762. https://doi.org/10.1039/C7RA02421E

Do, S., Kwon, W., Kim, Y.-H., Kang, S. R., Lee, T., Lee, T.-W., & Rhee, S.-W. (2016). N,S-Induced Electronic States of Carbon Nanodots Toward White Electroluminescence. *Advanced Optical Materials*, *4*(2), 276–284. https://doi.org/10.1002/adom.201500488

Efa, M. T., & Imae, T. (2019). Effects of carbon dots on ZnO nanoparticle-based dye-sensitized solar cells. *Electrochimica Acta*, *303*, 204–210. https://doi.org/10.1016/j.electacta.2019.02.012

Essner, J. B., & Baker, G. A. (2017). The emerging roles of carbon dots in solar photovoltaics: A critical review. *Environmental Science: Nano*, *4*(6), 1216–1263. https://doi.org/10.1039/C7EN00179G

Feng, Xiangyu, Jiang, K., Zeng, H., & Lin, H. (2019). A facile approach to solid-state white emissive carbon dots and their application in UV-excitable and single-component-based white LEDs. *Nanomaterials*, *9*(5), 725. https://doi.org/10.3390/nano9050725

Feng, Xiaoting, Zhao, Y., Yan, L., Zhang, Y., He, Y., Yang, Y., & Liu, X. (2015). Low-temperature hydrothermal synthesis of green luminescent Carbon Quantum Dots (CQD), and Optical Properties of Blends of the CQD with Poly(3-hexylthiophene). *Journal of Electronic Materials*, *44*(10), 3436–3443. https://doi.org/10.1007/s11664-015-3893-3

Fu, Y., Wu, Z., Yuan, Y., Chen, P., Yu, L., Yuan, L., Han, Q., Lan, Y., Bai, W., Kan, E., Huang, C., Ouyang, X., Wang, X., Zhu, J., & Lu, J. (2020). Switchable encapsulation of polysulfides in the transition between sulfur and lithium sulfide. *Nature Communications*, *11*(1), 845. https://doi.org/10.1038/s41467-020-14686-2

Gao, R., Li, Z., Zhang, X., Zhang, J., Hu, Z., & Liu, X. (2016). Carbon-dotted defective CoO with oxygen vacancies: A synergetic design of bifunctional cathode catalyst for Li–O 2 batteries. *ACS Catalysis*, *6*(1), 400–406. https://doi.org/10.1021/acscatal.5b01903

Han, J., Zhou, Y., Yin, X., Nan, H., Tai, M., Gu, Y., Li, J., Oron, D., & Lin, H. (2019). An excellent modifier: Carbon quantum dots for highly efficient carbon-electrode-based methylammonium lead iodide solar cells. *Solar RRL*, *3*(9), 1900146. https://doi.org/10.1002/solr.201900146

He, L., Bai, Y., Ge, C., Yang, H., Yu, X., & Zhang, X. (2020). Tunable luminescence and morphological evolution of facile synthesized zinc borate/carbon dots composites for NUV-WLEDs. *Journal of Alloys and Compounds*, *834*, 155021. https://doi.org/10.1016/j.jallcom.2020.155021

Hong, W., Zhang, Y., Yang, L., Tian, Y., Ge, P., Hu, J., Wei, W., Zou, G., Hou, H., & Ji, X. (2019). Carbon quantum dot micelles tailored hollow carbon anode for fast potassium and sodium storage. *Nano Energy*, *65*, 104038. https://doi.org/10.1016/j.nanoen.2019.104038

Hou, H., Cao, X., Yang, Y., Fang, L., Pan, C., Yang, X., Song, W., & Ji, X. (2014). NiSb alloy hollow nanospheres as anode materials for rechargeable lithium ion batteries. *Chem. Commun.*, *50*(60), 8201–8203. https://doi.org/10.1039/C4CC02875A

Hu, Y., Chen, W., Lei, T., Zhou, B., Jiao, Y., Yan, Y., Du, X., Huang, J., Wu, C., Wang, X., Wang, Y., Chen, B., Xu, J., Wang, C., & Xiong, J. (2019). Carbon quantum dots-modified interfacial interactions and ion conductivity for enhanced high current density performance in lithium-sulfur batteries. *Advanced Energy Materials*, 9(7), 1802955. https://doi.org/10.1002/aenm.201802955

Huang, P., Xu, S., Zhang, M., Zhong, W., Xiao, Z., & Luo, Y. (2020). Carbon quantum dots improving photovoltaic performance of CdS quantum dot-sensitized solar cells. *Optical Materials*, *110*, 110535. https://doi.org/10.1016/j.optmat.2020.110535

Inayat, A., Albalawi, K., Rehman, A.U., Adnan, Saad, A. Y., Saleh, E. A. M., Alamri, M. A., El-Zahhar, A. A., Haider, A., & Abbas, S. M. (2023). Tunable synthesis of carbon quantum dots from the biomass of spent tea leaves as supercapacitor electrode. *Materials Today Communications*, *34*, 105479. https://doi.org/10.1016/j.mtcomm.2023.105479

Javed, M., Saqib, A. N. S., Ata-ur-Rehman, Ali, B., Faizan, M., Anang, D. A., Iqbal, Z., & Abbas, S. M. (2019). Carbon quantum dots from glucose oxidation as a highly competent anode material for lithium and sodium-ion batteries. *Electrochimica Acta*, *297*, 250–257. https://doi.org/10.1016/j.electacta.2018.11.167

Ji, Z., Dai, W., Zhang, S., Wang, G., Shen, X., Liu, K., Zhu, G., Kong, L., & Zhu, J. (2020a). Bismuth oxide/nitrogen-doped carbon dots hollow and porous hierarchitectures for high-performance asymmetric supercapacitors. *Advanced Powder Technology*, *31*(2), 632–638. https://doi.org/10.1016/j.apt.2019.11.018

Ji, Z., Li, N., Xie, M., Shen, X., Dai, W., Liu, K., Xu, K., & Zhu, G. (2020b). High-performance hybrid supercapacitor realized by nitrogen-doped carbon dots modified cobalt sulfide and reduced graphene oxide. *Electrochimica Acta*, *334*, 135632. https://doi.org/10.1016/j.electacta.2020.135632

Ji, Z., Liu, K., Li, N., Zhang, H., Dai, W., Shen, X., Zhu, G., Kong, L., & Yuan, A. (2020c). Nitrogen-doped carbon dots anchored NiO/Co3O4 ultrathin nanosheets as advanced cathodes for hybrid supercapacitors. *Journal of Colloid and Interface Science*, *579*, 282–289. https://doi.org/10.1016/j.jcis.2020.06.070

Jian, X., Yang, H., Li, J., Zhang, E., Cao, L., & Liang, Z. (2017). Flexible all-solid-state high-performance supercapacitor based on electrochemically synthesized carbon quantum dots/polypyrrole composite electrode. *Electrochimica Acta*, *228*, 483–493. https://doi.org/10.1016/j.electacta.2017.01.082

Jing, M., Wang, J., Hou, H., Yang, Y., Zhang, Y., Pan, C., Chen, J., Zhu, Y., & Ji, X. (2015). Carbon quantum dot coated Mn 3 O 4 with enhanced performances for lithium-ion batteries. *Journal of Materials Chemistry A*, *3*(32), 16824–16830. https://doi.org/10.1039/C5TA03610K

Kandra, R., & Bajpai, S. (2020). Synthesis, mechanical properties of fluorescent carbon dots loaded nanocomposites chitosan film for wound healing and drug delivery. *Arabian Journal of Chemistry*, *13*(4), 4882–4894. https://doi.org/10.1016/j.arabjc.2019.12.010

Kaur, S., Krishnan, A., & Chakraborty, S. (2023). Recent advances and challenges of carbon nano onions (CNOs) for application in supercapacitor devices (SCDs). *Journal of Energy Storage*, *71*, 107928. https://doi.org/10.1016/j.est.2023.107928

Kim, J. K., Nguyen, D. N., Lee, J.-H., Kang, S., Kim, Y., Kim, S.-S., & Kim, H.-K. (2020). Carbon quantum dot-incorporated nickel oxide for planar p-i-n type perovskite solar cells with enhanced efficiency and stability. *Journal of Alloys and Compounds*, *818*, 152887. https://doi.org/10.1016/j.jallcom.2019.152887

Kokal, R. K., Naresh Kumar, P., Deepa, M., & Srivastava, A. K. (2015). Lead selenide quantum dots and carbon dots amplify solar conversion capability of a TiO 2 /CdS photoanode. *Journal of Materials Chemistry A*, *3*(41), 20715–20726. https://doi.org/10.1039/C5TA04393J

Kwon, W., Do, S., Won, D. C., & Rhee, S.-W. (2013). Carbon quantum dot-based field-effect transistors and their ligand length-dependent carrier mobility. *ACS Applied Materials & Interfaces*, *5*(3), 822–827. https://doi.org/10.1021/am3023898

Kwon, W., Lee, G., Do, S., Joo, T., & Rhee, S.-W. (2014). Size-controlled soft-template synthesis of carbon nanodots toward versatile photoactive materials. *Small*, *10*(3), 506–513. https://doi.org/10.1002/smll.201301770

Lee, C.-J., Chang, Y.-C., Wang, L.-W., & Wang, Y.-H. (2017). Nonvolatile resistive switching memory utilizing cobalt embedded in gelatin. *Materials*, *11*(1), 32. https://doi.org/10.3390/ma11010032

Lee, K., Cho, S., Kim, M., Kim, J., Ryu, J., Shin, K.-Y., & Jang, J. (2015). Highly porous nanostructured polyaniline/carbon nanodots as efficient counter electrodes for Pt-free dye-sensitized solar cells. *Journal of Materials Chemistry A*, *3*(37), 19018–19026. https://doi.org/10.1039/C5TA05522A

Lee, S.-W., Choi, K.-J., Kang, B.-H., Lee, J.-S., Kim, S.-W., Kwon, J.-B., Gopalan, S.-A., Bae, J.-H., Kim, E.-S., Kwon, D.-H., & Kang, S.-W. (2016). Low dark current and improved detectivity of hybrid ultraviolet photodetector based on carbon-quantum-dots/zinc-oxide-nanorod composites. *Organic Electronics*, *39*, 250–257. https://doi.org/10.1016/j.orgel.2016.10.003

Li, L., Jia, X., Zhang, Y., Qiu, T., Hong, W., Jiang, Y., Zou, G., Hou, H., Chen, X., & Ji, X. (2019a). Li 4 Ti 5 O 12 quantum dot decorated carbon frameworks from carbon dots for fast lithium ion storage. *Materials Chemistry Frontiers*, *3*(9), 1761–1767. https://doi.org/10.1039/C9QM00259F

Li, L., Li, M., Liang, J., Yang, X., Luo, M., Ji, L., Guo, Y., Zhang, H., Tang, N., & Wang, X. (2019b). Preparation of Core–Shell CQD@PANI nanoparticles and their electrochemical properties. *ACS Applied Materials & Interfaces*, *11*(25), 22621–22627. https://doi.org/10.1021/acsami.9b00963

Li, X., Wang, Z., Liu, Y., Zhang, W., Zhu, C., & Meng, X. (2020). Bright tricolor ultrabroadband emission carbon dots for white light-emitting diodes with a 96.5 high color rendering index. *Journal of Materials Chemistry C*, *8*(4), 1286–1291. https://doi.org/10.1039/C9TC06187H

Li, Z., Zhang, W., Tan, Y., Hu, J., He, S., Stein, A., & Tang, B. (2016). Three-dimensionally Ordered Macroporous β-Bi2O3 with Enhanced Electrochemical Performance in a Li-ion Battery. *Electrochimica Acta*, *214*, 103–109. https://doi.org/10.1016/j.electacta.2016.08.031

Li, Z., Zhang, X., Liu, C., Guo, J., Cui, H., Shen, L., & Guo, W. (2018). Toward efficient carbon-dots-based electron-extraction layer through surface charge engineering. *ACS Applied Materials & Interfaces*, *10*(46), 40255–40264. https://doi.org/10.1021/acsami.8b13523

Lim, H., Liu, Y., Kim, H. Y., & Son, D. I. (2018). Facile synthesis and characterization of carbon quantum dots and photovoltaic applications. *Thin Solid Films*, *660*, 672–677. https://doi.org/10.1016/j.tsf.2018.04.019

Lin, H., Yang, J., Liu, Y., Zeng, F., Tang, X.-S., Yao, Z., Guan, H., Xiong, Q., Zhou, J., Wu, D., & Du, J. (2020). Stable and efficient hybrid Ag-In-S/ZnS@SiO2-carbon quantum dots nanocomposites for white light-emitting diodes. *Chemical Engineering Journal*, *393*, 124654. https://doi.org/10.1016/j.cej.2020.124654

Lin, J., Yuan, Y., Su, Q., Pan, A., Dinesh, S., Peng, C., Cao, G., & Liang, S. (2018). Facile synthesis of Nb2O5/carbon nanocomposites as advanced anode materials for lithium-ion batteries. *Electrochimica Acta*, *292*, 63–71. https://doi.org/10.1016/j.electacta.2018.09.138

Lin, S., Lin, C., He, M., Yuan, R., Zhang, Y., Zhou, Y., Xiang, W., & Liang, X. (2017). Solvatochromism of bright carbon dots with tunable long-wavelength emission from green to red and their application as solid-state materials for warm WLEDs. *RSC Advances*, *7*(66), 41552–41560. https://doi.org/10.1039/C7RA07736J

Liu, C., Chang, K., Guo, W., Li, H., Shen, L., Chen, W., & Yan, D. (2014). Improving charge transport property and energy transfer with carbon quantum dots in inverted polymer solar cells. *Applied Physics Letters*, *105*(7). https://doi.org/10.1063/1.4893994

Liu, F., Wang, Y., Zhang, Y., Lin, J., Su, Q., Shi, J., Xie, X., Liang, S., & Pan, A. (2020a). A facile carbon quantum dot-modified reduction approach towards tunable Sb@CQDs nanoparticles for high performance sodium storage. *Batteries & Supercaps*, 3(5), 463–469. https://doi.org/10.1002/batt.201900167

Liu, L., Yu, X., Yi, Z., Chi, F., Wang, H., Yuan, Y., Li, D., Xu, K., & Zhang, X. (2019). High efficiency solar cells tailored using biomass-converted graded carbon quantum dots. *Nanoscale*, 11(32), 15083–15090. https://doi.org/10.1039/C9NR05957A

Liu, S., Cao, X., Zhang, Y., Wang, K., Su, Q., Chen, J., He, Q., Liang, S., Cao, G., & Pan, A. (2020b). Carbon quantum dot modified Na 3 V 2 (PO 4) 2 F 3 as a high-performance cathode material for sodium-ion batteries. *Journal of Materials Chemistry A*, 8(36), 18872–18879. https://doi.org/10.1039/D0TA04307A

Ma, Y., Zhang, H., Zhang, Y., Hu, R., Jiang, M., Zhang, R., Lv, H., Tian, J., Chu, L., Zhang, J., Xue, Q., Yip, H.-L., Xia, R., Li, X., & Huang, W. (2019). Enhancing the performance of inverted perovskite solar cells via grain boundary passivation with carbon quantum dots. *ACS Applied Materials & Interfaces*, 11(3), 3044–3052. https://doi.org/10.1021/acsami.8b18867

Margraf, J. T., Lodermeyer, F., Strauss, V., Haines, P., Walter, J., Peukert, W., Costa, R. D., Clark, T., & Guldi, D. M. (2016). Using carbon nanodots as inexpensive and environmentally friendly sensitizers in mesoscopic solar cells. *Nanoscale Horizons*, 1(3), 220–226. https://doi.org/10.1039/C6NH00010J

Meng, L., Ushakova, E. V., Zhou, Z., Liu, E., Li, D., Zhou, D., Tan, Z., Qu, S., & Rogach, A. L. (2020). Microwave-assisted in situ large scale synthesis of a carbon dots@g-C 3 N 4 composite phosphor for white light-emitting devices. *Materials Chemistry Frontiers*, 4(2), 517–523. https://doi.org/10.1039/C9QM00659A

Meng, Y., Zhang, Y., Sun, W., Wang, M., He, B., Chen, H., & Tang, Q. (2017). Biomass converted carbon quantum dots for all-weather solar cells. *Electrochimica Acta*, 257, 259–266. https://doi.org/10.1016/j.electacta.2017.10.086

Mirtchev, P., Henderson, E. J., Soheilnia, N., Yip, C. M., & Ozin, G. A. (2012). Solution phase synthesis of carbon quantum dots as sensitizers for nanocrystalline TiO 2 solar cells. *J. Mater. Chem.*, 22(4), 1265–1269. https://doi.org/10.1039/C1JM14112K

Lima, R.M. A. P., & de Oliveira, H. P. (2020). Carbon dots reinforced polypyrrole/ graphene nanoplatelets on flexible eggshell membranes as electrodes of all-solid flexible supercapacitors. *Journal of Energy Storage*, 28, 101284. https://doi.org/10.1016/j.est.2020.101284

Nan, H., Zhang, Y., Wei, H., Chen, H., Xue, C., Yang, G., Zou, S., Wang, G., & Lin, H. (2019). Low-cost and environmentally friendly synthesis of an Al 3+ and Mn 4+ co-doped Li 4 Ti 5 O 12 composite with carbon quantum dots as an anode for lithium-ion batteries. *RSC Advances*, 9(38), 22101–22105. https://doi.org/10.1039/C9RA03897C

Narayanan, R. (2017). Single step hydrothermal synthesis of carbon nanodot decorated V2O5 nanobelts as hybrid conducting material for supercapacitor application. *Journal of Solid State Chemistry*, 253, 103–112. https://doi.org/10.1016/j.jssc.2017.05.035

Narayanan, R., Deepa, M., & Srivastava, A. K. (2013). Förster resonance energy transfer and carbon dots enhance light harvesting in a solid-state quantum dot solar cell. *Journal of Materials Chemistry A*, 1(12), 3907. https://doi.org/10.1039/c3ta01601c

Pang, Y., Wei, J., Wang, Y., & Xia, Y. (2018). Synergetic protective effect of the ultralight MWCNTs/NCQDs modified separator for highly stable lithium-sulfur batteries. *Advanced Energy Materials*, 8(10), 1702288. https://doi.org/10.1002/aenm.201702288

Paulo, S., Stoica, G., Cambarau, W., Martinez-Ferrero, E., & Palomares, E. (2016). Carbon quantum dots as new hole transport material for perovskite solar cells. *Synthetic Metals*, 222, 17–22. https://doi.org/10.1016/j.synthmet.2016.04.025

Pelayo, E., Zazueta, A., Lopez, R., Saucedo, E., Ruelas, R., & Ayon, A. (2016). Silicon solar cell efficiency improvement employing the photoluminescent, down-shifting effects of carbon and CdTe quantum dots. *Materials for Renewable and Sustainable Energy*, 5(2), 5. https://doi.org/10.1007/s40243-016-0070-4

Permatasari, F. A., Irham, M. A., Bisri, S. Z., & Iskandar, F. (2021). Carbon-based quantum dots for supercapacitors: Recent advances and future challenges. *Nanomaterials, 11*(1), 91. https://doi.org/10.3390/nano11010091

Pholauyphon, W., Bulakhe, R. N., Manyam, J., In, I., & Paoprasert, P. (2022). High-performance supercapacitors using carbon dots/titanium dioxide composite electrodes and carbon dot-added sulfuric acid electrolyte. *Journal of Electroanalytical Chemistry, 910*, 116177. https://doi.org/10.1016/j.jelechem.2022.116177

Prasath, A., Athika, M., Duraisamy, E., Selva Sharma, A., Sankar Devi, V., & Elumalai, P. (2019). Carbon quantum dot-anchored bismuth oxide composites as potential electrode for lithium-ion battery and supercapacitor applications. *ACS Omega, 4*(3), 4943–4954. https://doi.org/10.1021/acsomega.8b03490

Privitera, A., Righetto, M., Mosconi, D., Lorandi, F., Isse, A. A., Moretto, A., Bozio, R., Ferrante, C., & Franco, L. (2016). Boosting carbon quantum dots/fullerene electron transfer via surface group engineering. *Physical Chemistry Chemical Physics, 18*(45), 31286–31295. https://doi.org/10.1039/C6CP05981C

Qi, C., Zhou, Y., Tao, X., Chen, H., Ouyang, Y., & Mo, X. (2020). Toward near-white electroluminescence with enhanced blue emission from carbon dots in PEDOT:PSS/ZnO organic/inorganic hybrid heterojunctions. *Journal of Luminescence, 224*, 117230. https://doi.org/10.1016/j.jlumin.2020.117230

Qi, M., Bai, L., Xu, H., Wang, Z., Kang, Z., Zhao, X., Liu, W., Ma, J., & Liu, Y. (2018). Oxidized carbon quantum dot–graphene oxide nanocomposites for improving data retention of resistive switching memory. *Journal of Materials Chemistry C, 6*(8), 2026–2033. https://doi.org/10.1039/C7TC04829G

Qu, S., Zhou, D., Li, D., Ji, W., Jing, P., Han, D., Liu, L., Zeng, H., & Shen, D. (2016). Toward efficient orange emissive carbon nanodots through conjugated sp 2 -domain controlling and surface charges engineering. *Advanced Materials, 28*(18), 3516–3521. https://doi.org/10.1002/adma.201504891

Quan, H., Zeng, W., Chen, W., Wang, Y., Tao, W., & Chen, D. (2023). Carbon quantum dot-induced robust ε-MnO2 electrode by synergistic engineering of oxygen vacancy and low crystallinity for high-performance flexible asymmetric supercapacitor. *Journal of Alloys and Compounds, 938*, 168524. https://doi.org/10.1016/j.jallcom.2022.168524

Raeis-Hosseini, N., Georgiadou, D. G., & Papavassiliou, C. (2023). High on/off ratio carbon quantum dot–chitosan biomemristors with coplanar nanogap electrodes. *ACS Applied Electronic Materials, 5*(1), 138–145. https://doi.org/10.1021/acsaelm.2c00979

Ren, J., Sun, J., Sun, X., Song, R., Xie, Z., & Zhou, S. (2018). Precisely controlled up/down-conversion liquid and solid state photoluminescence of carbon dots. *Advanced Optical Materials, 6*(14), 1800115. https://doi.org/10.1002/adom.201800115

Sahatiya, P., Jones, S. S., & Badhulika, S. (2018). 2D MoS2–carbon quantum dot hybrid based large area, flexible UV–vis–NIR photodetector on paper substrate. *Applied Materials Today, 10*, 106–114. https://doi.org/10.1016/j.apmt.2017.12.013

Sahoo, S., Satpati, A. K., Sahoo, P. K., & Naik, P. D. (2018). Incorporation of carbon quantum dots for improvement of supercapacitor performance of nickel sulfide. *ACS Omega, 3*(12), 17936–17946. https://doi.org/10.1021/acsomega.8b01238

Sarkar, K., Devi, P., Lata, A., Ghosh, R., & Kumar, P. (2019). Engineering carbon quantum dots for enhancing the broadband photoresponse in a silicon process-line compatible photodetector. *Journal of Materials Chemistry C, 7*(42), 13182–13191. https://doi.org/10.1039/C9TC04519H

Sharma, R., Alam, F., Sharma, A. K., Dutta, V., & Dhawan, S. K. (2015). Role of zinc oxide and carbonaceous nanomaterials in non-fullerene-based polymer bulk heterojunction solar cells for improved cost-to-performance ratio. *Journal of Materials Chemistry A, 3*(44), 22227–22238. https://doi.org/10.1039/C5TA06802A

Sharma, V.D., Vishal, V., Chandan, G., Bhatia, A., Chakrabarti, S., & Bera, M. K. (2022). Green, sustainable, and economical synthesis of fluorescent nitrogen-doped carbon quantum dots for applications in optical displays and light-emitting diodes. *Materials Today Sustainability*, *19*, 100184. https://doi.org/10.1016/j.mtsust.2022.100184

Sharma, V. D., Kansay, V., Chandan, G., Bhatia, A., Kumar, N., Chakrabarti, S., & Bera, M. K. (2023). Solid-state fluorescence based on nitrogen and calcium co-doped carbon quantum dots @ bioplastic composites for applications in optical displays and light-emitting diodes. *Carbon*, *201*, 972–983. https://doi.org/10.1016/j.carbon.2022.10.007

Shen, K., Wang, Z., Bi, X., Ying, Y., Zhang, D., Jin, C., Hou, G., Cao, H., Wu, L., Zheng, G., Tang, Y., Tao, X., & Lu, J. (2019). Magnetic field–suppressed lithium dendrite growth for stable lithium-metal batteries. *Advanced Energy Materials*, *9*(20), 1900260. https://doi.org/10.1002/aenm.201900260

Shi, Y., Na, Y., Su, T., Li, L., Yu, J., Fan, R., & Yang, Y. (2016). Fluorescent carbon quantum dots incorporated into dye-sensitized TiO 2 photoanodes with dual contributions. *ChemSusChem*, *9*(12), 1498–1503. https://doi.org/10.1002/cssc.201600067

Sikiru, S., Oladosu, T. L., Kolawole, S. Y., Mubarak, L. A., Soleimani, H., Afolabi, L. O., & Oluwafunke Toyin, A.-O. (2023). Advance and prospect of carbon quantum dots synthesis for energy conversion and storage application: A comprehensive review. *Journal of Energy Storage*, *60*, 106556. https://doi.org/10.1016/j.est.2022.106556

Sun, M., Ma, X., Chen, X., Sun, Y., Cui, X., & Lin, Y. (2014). A nanocomposite of carbon quantum dots and TiO 2 nanotube arrays: enhancing photoelectrochemical and photocatalytic properties. *RSC Adv.*, *4*(3), 1120–1127. https://doi.org/10.1039/C3RA45474F

Sun, W., & Lu, Q. (2023). Self-supported α-Ni(OH)2 nanosheet arrays modified with carbon quantum dots for high-performance supercapacitors. *Scripta Materialia*, *224*, 115119. https://doi.org/10.1016/j.scriptamat.2022.115119

Tian, Z., Tian, P., Zhou, X., Zhou, G., Mei, S., Zhang, W., Zhang, X., Li, D., Zhou, D., Guo, R., Qu, S., & Rogach, A. L. (2019). Ultraviolet-pumped white light emissive carbon dot based phosphors for light-emitting devices and visible light communication. *Nanoscale*, *11*(8), 3489–3494. https://doi.org/10.1039/C9NR00224C

Tian, Z., Zhang, X., Li, D., Zhou, D., Jing, P., Shen, D., Qu, S., Zboril, R., & Rogach, A. L. (2017). Full-color inorganic carbon dot phosphors for white-light-emitting diodes. *Advanced Optical Materials*, *5*(19), 1700416. https://doi.org/10.1002/adom.201700416

Verma, S., Arya, S., Gupta, V., Mahajan, S., Furukawa, H., & Khosla, A. (2021). Performance analysis, challenges and future perspectives of nickel based nanostructured electrodes for electrochemical supercapacitors. *Journal of Materials Research and Technology*, *11*, 564–599. https://doi.org/10.1016/j.jmrt.2021.01.027

Wang, A., Hou, Y.-L., Kang, F., Lyu, F., Xiong, Y., Chen, W.-C., Lee, C.-S., Xu, Z., Rogach, A. L., Lu, J., & Li, Y. Y. (2019a). Rare earth-free composites of carbon dots/metal–organic frameworks as white light emitting phosphors. *Journal of Materials Chemistry C*, *7*(8), 2207–2211. https://doi.org/10.1039/C8TC04171G

Wang, C., Wu, X., Li, X., Wang, W., Wang, L., Gu, M., & Li, Q. (2012). Upconversion fluorescent carbon nanodots enriched with nitrogen for light harvesting. *Journal of Materials Chemistry*, *22*(31), 15522. https://doi.org/10.1039/c2jm30935a

Wang, F., Chen, Y., Liu, C., & Ma, D. (2011). White light-emitting devices based on carbon dots' electroluminescence. *Chemical Communications*, *47*(12), 3502. https://doi.org/10.1039/c0cc05391k

Wang, J., Fang, Z., Li, T., ur Rehman, S., Luo, Q., Chen, P., Hu, L., Zhang, F., Wang, Q., & Bi, H. (2019b). Highly hydrophilic carbon dots' decoration on NiCo 2 O 4 nanowires for greatly increased electric conductivity, supercapacitance, and energy density. *Advanced Materials Interfaces*, *6*(9), 1900049. https://doi.org/10.1002/admi.201900049

Wang, Q., Wang, H., Liu, D., Du, P., & Liu, P. (2017a). Synthesis of flake-shaped nitrogen-doped carbon quantum dot/polyaniline (N-CQD/PANI) nanocomposites via rapid-mixing polymerization and their application as electrode materials in supercapacitors. *Synthetic Metals*, *231*, 120–126. https://doi.org/10.1016/j.synthmet.2017.06.018

Wang, S., Wang, H., Zhang, R., Zhao, L., Wu, X., Xie, H., Zhang, J., & Sun, H. (2018). Egg yolk-derived carbon: Achieving excellent fluorescent carbon dots and high performance lithium-ion batteries. *Journal of Alloys and Compounds*, *746*, 567–575. https://doi.org/10.1016/j.jallcom.2018.02.293

Wang, W., Xiao, Y., Li, X., Cheng, Q., & Wang, G. (2019c). Bismuth oxide self-standing anodes with concomitant carbon dots welded graphene layer for enhanced performance supercapacitor-battery hybrid devices. *Chemical Engineering Journal*, *371*, 327–336. https://doi.org/10.1016/j.cej.2019.04.048

Wang, Y., Yan, L., Ji, G., Wang, C., Gu, H., Luo, Q., Chen, Q., Chen, L., Yang, Y., Ma, C.-Q., & Liu, X. (2019d). Synthesis of N,S-Doped carbon quantum dots for use in organic solar cells as the ZnO modifier to eliminate the light-soaking effect. *ACS Applied Materials & Interfaces*, *11*(2), 2243–2253. https://doi.org/10.1021/acsami.8b17128

Wang, Y., Liu, H., Wang, K., Eiji, H., Wang, Y., & Zhou, H. (2009). Synthesis and electrochemical performance of nano-sized Li4Ti5O12 with double surface modification of Ti(III) and carbon. *Journal of Materials Chemistry*, *19*(37), 6789. https://doi.org/10.1039/b908025b

Wang, Z., Yuan, F., Li, X., Li, Y., Zhong, H., Fan, L., & Yang, S. (2017b). 53% efficient red emissive carbon quantum dots for high color rendering and stable warm white-light-emitting diodes. *Advanced Materials*, *29*(37), 1702910. https://doi.org/10.1002/adma.201702910

Wei, J.-S., Ding, H., Zhang, P., Song, Y.-F., Chen, J., Wang, Y.-G., & Xiong, H.-M. (2016). Carbon Dots/NiCo 2 O 4 Nanocomposites with Various Morphologies for High Performance Supercapacitors. *Small*, *12*(43), 5927–5934. https://doi.org/10.1002/smll.201602164

Wei, J.-S., Ding, C., Zhang, P., Ding, H., Niu, X., Ma, Y., Li, C., Wang, Y., & Xiong, H. (2018). Robust negative electrode materials derived from carbon dots and porous hydrogels for high-performance hybrid supercapacitors. *Advanced Materials*, 1806197. https://doi.org/10.1002/adma.201806197

Wei, J.-Y., Lou, Q., Zang, J., Liu, Z., Ye, Y., Shen, C., Zhao, W., Dong, L., & Shan, C. (2020). Scalable synthesis of green fluorescent carbon dot powders with unprecedented efficiency. *Advanced Optical Materials*, *8*(7), 1901938. https://doi.org/10.1002/adom.201901938

Wen, Y., Zhu, G., & Shao, Y. (2020). Improving the power conversion efficiency of perovskite solar cells by adding carbon quantum dots. *Journal of Materials Science*, *55*(7), 2937–2946. https://doi.org/10.1007/s10853-019-04145-9

Wu, M., Gao, Y., Hu, Y., Zhao, B., & Zhang, H. (2020). Boosting sodium storage of mesoporous TiO2 nanostructure regulated by carbon quantum dots. *Chinese Chemical Letters*, *31*(3), 897–902. https://doi.org/10.1016/j.cclet.2019.07.039

Wu, X., Zhao, B., Zhang, J., Xu, H., Xu, K., & Chen, G. (2019). Photoluminescence and photodetecting properties of the hydrothermally synthesized nitrogen-doped carbon quantum dots. *The Journal of Physical Chemistry C*, *123*(42), 25570–25578. https://doi.org/10.1021/acs.jpcc.9b06672

Xie, C., Nie, B., Zeng, L., Liang, F.-X., Wang, M.-Z., Luo, L., Feng, M., Yu, Y., Wu, C.-Y., Wu, Y., & Yu, S.-H. (2014). Core–Shell heterojunction of silicon nanowire arrays and carbon quantum dots for photovoltaic devices and self-driven photodetectors. *ACS Nano*, *8*(4), 4015–4022. https://doi.org/10.1021/nn501001j

Xu, L., Wang, H., Gao, J., & Jin, X. (2019). Electrochemical performance enhancement of flexible graphene supercapacitor electrodes by carbon dots modification and NiCo2S4 electrodeposition. *Journal of Alloys and Compounds*, *809*, 151802. https://doi.org/10.1016/j.jallcom.2019.151802

Xu, T., Wan, Z., Tang, H., Zhao, C., Lv, S., Chen, Y., Chen, L., Qiao, Q., & Huang, W. (2021). Carbon quantum dot additive engineering for efficient and stable carbon-based perovskite solar cells. *Journal of Alloys and Compounds, 859*, 157784. https://doi.org/10.1016/j.jallcom.2020.157784

Yan, F., Jiang, Y., Sun, X., Wei, J., Chen, L., & Zhang, Y. (2020). Multicolor carbon dots with concentration-tunable fluorescence and solvent-affected aggregation states for white light-emitting diodes. *Nano Research, 13*(1), 52–60. https://doi.org/10.1007/s12274-019-2569-3

Yang, G., & Park, S.-J. (2023). Nitrogen and iron co-doped carbon quantum dots/MnO2 nanowire composites for flexible solid-state supercapacitors with high areal capacitance. *Journal of Alloys and Compounds, 960*, 171021. https://doi.org/10.1016/j.jallcom.2023.171021

Yang, J., Tang, Q., Meng, Q., Zhang, Z., Li, J., He, B., & Yang, P. (2017). Photoelectric conversion beyond sunny days: all-weather carbon quantum dot solar cells. *Journal of Materials Chemistry A, 5*(5), 2143–2150. https://doi.org/10.1039/C6TA09261F

Yang, Y., Ji, X., Jing, M., Hou, H., Zhu, Y., Fang, L., Yang, X., Chen, Q., & Banks, C. E. (2015). Carbon dots supported upon N-doped TiO 2 nanorods applied into sodium and lithium ion batteries. *Journal of Materials Chemistry A, 3*(10), 5648–5655. https://doi.org/10.1039/C4TA05611F

Yang, Z., Li, G., Sun, J., Xie, L., Jiang, Y., Huang, Y., & Chen, S. (2020). High performance cathode material based on Na3V2(PO4)2F3 and Na3V2(PO4)3 for sodium-ion batteries. *Energy Storage Materials, 25*, 724–730. https://doi.org/10.1016/j.ensm.2019.09.014

Yuan, B., Guan, S., Sun, X., Li, X., Zeng, H., Xie, Z., Chen, P., & Zhou, S. (2018a). Highly efficient carbon dots with reversibly switchable green–red emissions for trichromatic white light-emitting diodes. *ACS Applied Materials & Interfaces, 10*(18), 16005–16014. https://doi.org/10.1021/acsami.8b02379

Yuan, F., Wang, Y.-K., Sharma, G., Dong, Y., Zheng, X., Li, P., Johnston, A., Bappi, G., Fan, J. Z., Kung, H., Chen, B., Saidaminov, M. I., Singh, K., Voznyy, O., Bakr, O. M., Lu, Z.-H., & Sargent, E. H. (2020). Bright high-colour-purity deep-blue carbon dot light-emitting diodes via efficient edge amination. *Nature Photonics, 14*(3), 171–176. https://doi.org/10.1038/s41566-019-0557-5

Yuan, F., Wang, Z., Li, X., Li, Y., Tan, Z., Fan, L., & Yang, S. (2017). Bright multicolor bandgap fluorescent carbon quantum dots for electroluminescent light-emitting diodes. *Advanced Materials, 29*(3), 1604436. https://doi.org/10.1002/adma.201604436

Yuan, F., Xi, Z., Shi, X., Li, Y., Li, X., Wang, Z., Fan, L., & Yang, S. (2019). Ultrastable and low-threshold random lasing from narrow-bandwidth-emission triangular carbon quantum dots. *Advanced Optical Materials, 7*(2), 1801202. https://doi.org/10.1002/adom.201801202

Yuan, F., Yuan, T., Sui, L., Wang, Z., Xi, Z., Li, Y., Li, X., Fan, L., Tan, Z., Chen, A., Jin, M., & Yang, S. (2018b). Engineering triangular carbon quantum dots with unprecedented narrow bandwidth emission for multicolored LEDs. *Nature Communications, 9*(1), 2249. https://doi.org/10.1038/s41467-018-04635-5

Yuan, T., Yuan, F., Sui, L., Zhang, Y., Li, Y., Li, X., Tan, Z., & Fan, L. (2023). Carbon quantum dots with near-unity quantum yield bandgap emission for electroluminescent light-emitting diodes. *Angewandte Chemie, 135*(20). https://doi.org/10.1002/ange.202218568

Zhang, X., Wang, J., Liu, J., Wu, J., Chen, H., & Bi, H. (2017). Design and preparation of a ternary composite of graphene oxide/carbon dots/polypyrrole for supercapacitor application: Importance and unique role of carbon dots. *Carbon, 115*, 134–146. https://doi.org/10.1016/j.carbon.2017.01.005

Zhang, X., Zhang, Y., Wang, Y., Kalytchuk, S., Kershaw, S. V., Wang, Y., Wang, P., Zhang, T., Zhao, Y., Zhang, H., Cui, T., Wang, Y., Zhao, J., Yu, W. W., & Rogach, A. L. (2013). Color-switchable electroluminescence of carbon dot light-emitting diodes. *ACS Nano, 7*(12), 11234–11241. https://doi.org/10.1021/nn405017q

Zhang, X., Li, Z., Zhang, Z., Li, S., Liu, C., Guo, W., Shen, L., Wen, S., Qu, S., & Ruan, S. (2016a). Efficiency improvement of organic solar cells via introducing combined anode buffer layer to facilitate hole extraction. *The Journal of Physical Chemistry C, 120*(26), 13954–13962. https://doi.org/10.1021/acs.jpcc.6b03697

Zhang, Y., Liu, Y., Li, Y., Yang, Z., & Liu, S. (Frank). (2016b). Perovskite CH 3 NH 3 Pb(Br x I 1−x) 3 single crystals with controlled composition for fine-tuned bandgap towards optimized optoelectronic applications. *Journal of Materials Chemistry C, 4*(39), 9172–9178. https://doi.org/10.1039/C6TC03592B

Zhao, C., Zhang, X., Shu, X., Liu, X., Fang, D., Song, Y., & Wang, J. (2018). Er-doped carbon dots broadening light absorption range and accelerating electron transport for enhancing photovoltaic performance of CdS quantum dots sensitized cells. *Optical Materials, 84*, 242–251. https://doi.org/10.1016/j.optmat.2018.07.016

Zhao, Z., & Xie, Y. (2017). Enhanced electrochemical performance of carbon quantum dots-polyaniline hybrid. *Journal of Power Sources, 337*, 54–64. https://doi.org/10.1016/j.jpowsour.2016.10.110

Zheng, J., Zhang, R., Wang, X., & Yu, P. (2019). Importance of carbon quantum dots for improving the electrochemical performance of MoS2@ZnS composite. *Journal of Materials Science, 54*(21), 13509–13522. https://doi.org/10.1007/s10853-019-03860-7

Zheng, Y., Zheng, J., Wang, J., Yang, Y., Lu, T., & Liu, X. (2020). Facile preparation of stable solid-state carbon quantum dots with multi-peak emission. *Nanomaterials, 10*(2), 303. https://doi.org/10.3390/nano10020303

Zhou, D., Li, D., Jing, P., Zhai, Y., Shen, D., Qu, S., & Rogach, A. L. (2017). Conquering aggregation-induced solid-state luminescence quenching of carbon dots through a carbon dots-triggered silica gelation process. *Chemistry of Materials, 29*(4), 1779–1787. https://doi.org/10.1021/acs.chemmater.6b05375

Zhou, J., Qin, J., Zhang, X., Shi, C., Liu, E., Li, J., Zhao, N., & He, C. (2015). 2D space-confined synthesis of few-layer MoS 2 anchored on carbon nanosheet for lithium-ion battery anode. *ACS Nano, 9*(4), 3837–3848. https://doi.org/10.1021/nn506850e

Zhou, Z., Tian, P., Liu, X., Mei, S., Zhou, D., Li, D., Jing, P., Zhang, W., Guo, R., Qu, S., & Rogach, A. L. (2018). Hydrogen peroxide-treated carbon dot phosphor with a bathochromic-shifted, aggregation-enhanced emission for light-emitting devices and visible light communication. *Advanced Science, 5*(8), 1800369. https://doi.org/10.1002/advs.201800369

Zhu, W., Zhao, Y., Duan, J., Duan, Y., Tang, Q., & He, B. (2017). Carbon quantum dot tailored counter electrode for 7.01%-rear efficiency in a bifacial dye-sensitized solar cell. *Chemical Communications, 53*(71), 9894–9897. https://doi.org/10.1039/C7CC05480G

Zhu, Y., Ji, X., Pan, C., Sun, Q., Song, W., Fang, L., Chen, Q., & Banks, C. E. (2013). A carbon quantum dot decorated RuO2 network: outstanding supercapacitances under ultrafast charge and discharge. *Energy & Environmental Science, 6*(12), 3665. https://doi.org/10.1039/c3ee41776j

16 Carbon Quantum Dots for Metal Detection

Karutha Pandian Divya and
Nagamony Ponpandian

16.1 INTRODUCTION

Carbon quantum dots (CQDs) have been regarded as one of the prominent probes for the effective sensing of metal ions with good selectivity and sensitivity due to the presence of oxygen moieties on their surface. This major property enables their coordination with several metal ions, resulting in photoluminescence quenching. Another important parameter responsible for the quenching property is the transfer of energy between metal ions and CQDs due to the functional group and surface interaction. The selectivity of metal ions is influenced through several factors such the size, morphology, functionalization, etc. It is to be noted that the optical and electronic properties of CQDs can be tuned through the process of doping. In order to construct a fluorescent sensor, several mechanisms like inner filter effect, Forster/fluorescence resonance energy transfer, fluorescence quenching and photoinduced electron transfer have been utilized which are either based on enhancement or attenuation of fluorescence. This chapter covers a wide range of natural sources for the preparation of CQDs that are used for the sensing of toxic metal ions utilizing photoluminescence technique. The sensing performance of different CQDs is evaluated by their limit of detection, linearity range and quantum yield.

16.2 DETECTION OF MERCURY (II)

Mercury is regarded as a toxic metal that pollutes the environment through large-scale agricultural and industrial processes. The +2 oxidation state of mercury is a non-biodegradable toxic threat to all living organisms especially aquatic animals. Even low-level consumption of Hg(II) polluted food/water may cause several health issues in our body such as renal failure, expiratory dyspnoea, lunacy, hyperspermia and so on. Hence it is important to monitor and detect the presence of Hg to avoid health hazards and protect the environment. The detection of Hg(II) by CQDs prepared from natural sources has been reported successfully. The first report was made by Lu et al. using Pomelo peel waste as a natural source for fluorescent CQD preparation. The prepared CQDs do not require further chemical modification which is cost-effective. Hg(II) was detected with a LOD value of 0.23 nM using a label-free method. A real sample analysis done using lake water proved the high selectivity of the sensor (Lu et al., 2012). An eco-friendly method utilizing crushed gingko leaves as a natural

DOI: 10.1201/9781003437857-18

source for CQD preparation was used for the detection of Hg(II). The fluorescence intensity study revealed a reduction in the signal only after adding Hg(II), whereas adding other metals did not show any change. The prepared CQDs were also proven to be biocompatible and permeable through cytotoxicity studies (Zhang et al., 2019). A 'off-on' fluorescence method based on CQDs prepared from the leaves of *Prosopis juliflora* was developed for the detection of Hg(II). A successful determination of Hg(II) in both spiked human serum and water samples containing numerous interfering materials was made. A LOD value of 1.26 ng mL^{-1} was achieved (Pourreza & Ghomi, 2019). A green synthetic approach was made using *Tamarindus indica* leaves for the preparation of CQDs by hydrothermal method and applied for Hg(II) detection. As the existing pH range of CQDs did not work out, the pH was tuned to 7. A stable emission of fluorescence was obtained at 433 nm at a reaction time of 5 min. A LOD value of 6 nM with high selectivity was achieved (Bano, Kumar, Singh, & Hasan, 2018). Ye at al. synthesized CQDs via hydrothermal reaction of dried eggshell membrane peeled from eggshells which showed long-term stability and applied for Hg(II) detection. The presence of Hg(II) decreased the intensity of fluorescence of the prepared CQDs at 420 nm. The increase in the concentration of Hg(II) resulted in the gradual decrease of the fluorescence intensity (Ye, Zhang, Li, & Li, 2020). A smart move of reducing the bagasse polluting the land and water after sugarcane cultivation by utilizing it as a carbon source for the synthesis of CQDs was reported by Kasinathan et al. The quenching of CQDs takes place by the electron transfer within CQDs and Hg(II). The sensor has showed LOD and LOQ values of 0.1 μM and 0.4 μM respectively with good selectivity (Kasinathan, Samayanan, Marimuthu, & Yim, 2022). Citrus lemon juice has been reported as a carbon source for the preparation of fluorescent nitrogen-doped CQDs via green method. They found that the prepared N-doped CQDs possess greater ionic stability, water solubility and resistance to photobleaching. It also showed good sensing behaviour towards the detection of Hg (II) with a LOD and LOQ value of 5.3 nM and 18.3 nM, respectively using fluorescence assay technique (Tadesse, Hagos, Ramadevi, Basavaiah, & Belachew, 2020). There are a lot of reports by various research groups for Hg(II) detection using CQDs synthesized from various natural sources as shown in Table 16.1.

16.3 DETECTION OF COPPER (II)

The industrial and human activities release a large amount of Cu(II) pollutant in the environment. Excess accumulation of Cu(II) in the human body causes several health hazards including myalgia, hepatomegaly, renal failure, lung disease, etc. So, it is important to develop sensitive methods for the detection of Cu(II). Highly fluorescent CQDs were obtained from banana juice using a simple hydrothermal method for the detection of Cu(II) with high selectivity. The CQDs were doped with nitrogen and sulphur (present in banana) and resulted in the formation of NS-CQDs. An excellent platform with negative surface charge and various functional groups was provided by the as-prepared NS-CQDs to bind with Cu(II). The charge transfer between NS-CQDs and Cu(II) and aggregation around Cu(II) by NS-CQDs resulted in non-radioactive recombination with a fall in fluorescence intensity. The sensor has resulted in good linearity of 1-800 μgmL^{-1} with a good recovery rate from

TABLE 16.1

Detection of Hg(II) using Various Green CQDs

Precursor	Quantum Yield (%)	Preparation Technique	Linearity Range (μM)	Limit of Detection (nM)	References
Lotus root	19	Microwave	0.1 to 60	18.7	Gu, Shang, Yu, and Shen (2016)
Strawberry juice	6.3	Hydrothermal	0.001 to 50	3	Huang et al. (2013)
Flour	5.4	Microwave	0.0005 to 0.01	0.5	Qin, Lu, Asiri, Al-Youbi, and Sun (2013)
Honey	–	Hydrothermal	0 to 10^{-3}	1.02	Srinivasan, Subramanian, Murugan, and Dinakaran, (2016)
Pineapple peel	42	Hydrothermal	0.1 to 100	–	Vandarkuzhali et al. (2018)
Cucumber juice	–	Hydrothermal	1 to 70	180	Chunfeng Wang, Sun, Zhuo, Zhang, and Wang, (2014)
Jinhua bergamot	50.7	Hydrothermal	0.01 to 100	5.5	J. Yu et al. (2015)
Hong caitai	12.1	Hydrothermal	0.2 to 15	60	L. S. Li et al. (2018)
Muskmelon	26.9	Acid oxidation	1 to 2.5	330	Desai et al. (2019)
Lemon juice	2.4	Hydrothermal	0 to 1.82×10^3	36×10^3	Gharat, Pal, and Dutta Choudhury (2019)
Dunaliella salina	8	Hydrothermal	0.03 to 0.1	0.018	Singh et al. (2019)
Dried rose petals	28	Hydrothermal	10 to 200×10^{-6}	81×10^{-6}	Das, Thakkar, Patel, and Thakore (2021)

spiked samples (Chaudhary, Gupta, Eremin, & Solanki, 2020). Xu et al. have prepared CQDs from waste wolfberry straw as the carbon source. A strong fluorescence emission was exhibited by the prepared CQDs when a concentration of 7.5 g L^{-1} of the wolfberry stem was taken, and the activation was performed for 24 h at 200 °C. After the introduction of Cu(II), there was an increase in the zeta potential from –24.8 mV to 4.7 mV due to the formation of the CQDs-Cu(II) complex. The reported sensor exhibited a linearity of 10 to 80 nM with a LOD value of 2.83 nM (Y. Xu et al., 2023). In another study, CQDs were synthesized from rice husks which serve as the carbon source and phosphorus is employed to CQDs for doping, resulting in phosphorus-doped carbon quantum dots (P-CQDs). By fine-tuning pH and temperature conditions, the obtained P-CQDs with green fluorescence are consistently monodisperse and spherical, exhibiting ±5.4 nm and an impressive quantum yield of 32.61%. Upon exposure to Cu(II) ions, the quenching of P-CQDs is due to the interaction between the two entities. This quenching is attributed to the enhanced electron

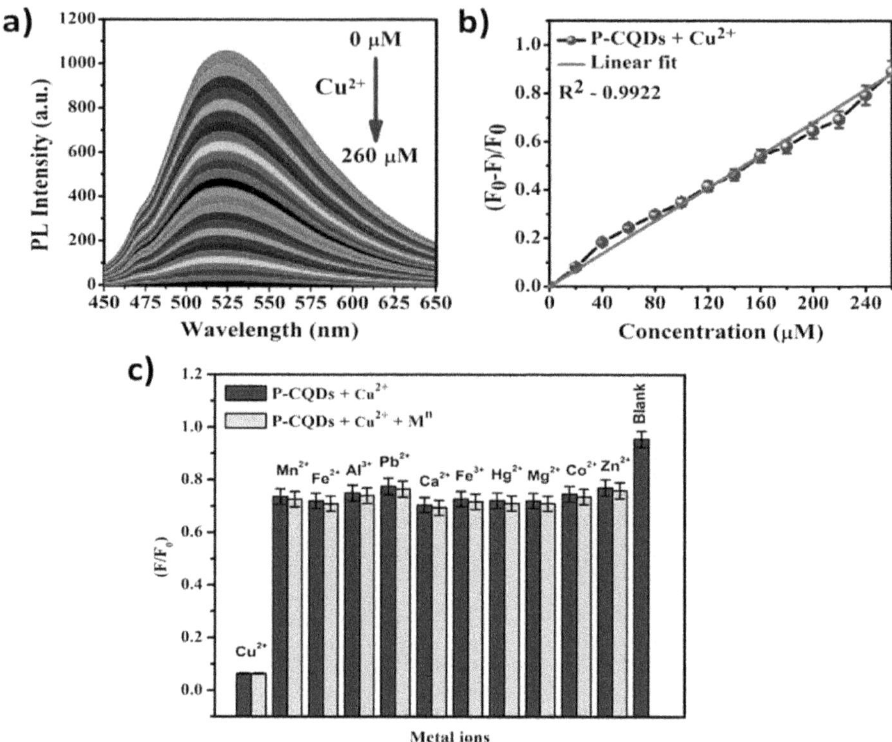

FIGURE 16.1 (a) Intensity variation study (b) Linear calibration plot (c) Selectivity study (M. Preethi et al., 2022).

Copyright 2022. Reproduced with permission from Elsevier.

transport facilitated by the integration of Cu(II) ions into P-CQDs, ultimately leading to fluorescence reduction under optimal conditions. This study reveals the capability to sense Cu(II) within a concentration range of 0 to 260 μM. The intensity variation and linear calibration plot could be seen from Figure 16.1(a & b) with a lower detection limit of 0.032 μM (M. Preethi, Viswanathan, & Ponpandian, 2022). The selectivity analysis has been done with various metal ions. The existence of metal ions has a minor impact on the quenching process involving P-CQDs (Figure 16.1c). This sensor exclusively responds to Cu(II) ions. Upon examining the graph, it became evident that Cu^{2+} ions exhibited the least quenching effect, underscoring the sensor's ability to detect them.

16.4 DETECTION OF IRON (II, III)

Iron is an important trace element essential for biological systems to function several mechanisms such as cellular metabolism, oxygen transport and nucleic acid synthesis due to its high affinity nature for oxygen and redox chemistry behaviour. However, several diseases such as hepatitis, diabetes, hemochromatosis, heart failure, arthritis and anaemia are caused due to the abnormal level of iron (Abbaspour, Hurrell, & Kelishadi, 2014). A lot of methods have been developed for the sensitive recognition of Fe ions. Four types of CQDs were prepared from biomass wastes such as orange peel, paulownias leaves, ginkgo biloba and magnolia flowers and were named as OP-CQDs, PL-CQDs, GB-CQDs and MF-CQDs, respectively. All the CQDs exhibited uniform size with monodispersed particles, bright blue-luminescence and good stability. When applied for the detection of Fe(III), all the CQDs resulted in good sensitivity and selectivity. In a concentration range of 0.2–100 µM, LODs of 0.073 µM, 0.099 µM, 0.080 µM and 0.088 µM were obtained. The excellent sensing ability is due to the carboxyl, amino and hydroxyl groups on the CQD surface. The practical application was examined using pond water. The biomass-derived CQDs were able to obtain 94.5 to 108% of recovery rate (Cunjin Wang et al., 2020). Another group reported CQDs prepared from natural biomass of water hyacinth via hydrothermal synthesis at 180 °C and named as wh-CQDs. The prepared Wh-CQDs possessed high water stability, uniform size, amorphous graphite structure, high photostability and excitation light-dependent characteristics. The linearity range obtained using the prepared Wh-CQDs is 0 to 330 µM. An excellent LOD of 0.084 µM much lower than the value (0.77 µM) specified by the WHO was detected in this work (P. Zhao et al., 2022).

Another study has evaluated an environmentally friendly method for producing CQDs in water. This process utilizes a variety of common agricultural residues as sources of carbon. These CQDs gets readily dispersed in water due to the presence of specific carboxyl and hydroxyl groups on their surface. Notably, among various CQDs created from different raw materials and conditions, those synthesized from corn stalks at a temperature of 140 °C exhibit the greatest fluorescence intensity when excited at 380 nm. Leveraging the energy transfer property and strong fluorescence, these synthesized CQDs serve as a fluorescent probe for accurately detecting Fe(III) ions with better analytical parameters, particularly within the concentration range of 0–500 µM (Ding, Gao, Ni, & Yang, 2021). Preethi et al. synthesized blue-fluorescent CQDs from coconut water with uniform spherical shape and with an average particle size of approximately 5 nm. Importantly, this preparation process avoids the need for any modification or functionalization, and various reaction parameters such as temperature and pH were carefully controlled during the synthesis (Manoharan Preethi, Viswanathan, & Ponpandian, 2021). The resulting CQDs emit blue light with a wavelength of around 487 nm. Furthermore, the CQDs exhibit the ability to detect Fe^{3+} ions within a concentration range from 0 to 700 µM. Notably, the limit of detection for Fe^{3+} ions using these CQDs is as low as 0.30 µM. The results demonstrated that the presence of various other metal ions has a negligible impact on the reduction of Fe^{3+} ions, which is due to the interaction between Fe^{3+} ions and the carboxylic or hydroxyl groups located on the surface periphery of the CQDs, and they play a pivotal role in the detection of Fe^{3+} ions. This interaction mechanism is believed to be the primary factor behind the ability to detect Fe^{3+} ions which is evident from photographic evidence (Figure 16.2).

In another study, a novel approach was employed to fabricate luminescent CQDs using Borassus flabellifer, commonly known as ice apple, as the carbon precursor through a simple one-step hydrothermal process (Nagaraj et al., 2022). The resulting

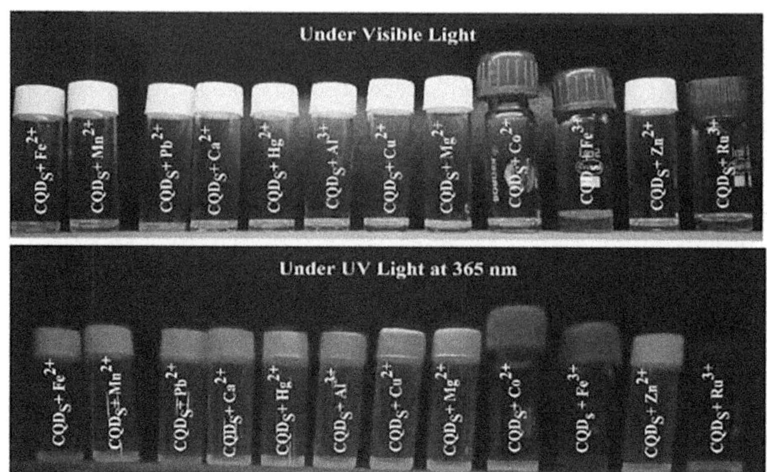

FIGURE 16.2   Photographic evidence of selectivity analysis (Manoharan Preethi et al., 2021). **Copyright 2021. Reproduced with permission from Elsevier.**

CQDs exhibited exceptional photoluminescent properties, boasting high photostability and enduring stability within aqueous environments. These CQDs also showcased a substantial quantum yield and remarkable stability under elevated pH conditions. The CQDs exhibit low limit of detection measured at 2.01 µM. Due to the selectivity of the engineered CQDs, an experiment was conducted by observing the quenching effects of several metal ions. Notably, the outcomes revealed that Fe(III) produced a significant fluorescence quenching effect, whereas the other metal ions have no interference on the signal. The mechanism underlying this phenomenon was illuminated by the role of functional groups present on the synthesized CQDs. These functional groups, functioning as electron donors, facilitated the formation of coordinate bonds with Fe(III) ions. Consequently, Fe(III) ions chelated with the tapered regions on the CQD surface, resulting in the noticeable quenching of fluorescence, as visually depicted in Figure 16.3.

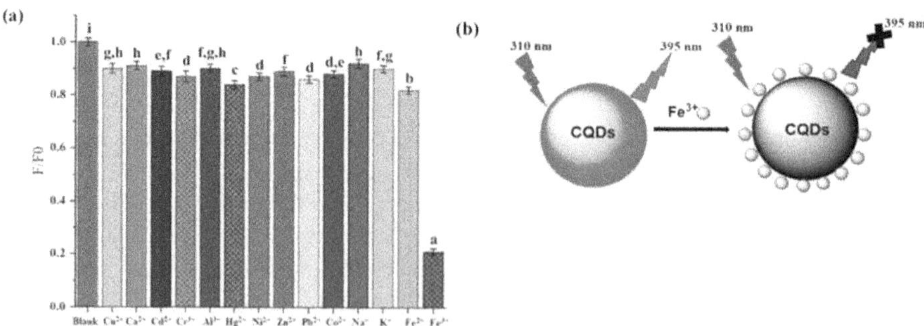

FIGURE 16.3   Fluorescence quenching study (Nagaraj et al., 2022). This is an open access article under the CC BY license (http://creativecommons.org/licenses/by/4.0/).

16.5 DETECTION OF LEAD (II)

Lead exists is three oxidation states. However, in the environment, it primarily exists as Pb(II). As Pb exists aqueous in nature it immediately forms a complex with hydroxyl ion in alkaline soil containing pH greater than 7. This can be transmitted through different levels of food chain and can possibly cause immense threat to living organisms. In the human body, Pb poisoning interrupts the normal functioning of kidney, nervous and cardiovascular systems leading to mortality (Raj & Das, 2023). Hence, it is of much importance to detect the presence of Pb in environmental and human samples. Though several aptamers, polymers, organic and inorganic nanomaterials have been used to detect the presence of Pb(II) ions, they suffer from limitations such as usage of toxic substances and high cost. Due to minimum cost and usage of green precursors, CQDs have sparkled the attention in the detection of Pb(II). The green precursor, quantum yield of CQDs, the preparation technique used, linearity and LOD values are provided in Table 16.2.

TABLE 16.2

Detection of Pb(II) using Various Green CQDs

Precursor	Quantum Yield (%)	Preparation Technique	Linearity Range (µM)	Limit of Detection (nM)	References
BSA	–	Acid Hydrolysis	0 to 6×10^{-3}	5.05×10^3	Wee, Ng, and Ng (2013)
Sago waste	–	Pyrolysis	0.2 to 0.8	7.49×10^3	Tan, Romainor, Chin, and Ng (2014)
Potato-dextrose agar	9.0	Microwave	0 to 20	0.11	Gupta et al. (2016)
Chocolate	–	Hydrothermal	0.033 to 1.67	12.7	Y. Liu, Zhou, Li, Lei, and Yan (2016)
Ocimum sanctum leaves	9.3	Hydrothermal	10 to 1000	0.59	Kumar et al. (2017)
Table sugar	2.5	Microwave	–	67	Ansi & Renuka (2018)
Ginkgo biloba leaves	16.1	Hydrothermal	0.1 to 20×10^{-3}	0.055	J. Xu et al. (2018)
Lantana camara berries and EDA	33.1	Hydrothermal	0 to 200×10^{-3}	9.64	Bandi, Dadigala, Gangapuram, and Guttena (2018)
Biomass	22.6	Hydrothermal	1.3 to 106.7	–	Jing, Zhao, Sun, Zhong, and Peng, (2019)
Bamboo leaves	–	Solvothermal	0.6 to 800×10^{-3}	0.14	Z. Liu et al. (2019)

Recently, picomolar level detection of Pb(II) has been achieved using functionally modified CQDs prepared from watermelon juice. The functional groups such as ethanolamine and ethylenediamine have been attached to the CQDs during preparation, and they exhibited an enormous increase in the fluorescence intensity. The ethylenediamine-modified CQDs showed greater selectivity towards Pb(II) sensing with a LOD of 190 pM, which is much lesser than that of the permissible amount (72 nM) in drinking water (Rawat et al., 2023).

16.6 DETECTION OF ALUMINIUM (III)

The WHO has recommended the safe limit of Al (III) as 3 to 10 mg per day and 7 mg /Kg per week. Although it is important to human body, it must not exceed the safe level as it may cause a lot of health hazards such as bone weakness, Parkinson's disease, Alzheimer's disease and even breast cancer (Darbre, 2005). There are conventional methods to detect Al (III) such as high-performance liquid chromatography and atomic absorption spectroscopy. Recently due to their rapid detection time, carbon-based nanoparticles have attracted much interest in the detection of heavy metal ions including Al (III). Without the use of any harmful chemicals and surfactants, Yu et al developed N-doped CQDs via hydrothermal technique using *Osmanthus fragrans* possessing a high quantum yield of 21.9 %. It also showed good optical stability and excellent water dispersity. The prepared N-CQDs have been used as an off-on fluorescent switch sensor for the detection of Al (III). It was able to provide a linearity response in the range of 0.1 to 100 μmol/L with an LOD value of 26 nmol/L (C. Yu, Qin, Jiang, Zheng, & Deng, 2021). Jigna et al developed a mechanism using 'turn on' chelation-enhanced FL (CHEF) for the detection of Al (III) with the help of CQDs prepared using *Pyrus pyrifolia* fruit via hydrothermal method. The mechanism of CHEF was elucidated with the interaction of hard acid and the donor group to form a Al(III)-CQDs complex. When the developed nanosensor was investigated for practical application in real samples, no signal interference in the presence of anions, cations and pesticides was reported (Bhamore, Jha, Singhal, Park, & Kailasa, 2018).

16.7 DETECTION OF ARSENIC (III)

Arsenic can be found in almost 200 minerals, some of which are volatile in nature and are soluble rapidly in water leading to arsenic leaching in ground water source. CQDs prepared from banana leaves were subjected to computational studies and the structure modified with chlorophyll functionalization contained a hydroxyl group for the attachment of As(III). A strong dependence on the temperature of graphitization and carbonization of CQDs was observed (Bayazeed Alam et al., 2022). Ramezani et al. developed highly stable and multicolour CQDs using *Cydonia oblonga* as a carbon source and microwave irradiation technique in one pot. When characterized using microscopic techniques, the sizes of the prepared CQDs were found to be between 4.85 and 0.07 nM. The maximum emission intensity of the CQDs was at 45 nm with 85% of quantum yield. Mn(II) was formed when As(III) was added to MnO_4^{-1} and the subsequent addition of CQDs resulted in an enhanced PL signal via electron-hole pair recombination mechanism (2018). Radhakrishnan et al. made efforts to introduce a new simple technique for the preparation of surface-passivated CQDs using prickly pear cactus fruit. The prepared material also exhibited good solubility, optical properties and sensitivity towards the sensing of As(III). The practical applicability when tested in real water samples was satisfactory. Using lifetime PL, it was identified that the PL quenching mechanism was static. An LOD of 2.3 nM for the detection of As(III) was achieved successfully (Radhakrishnan & Panneerselvam, 2018).

16.8 DETECTION OF CADMIUM (II)

Cadmium is regarded as one of the most hazardous and toxic metals which is widely used in cigarettes, batteries and plastic colorations. Cadmium greatly affects plants by destroying their cell membrane and organelles and disrupts their metabolism (Haider et al., 2021). It also leads to kidney failure and cancers in human. The disease called itai-itai in Japan has been reported due to the accumulation of cadmium in human body. So, it is very important to detect cadmium efficiently. The CQDs obtained from *Polyalthia longifolia* leaves using hydrothermal method via bottom-up approach was named as p-CQDs and utilized for the detection of cadmium. The sensing of cadmium was done at room temperature through fluorescence quenching method. A wide range of concentrations ranging from 7.3 nM to 12 µM of Cd (II) was taken to examine the p-CQDS's quenching mechanism. The intensity of PL was observed to be inversely related to the concentration of the analyte. The functional groups present at p-CQD surfaces were ascribed to the effective quenching mechanism. The p-CQDs demonstrated good sensitivity and selectivity with a LOD value of 2.4 nM. The real sample analysis done in tap water and industrial effluents showed a recovery of 98 to 101% (Sariga, Ayilliath Kolaprath, Benny, & Varghese, 2023).

16.9 DETECTION OF COBALT (II)

Cobalt is an important trace element that plays an essential role in the human metabolic system. It is capable of regulating the enzyme catalytic activities and stimulating the creation of red blood cells. But when consumed in excessive amount, it can lead to several diseases and conditions such as asthma, low blood pressure, diarrhoea, dermatitis and myocardial infarction (C. L. Li et al., 2015). As Co(II) is also used in batteries, paints, pigments, mining and others, it also causes several environmental problems. So the detection and monitoring of Co(II) is very important. A one-pot microwave irradiation method was established by Zhao et al. for the detection of Co(II) using a natural material kelp as the carbon source. Their method has been reported as a green, facile and economical method for the preparation of CQDs. The efficiency of quantum yield and size of the prepared CQDs was calculated to 23.5% and 3.7 nm, respectively. A good stability up to 2 months was established via fluorescence intensity study. A good linearity in the concentration range of 1 to 200 µmol/L with a LOD value of 0.39 µmol/L for the detection of Co(II) was observed. The real sample analysis in water samples proved that the prepared material possessed great potential prospects in the sensing of Co(II)(C. Zhao, Li, Cheng, & Yang,

2019a). Nitrogen-doped CQDs (N-CQDs) with improved efficiency was reported by Dutta et al. The N-CQDs were prepared from *Nerium Oleander* petals as the carbon source through hydrothermal method. The quenching of N-CQDs and Rhodamine 6G (Rh6G) takes place simultaneously due to the hindrance of the FRET process and the absorbance of metal ions through Brownian movement when Co(II) is added. The sensor showed good selectivity and sensitivity with a LOD of 6.45 nM towards the detection of Co(II)(Dutta, Rooj, Mondal, Mukherjee, & Mandal, 2020).

16.10   DETECTION OF ZINC (II)

Zinc (Zn) is a necessary trace element needed for the functioning of several biological processes such as immunity, inheritance, growth and incretion. Zn ions are used in various industrial processes, including galvanization and metal plating. Monitoring their presence and concentration ensures the quality and efficiency of these processes, preventing defects and minimizing waste. So, the analysis of content of zinc is inevitable. The impact of zinc ions on bio sourced cyanobacterial-derived blue-green fluorescent CQDs originating from camphor revealing a pronounced quenching phenomenon has been reported (Gaddam, Vasudevan, Narayan, & Raju, 2014).

16.11   DETECTION OF SILVER (I)

Silver in the form of Ag(I) stands out as a highly perilous and widespread pollutant, causing significant repercussions for both aquatic ecosystems and human well-being. Consequently, the identification of Ag(I) has emerged as a crucial undertaking, prompting endeavours employing diverse analytical methodologies. An environmentally friendly and cost-effective approach to synthesize water-soluble fluorescent CQDs has been reported in another study. These CQDs were designed for the specific identification of Ag(I) ions using a single-step hydrothermal process involving the edible green vegetable Broccoli (Arumugam & Kim, 2018). The developed CQDs were analysed both under exposure to ultraviolet and natural daylight. When illuminated by daylight, the solution of CQDs exhibited a transparent, light-brown appearance. Conversely, under ultraviolet light, the initial CQDs displayed vibrant blue luminescence without requiring any additional modifications. The CQDs that were prepared emitted a robust light at a wavelength of 450 nm, and their photoluminescence intensity decreased upon the addition of varying concentrations of Ag(I). This outcome can be attributed to the energy transfer occurring between Ag^+ ions and the oxygen functional groups situated on the CQDs' surface, leading to the formation of chelate complexes. As a result of these complexes, the luminescence of the CQDs is significantly quenched. Additionally, the CQDs exhibit substantial quenching behaviour towards Ag ions, with a notably low limit of detection (LOD) of 0.5 μM. Another unique type of CQDs, originating from biomass, was successfully created through a singular hydrothermal process involving purple perilla. These CQDs exhibit exceptional water solubility, intense fluorescence, and favourable biocompatibility. Employing the phenomenon of fluorescence quenching in CQDs, the freshly synthesized CQDs were ingeniously harnessed as an innovative 'signal-off' fluorescent tool. This tool is adept at discerning and sensitively identifying Ag^+, boasting two distinct linear measurement ranges: 0–10 and 10–3000 nM, with an impressively low detection threshold of 1.4 nM. The credibility of this fluorescent method's specificity and selectivity was further demonstrated by rigorous tests involving similar metallic cations and authentic water samples (X. Zhao, Liao, Wang, Liu, & Chen, 2019b).

Fluorescent carbon dots (CDs) doped with nitrogen and sulphur were successfully prepared with the help of caffeine as a raw material in a single-step, environmentally friendly and economical solid-state method. These CDs emitted a distinct blue fluorescence, boasting a quantum yield of 38%. Capitalizing on this robust blue fluorescence, the CDs produced in this research held promise as an efficient fluorescence tool for detecting Ag^+ ions, showcasing exceptional sensitivity and selectivity. In parallel, Ag^+ ions exhibited a strong attraction to and rapid interaction with the functional groups (amino, carboxyl and hydroxyl groups) present on the surface of the designated 'u-CDs.' This interaction led to alterations in the electronic makeup of the u-CDs, impacting the distribution of excitons. This, in turn, facilitated the non-radiative recombination of excitons through an efficient electron transfer process. Furthermore, as the concentration of Ag(I) ions was progressively elevated from 50 nM to 500 µM, a clear and linear decline in the photoluminescence (PL) intensity was observed. This conspicuous trend underscores the heightened sensitivity of the u-CDs towards Ag^+ ions. In another investigation, a green approach was employed to create nitrogen-doped carbon dots (NCDs) that are water soluble. This was achieved through a single-step hydrothermal process involving pomegranate juice and NH_4OH (Akhgari, Farhadi, Samadi, & Akhgari, 2020). These economical NCDs display strong fluorescence, peaking at 395 nm. When exposed to silver nanoparticles (AgNPs) in the presence of L-cysteine, they demonstrate a specific quenching effect due to an inner filter mechanism. The potential of this method was gauged by employing it to quantify AgNPs in environmental water samples through spiking. The straightforward nature of this approach, coupled with its reliable recovery outcomes, presents a fresh and ecologically sound technique for the swift and selective assessment of AgNPs in environmental water settings. It exhibits a detection limit 3.8×10^{-10} M.

16.12 DETECTION OF GOLD (III)

Au(I) and Au(II) are the two existing oxidation states of gold. Compared to the metallic gold, Au(III) serves as a potentially toxic material to the human body. A large amount of gold-containing waste products are released into the environment, which in turn results in adverse health hazards damaging the kidney, liver and peripheral nervous system. Apart from human health, it also affects the ecosystem. Hence, it is highly necessary to sense Au(III) (Kundu, Layek, Kuila, & Nandi, 2012). In another study, N-CQDs were prepared using a mixture of natural peach gum polysaccharide and EDA via one-pot hydrothermal technique for the detection of Au(III). The quantum yield efficiency Dots the prepared N-CQDs was found to be 28.46%. A strong fluorescence quenching effect was observed with high sensitivity and selectivity towards the detection of Au(III). The real sample analysis done in river water demonstrated its capability to be utilized in practical applications. The LOD value is found to be 6.4×10^{-8} M, which is quite comparable to other reports (Liao, Cheng, & Zhou, 2016). Water-soluble N-CQDs were prepared from a mixture of gum tragacanth and EDA.

The mechanism of fluorescence quenching was supported by both FRET and synergistic effect. A high sensitivity and selectivity towards Au(III) was reported with a linearity range of 1–100 µM and a LOD value of 2.69 µM (Rahmani & Ghaemy, 2019).

16.13   CHALLENGES AND FUTURE PERSPECTIVES

This chapter has summarized the recent progress of naturally derived green CQDs for the sensing of metal ions and their immense development in the last decade. But still, some challenges must be addressed for the application and possible scalability of CQDs as an economically viable senor probe. The major requirements for enhanced sensitivity of CQDs are narrow bandwidth of the fluorescence signal and emission from the complete visible spectrum. However, currently the stability and signal intensity of green CQDs are lower when compared to chemically synthesized CQDs. In recent days, researchers are trying to discover the possible inexpensively feasible technique for the purification of CQDs.

Though there have been lot of literatures citing the synthesis of green CQDs, there are still unexplored sustainable precursors such as bioresiduals, biomaterials and recycled wastes which may result in higher quantum yield. Though there is understanding towards the preparation mechanism of CQDs, it is important to recognize the reason behind the precursor-based specificity of CQDs towards the target metal ion sensing. Modification of the surface of CQDs through doping and functionalization with 2D and 3D nanomaterials can enhance the efficiency of the sensing probe in the UV-visible-NIR region. It is evident that the future exploration towards the development of CQDs using natural sources will gain attention in a variety of sensing applications owing to its simple, biocompatible and cost-effective nature.

16.14   STRATEGIES TO ENHANCE SELECTIVITY AND SENSITIVITY OF METAL IONS

The main disadvantage of using green precursors for the production of CQDs is that they are selective towards various metal ions for detection. It is necessary to enhance the sensitivity and selectivity of the prepared CQDs without compromising their chemical, optical and biological properties. On the other hand, development of genetically engineered biomass comprising specific metabolic mechanisms can improve the optical sensing responses. It is also necessary to improve the signal amplification for onsite real-time detections. This can be done by the passivation of CQDs with various polymer-based functionalizations. The combination of other nanomaterials and nanoparticles with CQDs can be done to improve their overall properties. Thus, the signal amplification, selectivity and sensitivity of CQDs can be improved.

REFERENCES

Abbaspour, N., Hurrell, R., & Kelishadi, R. (2014). Review on iron and its importance for human health. *Journal of Research in Medical Sciences* 2014;19, 164–74. *Journal of Research in Medical Sciences*, (February), 3–11.

Akhgari, F., Farhadi, K., Samadi, N., & Akhgari, M. (2020). Detection of silver nanoparticles using green synthesis of fluorescent nitrogen-doped carbon dots. *Iranian Journal of Science and Technology, Transaction A: Science, 44*(2), 379–387. doi:10.1007/s40995-020-00832-4

Ansi, V. A., & Renuka, N. K. (2018). Table sugar derived Carbon dot: A naked eye sensor for toxic Pb2+ ions. *Sensors and Actuators, B: Chemical, 264,* 67–75. doi:10.1016/j.snb.2018.02.167

Arumugam, N., & Kim, J. (2018). Synthesis of carbon quantum dots from Broccoli and their ability to detect silver ions. *Materials Letters, 219*(February), 37–40. doi:10.1016/j.matlet.2018.02.043

Bandi, R., Dadigala, R., Gangapuram, B. R., & Guttena, V. (2018). Green synthesis of highly fluorescent nitrogen: Doped carbon dots from Lantana camara berries for effective detection of lead(II) and bioimaging. *Journal of Photochemistry and Photobiology B: Biology, 178*(November 2017), 330–338. doi:10.1016/j.jphotobiol.2017.11.010

Bano, D., Kumar, V., Singh, V. K., & Hasan, S. H. (2018). Green synthesis of fluorescent carbon quantum dots for the detection of mercury(ii) and glutathione. *New Journal of Chemistry, 42*(8), 5814–5821. doi:10.1039/c8nj00432c

Bayazeed Alam, M., Hassan, N., Sahoo, K., Kumar, M., Sharma, M., Lahiri, J., & Singh Parmar, A. (2022). Deciphering interaction between chlorophyll functionalized carbon quantum dots with arsenic and mercury toxic metals in water as highly sensitive dual-probe sensor. *Journal of Photochemistry and Photobiology A: Chemistry, 431*(May), 114059. doi:10.1016/j.jphotochem.2022.114059

Bhamore, J. R., Jha, S., Singhal, R. K., Park, T. J., & Kailasa, S. K. (2018). Facile green synthesis of carbon dots from Pyrus pyrifolia fruit for assaying of Al3+ ion via chelation enhanced fluorescence mechanism. *Journal of Molecular Liquids, 264*(2017), 9–16. doi:10.1016/j.molliq.2018.05.041

Chaudhary, N., Gupta, P. K., Eremin, S., & Solanki, P. R. (2020). One-step green approach to synthesize highly fluorescent carbon quantum dots from banana juice for selective detection of copper ions. *Journal of Environmental Chemical Engineering, 8*(3), 103720. doi:10.1016/j.jece.2020.103720

Darbre, P. D. (2005). Aluminium, antiperspirants and breast cancer. *Journal of Inorganic Biochemistry, 99*(9 SPEC. ISS), 1912–1919. doi:10.1016/j.jinorgbio.2005.06.001

Das, M., Thakkar, H., Patel, D., & Thakore, S. (2021). Repurposing the domestic organic waste into green emissive carbon dots and carbonized adsorbent: A sustainable zero waste process for metal sensing and dye sequestration. *Journal of Environmental Chemical Engineering, 9*(5), 106312. doi:10.1016/j.jece.2021.106312

Desai, M. L., Jha, S., Basu, H., Singhal, R. K., Park, T. J., & Kailasa, S. K. (2019). Acid oxidation of muskmelon fruit for the fabrication of carbon dots with specific emission colors for recognition of Hg2+ ions and cell imaging. *ACS Omega, 4*(21), 19332–19340. doi:10.1021/acsomega.9b02730

Ding, S., Gao, Y., Ni, B., & Yang, X. (2021). Green synthesis of biomass-derived carbon quantum dots as fluorescent probe for Fe^{3+} detection. *Inorganic Chemistry Communications, 130*(February 2020), 108636. doi:10.1016/j.inoche.2021.108636

Dutta, A., Rooj, B., Mondal, T., Mukherjee, D., & Mandal, U. (2020). Detection of Co2+ via fluorescence resonance energy transfer between synthesized nitrogen-doped carbon quantum dots and Rhodamine 6G. *Journal of the Iranian Chemical Society, 17*(7), 1695–1704. doi:10.1007/s13738-020-01891-5

Gaddam, R. R., Vasudevan, D., Narayan, R., & Raju, K. V. S. N. (2014). Controllable synthesis of biosourced blue-green fluorescent carbon dots from camphor for the detection of heavy metal ions in water. *RSC Advances, 4*(100), 57137–57143. doi:10.1039/c4ra10471d

Gharat, P. M., Pal, H., & Dutta Choudhury, S. (2019). Photophysics and luminescence quenching of carbon dots derived from lemon juice and glycerol. *Spectrochimica Acta - Part A: Molecular and Biomolecular Spectroscopy, 209,* 14–21. doi:10.1016/j.saa.2018.10.029

Gu, D., Shang, S., Yu, Q., & Shen, J. (2016). Green synthesis of nitrogen-doped carbon dots from lotus root for Hg(II) ions detection and cell imaging. *Applied Surface Science, 390*(Ii), 38–42. doi:10.1016/j.apsusc.2016.08.012

Gupta, A., Verma, N. C., Khan, S., Tiwari, S., Chaudhary, A., & Nandi, C. K. (2016). Paper strip based and live cell ultrasensitive lead sensor using carbon dots synthesized from biological media. *Sensors and Actuators, B: Chemical, 232*, 107–114. doi:10.1016/j.snb.2016.03.110

Haider, F. U., Liqun, C., Coulter, J. A., Cheema, S. A., Wu, J., Zhang, R., … Farooq, M. (2021). Cadmium toxicity in plants: Impacts and remediation strategies. *Ecotoxicology and Environmental Safety, 211*, 111887. doi:10.1016/j.ecoenv.2020.111887

Huang, H., Lv, J. J., Zhou, D. L., Bao, N., Xu, Y., Wang, A. J., & Feng, J. J. (2013). One-pot green synthesis of nitrogen-doped carbon nanoparticles as fluorescent probes for mercury ions. *RSC Advances, 3*(44), 21691–21696. doi:10.1039/c3ra43452d

Jing, S., Zhao, Y., Sun, R. C., Zhong, L., & Peng, X. (2019). Facile and high-yield synthesis of carbon quantum dots from biomass-derived carbons at mild condition. *ACS Sustainable Chemistry and Engineering, 7*(8), 7833–7843. research-article. doi:10.1021/acssuschemeng.9b00027

Kasinathan, K., Samayanan, S., Marimuthu, K., & Yim, J. H. (2022). Green synthesis of multicolour fluorescence carbon quantum dots from sugarcane waste: Investigation of mercury (II) ion sensing, and bio-imaging applications. *Applied Surface Science, 601*(March), 154266. doi:10.1016/j.apsusc.2022.154266

Kumar, A., Chowdhuri, A. R., Laha, D., Mahto, T. K., Karmakar, P., & Sahu, S. K. (2017). Green synthesis of carbon dots from Ocimum sanctum for effective fluorescent sensing of Pb2+ ions and live cell imaging. *Sensors and Actuators, B: Chemical, 242*, 679–686. doi:10.1016/j.snb.2016.11.109

Kundu, A., Layek, R. K., Kuila, A., & Nandi, A. K. (2012). Highly fluorescent graphene oxide-poly(vinyl alcohol) hybrid: An effective material for specific Au^{3+} ion sensors. *ACS Applied Materials and Interfaces, 4*(10), 5576–5582. doi:10.1021/am301467z

Li, C. L., Huang, C. C., Periasamy, A. P., Roy, P., Wu, W. C., Hsu, C. L., & Chang, H. T. (2015). Synthesis of photoluminescent carbon dots for the detection of cobalt ions. *RSC Advances, 5*(3), 2285–2291. doi:10.1039/c4ra11704b

Li, L. S., Jiao, X. Y., Zhang, Y., Cheng, C., Huang, K., & Xu, L. (2018). Green synthesis of fluorescent carbon dots from Hongcaitai for selective detection of hypochlorite and mercuric ions and cell imaging. *Sensors and Actuators, B: Chemical, 263*, 426–435. doi:10.1016/j.snb.2018.02.141

Liao, J., Cheng, Z., & Zhou, L. (2016). Nitrogen-Doping enhanced fluorescent carbon dots: Green synthesis and their applications for bioimaging and label-free detection of Au3+ ions. *ACS Sustainable Chemistry and Engineering, 4*(6), 3053–3061. doi:10.1021/acssuschemeng.6b00018

Liu, Y., Zhou, Q., Li, J., Lei, M., & Yan, X. (2016). Selective and sensitive chemosensor for lead ions using fluorescent carbon dots prepared from chocolate by one-step hydrothermal method. *Sensors and Actuators, B: Chemical, 237*, 597–604. doi:10.1016/j.snb.2016.06.092

Liu, Z., Jin, W., Wang, F., Li, T., Nie, J., Xiao, W., … Zhang, Y. (2019). Ratiometric fluorescent sensing of Pb2+ and Hg2+ with two types of carbon dot nanohybrids synthesized from the same biomass. *Sensors and Actuators, B: Chemical, 296*(February), 126698. doi:10.1016/j.snb.2019.126698

Lu, W., Qin, X., Liu, S., Chang, G., Zhang, Y., Luo, Y., … Sun, X. (2012). Economical, green synthesis of fluorescent carbon nanoparticles and their use as probes for sensitive and selective detection of mercury(II) ions. *Analytical Chemistry, 84*(12), 5351–5357. doi:10.1021/ac3007939

Nagaraj, M., Ramalingam, S., Murugan, C., Aldawood, S., Jin, J. O., Choi, I., & Kim, M. (2022). Detection of Fe^{3+} ions in aqueous environment using fluorescent carbon quantum dots synthesized from endosperm of Borassus flabellifer. *Environmental Research, 212*(PB), 113273. doi:10.1016/j.envres.2022.113273

Pourreza, N., & Ghomi, M. (2019). Green synthesized carbon quantum dots from *Prosopis juliflora* leaves as a dual off-on fluorescence probe for sensing mercury (II) and chemet drug. *Materials Science and Engineering C, 98*(January), 887–896. doi:10.1016/j.msec.2018.12.141

Preethi, M., Viswanathan, C., & Ponpandian, N. (2022). Fluorescence quenching mechanism of P-doped carbon quantum dots as fluorescent sensor for Cu^{2+} ions. *Colloids and Surfaces A: Physicochemical and Engineering Aspects, 653*(August), 129942. doi:10.1016/j.colsurfa.2022.129942

Preethi, Manoharan, Viswanathan, C., & Ponpandian, N. (2021). A green path to extract carbon quantum dots by coconut water: Another fluorescent probe towards Fe^{3+} ions. *Particuology, 58*, 251–258. doi:10.1016/j.partic.2021.03.019

Qin, X., Lu, W., Asiri, A. M., Al-Youbi, A. O., & Sun, X. (2013). Microwave-assisted rapid green synthesis of photoluminescent carbon nanodots from flour and their applications for sensitive and selective detection of mercury(II) ions. *Sensors and Actuators, B: Chemical, 184*, 156–162. doi:10.1016/j.snb.2013.04.079

Radhakrishnan, K., & Panneerselvam, P. (2018). Green synthesis of surface-passivated carbon dots from the prickly pear cactus as a fluorescent probe for the dual detection of arsenic(iii) and hypochlorite ions from drinking water. *RSC Advances, 8*(53), 30455–30467. doi:10.1039/c8ra05861j

Rahmani, Z., & Ghaemy, M. (2019). One-step hydrothermal-assisted synthesis of highly fluorescent N-doped carbon dots from gum tragacanth: Luminescent stability and sensitive probe for Au3+ ions. *Optical Materials, 97*(August), 109356. doi:10.1016/j.optmat.2019.109356

Raj, K., & Das, A. P. (2023). Lead pollution: Impact on environment and human health and approach for a sustainable solution. *Environmental Chemistry and Ecotoxicology, 5*(February), 79–85. doi:10.1016/j.enceco.2023.02.001

Ramezani, Z., Qorbanpour, M., & Rahbar, N. (2018). Green synthesis of carbon quantum dots using quince fruit (Cydonia oblonga) powder as carbon precursor: Application in cell imaging and As3+ determination. *Colloids and Surfaces A: Physicochemical and Engineering Aspects, 549*, 58–66. doi:10.1016/j.colsurfa.2018.04.006

Rawat, K. S., Singh, V., Sharma, C. P., Vyas, A., Pandey, P., Singh, J., … Goel, A. (2023). Picomolar Detection of Lead Ions (Pb2+) by functionally modified fluorescent carbon quantum dots from watermelon juice and their imaging in cancer cells. *Journal of Imaging, 9*(1), 0–12. doi:10.3390/jimaging9010019

Sariga, Ayilliath Kolaprath, M. K., Benny, L., & Varghese, A. (2023). A facile, green synthesis of carbon quantum dots from *Polyalthia longifolia* and its application for the selective detection of cadmium. *Dyes and Pigments, 210*(December 2022), 111048. doi:10.1016/j.dyepig.2022.111048

Singh, A. K., Singh, V. K., Singh, M., Singh, P., Khadim, S. R., Singh, U., … Asthana, R. K. (2019). One pot hydrothermal synthesis of fluorescent NP-carbon dots derived from *Dunaliella salina* biomass and its application in on-off sensing of Hg (II), Cr (VI) and live cell imaging. *Journal of Photochemistry and Photobiology A: Chemistry, 376*(November 2018), 63–72. doi:10.1016/j.jphotochem.2019.02.023

Srinivasan, K., Subramanian, K., Murugan, K., & Dinakaran, K. (2016). Sensitive fluorescence detection of mercury(II) in aqueous solution by the fluorescence quenching effect of MoS2 with DNA functionalized carbon dots. *Analyst, 141*(22), 6344–6352. doi:10.1039/c6an00879h

Tadesse, A., Hagos, M., Ramadevi, D., Basavaiah, K., & Belachew, N. (2020). Fluorescent-Nitrogen-Doped carbon quantum dots derived from citrus lemon juice: Green Synthesis, Mercury(II) Ion Sensing, and Live Cell Imaging. *ACS Omega, 5*(8), 3889–3898. doi:10.1021/acsomega.9b03175

Tan, X. W., Romainor, A. N. B., Chin, S. F., & Ng, S. M. (2014). Carbon dots production via pyrolysis of sago waste as potential probe for metal ions sensing. *Journal of Analytical and Applied Pyrolysis, 105*, 157–165. doi:10.1016/j.jaap.2013.11.001

Vandarkuzhali, S. A. A., Natarajan, S., Jeyabalan, S., Sivaraman, G., Singaravadivel, S., Muthusubramanian, S., & Viswanathan, B. (2018). Pineapple peel-derived carbon dots: Applications as sensor, molecular keypad lock, and memory device. *ACS Omega, 3*(10), 12584–12592. research-article. doi:10.1021/acsomega.8b01146

Wang, Chunfeng, Sun, D., Zhuo, K., Zhang, H., & Wang, J. (2014). Simple and green synthesis of nitrogen-, sulfur-, and phosphorus-co-doped carbon dots with tunable luminescence properties and sensing application. *RSC Advances, 4*(96), 54060–54065. doi:10.1039/c4ra10885j

Wang, Cunjin, Shi, H., Yang, M., Yan, Y., Liu, E., Ji, Z., & Fan, J. (2020). Facile synthesis of novel carbon quantum dots from biomass waste for highly sensitive detection of iron ions. *Materials Research Bulletin, 124*, 110730. doi:10.1016/j.materresbull.2019.110730

Wee, S. S., Ng, Y. H., & Ng, S. M. (2013). Synthesis of fluorescent carbon dots via simple acid hydrolysis of bovine serum albumin and its potential as sensitive sensing probe for lead (II) ions. *Talanta, 116*, 71–76. doi:10.1016/j.talanta.2013.04.081

Xu, J., Jie, X., Xie, F., Yang, H., Wei, W., & Xia, Z. (2018). Flavonoid moiety-incorporated carbon dots for ultrasensitive and highly selective fluorescence detection and removal of Pb2+. *Nano Research, 11*(7), 3648–3657. doi:10.1007/s12274-017-1931-6

Xu, Y., Lan, J., Wang, B., Bo, C., Ou, J., & Gong, B. (2023). Simple fabrication of carbon quantum dots and activated carbon from waste wolfberry stems for detection and adsorption of copper ion. *RSC Advances, 13*(31), 21199–21210. doi:10.1039/d3ra04026g

Ye, Z., Zhang, Y., Li, G., & Li, B. (2020). Fluorescent Determination of Mercury(II) by green carbon quantum dots synthesized from eggshell membrane. *Analytical Letters, 53*(18), 2841–2853. doi:10.1080/00032719.2020.1759618

Yu, C., Qin, D., Jiang, X., Zheng, X., & Deng, B. (2021). N-doped carbon quantum dots from *Osmanthus fragrans* as a novel off-on fluorescent nanosensor for highly sensitive detection of quercetin and aluminium ion, and cell imaging. *Journal of Pharmaceutical and Biomedical Analysis, 192*. Elsevier B.V. doi:10.1016/j.jpba.2020.113673

Yu, J., Song, N., Zhang, Y. K., Zhong, S. X., Wang, A. J., & Chen, J. (2015). Green preparation of carbon dots by Jinhua bergamot for sensitive and selective fluorescent detection of Hg²⁺ and Fe³⁺. *Sensors and Actuators, B: Chemical, 214*(3), 29–35. doi:10.1016/j.snb.2015.03.006

Zhang, Q., Zhang, X., Bao, L., Wu, Y., Jiang, L., Zheng, Y., … Chen, Y. (2019). The application of green-synthesis-derived carbon quantum dots to bioimaging and the analysis of mercury(II). *Journal of Analytical Methods in Chemistry, 2019*(Ii). doi:10.1155/2019/8183134

Zhao, C., Li, X., Cheng, C., & Yang, Y. (2019a). Green and microwave-assisted synthesis of carbon dots and application for visual detection of cobalt(II) ions and pH sensing. *Microchemical Journal, 147*(January), 183–190. doi:10.1016/j.microc.2019.03.029

Zhao, P., Zhang, Q., Cao, J., Qian, C., Ye, J., Xu, S., … Li, Y. (2022). Facile and green synthesis of highly fluorescent carbon quantum dots from water hyacinth for the detection of ferric iron and cellular imaging. *Nanomaterials, 12*(9). doi:10.3390/nano12091528

Zhao, X., Liao, S., Wang, L., Liu, Q., & Chen, X. (2019b). Facile green and one-pot synthesis of purple perilla derived carbon quantum dot as a fluorescent sensor for silver ion. *Talanta, 201*(March), 1–8. doi:10.1016/j.talanta.2019.03.095

17 Environmental Issues Associated with Carbon Quantum Dots

S. Arun Sasi, Muhammed Shukkoor Kondengaden and Robert M. Pontrelli

17.1 INTRODUCTION

Carbon quantum dots (CQD) have good electrical and chemical properties, high stability, low toxicity, environmental friendliness nature, strong photoluminescence, and optical functions (Qu et al., 2018; Du & Guo, 2016). Recently, nontoxic, affordable, and biocompatible carbon nanoparticles have been developed to replace their poisonous counterparts. Due to their low cost and toxicity, CQDs are currently being researched as potential safe substitutes for metal-based nanostructures acting as environmental probes (Ahmed & Emam, 2020). Due to their distinctive features, quantum dots (QDs) have generated interest for a variety of environmental applications. Moreover, quantum dots have potential applications in technology, research, and medicine. The second-most mentioned nanoparticles in commercial products are carbon-based nanomaterials, which are produced on a massive scale and include graphene, graphene oxide, carbon nanotubes, fullerenes, and CQDs (Weinberg et al., 2011). As a result, there has been a lot of interest in the development, properties, and uses of CQDs. Large-scale production of carbon-based nanomaterials, such as graphene, graphene oxide, carbon nanotubes, fullerenes, and CQDs, makes them the second most mentioned type of nanomaterial in commercial goods. CQDs can be synthesized and functionalized quickly and easily Due to their high hydrophilicity, cell permeability, and a wide range of applications, the biosafety of CQDs needs attention. On the other hand, the ecological implications of CQDs are not well studied. Some early studies showed that CQDs were highly biocompatible and environmentally friendly. Before large-scale commercial use of CQDs, their toxicity and environmental effects must be thoroughly investigated to ensure biosafety (Li et al., 2020).

17.2 ROUTES OF EXPOSURE

Major routes of CQD exposure are environmental, workplace, and therapeutic administration (Hardman, 2006). Engineers and researchers, for example, may be exposed at work mostly by ingestion, skin contact, or inhalation. Larger aerosolized

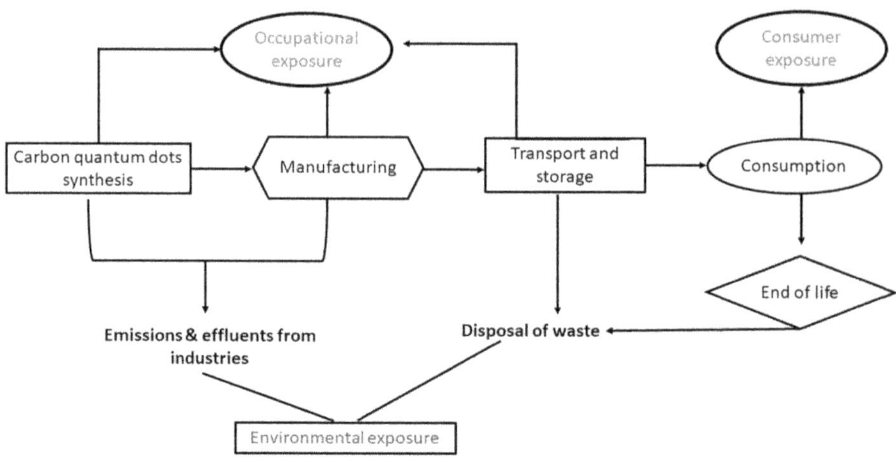

FIGURE 17.1   Life cycle of carbon quantum dot products and environmental exposure ways.

CQDs deposit in bronchial gaps, while CQDs larger than 2.5 nm may penetrate the lung deep and interact with the alveolar epithelium, according to studies. Inhalation exposure may pose potential risks due to QDs; it has been shown to participate by endocytosis according to several cell types (Figure 17.1).

17.3   ENVIRONMENTAL IMPACTS

Assessing QD exposure routes and potential toxicity is difficult because toxicity depends on multiple physicochemical and environmental factors (Hoet et al. 2004; Hardman 2006). As concerns grow about engineered nanoparticles, ecotoxicological and environmental risk assessment data of QDs are limited compared to other nanoparticles (Wang & Nowack, 2018).

Cadmium tellurium (CdTe) or cadmium selenium (CdSe) are frequently found in the core of QDs. Depending on the size of the QDs particle, these nanocrystalline cores offer broad emission spectra (Ahmad et al., 2012; Feswick et al., 2013). Other concerns included the materials' compatibility with capping agents, their capacity to hold particles larger than a particular size, biological magnification, and the inorganic materials' disintegration and dissolution (Bottrill & Green, 2011). However, it is well recognized that the environment and living things are negatively impacted by these commercial nanocrystalline cores. Comparing uses in sensors and electronics with those in biomedical and packaging, larger concentrations of QDs may be discharged into the environment (Wang & Nowack, 2018). Throughout the lifecycle of QDs or QD-enabled products, environmental emissions might happen at many stages, such as synthesis, manufacture, application, and end-of-life (Hardman, 2006; Gallagher et al., 2018). QDs have the potential to be released into the environment in product form or altered in products before, during, or after environmental release.

In manufacturing facilities and research labs, QDs may leak out during synthesis. Quantum dots can be released into the environment as they are used in products, or they can change while being released into the environment or thereafter. Environmental releases can occur at various phases of the QD's or QD-enabled product's lifecycle, including synthesis, manufacturing, application, and end-of-life (Hardman, 2006; Gallagher et al. 2018).

17.4 IMPACT OF CARBON QUANTUM DOTS ON AQUATIC ENVIRONMENT

Aqueous and marine environment has an enormous pool of biodiversity. Moreover, aquatic bio-organisms depict a diverse niche of ecosystem, which has a pivotal role in the ecosystem stability and food chain. Compared to freshwater, seawater allows QDs to agglomerate more easily and silt more readily. QDs are mostly accumulated and sediment easily and quickly in seawater compared to freshwater (Rocha et al., 2014). Concern over the ecotoxicological effects of QDs on aquatic life is developing, especially in light of their physicochemical changes in the environment and the release of hazardous metals (Rocha et al., 2016). Due to their innate physicochemical characteristics, nanomaterials have a direct impact on the living conditions of aquatic species. In 2016, another study by Silva and team reported the environmental implications of cadmium-based quantum dots towards aquatic environment. Comparison of the toxicity of CQDs to species at various trophic levels: effects on aquatic habitats has also been done (Yao et al., 2018). The primary cause of QD release during product storage and transit will be product breakage or mishandling (Lazareva & Keller, 2014). Our use-phase estimates indicate that, in comparison to uses in sensors and electronics, greater volumes of QDs may be released into the environment in biomedical and packaging applications (Wang & Nowack, 2018). Carbon quantum dots inevitably enter the natural environment and are widely distributed in water, their ecological impact on the natural environment, especially the aquatic environment, was studied (Sun et al., 2022). Within the range of solar energy that reaches the earth's surface, CQDs absorb it (Frank et al., 2020). Moreover, when sunlight reaches the surface of natural waterways, CQDs will rapidly photobleach (i.e., lose their distinctive fluorescence signal). Besides, several studies reported that, the final breakdown structurally stable carbon QDs reactions with hydroxyl radicals' solar radiation (Giroux et al., 2022; Sun et al., 2022). Tang et al. (2013) studied the CQD toxicity in freshwater zebra fish liver cell.

Compared to metal-based carbon dots carbon-based QDs have higher colloid stability in water systems due to their strong surface charge and low density. Depending on their structure, CQDs can degrade rapidly under the influence of sunlight or persist in water for decades (Pakarinen et al., 2013). Some of the byproducts of the reaction between hydroxyl radicals and carbon quantum dots can persist for decades (Chen et al., 2019). Conflicts between metals and carbon-based QD studies are probably due to newer one's tendency to produce and use carbon-based QDs, which are presumably less toxic than metal QDs (Giroux et al., 2022). Carbon quantum dots previously thought to be biocompatible or environmentally friendly can also stimulate prophecies due to the presence of light-activated redox species.

17.5 ECOTOXICOLOGY OF CARBON QUANTUM DOTS

Degraded CQDs may reach the bio-organisms through diverse pathways like food chain and aquatic pathways which may cause systemic and genotoxic effects (Rocha et al., 2014). Improved understanding of the mobility, bioavailability, and assessing the environmental risks associated with engineered nanomaterials is necessary to consider their ecotoxicity (Nowack & Bucheli, 2007). Carbon quantum dots are discharged into the atmosphere are influenced by elements in the environment as light, oxidants, or microorganisms. In the aquatic environment. Carbon quantum dots are discharged into the atmosphere and are influenced by elements in the environment as light, oxidants, or microorganisms. In the aquatic environment, CQDs will interact with the dissolved organic material (DOM), and this interaction will affect their presence in the water column. Carbon-based nanoparticles (e.g., single-walled carbon nanotubes) have also shown very limited acute toxicity to aquatic organisms (Parks et al., 2013; Freixa et al., 2018). Carbon quantum dots witness the environment difficult because toxicity varies widely chemical state of metals. Removal of CQD materials and the risk of leaks and spills during production and traffic are possible sources of concern. Testing CQDs in the environment is difficult because toxicity varies widely with the chemical state of metals and environment conversion/degradation. Ecotoxicological studies of carbon-based nanomaterials present a major difficulty because carbon nanomaterials have poor aqueous solubility (Ham et al., 2005) (Figure 17.2).

17.6 BIOACCUMULATION

Quantum dots (QDs) can be internalized and lead to oral exposure through food chain transfer (trophic transfer) at higher trophic levels. This process of QD transfer to higher trophic levels is reliant on environmental factors and QD uptake in food sources. Moreover, due to the robust encapsulation of QDs in products, QDs from commercial products in conditions similar to landfills exhibited low release of dissolved metals. When production and use of QDs increase, their environmental release remains comparatively low when compared to other artificial nanoparticles (Derfus et al., 2004). According to recent toxicological analyses, CQDs have been shown to be either low or harmless to mammalian cells and animals when used in bioimaging. The first *in vitro* and *in vivo* toxicity analyses of CQDs were published

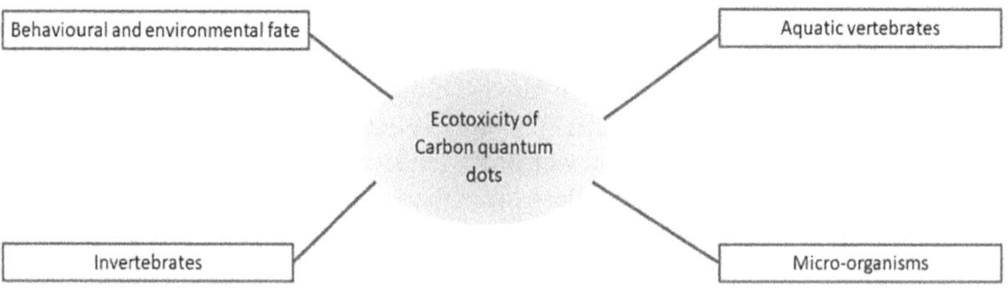

FIGURE 17.2 Ecotoxicology of carbon quantum dots.

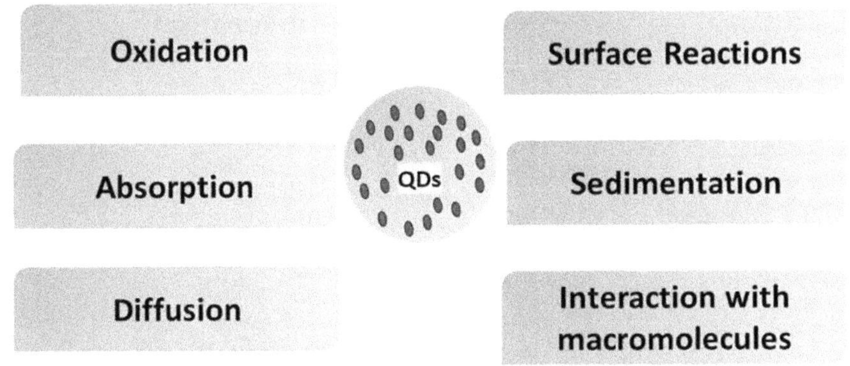

FIGURE 17.3   Different environmental interaction process of quantum dots.

in 2009 by Yang and colleagues. The surface chemistry of CQDs was mostly responsible for determining their cytotoxicological aspect. Cytotoxicity of QDs has been observed in several in vitro and in vivo studies affecting cell growth, viability and DNA damage. The level of QD toxicity was found to depend on size, type of coating and coating materials, and exposure concentration (Figure 17.3).

17.7   IN VITRO TOXICOLOGICAL EFFECTS

Numerous studies have been conducted to explore the potential toxicity of QDs in cells. These studies have utilized various cellular lines and QDs of different sizes and coatings. Consequently, it becomes exceedingly challenging to make accurate predictions regarding the adverse effects that QDs may have on cells. Indications of cytotoxicity are observed through alterations in cell growth, changes in cell motility, and modifications to cellular structure. Cytotoxicity studies have shown that QDs induce damage to the plasma membrane, mitochondrion, and nucleus, leading to apoptosis and may ultimately cause cell death (Tsay and Michalet 2005; Soenena et al. 2012). QDs have also been shown to accumulate in cell nuclei by passive diffusion after cell division (Dubertret et al., 2002) (Figure 17.4).

The ions utilized in the core of QDs, cadmium and selenium, are known to be cytotoxic (Alivisatos, 1996). The proliferation, mortality, and viability of human colorectal adenocarcinoma HT-29 and human breast cancer MCF-7 cells were used to evaluate the toxicity of C-Dots in vitro. All of these characteristics for both cell lines were not significantly impacted by C-Dots, nor were they impacted by the surface passivation agent PEG1500N. The carbon core of C-Dots is comparable to free carbon nanoparticles, which have not been found to have any major harmful effects in a variety of nanoscale forms (Long et al., 2014). Nurunnabi et al. (2013) studied in vivo biodistribution and toxicological impacts of carboxylated graphene QDs. Advances in the study of the environmental fate, transport, and ecotoxicological effects of engineered nanomaterials (ENMs) have been hampered by the lack of adequate techniques for the detection and quantification of ENMs at environmentally relevant concentrations in complex media (Von der Kammer et al., 2012). The

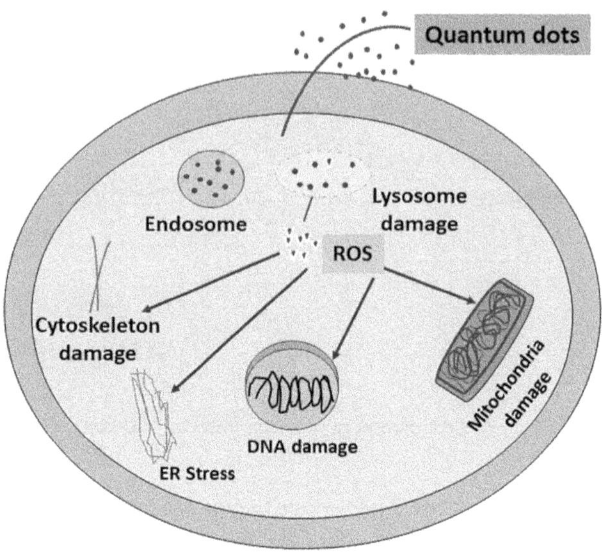

FIGURE 17.4   Cytotoxicity of quantum dots.

cytotoxicity and mechanism of CQDs should be quite different for various cell types. Recent studies by Fu et al. (2023) reported on both in vitro and in vivo toxicological evaluation of CQDs originating from *Spinacia oleracea.* CQDs found in processed Atlantic salmon accumulated in the brain, kidney, intestines, and liver of mice after oral feeding (Song et al., 2019).

17.8   SYSTEMATIC TOXICITIES OF CARBON DOTS

Furthermore, because of the QDs' highly crystalline structure, nanometric size, and bioactive surface coating, which enable easy skin penetration, bio-organisms can also ingest potentially dangerous QDs through dermal absorption (Wang et al., 2016). Exposed QDs and their constituents collected in important organs including the brain, heart, kidney, lungs, and intestines had toxic effects that could cause cancer and mutagenesis. Because of the QDs' highly crystalline structure, bioactive surface coating, and nanometric size, which enable easy skin penetration, bio-organisms can also ingest potentially dangerous QDs by dermal absorption. The systemic acute, chronic, and carcinogenic toxic consequences of these penetrated QDs could affect the blood flow and spread to other organs (Wang et al., 2016).

17.9   EFFECT OF QUANTUM DOTS ON PLANTS

Glutathione (GSH) levels have been found to be reduced compared to oxidized glutathione (GSSG) in plants. Therefore, QDs cause oxidative stress in plants. Specifically, it has been noted that QD toxicity results from factors arising from both the intrinsic physicochemical properties of QDs and environmental conditions and also, QD size, charge, concentration, bioactivity of the outer coating oxidative, photolytic and mechanical stability (Hardman, 2006). Environmental exposure to QDs is an important route and source. It depends on the extent of their use in society, half-life and interaction with nature. Zhang and their team (2021) studied the impact of fluorescent CQDs in fungi.

17.10 CONCLUSION

With the likely rise of QD products and their potential toxicity, it is important to understand the potential negative impacts of QD products, not only to protect human health and the environment but also to help industry and regulators to maximize the use of QD products. In order to safeguard people and the ecosystem against any potential negative effects of QD release into the environment, it may be necessary to close knowledge gaps regarding the mechanisms, routes, and causes of exposure as well as the potential toxicity of QDs.

REFERENCES

Ahmad, F., Pandey, A. K., Herzog, A. B., Rose, J. B., Gerba, C. P., & Hashsham, S. A. (2012). Environmental applications and potential health implications of quantum dots. *Journal of Nanoparticle Research*, 14, 1–24.

Ahmed, H. B., & Emam, H. E. (2020). Environmentally exploitable biocide/fluorescent metal marker carbon quantum dots. *RSC Advances*, 10(70), 42916–42929.

Alivisatos, A. P. (1996). Semiconductor clusters, nanocrystals, and quantum dots. *Science*, 271(5251), 933–937.

Bellanger, X., Billard, P., Schneider, R., Balan, L., & Merlin, C. (2015). Stability and toxicity of ZnO quantum dots: Interplay between nanoparticles and bacteria. *Journal of Hazardous Materials*, 283, 110–116.

Bottrill, M., & Green, M. (2011). Some aspects of quantum dot toxicity. *Chemical Communications*, 47(25), 7039–7050.

Chen, X., Fang, G., Liu, C., Dionysiou, D. D., Wang, X., Zhu, C., ... & Zhou, D. (2019). Cotransformation of carbon dots and contaminant under light in aqueous solutions: A mechanistic study. *Environmental Science & Technology*, 53(11), 6235–6244.

Chung, C. Y., Chen, Y. J., Kang, C. H., Lin, H. Y., Huang, C. C., Hsu, P. H., & Lin, H. J. (2021). Toxic or not toxic, that is the carbon quantum dot's question: A comprehensive evaluation with zebrafish embryo, eleutheroembryo, and adult models. *Polymers*, 13(10), 1598.

Derfus, A. M., Chan, W. C., & Bhatia, S. N. (2004). Probing the cytotoxicity of semiconductor quantum dots. *Nano Letters*, 4(1), 11–18.

Du, Y., & Guo, S. (2016). Chemically doped fluorescent carbon and graphene quantum dots for bioimaging, sensor, catalytic and photoelectronic applications. *Nanoscale*, 8(5), 2532–2543.

Dubertret, B., Skourides, P., Norris, D. J., Noireaux, V., Brivanlou, A. H., & Libchaber, A. (2002). In vivo imaging of quantum dots encapsulated in phospholipid micelles. *Science*, 298(5599), 1759–1762.

Feswick , A., Griffitt, R. J., Siebein, K., & Barber, D. S. (2013). Uptake, retention and internalization of quantum dots in Daphnia is influenced by particle surface functionalization. *Aquatic Toxicology*, 130, 210–218.

Frank, B. P., Sigmon, L. R., Deline, A. R., Lankone, R. S., Gallagher, M. J., Zhi, B., ... & Fairbrother, D. H. (2020). Photochemical transformations of carbon dots in aqueous environments. *Environmental Science & Technology*, 54(7), 4160–4170.

Freixa, A., Acuña, V., Sanchís, J., Farré, M., Barceló, D., & Sabater, S. (2018). Ecotoxicological effects of carbon based nanomaterials in aquatic organisms. *Science of the Total Environment*, 619, 328–337.

Fu, C., Qin, X., Zhang, J., Zhang, T., Song, Y., Yang, J., ... & Bikker, F. J. (2023). In vitro and in vivo toxicological evaluation of carbon quantum dots originating from Spinacia oleracea. *Heliyon*, 9(2).

Gallagher MJ, Buchman JT, Qiu TA, Zhi B, Lyons TY, Landy KM, et al. Release, detection and toxicity of fragments generated during artificial accelerated weathering of CdSe/ZnS and CdSe quantum dot polymer composites. *Environmental Science: Nano*. 2018;5(7): 1694–710.

Giroux, M. S., Zahra, Z., Salawu, O. A., Burgess, R. M., Ho, K. T., & Adeleye, A. S. (2022). Assessing the environmental effects related to quantum dot structure, function, synthesis and exposure. *Environmental Science: Nano*, 9(3), 867–910.

Gupta, M., & Gupta, S. (2017). An overview of selenium uptake, metabolism, and toxicity in plants. *Frontiers in Plant Science*, 7, 2074.

Ham, H. T., Choi, Y. S., & Chung, I. J. (2005). An explanation of dispersion states of single-walled carbon nanotubes in solvents and aqueous surfactant solutions using solubility parameters. *Journal of Colloid and Interface Science*, 286(1), 216–223.

Hardman, R. (2006). A toxicologic review of quantum dots: Toxicity depends on physicochemical and environmental factors. *Environmental Health Perspectives*, 114(2), 165–172.

Hoet, P. H., Brüske-Hohlfeld, I., & Salata, O. V. (2004). Nanoparticles–known and unknown health risks. *Journal of Nanobiotechnology*, 2, 1–15.

Holbrook, R. D., Murphy, K. E., Morrow, J. B., & Cole, K. D. (2008). Trophic transfer of nanoparticles in a simplified invertebrate food web. *Nature Nanotechnology*, 3(6), 352–355.

Kim, J., Park, Y., Yoon, T. H., Yoon, C. S., & Choi, K. (2010). Phototoxicity of CdSe/ZnSe quantum dots with surface coatings of 3-mercaptopropionic acid or tri-n-octylphosphine oxide/gum arabic in Daphnia magna under environmentally relevant UV-B light. *Aquatic Toxicology*, 97(2), 116–124.

Lazareva, A., & Keller, A. A. (2014). Estimating potential life cycle releases of engineered nanomaterials from wastewater treatment plants. *ACS Sustainable Chemistry & Engineering*, 2(7), 1656–1665.

Lee, W. M., & An, Y. J. (2015). Evidence of three-level trophic transfer of quantum dots in an aquatic food chain by using bioimaging. *Nanotoxicology*, 9(4), 407–412.

Li, Y., Sarvi, M., Khoshelham, K., & Haghani, M. (2020). Multi-view crowd congestion monitoring system based on an ensemble of convolutional neural network classifiers. *Journal of Intelligent Transportation Systems*, 24(5), 437–448.

Long, Y. M., Bao, L., Zhao, J. Y., Zhang, Z. L., & Pang, D. W. (2014). Revealing carbon nanodots as coreactants of the anodic electrochemiluminescence of Ru (bpy) 32+. *Analytical Chemistry*, 86(15), 7224–7228.

Moussa, H., Merlin, C., Dezanet, C., Balan, L., Medjahdi, G., Ben-Attia, M., & Schneider, R. (2016). Trace amounts of Cu2+ ions influence ROS production and cytotoxicity of ZnO quantum dots. *Journal of Hazardous Materials*, 304, 532–542.

Nikazar, S., Sivasankarapillai, V. S., Rahdar, A., Gasmi, S., Anumol, P. S., & Shanavas, M. S. (2020). Revisiting the cytotoxity of quantum dots: An in-depth overview. *Biophysical Reviews*, 12, 703–718.

Nowack, B., & Bucheli, T. D. (2007). Occurrence, behavior and effects of nanoparticles in the environment. *Environmental Pollution*, 150(1), 5–22.

Nurunnabi, M., Khatun, Z., Huh, K. M., Park, S. Y., Lee, D. Y., Cho, K. J., & Lee, Y. K. (2013). In vivo biodistribution and toxicology of carboxylated graphene quantum dots. *ACS Nano*, 7(8), 6858–6867.

Pakarinen, K., Petersen, E. J., Alvila, L., Waissi-Leinonen, G. C., Akkanen, J., Leppänen, M. T., & Kukkonen, J. V. (2013). A screening study on the fate of fullerenes (nC60) and their toxic implications in natural freshwaters. *Environmental Toxicology and Chemistry*, 32(6), 1224–1232.

Parks, A. N., Portis, L. M., Schierz, P. A., Washburn, K. M., Perron, M. M., Burgess, R. M., … & Ferguson, P. L. (2013). Bioaccumulation and toxicity of single-walled carbon nanotubes to benthic organisms at the base of the marine food chain. *Environmental Toxicology and Chemistry*, 32(6), 1270–1277.

Qu, J. H., Wei, Q., & Sun, D. W. (2018). Carbon dots: Principles and their applications in food quality and safety detection. *Critical Reviews in Food Science and Nutrition*, 58(14), 2466–2475.

Rahimzadeh, M. R., Rahimzadeh, M. R., Kazemi, S., & Moghadamnia, A. A. (2017). Cadmium toxicity and treatment: An update. *Caspian Journal of Internal Medicine*, 8(3), 135.

Rocha, T. L., Gomes, T., Cardoso, C., Letendre, J., Pinheiro, J. P., Sousa, V. S., … & Bebianno, M. J. (2014). Immunocytotoxicity, cytogenotoxicity and genotoxicity of cadmium-based quantum dots in the marine mussel *Mytilus galloprovincialis*. *Marine Environmental Research*, 101, 29–37.

Rocha, T. L., Gomes, T., Durigon, E. G., & Bebianno, M. J. (2016a). Subcellular partitioning kinetics, metallothionein response and oxidative damage in the marine mussel *Mytilus galloprovincialis* exposed to cadmium-based quantum dots. *Science of the Total Environment*, 554, 130–141.

Rocha, T. L., Sabóia-Morais, S. M. T., & Bebianno, M. J. (2016b). Histopathological assessment and inflammatory response in the digestive gland of marine mussel *Mytilus galloprovincialis* exposed to cadmium-based quantum dots. *Aquatic Toxicology*, 177, 306–315.

Silva, B. F., Andreani, T., Gavina, A., Vieira, M. N., Pereira, C. M., Rocha-Santos, T., & Pereira, R. (2016). Toxicological impact of cadmium-based quantum dots towards aquatic biota: Effect of natural sunlight exposure. *Aquatic Toxicology*, 176, 197–207.

Soenen, S. J., Demeester, J., De Smedt, S. C., & Braeckmans, K. (2012). The cytotoxic effects of polymer-coated quantum dots and restrictions for live cell applications. *Biomaterials*, 33(19), 4882–4888.

Song, Y., Wu, Y., Wang, H., Liu, S., Song, L., Li, S., & Tan, M. (2019). Carbon quantum dots from roasted Atlantic salmon (*Salmo salar* L.): Formation, biodistribution and cytotoxicity. *Food Chemistry*, 293, 387–395.

Sun, Y., Zhang, M., Bhandari, B., & Yang, C. (2022). Recent development of carbon quantum dots: Biological toxicity, antibacterial properties and application in foods. *Food Reviews International*, 38(7), 1513–1532.

Tang, S., Cai, Q., Chibli, H., Allagadda, V., Nadeau, J. L., & Mayer, G. D. (2013). Cadmium sulfate and CdTe-quantum dots alter DNA repair in zebrafish (Danio rerio) liver cells. *Toxicology and Applied Pharmacology*, 272(2), 443–452.

Tsay, J. M., & Michalet, X. (2005). New light on quantum dot cytotoxicity. *Chemistry & Biology*, 12(11), 1159–1161.

Von der Kammer, F., Ferguson, P. L., Holden, P. A., Masion, A., Rogers, K. R., Klaine, S. J., … & Unrine, J. M. (2012). Analysis of engineered nanomaterials in complex matrices (environment and biota): General considerations and conceptual case studies. *Environmental Toxicology and Chemistry*, 31(1), 32–49.

Wang, M., Wang, J., Sun, H., Han, S., Feng, S., Shi, L., … & Sun, Z. (2016). Time-dependent toxicity of cadmium telluride quantum dots on liver and kidneys in mice: Histopathological changes with elevated free cadmium ions and hydroxyl radicals. *International Journal of Nanomedicine*, 2319–2328.

Wang, Y., & Nowack, B. (2018a). Dynamic probabilistic material flow analysis of nano-SiO2, nano iron oxides, nano-CeO2, nano-Al2O3, and quantum dots in seven European regions. *Environmental Pollution*, 235, 589–601.

Wang, Y., & Nowack, B. (2018b). Environmental risk assessment of engineered nano-SiO2, nano iron oxides, nano-CeO2, nano-Al2O3, and quantum dots. *Environmental Toxicology and Chemistry*, 37(5), 1387–1395.

Weinberg, H., Galyean, A., & Leopold, M. (2011). Evaluating engineered nanoparticles in natural waters. *TrAC Trends in Analytical Chemistry*, 30(1), 72–83.

Xu, J., He, H., Wang, Y. Y., Yan, R., Zhou, L. J., Liu, Y. Z., … & Liu, Y. (2018). New aspects of the environmental risks of quantum dots: prophage activation. *Environmental Science: Nano*, 5(7), 1556–1566.

Yang, S. T., Wang, X., Wang, H., Lu, F., Luo, P. G., Cao, L., … & Sun, Y. P. (2009). Carbon dots as nontoxic and high-performance fluorescence imaging agents. *The Journal of Physical Chemistry C*, 113(42), 18110–18114.

Zhang, Q., Shi, R., Li, Q., Maimaiti, T., Lan, S., Ouyang, P., … & Yang, S. T. (2021). Low toxicity of fluorescent carbon quantum dots to white rot fungus *Phanerochaete chrysosporium*. *Journal of Environmental Chemical Engineering*, 9(1), 104633.

Yao, K., Lv, X., Zheng, G., Chen, Z., Jiang, Y., Zhu, X., … & Cai, Z. (2018). Effects of carbon quantum dots on aquatic environments: Comparison of toxicity to organisms at different trophic levels. *Environmental Science & Technology*, 52(24), 14445–14451.

Index

Pages in *italics* refer to figures.

A

acidic oxidation technique, 46
advanced batteries, 358, 365
aluminium, 402
animal-derived carbon source, 29
anode materials, 361–364
antibacterial effect, 101, 311
antibiofilm activity, 108
antifungal mechanisms, 107
antioxidant properties, 122
antiviral activity, 107, 111, 311
aquatic environment, 242
arsenic, 242–244
atomic force microscopy (AFM), 59–60, 62

B

bandages, 150, 199, 206
batteries, 12, 354, 358–365
bioaccumulation, 414
biofilm, 108–111
bioimaging, 44, 49, 54, 71, 75, 152, 175
biomedical imaging, 165–169
biosensing, 13
bottom-up approach methods, 46

C

cadmium, 143, 168, 403
cathode materials, 358
chemical oxidation, 9
chemiluminescence, 5
cobalt, 403
combustion method, 50
copper, 396
cosmetics, 140, 149–155
CQD-based spray, 206
crystal violet dye, 334

D

disinfecting agent, 344
drug delivery, 165, 303
dye removal, 325
dynamic light scattering (DLS), 66

E

ecotoxicology, 414
electrocatalysis, 14
electrochemical biosensing, 302
electroluminescent CQD, 377
energy dispersive spectroscopy (EDS), 84
environmental issues, 411

F

food toxins, 303
fourier transform infrared spectroscopy
    (FTIR), 59

G

gene delivery, 306
grain based carbon sources, 22
gram-negative bacteria, 202
gram-positive bacteria, 102

H

hemostasis, 196
hydrogel patches, 199
hydrolytic carbonization, 198
hydrophobic interactions, 102
hydrothermal synthesis, 10
hydrothermal technique, 227, 356, 358

I

in vitro imaging, 172
inflammation, 175, 195–196, 199, 216, 292–293, 296

L

laser ablation, 7, 8, 20

M

memory devices, 353, 379
metal detection, ix, 42, 59, 395–406
methyl orange dye, 336
methylene blue dye, 13, 327

For Product Safety Concerns and Information please contact our EU
representative GPSR@taylorandfrancis.com
Taylor & Francis Verlag GmbH, Kaufingerstraße 24, 80331 München, Germany